Cancer Development and Management: Impact of Bioactive Natural Products

Cancer Development and Management: Impact of Bioactive Natural Products

Edited by Chris Dalton

hayle medical

New York

Hayle Medical,
750 Third Avenue, 9th Floor,
New York, NY 10017, USA

Visit us on the World Wide Web at:
www.haylemedical.com

ISBN: 978-1-64647-521-6

Cataloging-in-Publication Data

Cancer development and management : impact of bioactive natural products / edited by Chris Dalton.
p. cm.
Includes bibliographical references and index.
ISBN 978-1-64647-521-6
1. Tumors--Growth. 2. Cancer--Treatment. 3. Cancer--Nutritional aspects. 4. Natural products--Biotechnology.
I. Dalton, Chris.

RC261 .C36 2023
616.994--dc23

Table of Contents

Preface VII

Chapter 1 **Bioactive Compounds: Multi-Targeting Silver Bullets for Preventing and Treating Breast Cancer** 1
Nethaji Muniraj, Sumit Siddharth and Dipali Sharma

Chapter 2 **Stable Isotope Tracing Metabolomics to Investigate the Metabolic Activity of Bioactive Compounds for Cancer Prevention and Treatment** 25
Feroza K. Choudhury, G. Lavender Hackman, Alessia Lodi and Stefano Tiziani

Chapter 3 **Bioactive Phenolic Compounds in the Modulation of Central and Peripheral Nervous System Cancers** 46
Lorena Perrone, Simone Sampaolo and Mariarosa Anna Beatrice Melone

Chapter 4 **EGCG Mediated Targeting of Deregulated Signaling Pathways and Non-Coding RNAs in Different Cancers: Focus on JAK/STAT, Wnt/β-Catenin, TGF/SMAD, NOTCH, SHH/GLI and TRAIL Mediated Signaling Pathways** 63
Ammad Ahmad Farooqi, Marina Pinheiro, Andreia Granja, Fulvia Farabegoli, Salette Reis, Rukset Attar, Uteuliyev Yerzhan Sabitaliyevich, Baojun Xu and Aamir Ahmad

Chapter 5 **Divergent Effects of Daidzein and its Metabolites on Estrogen-Induced Survival of Breast Cancer Cells** 84
Emiliano Montalesi, Manuela Cipolletti, Patrizio Cracco, Marco Fiocchetti and Maria Marino

Chapter 6 **Nobiletin and Derivatives: Functional Compounds from Citrus Fruit Peel for Colon Cancer Chemoprevention** 98
Joanna Xuan Hui Goh, Loh Teng Hern Tan, Joo Kheng Goh, Kok Gan Chan, Priyia Pusparajah, Learn-Han Lee and Bey-Hing Goh

Chapter 7 **Fatty Acid Synthase Inhibitor G28 Shows Anticancer Activity in EGFR Tyrosine Kinase Inhibitor Resistant Lung Adenocarcinoma Models** 132
Emma Polonio-Alcalá, Sònia Palomeras, Daniel Torres-Oteros, Joana Relat, Marta Planas, Lidia Feliu, Joaquim Ciurana, Santiago Ruiz-Martínez and Teresa Puig

Chapter 8 **Targeting Glucose Transporters for Breast Cancer Therapy: The Effect of Natural and Synthetic Compounds** 150
Ana M. Barbosa and Fátima Martel

Chapter 9 **Gigantol Targets Cancer Stem Cells and Destabilizes Tumors via the Suppression of the PI3K/AKT and JAK/STAT Pathways in Ectopic Lung Cancer Xenografts** 188
Nattanan Losuwannarak, Arnatchai Maiuthed, Nakarin Kitkumthorn, Asada Leelahavanichkul, Sittiruk Roytrakul and Pithi Chanvorachote

Chapter 10 **XIAP as a Target of New Small Organic Natural Molecules Inducing Human Cancer Cell Death** 208
Diego Muñoz, Martina Brucoli, Silvia Zecchini, Adrian Sandoval Hernandez, Gonzalo Arboleda, Fabian Lopez-Vallejo,Wilman Delgado, Matteo Giovarelli, Marco Coazzoli, Elisabetta Catalani, Clara De Palma, Cristiana Perrotta, Luis Cuca, Emilio Clementi and Davide Cervia

Permissions

List of Contributors

Index

Preface

Bioactive compounds are secondary metabolites that provide nutritional benefit as well as have therapeutic potential. They can be found in many foods including vegetables, whole grains, fruits and a variety of plants. Bioactive compounds are typically made up of amino acid residues and can have a variety of physical effects including antithrombotic, antioxidant and antihypertensive activities. They vary widely in terms of structures and functions, and could be used as chemopreventive and chemotherapeutic agents in cancer treatment. Various types of bioactive compounds include polyphenolic compounds, carotenoids, sulfur-containing compounds and terpenoids. Additionally, many pathways have been shown to mediate the influence of bioactive compounds on cancer and achieving positive outcomes in the cancer patients, through endoplasmic reticulum stress, regulation of oxidative stress and epigenetic changes. This book provides significant information to help develop a good understanding of cancer management using bioactive natural products. A number of latest researches have been included to keep the readers up-to-date.

After months of intensive research and writing, this book is the end result of all who devoted their time and efforts in the initiation and progress of this book. It will surely be a source of reference in enhancing the required knowledge of the new developments in the area. During the course of developing this book, certain measures such as accuracy, authenticity and research focused analytical studies were given preference in order to produce a comprehensive book in the area of study.

This book would not have been possible without the efforts of the authors and the publisher. I extend my sincere thanks to them. Secondly, I express my gratitude to my family and well-wishers. And most importantly, I thank my students for constantly expressing their willingness and curiosity in enhancing their knowledge in the field, which encourages me to take up further research projects for the advancement of the area.

Editor

1

Bioactive Compounds: Multi-Targeting Silver Bullets for Preventing and Treating Breast Cancer

Nethaji Muniraj, Sumit Siddharth and Dipali Sharma *

Department of Oncology, Johns Hopkins University School of Medicine and the Sidney Kimmel Comprehensive Cancer Center at Johns Hopkins, Baltimore, MD 21231, USA; nmunira1@jhmi.edu (N.M.); ssiddha2@jhmi.edu (S.S.)
* Correspondence: dsharma7@jhmi.edu

Abstract: Each cell in our body is designed with a self-destructive trigger, and if damaged, can happily sacrifice itself for the sake of the body. This process of self-destruction to safeguard the adjacent normal cells is known as programmed cell death or apoptosis. Cancer cells outsmart normal cells and evade apoptosis and it is one of the major hallmarks of cancer. The cardinal quest for anti-cancer drug discovery (bioactive or synthetic compounds) is to be able to re-induce the so called "programmed cell death" in cancer cells. The importance of bioactive compounds as the linchpin of cancer therapeutics is well known as many effective chemotherapeutic drugs such as vincristine, vinblastine, doxorubicin, etoposide and paclitaxel have natural product origins. The present review discusses various bioactive compounds with known anticancer potential, underlying mechanisms by which they induce cell death and their preclinical/clinical development. Most bioactive compounds can concurrently target multiple signaling pathways that are important for cancer cell survival while sparing normal cells hence they can potentially be the silver bullets for targeting cancer growth and metastatic progression.

Keywords: bioactive compounds; cancer; withaferin A; honokiol; BITC; resveratrol; curcumin; genistein; EGCG

---

1. Bioactive Compounds in Cancer

Breast cancer is one of the major health concerns for women and the second leading cause of cancer related mortality in the United States (https://www.cdc.gov/cancer/breast/statistics/ index.htm) [1]. In spite of major advancements in novel therapeutic strategies, development of drug resistance is common in all breast cancer subtypes. A significant number of cancers develop resistance towards drugs and relapse accounting for one of the most concerning issue with conventional therapies [2,3]. Conventional therapies mostly fail because of the dysregulation of the balance between cell growth and apoptosis [4]. Although the typical path of development of single target drugs for cancer has produced multiple successful targeted approaches, it has not been able to circumvent the problem of drug resistance and tumor recurrence. Cancer cells exhibit simultaneous activation of multiple cell surface receptors and signaling pathways hence targeting one node typically leads to the activation of alternative pathways. Development of novel anti-cancer drugs with low toxicity and improved efficacy is the need of the hour [5].

Also known as nutraceuticals, chemicals present in plants and certain foods as natural constituents are termed as bioactive compounds [6]. Bioactive compounds have been used for millennia in Ayurvedic and traditional Chinese therapy for various ailments [7] and have shown efficacy as anti-inflammatory, anti-depressant, anti-microbial as well as anti-cancer agents [5,8]. The discovery of bioactive compounds from plant sources not only established the basis of traditional medicine but is also proving to be an indispensable source of pharmacological agents for modern drug development [9]. Numerous research studies have provided substantial support over the decades for the suitability and effectiveness of several bioactive compounds against cancer [10]. Many successful drugs such as vincristine, vinblastine, doxorubicin, etoposide and paclitaxel have natural product origins. Several bioactive compounds have shown to increase apoptosis of cancer cells through different mechanisms of action [11] and many others have been reported to reduce cancer cell proliferation, induce apoptosis, inhibit invasion and migration and overcome chemo-resistance [5,12]. It has also been shown that several bioactive compounds isolated from medicinal plants delay metastasis and prevent angiogenesis [13,14]. Reports reveal that bioactive compounds affect intracellular signaling associated with carcinogenesis [14,15]. Together, these studies impart solid preclinical support for the clinical development of these bioactive compounds (Figure 1) [16].

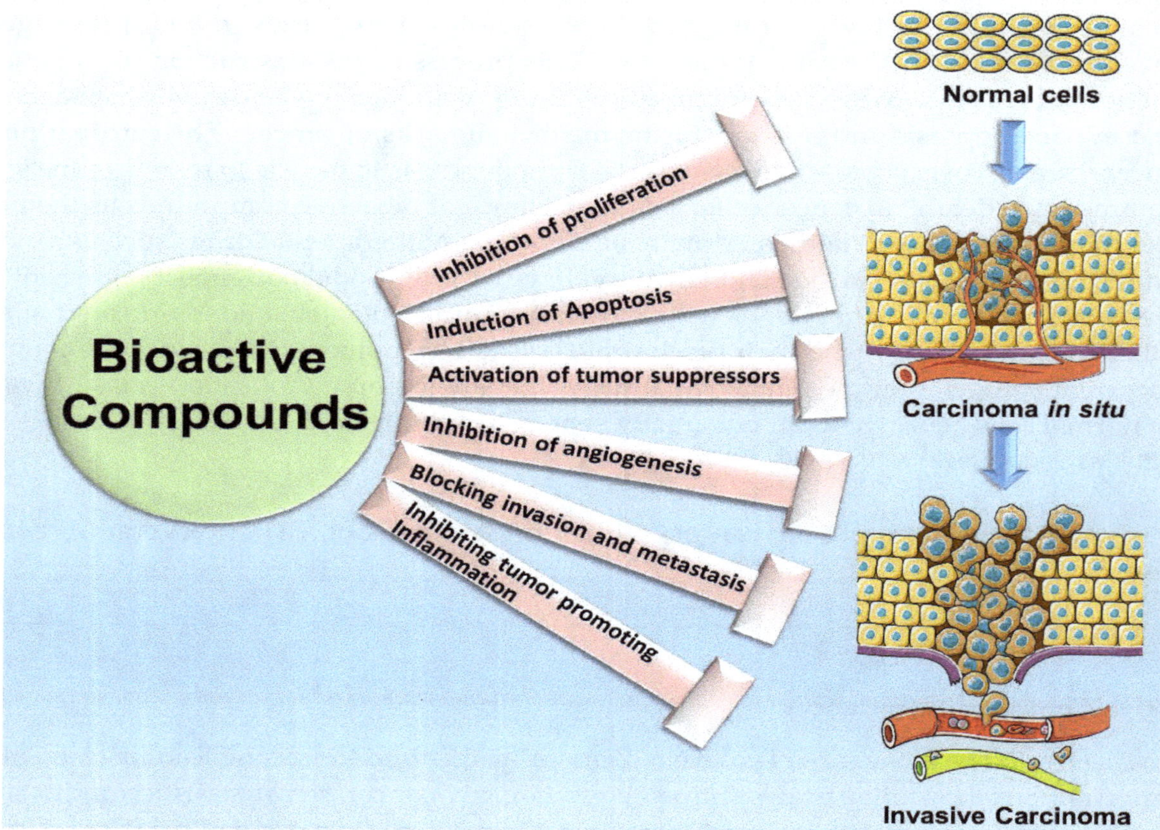

Figure 1. Schematic illustrating the anti-cancer potential of bioactive compounds. Bioactive compounds can inhibit cancer cell proliferation, induce apoptosis, activate multiple tumor suppressors, inhibit angiogenesis, inhibit invasion and migration potential of cancer cells and reduce/inhibit inflammation. Bioactive compounds are multifunctional.

Cancer therapeutics has seen a gradual paradigm shift from monotherapy towards combinational treatment approach and the synergistic effects of multiple bioactive compounds with standard chemotherapy supports this notion. The combination regimen involving bioactive compounds has shown decreased cell proliferation and clonogenicity of breast cancer cells [17]. Evidences suggest that bioactive compounds in combination with chemotherapy increases the efficacy and decreases the toxicity of chemotherapeutic agents [18]. The Dietary guidelines recommend the consumption of whole plant products as chemo preventive agents based on the health advantages observed in epidemiological studies [19] but achieving high levels of phytochemicals in target tissues is always a challenge. One advantage of developing bioactive compounds for cancer prevention and treatment is that these small molecules can be easily taken in effective doses with little or no toxicities. Recent mechanistic studies with various bioactive molecules have shown that most bioactive molecules do not target a single protein or pathway but exert pleiotropic effects concurrently affecting multiple pathways. While outwardly, this may seem like a shortcoming especially in light of the preference for single-target agents but this key characteristic allows bioactive compounds to evade the development of resistance due to the activation of supporting alternative pathways, a problem observed with most single-target drugs [20]. In addition, the effective doses of most bioactive agents do not exert any toxicities or side effects making them ideal preventative and anticancer agents. In this review, we discuss various bioactive compounds (Figure 2), their underlying mechanisms and their efficacy in breast cancer prevention and therapy.

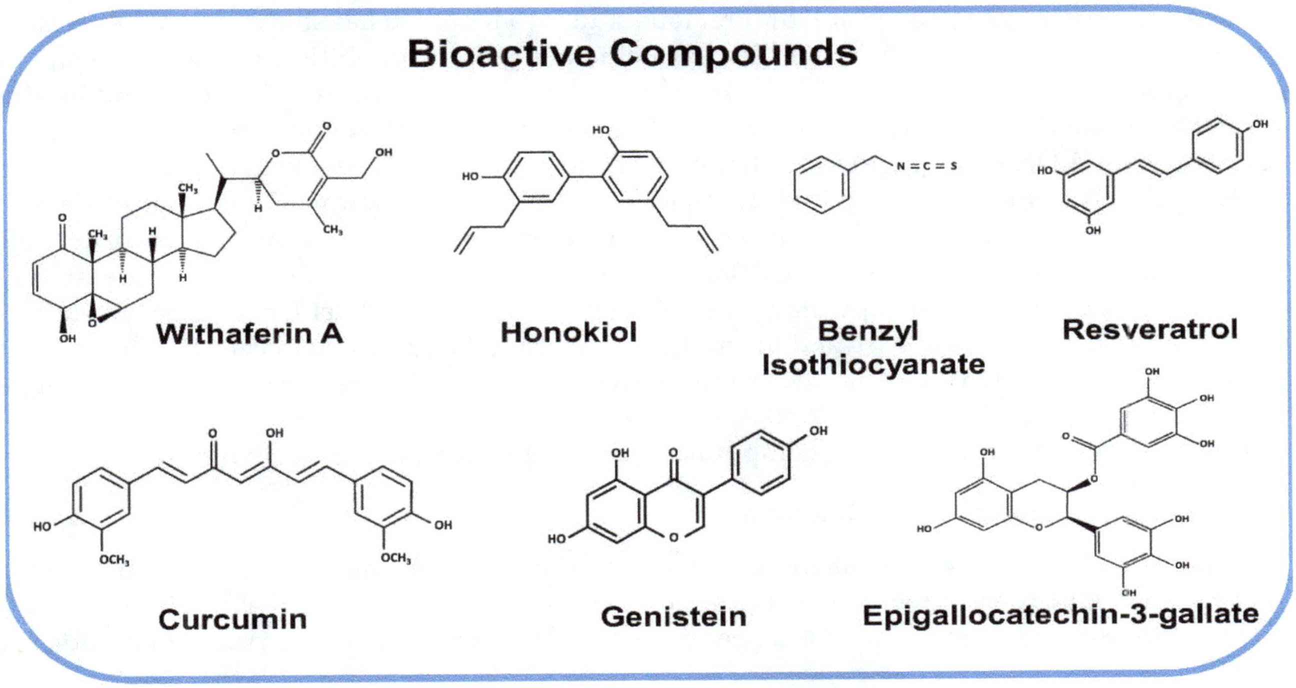

Figure 2. Structures of bioactive compounds. We discuss the anti-cancer potential, underlying molecular mechanisms and clinical development of these select bioactive compounds in this review.

2. Withaferin A, a Steroidal Lactone from Ashwagandha

Withaferin A (WFA), a steroidal lactone isolated from *Withania somnifera* commonly known as Ashwagandha, Indian ginseng or winter cherry, is the most potent bioactive compound among the 14 withanolides isolated from this plant. It has been known for its anti-inflammatory, anti-angiogenic, cardioprotective and anti-carcinogenic properties [21–23]. WFA modulates cell cycle in breast cancer cells and causes G2 and M phase arrest [24]. *In vivo* and *in vitro* studies from our group and others have revealed that WFA inhibits clonogenicity and induces apoptosis in breast cancer cells [25,26]. WFA administration is correlated with enhanced apoptosis, reduced mammary tumors and decreased pulmonary metastasis in the MMTV (mouse mammary tumor virus)-transgenic model [26]. Reports reveal that WFA-mediated apoptosis is dependent on Bcl-2 [22], ROS [27], Bax and Bak, respectively [28]. Involvement of ROS in WFA-induced cells death has also been shown in breast cancer cells [29,30]. WFA modulates multiple oncogenic signaling pathways in cancer cells to impart its anti-cancer effects. WFA induces anti-tumor effects via STAT3 inhibition in multiple myeloma and neuroblastoma [31]. Sehrawat et al., reported that WFA-mediated apoptosis is associated with the dysregulation of the mitochondrial dynamics in breast cancer cells [32]. In addition, FOXO3 regulates WFA mediated apoptosis in breast cancer cells with its transcriptional target, Bim, which causes reduced cell proliferation and increased tumor mass apoptosis in WFA-treated *in vivo* models [22]. Our recent findings demonstrate that WFA induces apoptosis by downregulating ATP levels and enhancing the activation of AMPK [33]. Importantly, combining 2-deoxyglucose (2-DG) and WFA synergistically enhances apoptosis in breast cancer cells proposing that a combinational regimen may prove more beneficial than either monotherapy [33]. Exhibiting the involvement of downstream effector molecules, Zhang et al., demonstrated that WFA induces caspase 3 and caspase7 leading to apoptosis in MCF-7 cells [34]. Several studies have reported the involvement of tumor suppressor p53 in WFA's biological functions. Hahm et al., reported that silencing of p53 attenuates WFA-induced apoptosis in breast cancer cells [35]. It has been demonstrated that the growth inhibitory effects of WFA are via induction of p53, p21 and phospho-p38MAPK, as well as by down regulation of ERα, RET and HSF1 [34]. On the contrary, p53-independent effects of WFA have also been demonstrated. WFA-induced apoptosis in breast cancer cells is associated with XIAP, c-IAP-2, and survivin suppression respectively, regardless of p53 or estrogen receptor [28]. Previous study from our lab has shown that WFA treatment activates death receptor 5 (DR5) which leads to efficient growth inhibition [25]. However, WFA has been reported to cause apoptosis in human breast cancer cells through intrinsic and extrinsic mechanism via modulating mitochondrial membrane potential, DNA condensation, cytoplasmic histone-associated DNA fragmentation that causes the degradation cytoskeletal protein and poly (ADP-Ribose) polymerase cleavage [22]. WFA treatment inhibits self-renewal of breast cancer stem cells *in vitro* and *in vivo* [36]. Treating breast cancer cells with a combination of WFA and sulforaphane (SFN) induces apoptosis via upregulation Bax/Bcl-2 ratio and downregulation of HDAC1 expression [37]. Combining WFA with chemotherapy may prove effective as WFA and cisplatin combination effectively inhibits ovarian cancer cells *in vitro* and *in vivo* by eliminating the cancer stem cells [38,39]. Cisplatin and WFA combination treatment has also shown benefit in triple negative breast cancer reducing the cellular proliferation and promoting apoptosis [40]. In summary, the polypharmaceutical effects of WFA holds promise as an anti-cancer compound and warrants further clinical exploration.

3. Honokiol, a Polyphenol from Magnolia

In traditional Asian medicine magnolia species have been used for many centuries to treat anxiety, nervous system disorders, fever, gastrointestinal symptoms, and stroke [41–45]. The potential of polyphenols as effective agents against cancer has been acknowledged for the past two decades [46]. Magnolol, one of the bioactive components of *Magnolia officianalis*, is demonstrated to possess inhibitory effects on multiple cancer cell lines [47–51]. Zhou et al., reported that magnolol induces apoptosis and G2/M arrest in MCF-7 cells [52]. Honokiol (HNK) is the major small molecule polyphonic compound derived from *Magnolia grandiflora* and it has been used in traditional Chinese and Japanese medicine. Preclinical *in vitro* and *in vivo* studies reveal anti-tumor, anti-angiogenic, anti-inflammatory and anti-oxidative properties of HNK [41,53,54]. HNK induces apoptosis and inhibits growth in breast and other cancer cells [41,55,56]. Our research group has shown that HNK inhibits breast cancer growth using various *in vitro* and *in vivo* models [54]. Hou et al., demonstrated that HNK induces apoptosis in mouse 4T1 breast cancer model and inhibits cancer cell proliferation *in vitro* and *in vivo* [57]. HNK inhibits nuclear translocation of NFkB and induces TNF-α mediated apoptosis [58]. Tumor microenvironment tend to be hypoxic in nature and HIF-1α helps the cancer cells to adapt to the low oxygen environment [59]. HNK decreases the expression level of HIF-1α and suppresses the hypoxia induced cancer-promoting pathway [60]. Our research group showed that HNK inhibits growth of breast cancer cells by inducing AMP-activated protein kinase in a LKB1-dependent manner [54] and inhibits epithelial-mesenchymal transition and stemness by modulating Stat3/Zeb1/E-Cadherin axis [61]. HNK treatment also effectively inhibits stemness in breast cancer by concurrent activation of tumor suppressor LKB1 and suppression of oncogenic Stat3 signaling [62]. Downregulation of Snail/slug by HNK targets EMT in breast cancer [63]. HNK synergistically induces apoptosis in combination with mTOR inhibitor, rapamycin, in breast cancer cells [64]. HNK modulates TNFα induced Nur77 expression in breast cancer cells [65]. HNK has also shown efficacy in hyperleptinemic obese state where oncogenic hyperactive leptin signaling drives tumor progression. HNK treatment inhibits Wnt1-MTA-1-β-catenin signaling and activates LKB1-miR34a axis leading to the inhibition of breast tumor progression [66,67]. We have shown that HNK impedes cell motility and stem-like breast cancer cell phenotype by decreasing mammosphere formation, OCT4, Nanog, SOX2, and ALDH1, respectively [62]. Studies have suggested that early progenitor cells in breast cancer preserve the capability of self-renewal and differentiation to repopulate the entire tumor [68]. In addition, breast cancer stem cells markers, like aldehyde dehydrogenase (ALDH1), CD24, CD166, CD47, and CD44 are present in abundance in the breast tumor samples [68,69]. HNK attenuates the self-renewal of oral cancer stem cells and reduces the expression of ALDH1 and CD44 cancer stem cell markers [70]. HNK is indeed an attractive bioactive compound with strong anti-cancer potential. Recently, a transdermal approach was developed to facilitate localized delivery of Honokiol that might prove beneficial [71]. Solid preclinical support for honokiol's anti-cancer potential and an understanding of underlying signaling mechanisms to guide the correlative biomarkers is already present, and now the field is awaiting clinical studies for further development of this promising bioactive compound.

4. Benzyl Isothiocyanate, an Isothiocynate from Cruciferous Vegetables

Epidemiological studies have reported that the consumption of cruciferous vegetables is associated with reduced cancer risk [72,73]. Cruciferous vegetables have a high content of glucosinolates and their metabolites, especially isothiocyanates [73–75]. Characteristically harboring the N=C=S group, the isothiocyanate class of chemicals is responsible for the well-established medicinal properties of isothiocyanate-rich vegetables and fruits. ITCs naturally occur in abundance in cruciferous vegetables such as broccoli, Brussels sprouts and cauliflower and play an important role in the chemoprevention properties of these vegetables. In a population-based study, broccoli intake inversely correlates with breast cancer in premenopausal women [76,77]. Over the past few decades, research has provided extensive preclinical evidence for the effectiveness of various ITCs against cancer progression [78–80]. Benzyl isothiocyanate (BITC), 1-naphthyl isothiocyanate (NITC), phenethyl isothiocyanate (PEITC) and sulforaphane (SFN) are the most significant ITCs that have been extensively researched against various cancers including breast cancer [79]. BITC and SFN reduce cell growth [79], induce apoptosis [81], inhibit spontaneous tumorigenesis in genetically-engineered models and significantly reduce tumor progression in xenografts models [82–84]. BITC administration reduces mammary tumor incidence and tumor progression in MMTV-neu mice and tumors in BITC treated group exhibit fewer Ki-67 positive cells and an increase in apoptotic bodies [85]. Yu et al., was first to demonstrate apoptosis induction by ITC in a caspase-3-dependent mechanism [86]. BITC mediated apoptotic-induction in breast cancer cells involves reactive oxygen species generation, increase in pro-apoptotic proteins such as Bax/Bak, reduction in anti-apoptotic proteins such as Bcl-2/Bcl-xL and activation of caspases including caspase 9, caspase 3, and caspase 8 [87]. BITC treatment leads to c-Jun N-terminal kinase (JNK) and p38 mitogen-activated protein kinase (p38 MAPK) activation that plays an important role in BITC's biological function as their inhibition abrogates BITC-mediated cell death [88]. JNK and p38 MAPK leads to increased Bax translocation from the cytosol to the mitochondria in breast cancer cells [88] and an ectopic expression of the catalytically inactive JNK kinase 2 mutant significantly suppresses the BITC medicated conformational change of Bax [88]. It is interesting to note that BITC can inhibit transcriptional activation of estrogen-responsive genes and disrupt estrogen-estrogen receptor axis in ER-positive breast cancer cells [89]. BITC treated breast cancer cells exhibit FoxO1-mediated autophagy and induces apoptosis via attenuation of mTOR activity *in vitro* and *in vivo* [90]. Inhibition of epithelial-mesenchymal transition (EMT) [91], stemness [92] as well as inhibition of various important oncogenic pathways including Wnt/catenin [93] in response to BITC has been observed. Both p53 dependent and –independent role of BITC has been shown [94,95]. Kim et al., showed that BITC-induced cell death is facilitated by down regulation of X-linked inhibitor of apoptosis (XIAP) in a p53-independent manner [94]. Our research group showed that BITC is effective in breast cancer cells harboring wild type p53 or mutant p53. In the presence of wild type p53, BITC increases p53 phosphorylation and decreases PRAS40 phosphorylation leading to accumulation of active p53 that acts as a transcription factor for tumor suppressor LKB1, and also tethers with LKB1 to upregulate p53-responsive genes. In breast cancer cells harboring mutant p53, BITC dissociates the mutant p53-p73 complex releasing p73 from sequestration. Upon release, p73 activates LKB1 expression and tethers with LKB1 to upregulate p53-responsive genes leading to growth inhibition [95]. Adipocytokine leptin has been shown to turn on an oncogenic signaling cascade and stimulate breast cancer growth in obese state [96–101]. Interestingly, BITC treatment can block leptin-induced breast cancer growth by directly inhibiting leptin-mediated Stat3 activation [102]. BITC treated breast cancer cells show decreased tumor progression and lower expression of epithelial-mesenchymal transition (EMT) markers [91]. BITC administration in the MMTV-*neu* mice reduces tumor progression and stemness [103]. Several studies have shown that BITC selectively affects cancer cells and exhibits minimal toxicity against normal cells. BITC effectively suppresses growth of breast cancer cells while normal mammary epithelial cells remain largely unaffected [87,93]. Similarly, human pancreatic cancer cells show increased apoptosis in response to BITC treatment whereas immortalized human pancreatic cells do not respond to BITC [104]. BITC is reported to inhibit growth and induce apoptosis in human oral cancer cells while exhibiting low toxicity to normal cells [105]. These preclinical studies have provided important insights into the anti-cancer efficacy of BITC however clinical validation is still pending.

5. Resveratrol, a Polyphenolic Phytoestrogen

Resveratrol (3,5,4′-trihydroxy-*trans*-stilbene) is a non-flavonoid, polyphenolic phytoestrogen majorly present in plants like grapes (*Vitis vinifera*), blueberries, mulberries, soy, pomegranate and peanuts [106–108]. Resveratrol was first appreciated in the context of "French Paradox" where resveratrol present in red wine was considered protective against heart disease and obesity in French population despite their high-fat French diet intake [109]. Although it is known today that the beneficial effects of French diet are because of the combination of resveratrol and various other plant-based components and not resveratrol alone, it is still well regarded for its health benefits. Multiple clinical trials have evaluated the efficacy of resveratrol for T2DM, obesity, prediabetes, diabetic neuropathy, NAFLD, fatty liver, brain function, memory, schizophrenia, and Parkinson's disease [110]. Many trials are currently undergoing to evaluate the benefits of resveratrol in various cancers including colon, colorectal, multiple myeloma and breast cancer [110]. Multiple studies have shown anti-tumor effects of resveratrol in many cancer types [111–115] and its efficacy as a chemopreventive and therapeutic agent is supported by epidemiological and preclinical research [116]. Activation of caspases is an important downstream event in apoptotic induction. Resveratrol has been shown to induce apoptotic death of cancer cells in a caspase-dependent as well as caspase-independent manner [117–119]. In estrogen receptor positive breast cancer cells, resveratrol mediates apoptotic cell death via Bcl-2 downregulation that is independent of cytochrome c release and cleavage of caspases 3/8 and PARP [117]. A caspase-3 activation dependent mechanism for apoptotic induction by resveratrol has been shown in estrogen receptor negative breast cancer cells [118]. Modulation of mitochondrial membrane potential, release of cytochrome c, activation of Second Mitochondria-derived Activator of Caspase/direct inhibitor of apoptosis-binding protein with low pI (Smac/DIABLO) and Ca2+-activated protease calpain have also been implicated in resveratrol-mediated apoptotic induction [120]. Interestingly, activation of upstream kinase ERK leads to Bcl-2 suppression in breast cancer cells treated with resveratrol resulting in apoptotic cell death [121]. Resveratrol is also known to inhibit Akt, mammalian target of rapamycin (mTOR), PI3K as well as Wnt/catenin pathway leading to decreased cancer cell growth [122,123]. Another study showed that resveratrol treatment decreases stem cell population in NOD/SCID mice and down-regulates Wnt/β-catenin self–renewal pathway [124]. Examining the involvement of signal transducer and activator of transcription 3 (Stat3) in resveratrol function, Kotha et al., showed that resveratrol inhibits the tyrosine kinase activity of Src leading to the inhibition of Stat3 in breast cancer cells [125]. Resveratrol treatment causes induction of p53, p21 and BRCA in breast cancer cells [126–128] via various pathways, one important mechanism being the modulation of epigenetic modulators protein arginine methyltransferase 5 (PRMT5) and enhancer of Zeste homolog 2 (EZH2) and causing changes in histone methylation marks [128]. Owing to its structural resemblance to diethylstilbestrol, a synthetic estrogen, resveratrol has been considered a phytoestrogen that binds to estrogen receptor-α and -β and modulates the expression of ER-responsive genes [129,130]. Multiple studies have evaluated the effectiveness of resveratrol in enhancing the efficacy of chemotherapy or re-sensitizing chemotherapy-resistance cells [131–133]. By modulating the SIRT1 and β-catenin axis, resveratrol sensitizes chemotherapy-resistant breast cancer cells to doxorubicin leading to effective inhibition of growth, migration, and EMT [131]. Involvement of miR-122-5p has also been shown in resveratrol-mediated chemo sensitization of Adriamycin-resistant breast cancer cells [132]. Owing to a large number of preclinical studies, the role and importance of resveratrol is already well-established in breast cancer therapeutics and chemoprevention. Multiple ongoing clinical trials will help propel this bioactive compound in clinical arena.

6. Curcumin, the Golden Spice

Curcumin is a hydrophobic, polyphenolic constituent of turmeric, the yellow spice extracted from the plant *Curcuma longa*. Curcuma longa grows naturally in Indian subcontinent and South East Asia. The use of turmeric dates to 1900 BCE as a major spice in Indian cuisine and it is commonly used in various homemade and Ayurvedic medicines [134]. Curcumin is the major curcuminoid found in turmeric [134] and has shown to be non-toxic, anti-oxidant, anti-inflammatory and anti-carcinogenic [135]. The contribution of curcumin in science is evident from the establishment of the Curcumin Resource Database (CRDB) incorporating 1186 curcumin analogs, 195 molecular targets, 9075 peer reviewed publications, 489 patents and 176 varieties of *C. longa* [136]. Curcumin inhibits the proliferation of both normal and malignant cells in a non-selective manner, although its apoptotic effect in malignant cells is more profound [137]. Curcumin treatment increases the expression as well as DNA-binding activity of p53 that culminates in modulation of Bax protein and apoptotic induction [138]. Breast cancer cells treated with curcumin show increased levels of pro-apoptotic protein Bax and decreased the expression of anti-apoptotic protein Bcl-2, resulting in an increase in ratio of Bax/Bcl-2 [139,140]. Curcumin derivative (MTH-3) follows extrinsic pathway of apoptosis by upregulating DR5 and FADD and down-regulating anti-apoptotic proteins [141]. Furthermore, MTH-3 shows a substantial rise in levels of CHOP and decreased the levels of IRE1α [141]. These findings indicate that MTH3 causes apoptosis in breast cancer cells via an ER-regulated mechanism through both extrinsic and intrinsic pathways [141]. Curcumin functions via modulating both extrinsic and intrinsic apoptosis pathways. Curcumin inhibits BCL-2 and XIAP resulting in enhanced expression of BAX and BAK members of the Bcl2 family of intrinsic apoptosis regulators [142]. Curcumin mediated cell cycle arrest at the G2/M phase and growth inhibition of breast cancer cells involves reduction in CDC25 and CDC2 expression. Inhibition of Akt phosphorylation, mTOR and Bcl2 along with increased BAX expression and caspase 3 cleavage are also involved in mediating apoptosis in curcumin treated breast cancer cells [143]. Interestingly, curcumin abrogates fatty acid synthase expression and activity in ER negative breast cancer cells exhibiting its potential as a FAS inhibitor [140]. High expression of FAS is observed in many tumor types and these results indicated that curcumin might inhibit multiple tumor types via FAS inhibition. AMPK activation in cancer cells is known to modulate downstream mTOR pathway leading to tumor growth inhibition. Curcumin activates AMPK in breast cancer cells including triple negative breast cancer cells and regulates ERK, p38, and COX-2 [144]. AMPK stimulation in response to curcumin also leads to activation of autophagy pathway and Akt degradation aiding in inhibition of proliferation and migration of breast cancer cells [145]. A study investigating the combined treatment of curcumin and β-interferon (IFN-β)/retinoic acid (RA) showed that curcumin synergistically increases the efficacy of β-interferon (IFN-β)/retinoic acid (RA) in breast cancer cells by upregulating GRIM-19 via Stat3-independent and –dependent pathways [146]. Although antitumor effects of curcumin are well documented in preclinical arena, its negative effect on the efficacy of chemotherapy has also been proposed [147]. Using *in vitro* and *in vivo* breast cancer models, it was shown that curcumin blocks camptothecin, mechlorethamine and doxorubicin induced apoptosis and lowers cyclophosphamide mediated tumor inhibition by inhibiting ROS generation and JNK pathway [147]. However, a plethora of studies showed that curcumin has the potential to function as a chemosensitizer and improves the efficacy of various chemotherapy drugs including bortezomib, paclitaxel, cisplatin, doxorubicin, gemcitabine, 5-FU, oxaliplatin, vincristine, butyrate, celecoxib, vinorelbine, etoposide, sulfinosine, thalidomide, and melphalan in multiple cancer types (reviewed in [148]). Also, curcumin is effective as a radiosensitizer for many cancer types [148]. Aggarwal, et al., revealed that curcumin potentiates paclitaxel cytotoxicity in breast cancer cells and inhibits lung metastasis in xenograft model [149]. Zhang et al., showed that the combination of curcumin and 5-FU increases apoptosis by blocking autophagy and downregulating AKT activity [150]. Combining curcumin and paclitaxel increases the effectiveness of paclitaxel leading to enhanced apoptosis and G2/M cell cycle arrest by increasing caspase-3/7 activity, PARP cleavage and decreasing nuclear factor (NF)-kB transcription factor [151]. Many chemotherapeutic drugs such as doxorubicin are associated with cardiotoxicity which can be successfully overcome by co-administration of curcumin [152]. HO-3867 (3,5-bis(4-fluoro-benzylidene)-1-[(2,2,5,5-tetramethyl-2,5-dihydro-1-hydroxypyrrol-3-yl)methyl] piperidin-4-one), a synthetic analog of curcumin, has been shown to reduce cardiotoxicity but maintain antitumor efficacy when combined with doxorubicin [152]. Mechanistically, curcumin treatment induces the crosstalk between p53 and p300 while alleviating SMAR1-p65NFkB activation leading to resensitization of doxorubicin-resistant cells to doxorubicin [153]. Curcumin treatment also inhibits doxorubicin-induced EMT by inhibiting TGF-β and PI3K/Akt pathways in TNBC and improves the efficacy of doxorubicin [154]. Multidrug resistance can be reversed with a combined treatment of curcumin and doxorubicin using poly(butyl cyanoacrylate) nanoparticles (PBCA-NPs) with co-encapsulated doxorubicin (DOX) and curcumin (CUR) [155]. Co-delivery of curcumin and doxorubicin using core-shell nanoparticles (NPs) with hydrophobic PLLA core loaded with curcumin (Cur) and hydrophilic heparin shell adsorbing doxorubicin (DOX) exhibits promising results for effective breast tumor inhibition [156]. Various research groups have developed nanoparticles containing curcumin alone or in combination with chemotherapies to enhance therapeutic efficacy and bioavailability [157–159]. Development of curcumin-loaded solid nanoparticles (Cur-SLN) [157], non-spherical mesoporous silica nanoparticles (MSNAs) [158], and HER2 aptamer-decorated curcumin-loaded human serum albumin nanoparticle (Apt-HSA/CCM NP) [159] are just few examples of nanoparticle approaches. There are multiple other formulations using liposomes, micelles, polymer nanoparticles, nanogels, cyclodextrin complexes, solid lipid nanoparticles (SLN), phytosomes, and gold nanoparticles being developed to further curcumin research [160,161].

7. Genistein, a Phytoestrogen from Soy

Genistein (5,7-dihydroxy-3-(4-hydroxyphenyl) chromen-4-one) is an isoflavone phytoestrogen compound present in soybeans and soy food products and is recognized for its beneficial health effects as well as for its chemopreventive and therapeutic properties against multiple cancers [162–165]. Genistein can effectively bind to estrogen receptors owing to its structural similarity to endogenous 17β-estradiol (E2) [166] raising concerns regarding its potential as a cancer-promoting agent especially for ER-positive breast cancer [167,168]. Additional factors such as genistein intake mode (minimally processed soy foods, MPSFs vs. soy protein isolates) and time of exposure along with individual's characteristics such as metabolic function, menopausal status, estrogen receptor expression and gene mutations also play an important role in mediating the chemo preventative or cancer-promoting functions of genistein [169]. It is interesting to note that level of soy exposure modulates its biological impact with higher intake of soy associated with lower breast cancer risk [170]. Importantly, clinical studies conducted in Asian population where the soy intake is much higher (5–20 mg/day) show a protective effect of soy on breast cancer risk whereas no correlation is observed in western population with low soy intake (0.8–0.15 mg per day) [170]. *In vitro* and *in vivo* studies support the dose-specific effect of genistein with low doses (≤10 μmol/L) increasing the estrogenic activity while the higher doses

(≥10 μmol/L) mediate anti-cancer effects [171,172]. Shim et al., reported that genistein treatment at micromolar concentrations stimulates apoptosis in breast cancer cells via activating calpain, caspase-7 and polymerase (ADP-ribose) in breast cancer cells. Additionally, genistein treated MCF7 cells exhibit enhanced phosphorylation of p38 mitogen-activated protein kinase and apoptosis signaling kinase 1 while ERK $\frac{1}{2}$ phosphorylation remained unaltered [173]. Another study revealed that genistein could block cell proliferation and induce apoptosis by inactivating the IGF-1R-PI3K/Akt pathway and decreasing the expression of Bcl-2/Bax [174]. Genistein treatment reduces the survival of breast cancer stem cells by blocking downstream hedgehog signaling leading to apoptosis [175]. Interestingly, genistein treatment increases the radiosensitivity of breast cancer cells. Breast cancer cells irradiated in the presence of genistein show increased DNA damage and cell cycle inhibition at G2/M phase via activation of ATM, Chk2, Cdc25C and Cdc2 checkpoint pathway. Breast cancer cells cotreated with genistein and radiation also exhibit upregulation of Bax and p73 and downregulation of Bcl2 [176]. Genistein-containing diet does not affect mammary gland proliferation but increases the apoptotic index and expression of PTEN in mammary glands of young adult rats [177]. Treatment with serum from these genistein-fed rats increases apoptosis and PTEN expression in MCF-7 breast cancer cells and, interestingly, silencing of PTEN abrogates the anti-cancer effects of serum from genistein-fed rats [177]. Investigating the chemopreventive potential of genistein, Katdare et al., showed that genistein can modulate cell cycle progression and induce apoptosis in 184-B5/HER breast epithelial cells, a model for comedo-form ductal carcinoma in situ (comedo-DCIS) via downregulation of Her2/neu signaling cascade, upregulation of p16INK4 and BCL2 [178]. This study showed that genistein administration can potentially prevent the progression of DCIS to invasive ductal carcinoma. Invasion and migration are important characteristics of an invasive cancer and genistein blocks invasion and migration of breast cancer cells by inhibiting S-phase kinase-associated protein 2 (Skp2), which is an important kinase frequently upregulated in multiple cancers [179]. Combined treatment with genistein and doxorubicin increases intracellular buildup of doxorubicin and increases efficacy of chemotherapy [180,181]. Inhibition of NK-kB has been implicated in synergistic effect of genistein on various chemotherapy drugs such as cisplatin, docetaxel and doxorubicin [181,182]. Contrasting with the synergistic or additive effect of genistein in potentiating the efficacy of chemotherapy, it has been shown that genistein interferes with the anti-tumor impact of cisplatin in breast cancer cells [172]. Importantly, anti-cisplatin effect of genistein is abrogated in the presence of estrogen in ER-positive breast cancer cells, an effect not observed in ER-negative breast cancer cells [172]. While mechanistic studies are still needed to fully decipher the pathways underlying the pro-tumor vs. anti-tumor effects of genistein, multiple studies have shown how the beneficial effects of genistein can be achieved by carefully titrating its dose in single as well as combination regimens.

8. Epigallocatechin-3-Gallate (EGCG), a Green Tea Polyphenol

Epidemiological studies conducted in Japan showed the chemopreventive effects of drinking green tea on breast cancer in women who consumed approximately 10 cups of green tea/day [183]. Many case control and cohort studies have evaluated the effect of green tea on breast cancer and have shown that green tea consumption is associated with a decreased risk of breast cancer [184,185]. Beneficial effects of green tea are associated with catechins class of phytochemicals such as epigallocatechin-3-gallate (EGCG), epicatechingallate (ECG), epigallocatechin (EGC), and epicatechin (EC). EGCG, the ester of epigallocatechin and gallic acid accounts for 40% of total catechins in green tea leaves and is the most important catechin with antioxidant, anti-inflammatory, and anti-carcinogenic potential [186]. Treatment with physiological concentrations of EGCG leads to growth inhibition in breast cancer cells mediated in part by ERα down-regulation, insulin-like growth factor binding protein-2 (IGFBP-2) reduction and p53/p21 upregulation [187]. Nude mice treated with EGCG exhibit inhibition of breast tumor progression and downregulation of multiple key effector molecules including Cyclin D, Cyclin E, CDK 4, CDK 1 and PCNA [188]. Deguchi et al., revealed that breast cancer cells treated with EGCG show increased phosphorylation of JNK/SAPK and p38 which in turn inhibit cdc2 phosphorylation and modulate the expression of Cyclin A, Cyclin Bl, and Cdks, resulting in G2 arrest [189]. Inhibition of Akt along with activation of caspase 3/9 and upregulation of p53 and PTEN leads to apoptotic induction in breast cancer cells treated with EGCG [190,191]. Another study investigating the involvement of Akt in EGCG function showed that EGCG induces growth-inhibition and apoptosis-induction through survivin suppression mediated by blockade of Akt pathway [192]. Induction of apoptosis upon EGCG treatment is associated with enhanced p53 expression, increased release of cytochrome c from mitochondria to cytosol, elevated expression of Apaf-1, and activation of caspase-3 and polymerase (ADP-Ribose) [191]. Also, mouse mammary epithelial cell 4T1 treated with EGCG showed increased p53, Apaf-1, caspase 3 cleavage and high cytochrome C release [193]. A study investigating the dose-dependent effect of EGCG shows that treatment with 50 μM EGCG increases oxidative stress, activation of JNK, and cleavage of caspase 3/9 leading to apoptotic induction while a higher concentration (100–400 μM) causes a necrotic cell death [194]. EGCG also functions through cell membrane-related signaling pathways and alters EGFR, LR, FAS, E-cadherin and β-catenin leading to suppression of cell proliferation, induction of apoptosis through nuclear condensation, and increased caspase-3 activity [195]. EGCG treatment inhibits telomerase activity by decreasing hTERT levels resulting in inhibition of cell growth and induction of apoptosis in MCF-7 breast cancer cells [196]. EGCG mediated growth inhibition and apoptotic induction involves downregulation of miR-25 whose restoration abrogates EGCG-induced apoptosis [197]. Therapeutic efficacy of EGCG has been well established and now efforts are being made to improve its bioavailability, stability and efficacy via utilizing various nanoparticles. Encapsulation of EGCG in the matrix of solid lipid nanoparticles and further conjugation with gastrin releasing peptide receptors (GRPR)-specific peptide not only provides stability to EGCG but also provides specificity towards GRPR overexpressed on breast cancer cells. Treatment with EGCG nanoparticles achieves significantly improved tumor growth inhibition in C57/BL6 mice [198]. EGCG loaded arginyl-glycyl-aspartic acid (RGD)-containing nanostructured lipid carriers (NLC) exhibit improved cytotoxicity and apoptosis in breast cancer cells proposing that EGCG-loaded NLC-RGD may prove beneficial for cancer treatment [199]. FA-NPS-PEG and FA-PEG-NPS also show anti-tumor efficacy in breast cancer cells [200]. Collectively, EGCG shows great potential as a chemopreventive and therapeutic agent.

9. Bioactive Compounds Based Anti-Cancer Drugs in Clinical Trials

It is important to note that many successful anti-cancer drugs such as taxol, Vinca alkaloids, combrestatin, epipodophyllotoxin, camptothecin, and their analogues have plant-based origins. Analogues of antimitotic agent paclitaxel/taxol including DHA-paclitaxel, ortataxel, taxol-HMPA polymer, and paclitaxel poliglumex are currently being evaluated in phase I-III clinical trials. Topoisomerase I/II inhibitor-camptothecin-based analogues and podophyllotoxin analogues as well as microtubule destabilizing agents—*Vinca* alkaloids (vinblastine, and vincristine)—analogues are being developed for the clinic (reviewed in [201]). In addition to these drugs with bioactive origins, there are multiple other bioactive compounds that have strong preclinical supporting data underlining their potential as chemopreventive and therapeutic agents against multiple cancers including breast cancer. Clinical development of some of these compounds has begun albeit with a focus on disease conditions other than cancer. (Table 1).

Table 1. Clinical Development of Bioactive Compounds.

Bioactive Compound	Clinical Trials	Phase	ClinicalTrials.Gov Identifier
Withania somnifera (Sensoril or Ashwagandha)	A randomized study conducted for schizophrenia	Interventional	NCT01793935
Curcumin and Ashwagandha extract	To study the safety and efficacy of Curcumin and Ashwagandha extract in osteosarcoma.	Phase 1 and Phase 2	NCT00689195

Table 1. *Cont.*

Bioactive Compound	Clinical Trials	Phase	ClinicalTrials.Gov Identifier
WFA	To evaluate the cognitive abilities in persons with bipolar disorder and to study the residual mood/anxiety symptoms	Phase 3	NCFT00761761
WFA	To study the safety and efficacy of the drug in patients having generalized anxiety disorder	Phase 2	NCT01311180
Resveratrol	Colon cancer patients were randomly given resveratrol at different concentration to study Wnt signaling pathway.	Phase 1	NCT00256334
Resveratrol	To study the effect of Notch signaling in neuroendocrine tumor treated with Resveratrol.	Interventional	NCT01476592
Resveratrol	To study the effect of resveratrol in colorectal cancer and also studied for tolerability, target tissue levels and pharmacodynamics.	Phase 1	NCT00433576
Resveratrol	A randomized trial to determine the disposition and characterize dietary polyphenols in normal and breast cancer patient.	Interventional	NCT03482401
Resveratrol	A randomized double-blind study, resveratrol was given for two weeks in non-diabetic obese subjects.	Phase 2	NCT02247596
Isothiocyanate	A randomized clinical trial, to study phenethyl isothiocyanate in lung cancer patients.	Phase 2	NCT00691132
Isothiocyanate	A randomized phase II study, patients received broccoli sprout extract through oral three times daily for 8 weeks to breast cancer patients, ductal carcinoma in situ and/or atypical ductal hyperplasia	Phase 2	NCT00843167 PMID:26511489 PMID:26329135
Curcumin	A randomized, double-blind, placebo-controlled study of curcumin for the prevention of acute radiation-induced dermatitis during postoperative radiotherapy for breast cancer.	Phase 2	NCT01042938
Curcumin	A randomized A randomized study treating docetaxel alone or together with curcumin in HER2 negative patients with metastatic breast cancer	Phase 2	NCT00852332
Genistein	A randomized study of genistein treatment in high risk of breast cancer patients.	Phase 2	NCT00290758 PMID: 22307566
Genistein	A randomized, phase 1 trial of genistein in preventing breast or endometrial cancer	Phase 1	NCT00099008 PMID:18446090
EGCG	A randomized phase 1 study, to find the effect of catechin extract in hormone negative stage I-III breast cancer patients	Phase 1	NCT00516243
EGCG	A phase 2 trial, to study the effect of green tea extract in breast cancer	Phase 2	NCT00917735 PMID 30926986, 28747487, 27806972, 26701796, 26581683

In a randomized, interventional clinical trial for schizophrenia patients, significant benefits were noted upon administration of a standardized extract of *Withania somnifera* (WSE) as compared to placebo control. This study successfully showed that a dose of WSE (1000 mg/day) provided beneficial effects with minimal side effects. Inflammatory markers and cytokine levels were also measured [202] (NCT01793935). Multiple other clinical trials have examined/are examining the clinical benefits of *Withania somnifera* extracts for schizophrenia (WSE 500 mg/day for 12 weeks; NCT03437668); cognitive impairment in elderly subjects (NCT03780621); periodontitis (Ashwagandha capsules 500 mg/day for

30 days; NCT03533972, NCT00010634); endurance exercise performance (NCT03596307), generalized anxiety disorder (NCT01311180); and bipolar disorder (Ashwagandha capsules 250/500 mg/day, NCT00761761). In a multicenter, observational, prospective study including patients with mood disorder, sleep disorder, anxiety or depression, the effects of soy isoflavones in combination with magnolia extract were studied (NCT01805674).

Bioactive compounds are being considered for cancer prevention in high risk population. Phenethyl isothiocyanate was given to the recruits orally 4 times a day for 30 days (NCT00005883) in a phase I trial to examine whether phenethyl isothiocyanate can prevent lung cancer in smokers. It is important to examine the bioavailability of bioactive compounds and a randomized early phase I trial examined bioavailability and absorption of bioactive compounds in broccoli (NCT01743924). In another phase II trial, women with breast cancer/precancerous state (ductal carcinoma in situ and atypical ductal hyperplasia) received broccoli sprout extract three times daily for 2–8 weeks with an aim to examine sulforaphane metabolism, HDAC activity, Ki-67 index and apoptosis (NCT00843167). Results from this trial showed that isothiocyanates, including sulforaphane, were present in urine samples in micromolar concentration along with changes in Ki-67 levels and HDAC activity in tumor samples of the patients in intervention arm.

Resveratrol has been examined for many clinical conditions, such as diabetes, heart failure, pulmonary disease and inflammation (NCT03762096, NCT02245932 and NCT02244879). In a phase I trial, resveratrol was given to colon cancer patients to examine the alteration in Wnt signaling pathway in response to resveratrol (NCT00256334). Resveratrol administration led to inhibition of Wnt pathway in normal colonic mucosa indicating a potential chemopreventive effect of resveratrol in colon cancer [203]. Patients with low-grade GI neuroendocrine tumors were treated with oral resveratrol (5 g/day) to determine the well-tolerated dose of resveratrol and its effect on tumor markers and Notch1 signaling pathway (NCT01476592). Another phase 1 clinical trial determined the safety, pharmacokinetics and modulation of insulin-like growth factor-1 (IGF-1) and IGF-binding protein-3 (IGFBP-3) in response to repeat dosing of resveratrol. Healthy participants received different doses of resveratrol once a day for 29 days. It was observed that 2.5/5 g of resveratrol treatment resulted in decreased IGF-1 and IGFBP-3 in the circulation albeit mild gastrointestinal symptoms were also observed (NCT00098969) [204].

More than 200 clinical trials have been conducted or are ongoing to evaluate the effect of curcumin on various disease conditions (*ClinicalTrials.gov*). An interventional, randomized double-blind study evaluated the efficacy of curcumin for the prevention of radiation-induced dermatitis in breast cancer patients. Breast cancer patients undergoing radiation treatment were given 2.0 g of curcumin thrice/daily for the course of radiation treatment (~4–7 weeks) (NCT01042938). Additional clinical trials (NCT02556632, NCT01246973) have also examined the effect of curcumin-based gel or oral-curcumin on radiation induced dermatitis. A phase II study examined the efficacy of curcumin intervention to reduce NF-kB DNA binding and IL6 levels in chemotherapy-treated breast cancer patients undergoing radiotherapy (NCT01740323). Chemopreventive effects of curcumin were examined in women with obesity and other high-risk factors for breast cancer development and levels of pro-inflammatory biomarkers in plasma and breast adipose tissues were examined (NCT01975363). Multiple clinical trials are currently evaluating the beneficial effects of curcumin for breast cancer prevention, combination-treatment (NCT03072992) and alleviating various breast cancer treatment-related side effects such as aromatase inhibitor-induced joint disease (NCT03865992).

10. Conclusions

Despite major advances in the development of novel cancer therapeutics, cancer is still the second leading cause of mortality world-wide with ~9.6 million people succumbing to cancer in 2018. Low and middle-income countries endure a bigger burden with 70% of cancer related deaths occurring in these parts of the world (https://www.who.int/en/news-room/fact-sheets/detail/cancer). Owing to these facts there is an urgent need to develop more affordable and effective therapeutic and preventive strategies to counteract the upsurge of cancer incidences. With the better understanding of molecular subtypes of various cancers, past few years have seen a dramatic increase in "one gene, one drug, one disease" approach to develop novel targeted therapeutic approaches. Although this approach has resulted in many effective drugs, the activation of alternative pathways often circumvents the inhibitory effect of 'the targeted gene' leading to the development of resistance. Resistant tumors are often more aggressive than the primary disease and are usually unresponsive to standard treatments owing to the heterogeneity within tumor and the presence of cancer stem cells. Combining various single target drugs is also being evaluated but these cocktails have not proven to be the 'silver bullets' either. Nature has performed the best combinatorial chemistry and blessed us with innumerable bioactive compounds that target various hallmarks of cancers simultaneously [205,206]. A plethora of epidemiological studies have shown the beneficial effects of bioactive compounds in various disease states including cancer. Most of these bioactive compounds have been successfully used in traditional medicines such as Ayurvedic, Chinese, Unani, and Homeopathy. As discussed in this review, large numbers of preclinical studies utilizing various in vitro and in vivo model systems have shown the chemopreventive and therapeutic role of various bioactive compounds laying a solid foundation for further clinical development (Table 2). Despite these evidences, clinical studies to evaluate the efficacy of bioactive compounds have been rather limited as the cancer research field has been focusing mainly on synthetic molecules targeting a single gene/protein. It is well known that cancer progression is mediated by an interaction of various signaling pathways but the very fact that bioactive compounds simultaneously modulate various pathways goes against them as the cancer research field remains too focused on single target drugs. Bioactive compounds can be optimal chemopreventive agents since they selectively target cancer cells with no or low toxicity to normal cells, many of them can be included in daily diet, are already part of the food system and are comparatively cheaper.

Table 2. Mechanistic Underpinnings of Bioactive Compounds.

Bioactive Compounds	Models	Specific Mechanism of Action	References
Withaferin A (WFA)	Human breast cancer, liver cancer	↑ PARP ↑expression of Bim-S and Bim EL ↓expression of Bcl2 ↑ generation of ROS ↑Bax and Bak ↓expression of XIAP G2/M arrest, ↓ PCNA and ↑apoptosis	[22,27,28,33,37]
Honokiol (HNK)	Human breast cancer	↑G2/M arrest ↑ AMPK	[52,54]
Benzyl Isothiocyanate (BITC)	Human breast cancer	↑ROS ↑Increased caspase 3 ↓mTOR ↓XIAP	[87,88,90,94]
Resveratrol	Human breast cancer	↓Bcl-2, ↓Bcl-XL, ↑Bax ↑Increased caspase 3	[117,118]
Curcumin	Human breast cancer	↓Bcl-2, ↑Bax, ↑Caspase 3, ↑AMPK, ↓AKT ↓pAKT/↓mTOR ↑PARP ↑Caspase3 and ↑caspase 7	[139,143,145,151]
Genistein	Human breast cancer	↑Caspase7, p38MAPK ↓Bcl2 ↑ATM/Chk2/Cdc25C/Cdc2	[173,174,176]
Epigallocatechin-3-gallate (EGCG)	Human breast cancer	↓Cdc ↑Bax, Bcl2, ↑ADP ribose, ↑Caspase 3 ↑hTERT	[189–191,196]

Author Contributions: N.M., S.S. and D.S. contributed to designing and writing of this review.

Acknowledgments: All figures have been constructed with the help of smart images from Servier medical art (https://smart.servier.com/).

References

1. Sauter, E.R. Breast Cancer Prevention: Current Approaches and Future Directions. *Eur. J. Breast Health* **2018**, *14*, 64–71. [CrossRef] [PubMed]
2. Doyle, L.A.; Yang, W.; Abruzzo, L.V.; Krogmann, T.; Gao, Y.; Rishi, A.K.; Ross, D.D. A multidrug resistance transporter from human MCF-7 breast cancer cells. *Proc. Natl. Acad. Sci. USA* **1998**, *95*, 15665–15670. [CrossRef] [PubMed]
3. Ju, J.; Zhu, A.J.; Yuan, P. Progress in targeted therapy for breast cancer. *Chronic Dis. Transl. Med.* **2018**, *4*, 164–175. [CrossRef]
4. Parton, M.; Dowsett, M.; Smith, I. Studies of apoptosis in breast cancer. *BMJ* **2001**, *322*, 1528–1532. [CrossRef] [PubMed]
5. Fridlender, M.; Kapulnik, Y.; Koltai, H. Plant derived substances with anti-cancer activity: From folklore to practice. *Front. Plant Sci.* **2015**, *6*, 799. [CrossRef] [PubMed]
6. Biesalski, H.K.; Dragsted, L.O.; Elmadfa, I.; Grossklaus, R.; Muller, M.; Schrenk, D.; Walter, P.; Weber, P. Bioactive compounds: Definition and assessment of activity. *Nutrition* **2009**, *25*, 1202–1205. [CrossRef]
7. Gali-Muhtasib, H.; Hmadi, R.; Kareh, M.; Tohme, R.; Darwiche, N. Cell death mechanisms of plant-derived anticancer drugs: Beyond apoptosis. *Apoptosis* **2015**, *20*, 1531–1562. [CrossRef]
8. Korkina, L.; Kostyuk, V. Biotechnologically produced secondary plant metabolites for cancer treatment and prevention. *Curr. Pharm. Biotechnol.* **2012**, *13*, 265–275. [CrossRef]
9. Newman, D.J.; Cragg, G.M. Natural products as sources of new drugs over the 30 years from 1981 to 2010. *J. Nat. Prod.* **2012**, *75*, 311–335. [CrossRef]
10. Teiten, M.H.; Gaascht, F.; Dicato, M.; Diederich, M. Anticancer bioactivity of compounds from medicinal plants used in European medieval traditions. *Biochem. Pharmacol.* **2013**, *86*, 1239–1247. [CrossRef]
11. George, B.P.; Abrahamse, H. Increased Oxidative Stress Induced by Rubus Bioactive Compounds Induce Apoptotic Cell Death in Human Breast Cancer Cells. *Oxidative Med. Cell. Longev.* **2019**, *2019*, 6797921. [CrossRef] [PubMed]
12. Shin, S.A.; Moon, S.Y.; Kim, W.Y.; Paek, S.M.; Park, H.H.; Lee, C.S. Structure-Based Classification and Anti-Cancer Effects of Plant Metabolites. *Int. J. Mol. Sci.* **2018**, *19*, 2651. [CrossRef] [PubMed]
13. Wang, H.; Khor, T.O.; Shu, L.; Su, Z.-Y.; Fuentes, F.; Lee, J.-H.; Kong, A.-N.T. Plants vs. Cancer: A Review on Natural Phytochemicals in Preventing and Treating Cancers and Their Druggability. *Anti-Cancer Agents Med. Chem.* **2012**, *12*, 1281–1305. [CrossRef]
14. Cianciosi, D.; Varela-Lopez, A.; Forbes-Hernandez, T.Y.; Gasparrini, M.; Afrin, S.; Reboredo-Rodriguez, P.; Zhang, J.; Quiles, J.L.; Nabavi, S.F.; Battino, M.; et al. Targeting molecular pathways in cancer stem cells by natural bioactive compounds. *Pharmacol. Res.* **2018**, *135*, 150–165. [CrossRef]
15. Wang, Y.; Li, Y.; Liu, X.; Cho, W.C. Genetic and epigenetic studies for determining molecular targets of natural product anticancer agents. *Curr. Cancer Drug Targets* **2013**, *13*, 506–518. [CrossRef]
16. Andrade, S.; Ramalho, M.J.; Loureiro, J.A.; Pereira, M.D.C. Natural Compounds for Alzheimer's Disease Therapy: A Systematic Review of Preclinical and Clinical Studies. *Int. J. Mol. Sci.* **2019**, *20*, 2313. [CrossRef]
17. Aumeeruddy, M.Z.; Mahomoodally, M.F. Combating breast cancer using combination therapy with 3 phytochemicals: Piperine, sulforaphane, and thymoquinone. *Cancer* **2019**, *125*, 1600–1611. [CrossRef]
18. Fu, B.; Wang, N.; Tan, H.Y.; Li, S.; Cheung, F.; Feng, Y. Multi-Component Herbal Products in the Prevention and Treatment of Chemotherapy-Associated Toxicity and Side Effects: A Review on Experimental and Clinical Evidences. *Front. Pharmacol.* **2018**, *9*, 1394. [CrossRef]
19. Kura, B.; Parikh, M.; Slezak, J.; Pierce, G.N. The Influence of Diet on MicroRNAs that Impact Cardiovascular Disease. *Molecules* **2019**, *24*, 1509. [CrossRef]

20. Mitra, S.; Dash, R. Natural Products for the Management and Prevention of Breast Cancer. *Evid. Based Complement. Altern. Med.* **2018**, *2018*, 8324696. [CrossRef]
21. Kaileh, M.; Vanden Berghe, W.; Heyerick, A.; Horion, J.; Piette, J.; Libert, C.; De Keukeleire, D.; Essawi, T.; Haegeman, G. Withaferin a strongly elicits IkappaB kinase beta hyperphosphorylation concomitant with potent inhibition of its kinase activity. *J. Biol. Chem.* **2007**, *282*, 4253–4264. [CrossRef] [PubMed]
22. Stan, S.D.; Hahm, E.R.; Warin, R.; Singh, S.V. Withaferin A causes FOXO3a- and Bim-dependent apoptosis and inhibits growth of human breast cancer cells in vivo. *Cancer Res.* **2008**, *68*, 7661–7669. [CrossRef] [PubMed]
23. Misra, L.; Mishra, P.; Pandey, A.; Sangwan, R.S.; Sangwan, N.S.; Tuli, R. Withanolides from Withania somnifera roots. *Phytochemistry* **2008**, *69*, 1000–1004. [CrossRef] [PubMed]
24. Stan, S.D.; Zeng, Y.; Singh, S.V. Ayurvedic medicine constituent withaferin a causes G2 and M phase cell cycle arrest in human breast cancer cells. *Nutr. Cancer* **2008**, *60* (Suppl. 1), 51–60. [CrossRef]
25. Nagalingam, A.; Kuppusamy, P.; Singh, S.V.; Sharma, D.; Saxena, N.K. Mechanistic elucidation of the antitumor properties of withaferin a in breast cancer. *Cancer Res.* **2014**, *74*, 2617–2629. [CrossRef]
26. Hahm, E.R.; Lee, J.; Kim, S.H.; Sehrawat, A.; Arlotti, J.A.; Shiva, S.S.; Bhargava, R.; Singh, S.V. Metabolic alterations in mammary cancer prevention by withaferin A in a clinically relevant mouse model. *J. Natl. Cancer Inst.* **2013**, *105*, 1111–1122. [CrossRef]
27. Hahm, E.R.; Moura, M.B.; Kelley, E.E.; Van Houten, B.; Shiva, S.; Singh, S.V. Withaferin A-induced apoptosis in human breast cancer cells is mediated by reactive oxygen species. *PLoS ONE* **2011**, *6*, e23354. [CrossRef]
28. Hahm, E.R.; Singh, S.V. Withaferin A-induced apoptosis in human breast cancer cells is associated with suppression of inhibitor of apoptosis family protein expression. *Cancer Lett.* **2013**, *334*, 101–108. [CrossRef]
29. Widodo, N.; Priyandoko, D.; Shah, N.; Wadhwa, R.; Kaul, S.C. Selective killing of cancer cells by Ashwagandha leaf extract and its component Withanone involves ROS signaling. *PLoS ONE* **2010**, *5*, e13536. [CrossRef]
30. Liu, X.; Li, Y.; Ma, Q.; Wang, Y.; Song, A.L. Withaferin-A Inhibits Growth of Drug-Resistant Breast Carcinoma by Inducing Apoptosis and Autophagy, Endogenous Reactive Oxygen Species (ROS) Production, and Inhibition of Cell Migration and Nuclear Factor kappa B (Nf-kappaB)/Mammalian Target of Rapamycin (m-TOR) Signalling Pathway. *Med. Sci. Monit.* **2019**, *25*, 6855–6863. [CrossRef]
31. Yco, L.P.; Mocz, G.; Opoku-Ansah, J.; Bachmann, A.S. Withaferin A Inhibits STAT3 and Induces Tumor Cell Death in Neuroblastoma and Multiple Myeloma. *Biochem. Insights* **2014**, *7*, 1–13. [CrossRef] [PubMed]
32. Sehrawat, A.; Samanta, S.K.; Hahm, E.R.; Croix, C.; Watkins, S.; Singh, S.V. Withaferin A-mediated apoptosis in breast cancer cells is associated with alterations in mitochondrial dynamics. *Mitochondrion* **2019**, *47*, 282–293. [CrossRef] [PubMed]
33. Muniraj, N.; Siddharth, S.; Nagalingam, A.; Walker, A.; Woo, J.; Gyorffy, B.; Gabrielson, E.; Saxena, N.K.; Sharma, D. Withaferin A inhibits lysosomal activity to block autophagic flux and induces apoptosis via energetic impairment in breast cancer cells. *Carcinogenesis* **2019**, *40*, 1110–1120. [CrossRef] [PubMed]
34. Zhang, X.; Mukerji, R.; Samadi, A.K.; Cohen, M.S. Down-regulation of estrogen receptor-alpha and rearranged during transfection tyrosine kinase is associated with withaferin a-induced apoptosis in MCF-7 breast cancer cells. *BMC Complement. Altern. Med.* **2011**, *11*, 84. [CrossRef]
35. Hahm, E.R.; Lee, J.; Huang, Y.; Singh, S.V. Withaferin a suppresses estrogen receptor-alpha expression in human breast cancer cells. *Mol. Carcinog.* **2011**, *50*, 614–624. [CrossRef] [PubMed]
36. Kim, S.H.; Singh, S.V. Mammary cancer chemoprevention by withaferin A is accompanied by in vivo suppression of self-renewal of cancer stem cells. *Cancer Prev. Res.* **2014**, *7*, 738–747. [CrossRef] [PubMed]
37. Royston, K.J.; Udayakumar, N.; Lewis, K.; Tollefsbol, T.O. A Novel Combination of Withaferin A and Sulforaphane Inhibits Epigenetic Machinery, Cellular Viability and Induces Apoptosis of Breast Cancer Cells. *Int. J. Mol. Sci.* **2017**, *18*, 1092. [CrossRef]
38. Kakar, S.S.; Ratajczak, M.Z.; Powell, K.S.; Moghadamfalahi, M.; Miller, D.M.; Batra, S.K.; Singh, S.K. Withaferin a alone and in combination with cisplatin suppresses growth and metastasis of ovarian cancer by targeting putative cancer stem cells. *PLoS ONE* **2014**, *9*, e107596. [CrossRef]
39. Kakar, S.S.; Jala, V.R.; Fong, M.Y. Synergistic cytotoxic action of cisplatin and withaferin A on ovarian cancer cell lines. *Biochem. Biophys. Res. Commun.* **2012**, *423*, 819–825. [CrossRef]
40. Hahm, E.R.; Lee, J.; Abella, T.; Singh, S.V. Withaferin A inhibits expression of ataxia telangiectasia and Rad3-related kinase and enhances sensitivity of human breast cancer cells to cisplatin. *Mol. Carcinog.* **2019**, *58*, 2139–2148. [CrossRef]

41. Fried, L.E.; Arbiser, J.L. Honokiol, a multifunctional antiangiogenic and antitumor agent. *Antioxid Redox Signal.* **2009**, *11*, 1139–1148. [CrossRef]
42. Amblard, F.; Govindarajan, B.; Lefkove, B.; Rapp, K.L.; Detorio, M.; Arbiser, J.L.; Schinazi, R.F. Synthesis, cytotoxicity, and antiviral activities of new neolignans related to honokiol and magnolol. *Bioorg. Med. Chem. Lett.* **2007**, *17*, 4428–4431. [CrossRef] [PubMed]
43. Li, N.; Song, Y.; Zhang, W.; Wang, W.; Chen, J.; Wong, A.W.; Roberts, A. Evaluation of the in vitro and in vivo genotoxicity of magnolia bark extract. *Regul. Toxicol. Pharmacol. RTP* **2007**, *49*, 154–159. [CrossRef] [PubMed]
44. Liu, Z.; Zhang, X.; Cui, W.; Zhang, X.; Li, N.; Chen, J.; Wong, A.W.; Roberts, A. Evaluation of short-term and subchronic toxicity of magnolia bark extract in rats. *Regul. Toxicol. Pharmacol. RTP* **2007**, *49*, 160–171. [CrossRef] [PubMed]
45. Lee, Y.J.; Lee, Y.M.; Lee, C.K.; Jung, J.K.; Han, S.B.; Hong, J.T. Therapeutic applications of compounds in the Magnolia family. *Pharmacol. Ther.* **2011**, *130*, 157–176. [CrossRef] [PubMed]
46. Manach, C.; Scalbert, A.; Morand, C.; Remesy, C.; Jimenez, L. Polyphenols: Food sources and bioavailability. *Am. J. Clin. Nutr.* **2004**, *79*, 727–747. [CrossRef] [PubMed]
47. Ikai, T.; Akao, Y.; Nakagawa, Y.; Ohguchi, K.; Sakai, Y.; Nozawa, Y. Magnolol-induced apoptosis is mediated via the intrinsic pathway with release of AIF from mitochondria in U937 cells. *Biol. Pharm. Bull.* **2006**, *29*, 2498–2501. [CrossRef]
48. Rasul, A.; Yu, B.; Khan, M.; Zhang, K.; Iqbal, F.; Ma, T.; Yang, H. Magnolol, a natural compound, induces apoptosis of SGC-7901 human gastric adenocarcinoma cells via the mitochondrial and PI3K/Akt signaling pathways. *Int. J. Oncol.* **2012**, *40*, 1153–1161. [CrossRef]
49. Fong, W.F.; Tse, A.K.; Poon, K.H.; Wang, C. Magnolol and honokiol enhance HL-60 human leukemia cell differentiation induced by 1,25-dihydroxyvitamin D3 and retinoic acid. *Int. J. Biochem. Cell Biol.* **2005**, *37*, 427–441. [CrossRef]
50. Lee, S.J.; Cho, Y.H.; Park, K.; Kim, E.J.; Jung, K.H.; Park, S.S.; Kim, W.J.; Moon, S.K. Magnolol elicits activation of the extracellular signal-regulated kinase pathway by inducing p27KIP1-mediated G2/M-phase cell cycle arrest in human urinary bladder cancer 5637 cells. *Biochem. Pharmacol.* **2008**, *75*, 2289–2300. [CrossRef]
51. Park, J.B.; Lee, M.S.; Cha, E.Y.; Lee, J.S.; Sul, J.Y.; Song, I.S.; Kim, J.Y. Magnolol-induced apoptosis in HCT-116 colon cancer cells is associated with the AMP-activated protein kinase signaling pathway. *Biol. Pharm. Bull.* **2012**, *35*, 1614–1620. [CrossRef] [PubMed]
52. Zhou, Y.; Bi, Y.; Yang, C.; Yang, J.; Jiang, Y.; Meng, F.; Yu, B.; Khan, M.; Ma, T.; Yang, H. Magnolol induces apoptosis in MCF-7 human breast cancer cells through G2/M phase arrest and caspase-independent pathway. *Pharmazie* **2013**, *68*, 755–762. [PubMed]
53. Bai, X.; Cerimele, F.; Ushio-Fukai, M.; Waqas, M.; Campbell, P.M.; Govindarajan, B.; Der, C.J.; Battle, T.; Frank, D.A.; Ye, K.; et al. Honokiol, a small molecular weight natural product, inhibits angiogenesis in vitro and tumor growth in vivo. *J. Biol. Chem.* **2003**, *278*, 35501–35507. [CrossRef] [PubMed]
54. Nagalingam, A.; Arbiser, J.L.; Bonner, M.Y.; Saxena, N.K.; Sharma, D. Honokiol activates AMP-activated protein kinase in breast cancer cells via an LKB1-dependent pathway and inhibits breast carcinogenesis. *Breast Cancer Res.* **2012**, *14*, R35. [CrossRef] [PubMed]
55. Wolf, I.; O'Kelly, J.; Wakimoto, N.; Nguyen, A.; Amblard, F.; Karlan, B.Y.; Arbiser, J.L.; Koeffler, H.P. Honokiol, a natural biphenyl, inhibits in vitro and in vivo growth of breast cancer through induction of apoptosis and cell cycle arrest. *Int. J. Oncol.* **2007**, *30*, 1529–1537. [CrossRef]
56. Garcia, A.; Zheng, Y.; Zhao, C.; Toschi, A.; Fan, J.; Shraibman, N.; Brown, H.A.; Bar-Sagi, D.; Foster, D.A.; Arbiser, J.L. Honokiol suppresses survival signals mediated by Ras-dependent phospholipase D activity in human cancer cells. *Clin. Cancer Res.* **2008**, *14*, 4267–4274. [CrossRef]
57. Hou, W.; Chen, L.; Yang, G.; Zhou, H.; Jiang, Q.; Zhong, Z.; Hu, J.; Chen, X.; Wang, X.; Yuan, Y.; et al. Synergistic antitumor effects of liposomal honokiol combined with adriamycin in breast cancer models. *Phytother. Res.* **2008**, *22*, 1125–1132. [CrossRef]
58. Tse, A.K.; Wan, C.K.; Shen, X.L.; Yang, M.; Fong, W.F. Honokiol inhibits TNF-alpha-stimulated NF-kappaB activation and NF-kappaB-regulated gene expression through suppression of IKK activation. *Biochem. Pharmacol.* **2005**, *70*, 1443–1457. [CrossRef]
59. Samarajeewa, N.U.; Yang, F.; Docanto, M.M.; Sakurai, M.; McNamara, K.M.; Sasano, H.; Fox, S.B.; Simpson, E.R.; Brown, K.A. HIF-1alpha stimulates aromatase expression driven by prostaglandin E2 in breast adipose stroma. *Breast Cancer Res.* **2013**, *15*, R30. [CrossRef]

60. Lan, K.L.; Lan, K.H.; Sheu, M.L.; Chen, M.Y.; Shih, Y.S.; Hsu, F.C.; Wang, H.M.; Liu, R.S.; Yen, S.H. Honokiol inhibits hypoxia-inducible factor-1 pathway. *Int. J. Radiat. Biol.* **2011**, *87*, 579–590. [CrossRef]
61. Avtanski, D.B.; Nagalingam, A.; Bonner, M.Y.; Arbiser, J.L.; Saxena, N.K.; Sharma, D. Honokiol inhibits epithelial-mesenchymal transition in breast cancer cells by targeting signal transducer and activator of transcription 3/Zeb1/E-cadherin axis. *Mol. Oncol.* **2014**, *8*, 565–580. [CrossRef] [PubMed]
62. Sengupta, S.; Nagalingam, A.; Muniraj, N.; Bonner, M.Y.; Mistriotis, P.; Afthinos, A.; Kuppusamy, P.; Lanoue, D.; Cho, S.; Korangath, P.; et al. Activation of tumor suppressor LKB1 by honokiol abrogates cancer stem-like phenotype in breast cancer via inhibition of oncogenic Stat3. *Oncogene* **2017**, *36*, 5709–5721. [CrossRef] [PubMed]
63. Wang, W.D.; Shang, Y.; Li, Y.; Chen, S.Z. Honokiol inhibits breast cancer cell metastasis by blocking EMT through modulation of Snail/Slug protein translation. *Acta Pharmacol. Sin.* **2019**, *40*, 1219–1227. [CrossRef] [PubMed]
64. Liu, H.; Zang, C.; Emde, A.; Planas-Silva, M.D.; Rosche, M.; Kuhnl, A.; Schulz, C.O.; Elstner, E.; Possinger, K.; Eucker, J. Anti-tumor effect of honokiol alone and in combination with other anti-cancer agents in breast cancer. *Eur. J. Pharmacol.* **2008**, *591*, 43–51. [CrossRef]
65. Xie, L.; Jiang, F.; Zhang, X.; Alitongbieke, G.; Shi, X.; Meng, M.; Xu, Y.; Ren, A.; Wang, J.; Cai, L.; et al. Honokiol sensitizes breast cancer cells to TNF-alpha induction of apoptosis by inhibiting Nur77 expression. *Br. J. Pharmacol.* **2016**, *173*, 344–356. [CrossRef]
66. Avtanski, D.B.; Nagalingam, A.; Bonner, M.Y.; Arbiser, J.L.; Saxena, N.K.; Sharma, D. Honokiol activates LKB1-miR-34a axis and antagonizes the oncogenic actions of leptin in breast cancer. *Oncotarget* **2015**, *6*, 29947–29962. [CrossRef]
67. Avtanski, D.B.; Nagalingam, A.; Kuppusamy, P.; Bonner, M.Y.; Arbiser, J.L.; Saxena, N.K.; Sharma, D. Honokiol abrogates leptin-induced tumor progression by inhibiting Wnt1-MTA1-beta-catenin signaling axis in a microRNA-34a dependent manner. *Oncotarget* **2015**, *6*, 16396–16410. [CrossRef]
68. Ginestier, C.; Hur, M.H.; Charafe-Jauffret, E.; Monville, F.; Dutcher, J.; Brown, M.; Jacquemier, J.; Viens, P.; Kleer, C.G.; Liu, S.; et al. ALDH1 is a marker of normal and malignant human mammary stem cells and a predictor of poor clinical outcome. *Cell Stem Cell* **2007**, *1*, 555–567. [CrossRef]
69. Kagara, N.; Huynh, K.T.; Kuo, C.; Okano, H.; Sim, M.S.; Elashoff, D.; Chong, K.; Giuliano, A.E.; Hoon, D.S. Epigenetic regulation of cancer stem cell genes in triple-negative breast cancer. *Am. J. Pathol.* **2012**, *181*, 257–267. [CrossRef]
70. Chang, M.T.; Lee, S.P.; Fang, C.Y.; Hsieh, P.L.; Liao, Y.W.; Lu, M.Y.; Tsai, L.L.; Yu, C.C.; Liu, C.M. Chemosensitizing effect of honokiol in oral carcinoma stem cells via regulation of IL-6/Stat3 signaling. *Environ. Toxicol.* **2018**, *33*, 1105–1112. [CrossRef]
71. Gao, X.; Patel, M.G.; Bakshi, P.; Sharma, D.; Banga, A.K. Enhancement in the Transdermal and Localized Delivery of Honokiol Through Breast Tissue. *AAPS PharmSciTech* **2018**, *19*, 3501–3511. [CrossRef] [PubMed]
72. Verhoeven, D.T.; Goldbohm, R.A.; van Poppel, G.; Verhagen, H.; van den Brandt, P.A. Epidemiological studies on brassica vegetables and cancer risk. *Cancer Epidemiol. Biomark. Prev.* **1996**, *5*, 733–748.
73. Kelloff, G.J.; Boone, C.W.; Crowell, J.A.; Steele, V.E.; Lubet, R.A.; Doody, L.A.; Malone, W.F.; Hawk, E.T.; Sigman, C.C. New agents for cancer chemoprevention. *J. Cell. Biochem. Suppl.* **1996**, *26*, 1–28. [CrossRef]
74. Conaway, C.C.; Yang, Y.M.; Chung, F.L. Isothiocyanates as cancer chemopreventive agents: Their biological activities and metabolism in rodents and humans. *Curr. Drug Metab.* **2002**, *3*, 233–255. [CrossRef] [PubMed]
75. Shapiro, T.A.; Fahey, J.W.; Wade, K.L.; Stephenson, K.K.; Talalay, P. Human metabolism and excretion of cancer chemoprotective glucosinolates and isothiocyanates of cruciferous vegetables. *Cancer Epidemiol. Biomark. Prev.* **1998**, *7*, 1091–1100.
76. Ambrosone, C.B.; McCann, S.E.; Freudenheim, J.L.; Marshall, J.R.; Zhang, Y.; Shields, P.G. Breast cancer risk in premenopausal women is inversely associated with consumption of broccoli, a source of isothiocyanates, but is not modified by GST genotype. *J. Nutr.* **2004**, *134*, 1134–1138. [CrossRef]
77. Singh, S.V.; Singh, K. Cancer chemoprevention with dietary isothiocyanates mature for clinical translational research. *Carcinogenesis* **2012**, *33*, 1833–1842. [CrossRef]
78. Rao, C.V. Benzyl isothiocyanate: Double trouble for breast cancer cells. *Cancer Prev. Res.* **2013**, *6*, 760–763. [CrossRef]
79. Tseng, E.; Scott-Ramsay, E.A.; Morris, M.E. Dietary organic isothiocyanates are cytotoxic in human breast cancer MCF-7 and mammary epithelial MCF-12A cell lines. *Exp. Biol. Med.* **2004**, *229*, 83–842. [CrossRef]

80. Nakamura, Y.; Miyoshi, N. Cell death induction by isothiocyanates and their underlying molecular mechanisms. *BioFactors* **2006**, *26*, 123–134. [CrossRef]
81. Jeong, Y.J.; Cho, H.J.; Chung, F.L.; Wang, X.; Hoe, H.S.; Park, K.K.; Kim, C.H.; Chang, H.W.; Lee, S.R.; Chang, Y.C. Isothiocyanates suppress the invasion and metastasis of tumors by targeting FAK/MMP-9 activity. *Oncotarget* **2017**, *8*, 63949–63962. [CrossRef] [PubMed]
82. Warin, R.; Xiao, D.; Arlotti, J.A.; Bommareddy, A.; Singh, S.V. Inhibition of human breast cancer xenograft growth by cruciferous vegetable constituent benzyl isothiocyanate. *Mol. Carcinog.* **2010**, *49*, 500–507. [CrossRef] [PubMed]
83. Hecht, S.S. Inhibition of carcinogenesis by isothiocyanates. *Drug Metab. Rev.* **2000**, *32*, 395–411. [CrossRef] [PubMed]
84. Kim, E.J.; Hong, J.E.; Eom, S.J.; Lee, J.Y.; Park, J.H. Oral administration of benzyl-isothiocyanate inhibits solid tumor growth and lung metastasis of 4T1 murine mammary carcinoma cells in BALB/c mice. *Breast Cancer Res. Treat.* **2011**, *130*, 61–71. [CrossRef] [PubMed]
85. Warin, R.; Chambers, W.H.; Potter, D.M.; Singh, S.V. Prevention of mammary carcinogenesis in MMTV-neu mice by cruciferous vegetable constituent benzyl isothiocyanate. *Cancer Res.* **2009**, *69*, 9473–9480. [CrossRef]
86. Yu, R.; Mandlekar, S.; Harvey, K.J.; Ucker, D.S.; Kong, A.N. Chemopreventive isothiocyanates induce apoptosis and caspase-3-like protease activity. *Cancer Res.* **1998**, *58*, 402–408.
87. Xiao, D.; Vogel, V.; Singh, S.V. Benzyl isothiocyanate-induced apoptosis in human breast cancer cells is initiated by reactive oxygen species and regulated by Bax and Bak. *Mol. Cancer Ther.* **2006**, *5*, 2931–2945. [CrossRef]
88. Xiao, D.; Powolny, A.A.; Singh, S.V. Benzyl isothiocyanate targets mitochondrial respiratory chain to trigger reactive oxygen species-dependent apoptosis in human breast cancer cells. *J. Biol. Chem.* **2008**, *283*, 30151–30163. [CrossRef]
89. Kang, L.; Ding, L.; Wang, Z.Y. Isothiocyanates repress estrogen receptor alpha expression in breast cancer cells. *Oncol. Rep.* **2009**, *21*, 185–192.
90. Xiao, D.; Bommareddy, A.; Kim, S.H.; Sehrawat, A.; Hahm, E.R.; Singh, S.V. Benzyl isothiocyanate causes FoxO1-mediated autophagic death in human breast cancer cells. *PLoS ONE* **2012**, *7*, e32597. [CrossRef]
91. Sehrawat, A.; Singh, S.V. Benzyl isothiocyanate inhibits epithelial-mesenchymal transition in cultured and xenografted human breast cancer cells. *Cancer Prev. Res.* **2011**, *4*, 1107–1117. [CrossRef] [PubMed]
92. Kim, S.H.; Singh, S.V. Role of Kruppel-like Factor 4-p21(CIP1) Axis in Breast Cancer Stem-like Cell Inhibition by Benzyl Isothiocyanate. *Cancer Prev. Res.* **2019**, *12*, 125–134. [CrossRef] [PubMed]
93. Xie, B.; Zhao, L.; Guo, L.; Liu, H.; Fu, S.; Fan, W.; Lin, L.; Chen, J.; Wang, B.; Fan, L.; et al. Benzyl isothiocyanate suppresses development and metastasis of murine mammary carcinoma by regulating the Wnt/betacatenin pathway. *Mol. Med. Rep.* **2019**, *20*, 1808–1818. [CrossRef] [PubMed]
94. Kim, S.H.; Singh, S.V. p53-Independent apoptosis by benzyl isothiocyanate in human breast cancer cells is mediated by suppression of XIAP expression. *Cancer Prev. Res.* **2010**, *3*, 718–726. [CrossRef] [PubMed]
95. Xie, B.; Nagalingam, A.; Kuppusamy, P.; Muniraj, N.; Langford, P.; Gyorffy, B.; Saxena, N.K.; Sharma, D. Benzyl Isothiocyanate potentiates p53 signaling and antitumor effects against breast cancer through activation of p53-LKB1 and p73-LKB1 axes. *Sci. Rep.* **2017**, *7*, 40070. [CrossRef]
96. Saxena, N.K.; Vertino, P.M.; Anania, F.A.; Sharma, D. leptin-induced growth stimulation of breast cancer cells involves recruitment of histone acetyltransferases and mediator complex to CYCLIN D1 promoter via activation of Stat3. *J. Biol. Chem.* **2007**, *282*, 13316–13325. [CrossRef]
97. Saxena, N.K.; Taliaferro-Smith, L.; Knight, B.B.; Merlin, D.; Anania, F.A.; O'Regan, R.M.; Sharma, D. Bidirectional crosstalk between leptin and insulin-like growth factor-I signaling promotes invasion and migration of breast cancer cells via transactivation of epidermal growth factor receptor. *Cancer Res.* **2008**, *68*, 9712–9722. [CrossRef]
98. Knight, B.B.; Oprea-Ilies, G.M.; Nagalingam, A.; Yang, L.; Cohen, C.; Saxena, N.K.; Sharma, D. Survivin upregulation, dependent on leptin-EGFR-Notch1 axis, is essential for leptin-induced migration of breast carcinoma cells. *Endocr. Relat. Cancer* **2011**, *18*, 413–428. [CrossRef]
99. Yan, D.; Avtanski, D.; Saxena, N.K.; Sharma, D. Leptin-induced epithelial-mesenchymal transition in breast cancer cells requires beta-catenin activation via Akt/GSK3- and MTA1/Wnt1 protein-dependent pathways. *J. Biol. Chem.* **2012**, *287*, 8598–8612. [CrossRef]

100. Saxena, N.K.; Sharma, D. Multifaceted leptin network: The molecular connection between obesity and breast cancer. *J. Mammary Gland. Biol. Neoplasia* **2013**, *18*, 309–320. [CrossRef]
101. Taliaferro-Smith, L.; Nagalingam, A.; Knight, B.B.; Oberlick, E.; Saxena, N.K.; Sharma, D. Integral role of PTP1B in adiponectin-mediated inhibition of oncogenic actions of leptin in breast carcinogenesis. *Neoplasia* **2013**, *15*, 23–38. [CrossRef] [PubMed]
102. Kim, S.H.; Nagalingam, A.; Saxena, N.K.; Singh, S.V.; Sharma, D. Benzyl isothiocyanate inhibits oncogenic actions of leptin in human breast cancer cells by suppressing activation of signal transducer and activator of transcription 3. *Carcinogenesis* **2011**, *32*, 359–367. [CrossRef] [PubMed]
103. Kim, S.H.; Sehrawat, A.; Singh, S.V. Dietary chemopreventative benzyl isothiocyanate inhibits breast cancer stem cells in vitro and in vivo. *Cancer Prev. Res.* **2013**, *6*, 782–790. [CrossRef] [PubMed]
104. Sahu, R.P.; Srivastava, S.K. The role of STAT-3 in the induction of apoptosis in pancreatic cancer cells by benzyl isothiocyanate. *J. Natl. Cancer Inst.* **2009**, *101*, 176–193. [CrossRef] [PubMed]
105. Yeh, Y.T.; Hsu, Y.N.; Huang, S.Y.; Lin, J.S.; Chen, Z.F.; Chow, N.H.; Su, S.H.; Shyu, H.W.; Lin, C.C.; Huang, W.T.; et al. Benzyl isothiocyanate promotes apoptosis of oral cancer cells via an acute redox stress-mediated DNA damage response. *Food Chem. Toxicol.* **2016**, *97*, 336–345. [CrossRef] [PubMed]
106. Pezzuto, J.M. Grapes and human health: A perspective. *J. Agric. Food Chem.* **2008**, *56*, 6777–6784. [CrossRef] [PubMed]
107. Rimando, A.M.; Kalt, W.; Magee, J.B.; Dewey, J.; Ballington, J.R. Resveratrol, pterostilbene, and piceatannol in vaccinium berries. *J. Agric. Food Chem.* **2004**, *52*, 4713–4719. [CrossRef]
108. Sales, J.M.; Resurreccion, A.V. Resveratrol in peanuts. *Crit. Rev. Food Sci. Nutr.* **2014**, *54*, 734–770. [CrossRef]
109. Sun, A.Y.; Simonyi, A.; Sun, G.Y. The "French Paradox" and beyond: Neuroprotective effects of polyphenols. *Free Radic. Biol. Med.* **2002**, *32*, 314–318. [CrossRef]
110. Singh, A.P.; Singh, R.; Verma, S.S.; Rai, V.; Kaschula, C.H.; Maiti, P.; Gupta, S.C. Health benefits of resveratrol: Evidence from clinical studies. *Med. Res. Rev.* **2019**, *39*, 1851–1891. [CrossRef]
111. Bhat, K.P.; Lantvit, D.; Christov, K.; Mehta, R.G.; Moon, R.C.; Pezzuto, J.M. Estrogenic and antiestrogenic properties of resveratrol in mammary tumor models. *Cancer Res.* **2001**, *61*, 7456–7463. [PubMed]
112. Dong, Z. Molecular mechanism of the chemopreventive effect of resveratrol. *Mutat. Res.* **2003**, *523–524*, 145–150. [CrossRef]
113. Le Corre, L.; Chalabi, N.; Delort, L.; Bignon, Y.J.; Bernard-Gallon, D.J. Resveratrol and breast cancer chemoprevention: Molecular mechanisms. *Mol. Nutr. Food Res.* **2005**, *49*, 462–471. [CrossRef] [PubMed]
114. Kundu, J.K.; Surh, Y.J. Cancer chemopreventive and therapeutic potential of resveratrol: Mechanistic perspectives. *Cancer Lett.* **2008**, *269*, 243–261. [CrossRef]
115. Shukla, Y.; Singh, R. Resveratrol and cellular mechanisms of cancer prevention. *Ann. N. Y. Acad. Sci.* **2011**, *1215*, 1–8. [CrossRef]
116. Ko, J.H.; Sethi, G.; Um, J.Y.; Shanmugam, M.K.; Arfuso, F.; Kumar, A.P.; Bishayee, A.; Ahn, K.S. The Role of Resveratrol in Cancer Therapy. *Int. J. Mol. Sci.* **2017**, *18*, 2589. [CrossRef]
117. Pozo-Guisado, E.; Merino, J.M.; Mulero-Navarro, S.; Lorenzo-Benayas, M.J.; Centeno, F.; Alvarez-Barrientos, A.; Fernandez-Salguero, P.M. Resveratrol-induced apoptosis in MCF-7 human breast cancer cells involves a caspase-independent mechanism with downregulation of Bcl-2 and NF-kappaB. *Int. J. Cancer* **2005**, *115*, 74–84. [CrossRef]
118. Alkhalaf, M.; El-Mowafy, A.; Renno, W.; Rachid, O.; Ali, A.; Al-Attyiah, R. Resveratrol-induced apoptosis in human breast cancer cells is mediated primarily through the caspase-3-dependent pathway. *Arch. Med. Res.* **2008**, *39*, 162–168. [CrossRef]
119. Chen, F.P.; Chien, M.H. Phytoestrogens induce apoptosis through a mitochondria/caspase pathway in human breast cancer cells. *Climacteric* **2014**, *17*, 385–392. [CrossRef]
120. Sareen, D.; Darjatmoko, S.R.; Albert, D.M.; Polans, A.S. Mitochondria, calcium, and calpain are key mediators of resveratrol-induced apoptosis in breast cancer. *Mol. Pharmacol.* **2007**, *72*, 1466–1475. [CrossRef]
121. Nguyen, T.H.; Mustafa, F.B.; Pervaiz, S.; Ng, F.S.; Lim, L.H. ERK1/2 activation is required for resveratrol-induced apoptosis in MDA-MB-231 cells. *Int. J. Oncol.* **2008**, *33*, 81–92. [CrossRef] [PubMed]
122. Tsai, J.H.; Hsu, L.S.; Lin, C.L.; Hong, H.M.; Pan, M.H.; Way, T.D.; Chen, W.J. 3,5,4′-Trimethoxystilbene, a natural methoxylated analog of resveratrol, inhibits breast cancer cell invasiveness by downregulation of PI3K/Akt and Wnt/beta-catenin signaling cascades and reversal of epithelial-mesenchymal transition. *Toxicol. Appl. Pharmacol.* **2013**, *272*, 746–756. [CrossRef] [PubMed]

123. Castillo-Pichardo, L.; Dharmawardhane, S.F. Grape polyphenols inhibit Akt/mammalian target of rapamycin signaling and potentiate the effects of gefitinib in breast cancer. *Nutr. Cancer* **2012**, *64*, 1058–1069. [CrossRef] [PubMed]
124. Fu, Y.; Chang, H.; Peng, X.; Bai, Q.; Yi, L.; Zhou, Y.; Zhu, J.; Mi, M. Resveratrol inhibits breast cancer stem-like cells and induces autophagy via suppressing Wnt/beta-catenin signaling pathway. *PLoS ONE* **2014**, *9*, e102535. [CrossRef]
125. Kotha, A.; Sekharam, M.; Cilenti, L.; Siddiquee, K.; Khaled, A.; Zervos, A.S.; Carter, B.; Turkson, J.; Jove, R. Resveratrol inhibits Src and Stat3 signaling and induces the apoptosis of malignant cells containing activated Stat3 protein. *Mol. Cancer Ther.* **2006**, *5*, 621–629. [CrossRef] [PubMed]
126. She, Q.B.; Bode, A.M.; Ma, W.Y.; Chen, N.Y.; Dong, Z. Resveratrol-induced activation of p53 and apoptosis is mediated by extracellular-signal-regulated protein kinases and p38 kinase. *Cancer Res.* **2001**, *61*, 1604–1610.
127. Hsieh, T.C.; Wong, C.; John Bennett, D.; Wu, J.M. Regulation of p53 and cell proliferation by resveratrol and its derivatives in breast cancer cells: An in silico and biochemical approach targeting integrin alphavbeta3. *Int. J. Cancer* **2011**, *129*, 2732–2743. [CrossRef]
128. Chatterjee, B.; Ghosh, K.; Kanade, S.R. Resveratrol modulates epigenetic regulators of promoter histone methylation and acetylation that restores BRCA1, p53, p21(CIP1) in human breast cancer cell lines. *BioFactors* **2019**. [CrossRef]
129. Gehm, B.D.; McAndrews, J.M.; Chien, P.Y.; Jameson, J.L. Resveratrol, a polyphenolic compound found in grapes and wine, is an agonist for the estrogen receptor. *Proc. Natl. Acad. Sci. USA* **1997**, *94*, 14138–14143. [CrossRef]
130. Bowers, J.L.; Tyulmenkov, V.V.; Jernigan, S.C.; Klinge, C.M. Resveratrol acts as a mixed agonist/antagonist for estrogen receptors alpha and beta. *Endocrinology* **2000**, *141*, 3657–3667. [CrossRef]
131. Jin, X.; Wei, Y.; Liu, Y.; Lu, X.; Ding, F.; Wang, J.; Yang, S. Resveratrol promotes sensitization to Doxorubicin by inhibiting epithelial-mesenchymal transition and modulating SIRT1/beta-catenin signaling pathway in breast cancer. *Cancer Med.* **2019**, *8*, 1246–1257. [CrossRef] [PubMed]
132. Zhang, W.; Jiang, H.; Chen, Y.; Ren, F. Resveratrol chemosensitizes adriamycin-resistant breast cancer cells by modulating miR-122-5p. *J. Cell. Biochem.* **2019**, *120*, 16283–16292. [CrossRef] [PubMed]
133. Hallajian, F.; Ghasmi, M.; Abedi, S.M.; Behzadi, R.; Hayati, E.; Sadeghzadeh, N.; Rezazadeh, F.; Karimi, H. Evaluation of the Effect of Resveratrol and Doxorubicin on (99m)Tc-MIBI Uptake in Breast Cancer Cell Xenografts in Mice. *Cancer Biother. Radiopharm.* **2018**, *33*, 403–410. [CrossRef] [PubMed]
134. Sinha, D.; Biswas, J.; Sung, B.; Aggarwal, B.B.; Bishayee, A. Chemopreventive and chemotherapeutic potential of curcumin in breast cancer. *Curr. Drug Targets* **2012**, *13*, 1799–1819. [CrossRef] [PubMed]
135. Basnet, P.; Skalko-Basnet, N. Curcumin: An anti-inflammatory molecule from a curry spice on the path to cancer treatment. *Molecules* **2011**, *16*, 4567–4598. [CrossRef] [PubMed]
136. Kumar, A.; Chetia, H.; Sharma, S.; Kabiraj, D.; Talukdar, N.C.; Bora, U. Curcumin Resource Database. *Database* **2015**, *2015*, bav070. [CrossRef]
137. Ramachandran, C.; You, W. Differential sensitivity of human mammary epithelial and breast carcinoma cell lines to curcumin. *Breast Cancer Res. Treat.* **1999**, *54*, 269–278. [CrossRef]
138. Choudhuri, T.; Pal, S.; Agwarwal, M.L.; Das, T.; Sa, G. Curcumin induces apoptosis in human breast cancer cells through p53-dependent Bax induction. *FEBS Lett.* **2002**, *512*, 334–340. [CrossRef]
139. Lv, Z.D.; Liu, X.P.; Zhao, W.J.; Dong, Q.; Li, F.N.; Wang, H.B.; Kong, B. Curcumin induces apoptosis in breast cancer cells and inhibits tumor growth in vitro and in vivo. *Int. J. Clin. Exp. Pathol.* **2014**, *7*, 2818–2824.
140. Fan, H.; Liang, Y.; Jiang, B.; Li, X.; Xun, H.; Sun, J.; He, W.; Lau, H.T.; Ma, X. Curcumin inhibits intracellular fatty acid synthase and induces apoptosis in human breast cancer MDA-MB-231 cells. *Oncol. Rep.* **2016**, *35*, 2651–2656. [CrossRef]
141. Chang, L.C.; Hsieh, M.T.; Yang, J.S.; Lu, C.C.; Tsai, F.J.; Tsao, J.W.; Chiu, Y.J.; Kuo, S.C.; Lee, K.H. Effect of bis(hydroxymethyl) alkanoate curcuminoid derivative MTH-3 on cell cycle arrest, apoptotic and autophagic pathway in triple-negative breast adenocarcinoma MDA-MB-231 cells: An in vitro study. *Int. J. Oncol.* **2018**, *52*, 67–76. [CrossRef] [PubMed]
142. Ravindran, J.; Prasad, S.; Aggarwal, B.B. Curcumin and cancer cells: How many ways can curry kill tumor cells selectively? *AAPS J.* **2009**, *11*, 495–510. [CrossRef] [PubMed]
143. Hu, S.; Xu, Y.; Meng, L.; Huang, L.; Sun, H. Curcumin inhibits proliferation and promotes apoptosis of breast cancer cells. *Exp. Ther. Med.* **2018**, *16*, 1266–1272. [CrossRef] [PubMed]

144. Lee, Y.K.; Lee, W.S.; Hwang, J.T.; Kwon, D.Y.; Surh, Y.J.; Park, O.J. Curcumin exerts antidifferentiation effect through AMPKalpha-PPAR-gamma in 3T3-L1 adipocytes and antiproliferatory effect through AMPKalpha-COX-2 in cancer cells. *J. Agric. Food Chem.* **2009**, *57*, 305–310. [CrossRef]
145. Guan, F.; Ding, Y.; Zhang, Y.; Zhou, Y.; Li, M.; Wang, C. Curcumin Suppresses Proliferation and Migration of MDA-MB-231 Breast Cancer Cells through Autophagy-Dependent Akt Degradation. *PLoS ONE* **2016**, *11*, e0146553. [CrossRef]
146. Ren, M.; Wang, Y.; Wu, X.; Ge, S.; Wang, B. Curcumin synergistically increases effects of beta-interferon and retinoic acid on breast cancer cells in vitro and in vivo by up-regulation of GRIM-19 through STAT3-dependent and STAT3-independent pathways. *J. Drug Target.* **2017**, *25*, 247–254. [CrossRef]
147. Somasundaram, S.; Edmund, N.A.; Moore, D.T.; Small, G.W.; Shi, Y.Y.; Orlowski, R.Z. Dietary curcumin inhibits chemotherapy-induced apoptosis in models of human breast cancer. *Cancer Res.* **2002**, *62*, 3868–3875.
148. Goel, A.; Aggarwal, B.B. Curcumin, the golden spice from Indian saffron, is a chemosensitizer and radiosensitizer for tumors and chemoprotector and radioprotector for normal organs. *Nutr. Cancer* **2010**, *62*, 919–930. [CrossRef]
149. Aggarwal, B.B.; Shishodia, S.; Takada, Y.; Banerjee, S.; Newman, R.A.; Bueso-Ramos, C.E.; Price, J.E. Curcumin suppresses the paclitaxel-induced nuclear factor-kappaB pathway in breast cancer cells and inhibits lung metastasis of human breast cancer in nude mice. *Clin. Cancer Res.* **2005**, *11*, 7490–7498. [CrossRef]
150. Zhang, P.; Lai, Z.L.; Chen, H.F.; Zhang, M.; Wang, A.; Jia, T.; Sun, W.Q.; Zhu, X.M.; Chen, X.F.; Zhao, Z.; et al. Curcumin synergizes with 5-fluorouracil by impairing AMPK/ULK1-dependent autophagy, AKT activity and enhancing apoptosis in colon cancer cells with tumor growth inhibition in xenograft mice. *J. Exp. Clin. Cancer Res. CR* **2017**, *36*, 190. [CrossRef]
151. Calaf, G.M.; Ponce-Cusi, R.; Carrion, F. Curcumin and paclitaxel induce cell death in breast cancer cell lines. *Oncol. Rep.* **2018**, *40*, 2381–2388. [CrossRef] [PubMed]
152. Dayton, A.; Selvendiran, K.; Meduru, S.; Khan, M.; Kuppusamy, M.L.; Naidu, S.; Kalai, T.; Hideg, K.; Kuppusamy, P. Amelioration of doxorubicin-induced cardiotoxicity by an anticancer-antioxidant dual-function compound, HO-3867. *J. Pharmacol. Exp. Ther.* **2011**, *339*, 350–357. [CrossRef] [PubMed]
153. Sen, G.S.; Mohanty, S.; Hossain, D.M.; Bhattacharyya, S.; Banerjee, S.; Chakraborty, J.; Saha, S.; Ray, P.; Bhattacharjee, P.; Mandal, D.; et al. Curcumin enhances the efficacy of chemotherapy by tailoring p65NFkappaB-p300 cross-talk in favor of p53-p300 in breast cancer. *J. Biol. Chem.* **2011**, *286*, 42232–42247. [CrossRef] [PubMed]
154. Chen, W.C.; Lai, Y.A.; Lin, Y.C.; Ma, J.W.; Huang, L.F.; Yang, N.S.; Ho, C.T.; Kuo, S.C.; Way, T.D. Curcumin suppresses doxorubicin-induced epithelial-mesenchymal transition via the inhibition of TGF-beta and PI3K/AKT signaling pathways in triple-negative breast cancer cells. *J. Agric. Food Chem.* **2013**, *61*, 11817–11824. [CrossRef] [PubMed]
155. Duan, J.; Mansour, H.M.; Zhang, Y.; Deng, X.; Chen, Y.; Wang, J.; Pan, Y.; Zhao, J. Reversion of multidrug resistance by co-encapsulation of doxorubicin and curcumin in chitosan/poly(butyl cyanoacrylate) nanoparticles. *Int. J. Pharm.* **2012**, *426*, 193–201. [CrossRef] [PubMed]
156. Guo, O.; Li, X.; Yang, Y.; Wei, J.; Zhao, Q.; Luo, F.; Qian, Z. Enhanced 4T1 breast carcinoma anticancer activity by co-delivery of doxorubicin and curcumin with core-shell drug-carrier based on heparin modified poly(L-lactide) grafted polyethylenimine cationic nanoparticles. *J. Biomed. Nanotechnol.* **2014**, *10*, 227–237. [CrossRef]
157. Minafra, L.; Porcino, N.; Bravata, V.; Gaglio, D.; Bonanomi, M.; Amore, E.; Cammarata, F.P.; Russo, G.; Militello, C.; Savoca, G.; et al. Radiosensitizing effect of curcumin-loaded lipid nanoparticles in breast cancer cells. *Sci. Rep.* **2019**, *9*, 11134. [CrossRef]
158. Harini, L.; Srivastava, S.; Gnanakumar, G.P.; Karthikeyan, B.; Ross, C.; Krishnakumar, V.; Kannan, V.R.; Sundar, K.; Kathiresan, T. An ingenious non-spherical mesoporous silica nanoparticle cargo with curcumin induces mitochondria-mediated apoptosis in breast cancer (MCF-7) cells. *Oncotarget* **2019**, *10*, 1193–1208. [CrossRef]
159. Saleh, T.; Soudi, T.; Shojaosadati, S.A. Aptamer functionalized curcumin-loaded human serum albumin (HSA) nanoparticles for targeted delivery to HER-2 positive breast cancer cells. *Int. J. Biol. Macromol.* **2019**, *130*, 109–116. [CrossRef]
160. Wong, K.E.; Ngai, S.C.; Chan, K.G.; Lee, L.H.; Goh, B.H.; Chuah, L.H. Curcumin Nanoformulations for Colorectal Cancer: A Review. *Front. Pharmacol.* **2019**, *10*, 152. [CrossRef]

161. Feng, T.; Wei, Y.; Lee, R.J.; Zhao, L. Liposomal curcumin and its application in cancer. *Int. J. Nanomed.* **2017**, *12*, 6027–6044. [CrossRef] [PubMed]
162. Pavese, J.M.; Krishna, S.N.; Bergan, R.C. Genistein inhibits human prostate cancer cell detachment, invasion, and metastasis. *Am. J. Clin. Nutr.* **2014**, *100* (Suppl. 1), 431S–436S. [CrossRef]
163. Lee, J.Y.; Kim, H.S.; Song, Y.S. Genistein as a Potential Anticancer Agent against Ovarian Cancer. *J. Tradit. Complementary Med.* **2012**, *2*, 96–104. [CrossRef]
164. Ziegler, R.G. Phytoestrogens and breast cancer. *Am. J. Clin. Nutr.* **2004**, *79*, 183–184. [CrossRef] [PubMed]
165. Rietjens, I.; Louisse, J.; Beekmann, K. The potential health effects of dietary phytoestrogens. *Br. J. Pharmacol.* **2017**, *174*, 1263–1280. [CrossRef] [PubMed]
166. Vitale, D.C.; Piazza, C.; Melilli, B.; Drago, F.; Salomone, S. Isoflavones: Estrogenic activity, biological effect and bioavailability. *Eur. J. Drug Metab. Pharm.* **2013**, *38*, 15–25. [CrossRef]
167. Wu, Q.; Yang, Y.; Yu, J.; Jin, N. Soy isoflavone extracts stimulate the growth of nude mouse xenografts bearing estrogen-dependent human breast cancer cells (MCF-7). *J. Biomed. Res.* **2012**, *26*, 44–52. [CrossRef]
168. Hsieh, C.Y.; Santell, R.C.; Haslam, S.Z.; Helferich, W.G. Estrogenic effects of genistein on the growth of estrogen receptor-positive human breast cancer (MCF-7) cells in vitro and in vivo. *Cancer Res.* **1998**, *58*, 3833–3838.
169. Liu, R.; Yu, X.; Chen, X.; Zhong, H.; Liang, C.; Xu, X.; Xu, W.; Cheng, Y.; Wang, W.; Yu, L.; et al. Individual factors define the overall effects of dietary genistein exposure on breast cancer patients. *Nutr. Res.* **2019**, *67*, 1–16. [CrossRef]
170. Wu, A.H.; Yu, M.C.; Tseng, C.C.; Pike, M.C. Epidemiology of soy exposures and breast cancer risk. *Br. J. Cancer* **2008**, *98*, 9–14. [CrossRef]
171. Ahn, S.Y.; Jo, M.S.; Lee, D.; Baek, S.E.; Baek, J.; Yu, J.S.; Jo, J.; Yun, H.; Kang, K.S.; Yoo, J.E.; et al. Dual effects of isoflavonoids from Pueraria lobata roots on estrogenic activity and anti-proliferation of MCF-7 human breast carcinoma cells. *Bioorg. Chem.* **2019**, *83*, 135–144. [CrossRef] [PubMed]
172. Hu, X.J.; Xie, M.Y.; Kluxen, F.M.; Diel, P. Genistein modulates the anti-tumor activity of cisplatin in MCF-7 breast and HT-29 colon cancer cells. *Arch. Toxicol.* **2014**, *88*, 625–635. [CrossRef] [PubMed]
173. Shim, H.Y.; Park, J.H.; Paik, H.D.; Nah, S.Y.; Kim, D.S.; Han, Y.S. Genistein-induced apoptosis of human breast cancer MCF-7 cells involves calpain-caspase and apoptosis signaling kinase 1-p38 mitogen-activated protein kinase activation cascades. *Anticancer Drugs* **2007**, *18*, 649–657. [CrossRef] [PubMed]
174. Chen, J.; Duan, Y.; Zhang, X.; Ye, Y.; Ge, B.; Chen, J. Genistein induces apoptosis by the inactivation of the IGF-1R/p-Akt signaling pathway in MCF-7 human breast cancer cells. *Food Funct.* **2015**, *6*, 995–1000. [CrossRef]
175. Fan, P.; Fan, S.; Wang, H.; Mao, J.; Shi, Y.; Ibrahim, M.M.; Ma, W.; Yu, X.; Hou, Z.; Wang, B.; et al. Genistein decreases the breast cancer stem-like cell population through Hedgehog pathway. *Stem Cell Res. Ther.* **2013**, *4*, 146. [CrossRef]
176. Liu, X.; Sun, C.; Jin, X.; Li, P.; Ye, F.; Zhao, T.; Gong, L.; Li, Q. Genistein enhances the radiosensitivity of breast cancer cells via G(2)/M cell cycle arrest and apoptosis. *Molecules* **2013**, *18*, 13200–13217. [CrossRef]
177. Dave, B.; Eason, R.R.; Till, S.R.; Geng, Y.; Velarde, M.C.; Badger, T.M.; Simmen, R.C. The soy isoflavone genistein promotes apoptosis in mammary epithelial cells by inducing the tumor suppressor PTEN. *Carcinogenesis* **2005**, *26*, 1793–1803. [CrossRef]
178. Katdare, M.; Osborne, M.; Telang, N.T. Soy isoflavone genistein modulates cell cycle progression and induces apoptosis in HER-2/neu oncogene expressing human breast epithelial cells. *Int. J. Oncol.* **2002**, *21*, 809–815. [CrossRef]
179. Ye, D.; Li, Z.; Wei, C. Genistein inhibits the S-phase kinase-associated protein 2 expression in breast cancer cells. *Exp. Ther. Med.* **2018**, *15*, 1069–1075. [CrossRef]
180. Xue, J.P.; Wang, G.; Zhao, Z.B.; Wang, Q.; Shi, Y. Synergistic cytotoxic effect of genistein and doxorubicin on drug-resistant human breast cancer MCF-7/Adr cells. *Oncol. Rep.* **2014**, *32*, 1647–1653. [CrossRef]
181. Satoh, H.; Nishikawa, K.; Suzuki, K.; Asano, R.; Virgona, N.; Ichikawa, T.; Hagiwara, K.; Yano, T. Genistein, a soy isoflavone, enhances necrotic-like cell death in a breast cancer cell treated with a chemotherapeutic agent. *Res. Commun. Mol. Pathol. Pharmacol.* **2003**, *113–114*, 149–158.
182. Li, Y.; Ahmed, F.; Ali, S.; Philip, P.A.; Kucuk, O.; Sarkar, F.H. Inactivation of nuclear factor kappaB by soy isoflavone genistein contributes to increased apoptosis induced by chemotherapeutic agents in human cancer cells. *Cancer Res.* **2005**, *65*, 6934–6942. [CrossRef] [PubMed]

183. Imai, K.; Suga, K.; Nakachi, K. Cancer-preventive effects of drinking green tea among a Japanese population. *Prev. Med.* **1997**, *26*, 769–775. [CrossRef] [PubMed]
184. Li, M.; Tse, L.A.; Chan, W.C.; Kwok, C.H.; Leung, S.L.; Wu, C.; Yu, W.C.; Yu, I.T.; Yu, C.H.; Wang, F.; et al. Evaluation of breast cancer risk associated with tea consumption by menopausal and estrogen receptor status among Chinese women in Hong Kong. *Cancer Epidemiol.* **2016**, *40*, 73–78. [CrossRef] [PubMed]
185. Wu, A.H.; Yu, M.C.; Tseng, C.C.; Hankin, J.; Pike, M.C. Green tea and risk of breast cancer in Asian Americans. *Int. J. Cancer* **2003**, *106*, 574–579. [CrossRef] [PubMed]
186. Xiang, L.P.; Wang, A.; Ye, J.H.; Zheng, X.Q.; Polito, C.A.; Lu, J.L.; Li, Q.S.; Liang, Y.R. Suppressive Effects of Tea Catechins on Breast Cancer. *Nutrients* **2016**, *8*, 458. [CrossRef]
187. Zeng, L.; Holly, J.M.; Perks, C.M. Effects of physiological levels of the green tea extract epigallocatechin-3-gallate on breast cancer cells. *Front. Endocrinol.* **2014**, *5*, 61. [CrossRef]
188. Thangapazham, R.L.; Singh, A.K.; Sharma, A.; Warren, J.; Gaddipati, J.P.; Maheshwari, R.K. Green tea polyphenols and its constituent epigallocatechin gallate inhibits proliferation of human breast cancer cells in vitro and in vivo. *Cancer Lett.* **2007**, *245*, 232–241. [CrossRef]
189. Deguchi, H.; Fujii, T.; Nakagawa, S.; Koga, T.; Shirouzu, K. Analysis of cell growth inhibitory effects of catechin through MAPK in human breast cancer cell line T47D. *Int. J. Oncol.* **2002**, *21*, 1301–1305. [CrossRef]
190. Moradzadeh, M.; Hosseini, A.; Erfanian, S.; Rezaei, H. Epigallocatechin-3-gallate promotes apoptosis in human breast cancer T47D cells through down-regulation of PI3K/AKT and Telomerase. *Pharmacol. Rep.* **2017**, *69*, 924–928. [CrossRef]
191. Roy, A.M.; Baliga, M.S.; Katiyar, S.K. Epigallocatechin-3-gallate induces apoptosis in estrogen receptor-negative human breast carcinoma cells via modulation in protein expression of p53 and Bax and caspase-3 activation. *Mol. Cancer Ther.* **2005**, *4*, 81–90. [PubMed]
192. Tang, Y.; Zhao, D.Y.; Elliott, S.; Zhao, W.; Curiel, T.J.; Beckman, B.S.; Burow, M.E. Epigallocatechin-3 gallate induces growth inhibition and apoptosis in human breast cancer cells through survivin suppression. *Int. J. Oncol.* **2007**, *31*, 705–711. [CrossRef] [PubMed]
193. Baliga, M.S.; Meleth, S.; Katiyar, S.K. Growth inhibitory and antimetastatic effect of green tea polyphenols on metastasis-specific mouse mammary carcinoma 4T1 cells in vitro and in vivo systems. *Clin. Cancer Res.* **2005**, *11*, 1918–1927. [CrossRef] [PubMed]
194. Hsuuw, Y.D.; Chan, W.H. Epigallocatechin gallate dose-dependently induces apoptosis or necrosis in human MCF-7 cells. *Ann. N. Y. Acad. Sci.* **2007**, *1095*, 428–440. [CrossRef] [PubMed]
195. Hsu, Y.C.; Liou, Y.M. The anti-cancer effects of (-)-epigallocatechin-3-gallate on the signaling pathways associated with membrane receptors in MCF-7 cells. *J. Cell. Physiol.* **2011**, *226*, 2721–2730. [CrossRef]
196. Mittal, A.; Pate, M.S.; Wylie, R.C.; Tollefsbol, T.O.; Katiyar, S.K. EGCG down-regulates telomerase in human breast carcinoma MCF-7 cells, leading to suppression of cell viability and induction of apoptosis. *Int. J. Oncol.* **2004**, *24*, 703–710. [CrossRef]
197. Zan, L.; Chen, Q.; Zhang, L.; Li, X. Epigallocatechin gallate (EGCG) suppresses growth and tumorigenicity in breast cancer cells by downregulation of miR-25. *Bioengineered* **2019**, *10*, 374–382. [CrossRef]
198. Radhakrishnan, R.; Pooja, D.; Kulhari, H.; Gudem, S.; Ravuri, H.G.; Bhargava, S.; Ramakrishna, S. Bombesin conjugated solid lipid nanoparticles for improved delivery of epigallocatechin gallate for breast cancer treatment. *Chem. Phys. Lipids* **2019**, *224*, 104770. [CrossRef]
199. Hajipour, H.; Hamishehkar, H.; Nazari Soltan Ahmad, S.; Barghi, S.; Maroufi, N.F.; Taheri, R.A. Improved anticancer effects of epigallocatechin gallate using RGD-containing nanostructured lipid carriers. *Artif. Cells Nanomed. Biotechnol.* **2018**, *46*, 283–292. [CrossRef]
200. Zeng, L.; Yan, J.; Luo, L.; Ma, M.; Zhu, H. Preparation and characterization of (-)-Epigallocatechin-3-gallate (EGCG)-loaded nanoparticles and their inhibitory effects on Human breast cancer MCF-7 cells. *Sci. Rep.* **2017**, *7*, 45521. [CrossRef]
201. Saklani, A.; Kutty, S.K. Plant-derived compounds in clinical trials. *Drug Discov. Today* **2008**, *13*, 161–171. [CrossRef] [PubMed]
202. Chengappa, K.N.R.; Brar, J.S.; Gannon, J.M.; Schlicht, P.J. Adjunctive Use of a Standardized Extract of Withania somnifera (Ashwagandha) to Treat Symptom Exacerbation in Schizophrenia: A Randomized, Double-Blind, Placebo-Controlled Study. *J. Clin. Psychiatry* **2018**, *79*. [CrossRef] [PubMed]

203. Nguyen, A.V.; Martinez, M.; Stamos, M.J.; Moyer, M.P.; Planutis, K.; Hope, C.; Holcombe, R.F. Results of a phase I pilot clinical trial examining the effect of plant-derived resveratrol and grape powder on Wnt pathway target gene expression in colonic mucosa and colon cancer. *Cancer Manag. Res.* **2009**, *1*, 25–37. [PubMed]
204. Brown, V.A.; Patel, K.R.; Viskaduraki, M.; Crowell, J.A.; Perloff, M.; Booth, T.D.; Vasilinin, G.; Sen, A.; Schinas, A.M.; Piccirilli, G.; et al. Repeat dose study of the cancer chemopreventive agent resveratrol in healthy volunteers: Safety, pharmacokinetics, and effect on the insulin-like growth factor axis. *Cancer Res.* **2010**, *70*, 9003–9011. [CrossRef] [PubMed]
205. Kris-Etherton, P.M.; Hecker, K.D.; Bonanome, A.; Coval, S.M.; Binkoski, A.E.; Hilpert, K.F.; Griel, A.E.; Etherton, T.D. Bioactive compounds in foods: Their role in the prevention of cardiovascular disease and cancer. *Am. J. Med.* **2002**, *113* (Suppl. 9B), 71S–88S. [CrossRef]
206. Liu, R.H. Dietary bioactive compounds and their health implications. *J. Food Sci.* **2013**, *78* (Suppl. 1), A18–A25. [CrossRef]

2

Stable Isotope Tracing Metabolomics to Investigate the Metabolic Activity of Bioactive Compounds for Cancer Prevention and Treatment

Feroza K. Choudhury [1,2], G. Lavender Hackman [1,2], Alessia Lodi [1,2] and Stefano Tiziani [1,2,3,*]

1 Department of Nutritional Sciences, College of Natural Sciences, The University of Texas at Austin, Austin, TX 78712, USA; feroza.choudhury@austin.utexas.edu (F.K.C.); lavenderhackman@utexas.edu (G.L.H.); alessia@austin.utexas.edu (A.L.)
2 Department of Pediatrics, Dell Medical School, The University of Texas at Austin, Austin, TX 78723, USA
3 Department of Oncology, Dell Medical School, The University of Texas at Austin, Austin, TX 78723, USA
* Correspondence: tiziani@austin.utexas.edu

Abstract: A major hallmark of cancer is the metabolic reprogramming of cancer cells to fuel tumor growth and proliferation. Various plant-derived bioactive compounds efficiently target the metabolic vulnerabilities of cancer cells and exhibit potential as emerging therapeutic agents. Due to their safety and common use as dietary components, they are also ideal for cancer prevention. However, to render their use as efficient as possible, the mechanism of action of these phytochemicals needs to be well characterized. Stable isotope tracing is an essential technology to study the molecular mechanisms by which nutraceuticals modulate and target cancer metabolism. The use of positionally labeled tracers as exogenous nutrients and the monitoring of their downstream metabolites labeling patterns enable the analysis of the specific metabolic pathway activity, via the relative production and consumption of the labeled metabolites. Although stable isotope tracing metabolomics is a powerful tool to investigate the molecular activity of bioactive compounds as well as to design synergistic nutraceutical combinations, this methodology is still underutilized. This review aims to investigate the research efforts and potentials surrounding the use of stable isotope tracing metabolomics to examine the metabolic alterations mediated by bioactive compounds in cancer.

Keywords: bioactive compounds; natural products; metabolic pathways; stable isotope tracing; cancer prevention; cancer metabolism

---

1. Introduction

In co-ordination with deregulated cell proliferation in cancer, the energy metabolism is adjusted to the increased demand to fuel cell growth and division as well as to maintain the redox balance. Reprogramming energy metabolism is one of the major hallmarks of cancer [1–3]. Reprogrammed metabolism in cancer cells presents as important target for developing therapeutic regimens and preventative measures against cancer. Due to their diverse structure and the ability to target different aspects of the metabolism, plant-derived natural bioactive compounds have gained increasing interest over the years for combating cancer [4]. They have inspired the successful development of new drugs in the pharmaceutical industry [5]. Their diverse biological activity, bioavailability and tolerability have proven them to be potential therapeutic agents and a safe option for preventing cancer [6,7]. For their successful utilization against cancer, their mechanism of action needs to be well characterized. In this review, we discuss the natural bioactive compounds that target different aspects of cancer metabolism and techniques to investigate their mechanism of action.

2. Bioactive Compounds

Different components of the altered metabolism in cancer can be targeted by bioactive compounds (Table 1, Figure 1). They can be used for treatment in various cancers and some have proven their efficacy in clinical trials. Preliminary studies have been done in cell culture experiments to analyze cytotoxic potential and mechanisms of action, followed by experiments in animal models to study tumor growth inhibitory potential. A few studies have been done in patients to determine therapeutic efficacy; however, additional patient data are necessary to fully elucidate the metabolic activity of these compounds in humans and more clinical studies should be performed in the future. The main principle by which these compounds work against cancer is by producing energy deficiency or by limiting the components needed for cell growth and proliferation. The combination of two compounds can have synergism and can be more effective in treatment against cancer. Ursolic acid in combination with curcumin and resveratrol has a synergistic effect and shows more potency in reducing tumor size in mouse allograft model of prostate cancer than when administered individually [8].

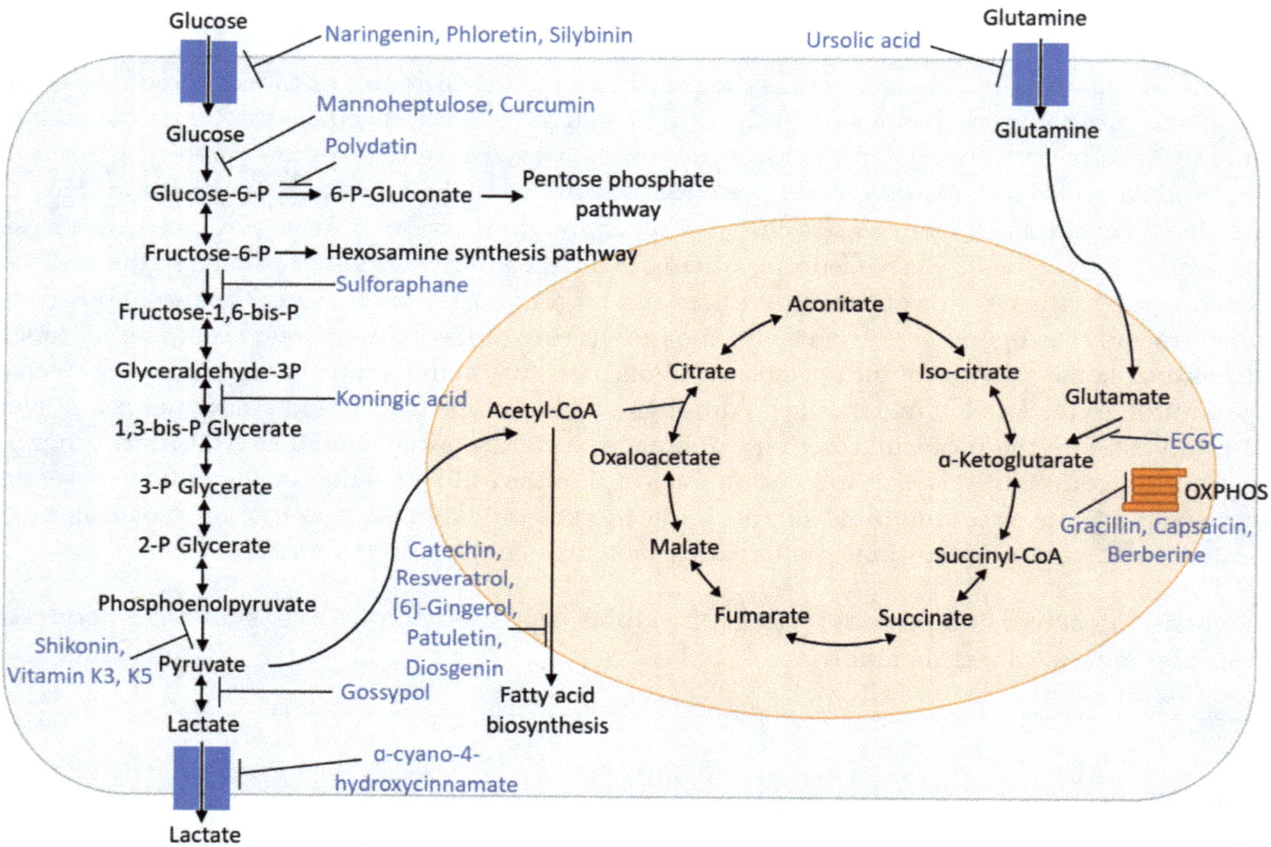

Figure 1. Different bioactive compounds that target metabolic processes. The primary target step of the bioactive compounds is shown and numbered in red color. 1. Glucose transporter (GLUT), 2. hexokinase, 3. glucose-6-phosphate dehydrogenase, 4. phosphofructokinase, 5. gyceraldehyde-3-phosphate dehydrogenase, 6. pyruvate kinase M2, 7. lactate dehydrogenase, 8. monocarboxylate transporter, 9. glutamine transporter, 10. glutamate dehydrogenase, 11. fatty acid synthase.

Table 1. Effect of bioactive compounds on different metabolic processes.

Bioactive Compounds	Source	Effect	Cancers	Ref.
Naringenin (a flavonoid)	Citrus fruits, tomatoes, figs	Inhibit insulin stimulated glucose uptake	Breast, prostate, melanoma, liver	[9–19]
Myricetin, Fisetin, Quercetin, Isoquercitin (flavonoid)	Tomatoes, oranges, nuts, berries, tea	Inhibit GLUT2		[20]
Phloretin (dihydrochalcone)	Apple tree leaves, apple	Inhibit GLUT1 and GUT2, induce glutathione biosynthesis	Lung, liver, colon, gastric, esophageal, breast epithelial, prostate, glioblastoma	[21–35]
Silybinin (flavonoid)	Milk thistle	Interact with GLUT1 and GLUT4	Prostate, breast, ovary, colon, lung, bladder	[36–42]
Curcumin	Turmeric	Decrease GLUT1 and hexokinase II protein level	Liver, breast, pancreatic, hepatic, gastric, colorectal, prostate	[43–49]
Mannoheptulose	Avocado	Inhibit hexokinase		[38,50]
Sulforaphane (isothiocyanate derivative)	Cruciferous vegetables, such as broccoli	Inhibit phosphofructokinase	breast, prostate, colon, skin, lung, gastric, bladder	[51–55]
Koningic acid	Fungi	Inhibit glyceraldehyde-3-phohohate dehydrogenase	Neuroblastoma	[56–58]
Shikonin (naphthoquinone derivative)	Dried root of the plant *Lithospermum erythrorhizon*	Inhibit pyruvate kinase M2	Lung, leukemia, breast, melanoma, bladder, esophageal	[59–63]
Vitamin K3 and K5		Inhibit pyruvate kinase M2	Cervix	[64]
Oleanolic acid	Olive oil, garlic	Switch PKM2 to PKM1		[65]
Gossypol (polyphenolic aldehyde)	Cotton seeds	Non-selective lactate dehydrogenase inhibitor that competes with NADH	Melanoma, lung, breast, cervix, leukemia, glioblastoma, myeloma, colon, prostate	[66–73]
α-cyano-4-hydroxycinnamate (Cinnamic acid derivative)		Inhibit monocarboxylate transporter	Glioma, pancreatic, Dalton's lymphoma	[74–81]
Polydatin	Grape, peanut, hop cones, red wines, hop pellets, cocoa-containing products	Inhibit glucose-6-phosphate dehydrogenase	Cervix, hepatoma, epidermal carcinoma, nasopharyngeal carcinoma	[82,83]
Ursolic acid	Apples, basil, cranberries, peppermint, rosemary, lavender, oregano, thyme, prunes	Inhibit ASCT2- glutamine transporter	Prostate, breast, cervix	[8,84–86]
Gracillin		Inhibit mitochondrial complex II	Lung, colorectum, prostate, pharynx, liver	[87]

Table 1. *Cont.*

Bioactive Compounds	Source	Effect	Cancers	Ref.
Capsaicin	Peppers	Inhibit mitochondrial respiration	Cutaneous squamous cell carcinoma	[88]
Berberine	Root, rhizome, and stem bark of barberry, goldenseal, Oregon grape, and tree turmeric	Inhibit mitochondrial respiration		[89]
(-)-epigallocatechin-3- gallate (EGCG)	Tea	Inhibit expression of fatty acid synthase	Colorectal, breast	[90–95]
Resveratrol	Peels and seeds of grape	Inhibit fatty acid synthase	Breast, uterine, blood, kidney, liver, eye, bladder, thyroid, esophageal, prostate, brain, lung, skin, gastric, colon, head and neck, bone, ovarian, cervix	[90,96–99]
Patuletin	Pipeworts	Inhibit expression of fatty acid synthase	Breast	[100]
Sea buckthorn procyanidins	Sea buckthorn	Inhibit fatty acid synthase	Breast	[101]
Diosgenin	Fenugreek, wild yam	Inhibit fatty acid synthase	HER2 overexpressing breast	[102]
[6]-Gingerol	Ginger	Suppress fatty acid β-oxidation	Liver	[103]

3. Inhibitors of Glucose Uptake

Naringenin inhibits insulin-stimulated glucose uptake in breast cancer cells by binding to estrogen receptor beta. It disrupts the insulin-induced GLUT4 translocation from intracellular compartment to the plasma membrane [9]. Naringenin has therapeutic potential as it reduced insulin-mediated glucose uptake and suppressed proliferation at a dose of 10μM [10]. Naringenin has anti-proliferative, proapoptotic anti-cancerous role in several cancer cell lines, such as breast (MDA-MB-231) [11], prostate (PC3, LNCaP) [12], melanoma (B16F10) [13], liver (HepG2) [14], HER2 positive breast cancer cell line [15] and mammary tumor cells (E0771) [16]. In rats bearing Walker 256 carcinosarcoma (W256), a dose of 25 mg/kg of naringenin inhibited tumor growth by around 75% [17]. The therapeutic potential of naringenin is greatly limited due to its low aqueous solubility and inefficient transport across biological membrane causing lower bioavailability in tumor sites [18]. D- α-tocopheryl polyethelene glycol succinate 1000 (TPGS)-coated naringenin nanosuspension can reverse the drug resistance and have higher cytotoxic potential in MCF-7 cells [19].

Flavonoids, such as myricetin, fisetin, quercetin, and its glucoside analog isoquercitin, inhibit GLUT2 present in the intestine. The non-competitive inhibition was observed at IC_{50} for quercetin, myricetin and isoquercitin that is approximately 200- to 1000- fold less than glucose and fructose concentration [20].

Phloretin, a dihydrochalcone, retarded tumor growth in vitro and in vivo by inhibiting glucose transporter GLUT1 and GLUT2 [21–23]. Phloretin can sensitize cancer cells to chemotherapeutic agents, such as daunorubicin, and mediates apoptosis to overcome drug resistance in colon cancer and leukemia cells in hypoxia [24]. In HepG2 xenografted mice, tumor growth was inhibited following combined treatment with phloretin and paclitaxel [25]. Phloretin inhibited proliferation and induced apoptosis in Calu-1, H838 and H520 cells and suppress the migration and invasion of NSCLC cells and enhanced the effect of cisplatin [26]. Phloretin increased the efficacy of HSP70 penetration and thus its anticancer activity in B16 mouse melanoma cells and K-562 human erythroblasts [27]. Phloretin showed anticancer activity in several human cancer cell lines, including lung (A549), liver (HepG2), colon (HT-29) [28], gastric (AGS) [29], esophageal (EC-109) [30], breast (MDA-MB-231) [31], prostate (LNCaP) [32] and glioblastoma cells [33]. Phloretin has a cancer preventative role by its activity in reducing oxidative DNA damage, as observed in human colon cancer cell lines (Caco-2 and HT-29) [34]. The preventative action is mainly mediated by elevated glutathione level by inducing rate limiting enzyme of glutathione biosynthesis, gamma-glutamyl cysteine ligase [35].

Sylibinin and its oxidized form 2,3-dihydrosilybinin inhibit cellular glucose uptake in different cancer cells by means of interaction with GLUT4, rendering an inhibitory effect on their proliferation and survival. 2,3-dihydrosilybinin has a stronger inhibition on glucose uptake. Sylibinin and 2,3-dihydrosilybinin inhibit GLUT4-mediated glucose transport in a competitive manner with $K_i = 60$ and 116 μM, respectively [36]. Sylibinin was found to be effective in clinical trials in prostate cancer patients [37,38]. Sylimarin, a family of flavonoids including sylibinin, can suppress the proliferation of several cancer cell lines, such as prostate, breast, ovary, colon, lung and bladder cancer cell lines, by arresting the cell cycle at G1/S- phase, through the induction of cyclin-dependent kinase inhibitors (such as p15, p21 and p27), down-regulation of anti-apoptotic gene products (e.g., Bcl-2 and Bcl-xL) and inhibition of cell-survival kinases (AKT, PKC and MAPK) [39–41]. Silymarin's chemo preventive role has been associated with the inhibition of ultraviolet B radiation or chemically initiated carcinogenesis in skin cancer. Moreover, silymarin suppressed 3, 2-dimethyl-4-aminobiphenyl-induced carcinogenesis in prostate cancer and the growth of advanced prostate tumor xenografts in athymic nude mice [42].

Curcumin causes decreased protein levels of GLUT1 in breast and lung cancer cells and hexokinase II in colorectal cancer cells, which causes a decrease in glucose uptake, lactate production, and ATP generation [43,44]. Curcumin also caused dissociation of hexokinase II from mitochondria, causing mitochondria-mediated apoptosis [44]. Curcumin helped to overcome the resistance of triple negative breast cancer to 4-hydroxytamoxifen by inhibiting hexokinase II expression and promoting mitochondrion-mediated apoptosis [45]. It also induces apoptosis in HepG2 and MDA-MB-231 cells via inhibiting fatty acid synthase [46,47]. Apart from these, curcumin has shown anticancer potential in several other cancers, like pancreatic, hepatic, gastric, colorectal, prostate cancer [48,49].

4. Inhibitor of Glycolysis

Mannoheptulose is a seven-carbon sugar that inhibits hexokinase, thus reducing glycolysis, and could be used as a potential anti-cancer treatment [38,50].

Sulforaphane has anti-cancer activity in several cancer cell lines. The anti-cancer activity is mediated by down-regulation of 6-phosphofructo-2-kinase/fructose-2,6-biphosphatase4 (PFKFB4) protein, which is a key modulator of glycolysis. Sulforaphane also down regulates the expression of transcription factor, hypoxia inducible factor- 1α (HIF-1α), which regulates the expression of PFKFB4 [51]. The anti-cancer activity of sulforaphane is not mediated by direct inhibition of phosphofructokinase, but through the inhibition of the PFKFB4 pathway. It inhibits the growth of several cancer cell lines, including breast, prostate, colon, skin, lung, gastric and bladder cancer cell lines, by inducing cell cycle arrest and apoptosis [52]. It also has a cytoprotective role by activating Nrf2 mediated signaling pathway required for response to oxidative stress [53]. A phase II study with sulforaphane in men with recurrent prostate cancer showed moderate improvement in outcomes, and given the safety of the compound, higher doses were proposed to further improve treatment outcome [54]. In patients with advanced pancreatic ductal carcinoma, 90 mg/day of sulforaphane inhibited tumor growth and increased the sensitivity of cancer cells to chemotherapeutics [55].

Koningic acid is an inhibitor of glyceraldehyde 3-phosphate dehydrogenase (GAPDH) and the inhibition of its activity in NG108-15 cells leads to apoptosis [56]. It is a potent cytotoxic agent in both hypoxic and normoxic condition [57]. Inhibition of GAPDH and thus glycolysis by koningic acid can be effective against glycolytic cancer cells, which are more sensitive to glycolytic inhibition than their healthy counterparts [58].

Shikonin and its enantiomer alkannin are both potent inhibitors of pyruvate kinase M2 (PKM2) isoform with IC_{50} values of 0.8 and 0.9 μM, respectively. They are the most potent and specific inhibitors of PKM2 reported. In cell lines such as MCF7 and A549 tumor cells, which predominantly express PKM2, shikonin and alkannin caused decrease in both glucose consumption and lactate production, with significantly lower PKM2 activity in the cell lysate, which in total represent lower glycolytic flux [59]. Shikonin dose-dependently inhibited glucose uptake and lactate production in pre-B cell acute lymphoblastic leukemia (BCP-ALL) [60], Lewis lung carcinoma (LLC) and B16 melanoma cells and suppressed cellular aerobic glycolysis through inhibiting PKM2 by reducing PKM2 phosphorylation. Shikonin promoted tumor cell (B16) apoptosis in vitro and in vivo [61]. PKM2 is strongly upregulated in bladder cancer, which contributes to cisplatin resistance. Administration of shikonin to cisplatin resistant T24 cells inhibited PKM2 and re-sensitized them to cisplatin treatment [62]. Higher expression of PKM2 is also observed in esophageal cancer cells, which go through apoptosis and have reduced tumor burden when treated with shikonin [63].

Vitamin K3 and K5 mediates their anticancer effect by inhibiting PKM2, among them vitamin K5 is more potent. They both caused lower glycolytic flux and decreased survival of Hela cells [64].

Oleanolic acid is a potential anticancer agent as it induces a switch from PKM2, which is responsible for enhanced aerobic glycolysis in cancer cells, to PKM1 and thus abrogate the Warburg effect in cancer cells [65].

Gossypol is a non-selective inhibitor of lactate dehydrogenase (LDH) which competes with NADH. It has K_i of 1.9 and 1.4 μM for LDH-A and LDH-B, respectively. It also inhibits other NAD^+ dependent enzymes, such as GAPDH [66]. The (R)-(-)-gossypol is a more potent cytotoxic agent with a mean IC_{50} value of 20 μM compared to (S)-(-)-gossypol. It exerts its cytotoxic effect on several cancer cell lines, including melanoma, lung, breast, cervix and leukemia [67]. Gossypol suppressed the growth of temozolomide-resistant glioblastoma cells [68]. It induced apoptosis in multiple myeloma [69], colon cancer (HT-29) [70], chronic lymphocytic leukemia [71] and prostate cancer (LAPC4, PC3, and DU145) with an IC_{50} between 35– μM and inhibited prostate tumor growth in a xenograft model [72]. Gossypol also inhibited the adhesion and invasion of human breast cancer cell lines [73].

α-cyano-4-hydroxycinnamate (αCHC) and other cinnamic acid derivatives are most studied monocarboxylate transporter (MCT) inhibitors [74,75]. αCHC inhibits MCT1 with a K_i of 166 μM, MCT2 with a K_i of 24 μM and MCT4 with a K_i of 991 μM [76]. Human melanoma cells, when treated with αCHC, had reduced intracellular pH at low extracellular pH, which resulted in reduced survival of these cells [77]. Treatment of malignant glioma cells with αCHC resulted in altered glycolytic metabolism, making them more radiosensitive [78] and adversely impacting the invasiveness and proliferative ability [79]. In human pancreatic cancer cells, αCHC inhibited migration and proliferation and induced cell death, performing better when applied in combination with metformin [80]. αCHC treatment of Dalton's lymphoma cells resulted in modulation of the biophysical parameters of the tumor cell culture medium with respect to pH, nitric oxide, glucose, and lactate, inducing apoptosis and decreased cell survival [81].

5. Inhibitor of Pentose Phosphate Pathway

Polydatin inhibits glucose-6-phosphate dehydrogenase, the entry enzyme in the pentose phosphate pathway (PPP) causing the inhibition of NADPH production and accumulation of reactive oxygen species, inducing apoptosis. In an orthopedic metastatic model of tongue cancer, it reduced tumor size by 30% and metastasis by 80%. In a phase II clinical trial it has been proven to be safe in humans [82]. It has an anti-proliferative effect on several human tumor cell lines, such as human cervical carcinoma HeLa cells, hepatoma cell line SMMC-7721 cells, epidermal carcinoma A-431 cells and nasopharyngeal carcinoma CNE cells [83].

6. Inhibitor of Glutamine Metabolism

Ursolic acid is an inhibitor of ASCT2 transporters, which is a neutral transporter in the plasma membrane that preferably transports glutamine [8,84]. It is a potent anti-cancer agent for prostate cancer reducing tumor size in mouse allograft model and performed better in combination with resveratrol and curcumin [8]. It inhibited breast cancer cell proliferation by inducing G1/G2 cell cycle arrest and apoptosis through intrinsic and extrinsic apoptosis pathways [85]. In cervical cancer cell TC-1, ursolic acid activated autophagy and reduced tumor growth in vivo [86].

7. Inhibitor of Mitochondrial Metabolism

Gracillin, a steroidal saponin, disrupts mitochondrial complex II function by abrogating succinate dehydrogenase (SDH) activity. It induced apoptosis, suppressed ATP synthesis, and increased reactive oxygen species in several cancer cell lines derived from the lung, colorectum, prostate, pharynx, and liver with IC_{50} values of 1–5 μM. It also suppresses mutant-Kras-driven lung tumorigenesis and the growth of xenograft tumors [87].

Capsaicin and resiniferatoxin are vanilloids that induced apoptosis in human cutaneous squamous cell carcinoma (SCC) cell lines by the inhibition of mitochondrial respiration via increasing the permeability of inner mitochondrial membrane [88].

Berberine arrested cell cycle of several malignant cell lines by accumulating in mitochondria and causing mitochondrial fragmentation and depolarization and inhibiting respiration [89].

8. Inhibitor of Fatty Acid Synthesis

(-)-epigallocatechin-3- gallate (EGCG) the most abundant catechin compound in tea, inhibits fatty acid synthase with an IC_{50} value of 42.0 μg/mL [90]. It induced cell cycle arrest in the G1 phase and apoptosis in human colorectal cancer cells HCT-116 and SW-480 [91]. A mixture of catechins exerted a synergistic cancer cell growth inhibitory effect and antioxidant potential [92]. Catechins in combination with anticancer drugs, such as tamoxifen, COX-2 inhibitors, and retinoids showed enhanced efficacy in inducing apoptosis [93]. EGCG significantly reduced the mRNA level and activity of glycolytic enzymes and reduced breast cancer cell 4T1 growth and breast tumor weight in a dose dependent manner [94]. EGCG is also a potent inhibitor of glutamate dehydrogenase, a key enzyme in glutaminolysis process [95].

Resveratrol inhibits fatty acid synthase reversibly with IC_{50} value 6.1 μg/mL and having competitive inhibition with acetyl CoA and non-competitive inhibition with malonyl CoA [90]. It has an anti-cancer effect on several human cancers, including breast, uterine, blood, kidney, liver, eye, bladder, thyroid, esophageal, prostate, brain, lung, skin, gastric, colon, head and neck, bone, ovarian, and cervical cancer [96]. It induced apoptosis by the down-regulation of fatty acid synthase and upregulation of proapoptotic genes and suppressed growth in a xenograft model of breast cancer [97]. In some cancer cells, resveratrol exerts its cytotoxic effect by inducing intracellular palmitate accumulation that triggers lipid-mediated cell death [98]. It also acts as a radio sensitizing agent [99].

Patuletin inhibited the gene expression and activity of fatty acid synthase and induced the apoptosis of human breast cancer cell line SK-BR-3 [100].

Sea buckthorn procyanidins inhibit fatty acid synthase with a IC_{50} value of 0.087 μg/mL and reduced MDA-MB-231 cell viability with a IC_{50} value of 37.5 μg/mL [101].

Diosgenin suppresses fatty acid synthase in HER2 overexpressing breast cancer cell line, thus inducing apoptosis and enhancing paclitaxel-induced cytotoxicity [102].

[6]-Gingerol exhibits therapeutic potential by the suppression of fatty acid β-oxidation via the inhibition of fatty acid synthase and cartinitne palmitoyltranferase-1 activity in HepG2 cells [103].

Apart from these, osthole [104], amentoflavone [105], cacalol [106], cerulenin [107], gingkolic acid [108] and constituents of extra virgin olive oil (phenols, phenolic acids, flavonoids, secoirodoids) [109] have shown potential for inhibiting fatty acid synthase.

9. Metabolic Pathway Analysis

The mechanism of action of plant-derived compounds and their ability to modulate metabolic pathways needs to be elucidated to render them more efficacious for use as cancer therapeutics. When a compound is administered, the modulation of one component of metabolism may reprogram the whole metabolism reflected in the change of the activity of different pathways. Inhibition of glucose or glutamine transporter results in decreased uptake of the respective molecule. When glutamine transport is inhibited by ursolic acid, the cells may increase their glycolytic flux, compensating for decreased glutaminolysis, and on the other hand, inhibition of glucose uptake or glycolysis may make the cell more dependent on glutamine for energy production. Different flavonoids in conjugation with the inhibition of glucose uptake may also act as an antioxidant and have an effect on NADPH biosynthesis. Compounds such as polydatin inhibit NADPH production in the pentose phosphate pathway, and so other NADPH-producing pathways may have higher activity. Decreased pentose phosphate pathway activity may also result in decreased nucleotide biosynthesis. Agents that affect mitochondrial metabolism, such as gracillin, may induce reductive carboxylation. For this, different pathways' activity needs to be analyzed to get an idea about the mechanism of action of a given compound.

9.1. Stable Isotope Tracing

Conventional metabolomics experiments are done by analyzing metabolite abundances. This has very limited implications in studying pathway activity. The abundance of a specific metabolite depends on its consumption and production. Higher abundance may indicate higher activity of the producing pathways or decreased activity of the consumption pathways. The metabolite abundance may stay the same if the rate of production complements the rate of consumption and both can have higher activity. To distinguish specific pathway activity, metabolic tracers are very useful. Stable isotope tracing or stable isotope resolved metabolomics are powerful approaches in which isotopically enriched precursors are administered as a metabolic tracer in a biological system. Introducing a metabolic tracer and analyzing the labeling pattern of downstream metabolites by mass spectrometry

(MS) or nuclear magnetic resonance (NMR) spectroscopy provides information about the activity of the metabolic pathways [110]. Carefully choosing positionally labeled tracers is useful in distinguishing the activity of a specific pathway. When analyzing the activity of a specific pathway, the enrichment of the metabolic intermediates is analyzed at an isotopic steady state, where label enrichment of the metabolites is constant over time upon introduction of the tracer. Duration of the tracer incubation depends on the pathway of interest; in cultured cells, the isotopic steady state is achieved for glycolysis within just 10 min, and for TCA cycle it takes over 2 h [111]. The bioactive compounds may have multiple targets, which can make them more suitable for cancer treatment. A benefit of using stable isotope tracing metabolomics is that it can elucidate the multiple targets of a single bioactive compound. Therefore, this approach will be useful in analyzing the overall mechanism of action of a bioactive compound. The analytical methods and tools used for stable isotope tracing metabolomics have been extensively reviewed previously [110,111], and are not the focus of our review. In this review, the main focus is on how the modulation of different metabolic pathways upon administration of bioactive compounds can be analyzed using these tools. Below, we discuss the metabolic tracers used to analyze different pathways, how the results are interpreted and what the limitations are to their use. Table 2 includes information on the appropriate stable isotope tracers to employ to investigate the metabolic effects of the natural products described previously.

9.2. *Glycolysis*

Otto Warburg first observed cancer cell performing aerobic glycolysis, where even in the presence of oxygen, cancer cells limit their energy metabolism largely to glycolysis [112]. To compensate for the increased energy demand and lower energy yield of glycolysis, cancer cells increase their glucose uptake as well as glycolytic flux [113–116]. The flux of glycolysis can be measured by introducing U-^{13}C glucose and measuring the percentage of incorporation of glycolysis precursors, such as fructose-1,6-bis-P, dihydroxyacetone phosphate, 3-phosphoglycerate and phosphoenolpyruvate. Compounds which inhibit glucose uptake, such as naringenin, phloretin, sylibinin, cytochalasin, curcumin, and compounds which impact different steps of glycolysis, such as mannoheptulose, sulforaphane, gossypol, konningic acid and shikonin, would directly impair glycolytic flux, which would be reflected in a lower percentage of incorporation of the glycolytic intermediates upon the introduction of U-^{13}C glucose. When a specific step of glycolysis is blocked by a compound, the precursors will have higher enrichment and ^{13}C incorporation will be stopped in the succeeding steps.

9.3. *TCA Cycle*

Uniformly labeled glucose (U-^{13}C glucose) is usually introduced to measure the contribution of glucose to the TCA cycle intermediates, including citrate, malate, fumarate, succinate. Glucose contributes to TCA cycle via generating acetyl CoA. In the first round of the TCA cycle, M+2 intermediates will be generated. In each succeeding round, M+4 and M+6 intermediates will be generated. An alternate way of representing the oxidative TCA cycle flux from glucose is measuring M+4/M+2 ratio of citrate or other TCA cycle intermediates. Compounds that impact glucose uptake and steps of the glycolysis will limit the contribution of acetyl-CoA to the TCA cycle and thus the TCA cycle flux will be lower.

The contribution of glutamine to TCA cycle is measured by introducing U-^{13}C glutamine, where glutamine is converted to alpha-ketoglutarate, which then goes through oxidative metabolism in the TCA cycle contributing 4-carbon to the TCA cycle intermediates (Figure 2). When glucose uptake or glycolysis is blocked, cells might get more dependent on glutamine and oxidative glutamine metabolism as an energy source. Glutamine can be partially oxidized in a process called glutaminolysis and add to the cellular production of NADPH and lactate. In doing so, it uses several steps of the TCA cycle and acts as a source of energy for proliferating cells. Glutamine has been proven to be a major anaplerotic precursor in proliferating glioma cells [117].

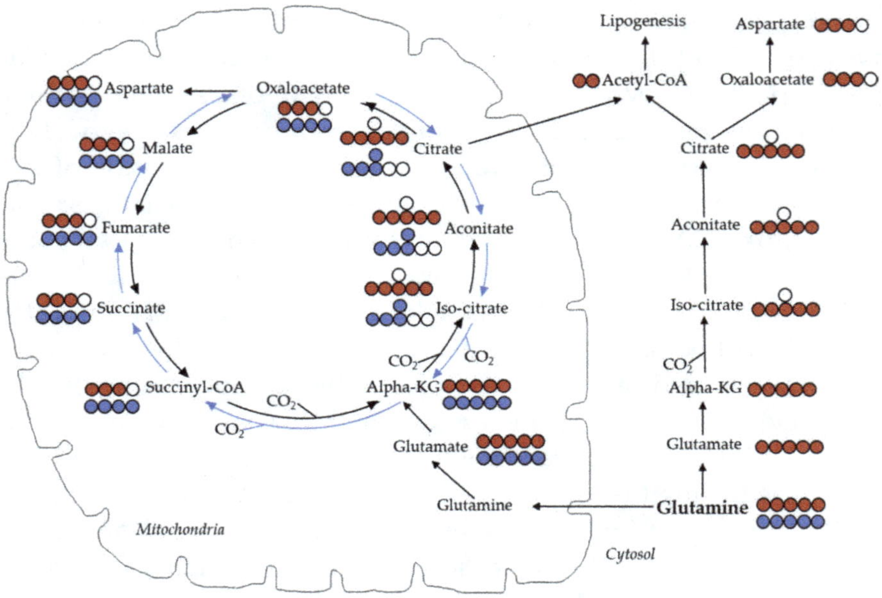

Figure 2. Carbon labelling TCA cycle intermediates and aspartate from U-^{13}C glutamine via oxidative (carbon marked with blue) and reductive carboxylation (carbon marked with red) pathway. Oxidative glutaminolysis generates M+4-labeled TCA cycle intermediates while reductive carboxylation generates M+5 citrate followed by M+3 malate, fumarate, succinate and aspartate.

Another important pathway for metabolizing glutamine is through reductive carboxylation, where it provides carbon for lipid biosynthesis [118]. An important function of reductive carboxylation is maintaining the redox balance of mitochondria, especially during anchorage-independent growth [119]. The reductive carboxylation pathway or reverse TCA cycle can generate M+5 citrate, where U-^{13}C glutamine produces alpha-ketoglutarate, which goes through the carboxylation reaction to produce M+5 isocitrate and citrate (Figure 2). This pathway can happen in both cytosol [118] or in mitochondria [120]. Generation of M+5 citrate in this pathway can later produce M+3 malate, fumarate and aspartate. A useful way of representing reductive carboxylation relative to oxidative TCA cycle activity is by measuring M+5/M+4 citrate ratio. Another way of confirming the contribution of reductive carboxylation pathway is by introducing glutamine labeled selectively at its first carbon ([1-^{13}C] glutamine). If glutamine is converted to alpha-ketoglutarate and that goes through oxidative metabolism, then this carbon is lost. This carbon will only be retained in the reductive carboxylation pathway and will generate M+1 citrate and other TCA cycle intermediates. Gracillin impacts mitochondrial metabolism and thus may induce reductive carboxylation, as this is a predominant pathway in cells with impaired mitochondria for citrate synthesis [121]. Agents that block glutamine uptake, such as ursolic acid, and glutamine utilization, such as EGCG, will impair glutamine's contribution via both oxidative and reductive carboxylation pathway.

9.4. Pentose Phosphate Pathway (PPP)

For increased demand of nucleotide biosynthesis and maintaining redox balance, the pentose phosphate pathway plays a vital role in proliferating cells [122]. One of the most widely used positionally labeled tracer is glucose labeled selectively at carbon 1 and 2 ([1,2-U-^{13}C] glucose). Oxidative pentose phosphate pathway (oxPPP) will cause the release of carbon at position 1 of glucose as CO_2 and subsequently generate M+1 ribose-5-P or M+1 intermediates of PPP, which can give rise to M+1 glycolytic intermediates generating M+1 lactate. If glucose goes through glycolysis that can only generate M+2 glycolytic intermediates and M+2 lactate. The flux trough PPP relative to glycolysis can be represented by the ratio of M+1 lactate/ M+1 + M+2 lactate, and this should be normalized for glucose consumption rate [123]. One limitation of this calculation is that it takes the assumption that most PPP-generated M+1 intermediates are recycled back to glycolysis, rather than being exported for nucleotide synthesis. For measuring the relative rate of oxidative to non-oxidative PPP, the ribose 5-P M+1/M+2 ratio is calculated. One limitation of this approach is that the reversibility of the PPP can generate M+2 ribose-5-P, even if it is produced via oxPPP initially. An alternative approach for measuring activity of oxPPP is the introduction of U-^{13}C glucose and analyzing the sedoheptulose-7-P labeling pattern. The conjugation of labeled ribose-5-P with unlabeled xylulose-5-P can only give rise to M+5 or M+2 label enrichment in sedoheptulose-7-P in the forward direction of PPP from oxPPP generated ribose-5-P. This can estimate the ribose-5-P coming from oxPPP and hence the activity of oxPPP. Since sedoheptulose-7-P is a unique intermediate of PPP, it would provide a reliable result. The reversibility of PPP can also give rise to M+5 or M+2 sedoheptulose-7-P, but the initial direct production via oxPPP would have a major influence on percentage of incorporation.

Another way of measuring PPP is by introducing 1-^{14}C glucose or 6-^{14}C glucose in two separate experiments and measuring the excretion of radioactive CO_2. Carbon number 1 of glucose is selectively released in oxPPP. Therefore, the radioactive CO_2 released from 1-^{14}C glucose relative to 6-^{14}C glucose labelling experiment would indicate the flux of oxPPP. Similar results can be derived by introducing 1-^{13}C glucose or 6-^{13}C glucose in two separate experiments and measuring M+1 ribose-5-P. The 6-^{13}C glucose would produce M+1 ribose-5-P by oxPPP, while labeled carbon number 1 of 1-^{13}C glucose is lost. Comparing the enrichment of M+1 ribose-5-P from 6-^{13}C glucose relative to 1-^{13}C glucose would indicate oxPPP activity [124]. Polydatin blocks the initial step of oxPPP and will result in lower activity of this pathway. Agents that block glucose uptake will limit the carbon entering in the PPP and will cause reduction in its activity for the production of NADPH and nucleotides.

9.5. *Pyruvate Carboxylase Activity*

The activity of pyruvate carboxylase is strongly associated with tumorigenesis in several cancers, including breast, non-small cell lung cancer, glioblastoma, renal carcinoma, and gall bladder, and feeds the carbon skeleton of down-stream metabolites of oxaloacetate for the biosynthesis of cellular components, such as amino acid, nucleotides, and membrane lipids [125]. Heterogeneity exists, as in some cancer cells, such as MCF-7, suppression of pyruvate carboxylase activity by estrogen is associated with proliferation [126]. When U-^{13}C- glucose is introduced, by the action of pyruvate dehydrogenase, labeled two carbon is incorporated in the TCA cycle via acetyl CoA and produces M+2 and M+4 TCA cycle intermediates in the first and second round of TCA cycle, respectively. Pyruvate carboxylase can incorporate one unlabeled carbon in the uniformly labeled pyruvate and generate M+3 oxaloacetate. This can go to the TCA cycle and generate M+3-labeled TCA cycle intermediates in the first round, while generating M+5 intermediates in the second round of TCA cycle. The activity of pyruvate carboxylase can be further monitored by introducing 3,4-^{13}C glucose. The first carbon of pyruvate come from carbon of the 3 or 4 position of glucose. While this carbon is lost when acetyl CoA is produced from pyruvate, it can be retained if pyruvate goes through carboxylation by pyruvate carboxylase and produces M+1 oxaloacetate. This can give rise to M+1 TCA cycle intermediates, such as M+1 malate, citrate and aspartate [110]. Compounds that block glucose uptake and those which impact steps of the glycolysis pathway producing pyruvate may reduce pyruvate carboxylase activity.

9.6. *Malic Enzyme Activity*

Malic enzyme catalyzed the production of pyruvate from malate while producing NAD(P)H at the same time. There are three isoenzymes of malic enzyme—malic enzyme 1 is in the cytosol, and 2 and 3 are in the mitochondria. The malic enzyme activity can be measures by introducing U-^{13}C glutamine and measuring the ratio of M+3 pyruvate/M+4 malate. Instead of pyruvate, an alternate option is to measure M+3 lactate / M+4 malate ratio. However, this gives an overall estimation of the activity of three forms of malic enzyme [124]. The activity of mitochondrial malic enzyme can be measured by isolating mitochondria and labelling with U-^{13}C- glutamine or U-^{13}C- malate and measuring the ratio of M+3 pyruvate or M+3 lactate/ M+4 malate. Agents that impact NADPH production via the oxPPP will induce malic enzyme for compensating the production of NADPH.

9.7. NAD^+/NADH Redox State

The production of NADH can be tracked by introducing 4-^{2}H-glucose, which goes through glycolysis and produce deuterium labeled NADH via the activity of glyceraldehyde-3-phosphate dehydrogenase. The ^{2}H from NADH can be transferred to lactate or malate. So, the production of deuterium-labeled NADH can be monitored by measuring the M+1 enrichment in malate and lactate [127]. Koningic acid specifically block this step and will result in lower NADH level.

9.8. $NADP^+$/NADPH Redox State

The production of NADPH can be tracked by introducing 1-^{2}H-glucose, which produces deuterium-labeled NADPH in the first reaction of oxPPP catalyzed by glucose-6-phosphate dehydrogenase [123]. Another way is by introducing 3-^{2}H-glucose, which produces deuterium-labeled NADPH in the second reaction of oxPPP catalyzed by phosphogluconate dehydrogenase. Lewis et al. [128] showed that the production of the deuterium labeled NADPH by introducing 3-^{2}H-glucose can be tracked by creating mutant IDH cells producing 2-HG and measuring the production of deuterium labeled 2-HG transferred from labeled NADPH. One limitation in using this approach is that 3-^{2}H-glucose, instead of going through oxPPP, can also go through glycolysis and produce deuterium-labeled dihydroxyacetone phosphate (DHAP) intermediate (Figure 3). The hydrogen in the 3 position of DHAP is shuffled by triose phosphate isomerase enzyme and can end up in the 2 or 3 position of glyceraldehyde-3-phosphate. If 3-^{2}H-DHAP produce 2-^{2}H-glyceraldehyde-3-P then the deuterium labeled hydrogen is transferred in water. On the other hand, if 3-^{2}H-DHAP produces 3-^{2}H-glyceraldehyde-3-P then the deuterium-labeled hydrogen is transferred to NAD by the action of gyceraldehyde-3-phosphate dehydrogenase. So, the 3-^{2}H-glucose can produce deuterium-labeled NADH and water through glycolysis in parallel with producing NADPH. 1-^{2}H-glucose should be the preferred tracer for labelling NADPH via oxPPP. The production of NADPH from malic enzyme and isocitrate dehydrogenase can be tracked by introducing 4-^{2}H-glucose, which can label malate and isocitrate and hence deuterium labeled NADPH is produced. 2,3,3-^{2}H- serine can be introduced to measure deuterium labeled NADPH produced in the folate pathway. The production of deuterium-labeled NADPH can be tracked by measuring M+1 enrichment of the fatty acids. Several bioactive compounds exert their cytotoxic effect through the generation of reactive oxygen species which would present increased need for NADPH generation and different NADPH producing pathways would have higher flux for meeting the increased demand.

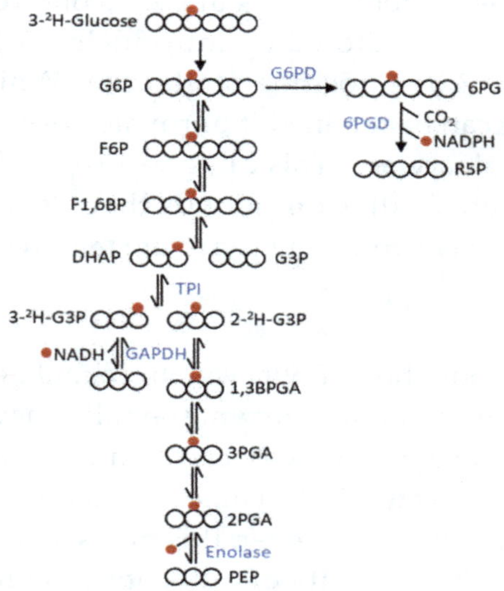

Figure 3. Fate of ^{2}H at position 3 of glucose. 3-^{2}H-glucose can produce deuterium labeled NADPH when processed through oxPPP and NADH and water when processed through glycolysis. The deuterium-labeled hydrogen is marked with a red dot. Abbreviation: G6P: glucose-6-phosphate; G6PD:

glucose-6-phosphate dehydrogenase; 6PG: 6-phosphogluconate; 6PGD: 6-phosphogluconate dehydrogenase; R5P: ribose-5-phosphate; F6P: fructose-6-phosphate; F1,6BP: fructose-1,6-bis-phosphate, DHAP: dihydroxyacetone phosphate; G3P: glyceraldehyde-3-phosphate; 1,3BPGA: 1,3-bisphosphoglycerate; 3PGA: 3-phosphoglycerate; 2PGA: 2-phosphoglycerate; PEP: phosphoenolpyruvate.

9.9. Glutathione Biosynthesis

Glutathione is produced from precursor- glutamate, glycine and cysteine. The production of glutathione can be monitored by introducing U-^{13}C- glutamine (main source of glutamate) or U-^{13}C-glycine. Bioactive compounds which stimulate the production of reactive oxygen species might cause increased biosynthesis of glutathione to neutralize it. Phloretin induces the biosynthesis of glutathione.

9.10. CoQ Biosynthesis

Coenzyme Q (CoQ) is a redox active molecule that plays a key role in the mitochondrial electron transport chain. Biosynthesis of CoQ is an important marker for mitochondrial dysfunction and oxidative stress [129]. The head group of CoQ comes from phenylalanine or tyrosine. So, the biosynthesis of CoQ can be monitored by introducing uniformly labeled phenylalanine or tyrosine. U-^{13}C- glucose can also be given and label incorporation in the fatty acid chain of CoQ can be monitored, which is also an indicator of CoQ biosynthesis [130]. Compounds that impair mitochondrial oxydative phophorylation, such as gracillin, may impair CoQ biosynthesis.

9.11. Nucleotide Biosynthesis

Figure 4 shows the source of the carbon and nitrogen in the purine ring. Purine biosynthesis can be analyzed by introducing U-^{13}C- glycine which can contribute up to four ^{13}C to the purine ring, with two ^{13}C derived from the direct incorporation of glycine and up to two additional ^{13}C from glycine derived one carbon units.

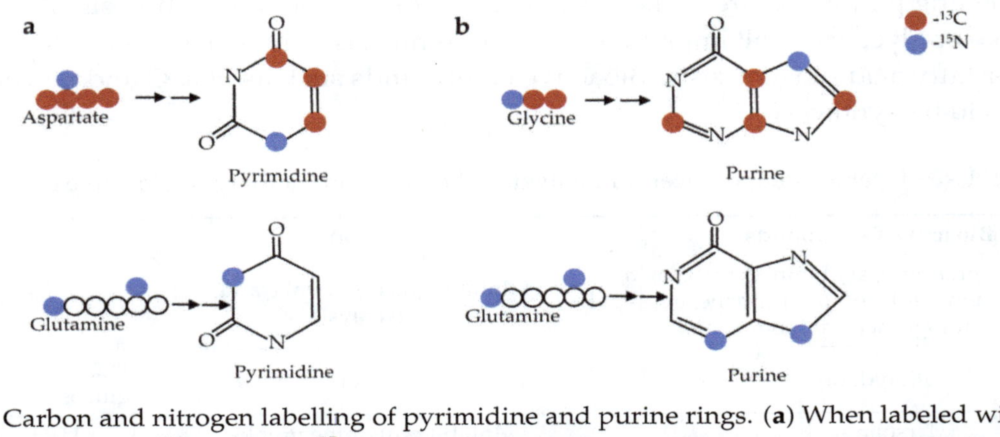

Figure 4. Carbon and nitrogen labelling of pyrimidine and purine rings. (**a**) When labeled with 1-^{15}N, 4-^{13}C- aspartate, three ^{13}C and one ^{15}N are incorporated into the pyrimidine ring, and when labeled with 2-^{15}N- glutamine, one ^{15}N is incorporated into the pyrimidine ring. (**b**) When labeled with 1-^{15}N, 2-^{13}C- glycine, up to four ^{13}C and one ^{15}N are incorporated into the purine ring, and when labeled with 2-^{15}N- glutamine, two ^{15}N are incorporated into the purine ring. ^{13}C and ^{15}N are represented with red and blue dots respectively.

Pyrimidine biosynthesis can be analyzed by introducing U-^{13}C- aspartate and measuring M+3 uridine or UMP. Pyrimidine and purine ring biosynthesis can also be analyzed by introducing 2-^{15}N-glutamine, which will contribute one and two ^{15}N in the pyrimidine and purine ring, respectively. Agents that block glucose uptake or PPP will impair nucleotide biosynthesis. Agents that block TCA cycle and thus the production of aspartate will inhibit pyrimidine biosynthesis.

9.12. Folate Pathway

The biosynthesis of the 1C unit via the folate pathway can be analyzed via different ways. One important fact based on which biosynthesis of the 1C unit can be analyzed is that the dTTP contains 1C from cytosolic methylene THF. For analyzing the production of 1C unit in the cytosol from serine, 3-^{13}C- serine is introduced and M+1 dTTP is analyzed. The third carbon of serine goes on to produce 5,10 methylene tetrahydrofolate via the action of serine hydroxymethyl transferase (SHMT). SHMT has two isoenzymes—SHMT1 is in the cytosol and SHMT2 is in the mitochondria. To distinguish the contribution of SHMT1 and SHMT2, 2,3,3-^{2}H- serine is introduced. Here, M+2 dTTP is generated via the action of SHMT1 and M+1 dTTP is generated via the action of SHMT2 via a more cyclic route, where serine is cleaved in mitochondria, goes through dehydrogenation and transported to cytosol to produce 5, 10 methylene THF to get incorporated in dTTP [131]. U-^{13}C- glycine can be introduced and measure M+1, M+2, M+3, M+4 ATP. Glycine can be incorporated in the purine ring generating M+2 ATP. Glycine is cleaved by the glycine cleavage system and generates 1C units in the folate pathway. The purine ring contains 1C unit from cytosolic 10-formyl-THF generating different labelling patterns in ATP. The generation of mitochondrial 1C unit can be monitored by measuring formyl-methionine M+1, as it contains 1C from mitochondrial 10-formyl-THF. Formate M+1 is also an indicator of the folate pathway activity. U-^{13}C- sarcosine and U-^{13}C- formate can also be introduced to measure flux through the folate pathway. When NADPH production is blocked via the oxPPP, folate pathway activity might get stimulated for compensating NADPH production.

9.13. Fatty Acid Biosynthesis

Fatty acid biosynthesis can happen using both glucose and glutamine as a carbon source. Using U-^{13}C- glucose or U-^{13}C- glutamine fatty acid biosynthesis can be monitored as they contribute to fatty acid biosynthesis via producing labeled acetyl CoA generating fatty acids labelling pattern in even numbers (M+2, 4, 6 etc). To analyze the contribution of glutamine to fatty acid biosynthesis via reductive carboxylation, 5-^{13}C- glutamine is introduced. It contributes to fatty acid biosynthesis via generating M+1 acetyl CoA, resulting in labelling patterns with odd numbers in fatty acid [118]. Palmitate labelling pattern is often taken as a read out of fatty acid biosynthesis. Agents that block glucose uptake or glycolysis will impair fatty acid biosynthesis or may make cells more dependent on glutamine for fatty acid biosynthesis. Bioactive compounds such as EGCG and resveratrol directly inhibit fatty acid biosynthesis.

Table 2. Use of stable isotope tracer for analyzing the metabolic activity of bioactive compounds.

Bioactive Compounds	Target	Stable Isotope Tracer
Naringenin, phloretin, sylibinin, cytochalasin, curcumin, mannoheptulose, sulforaphane, gossypol, konningic acid, shikonin	Inhibit glucose uptake and glycolysis	U-^{13}C glucose
Polydatin	Inhibit PPP	[1,2-U-^{13}C] glucose, 1-^{13}C glucose and 6-^{13}C glucose
Ursolic acid	Inhibit glutamine uptake	U-^{13}C glutamine
Koningic acid	Inhibit GAPDH	4-^{2}H-glucose
Phloretin	Induce glutathione biosynthesis	U-^{13}C- glutamine or U-^{13}C-glycine
EGCG, resveratrol, patuletin, diosgenin, [6]-gingerol	Inhibit fatty acid biosynthesis	U-^{13}C glucose, U-^{13}C glutamine

10. Conclusions

Bioactive compounds that targets different components of the metabolic process hold great potential as a safer option for the treatment of cancer. They need to be studied further in terms of how they reprogram the metabolism for their efficient use as cancer therapeutics. Carefully choosing positionally labeled stable isotope tracers could show how these compounds modulate the activity of different pathways. This will reveal their mechanism of action in cancer cells. Metabolic flux analysis in animal models and patients upon treatment with bioactive compounds could provide valuable information about the metabolic activity of bioactive compounds in a physiological state. Currently, there is lack of such studies and this could be a promising avenue of research in the future.

Author Contributions: Conceptualization, F.K.C. and S.T.; writing—original draft preparation, F.K.C., G.L.H., A.L., and S.T.; writing—review and editing, F.K.C., G.L.H., A.L., and S.T.; visualization, F.K.C., G.L.H., A.L., and S.T.; supervision S.T.; funding acquisition, S.T. All authors have read and agreed to the published version of the manuscript.

References

1. Hanahan, D.; Weinberg, R.A. Hallmarks of cancer: The next generation. *Cell* **2011**, *144*, 646–674. [CrossRef]
2. Hsu, P.P.; Sabatini, D.M. Cancer cell metabolism: Warburg and beyond. *Cell* **2008**, *134*, 703–707. [CrossRef] [PubMed]
3. Vander Heiden, M.G.; Deberardinis, R.J. Understanding the intersections between metabolism and cancer biology. *Cell* **2017**, *168*, 657–669. [CrossRef]
4. Guerra, A.R.; Duarte, M.F.; Duarte, I.F. Targeting tumor metabolism with plant-derived natural products: Emerging trends in cancer therapy. *J. Agric. Food Chem.* **2018**, *66*, 10663–10685. [CrossRef] [PubMed]
5. Cragg, G.M.; Pezzuto, J.M. Natural products as a vital source for the discovery of cancer chemotherapeutic and chemopreventive agents. *Med. Princ. Pract.* **2015**, *25*, 41–59. [CrossRef] [PubMed]
6. Dutta, S.; Mahalanobish, S.; Saha, S.; Ghosh, S.; Sil, P.C. Natural products: An upcoming therapeutic approach to cancer. *Food Chem. Toxicol.* **2019**, *128*, 240–255. [CrossRef]
7. Lin, S.R.; Chang, C.H.; Hsu, C.F.; Tsai, M.J.; Cheng, H.; Leong, M.K.; Sung, P.J.; Chen, J.C.; Weng, C.F. Natural compounds as potential adjuvants to cancer therapy: Preclinical evidence. *Br. J. Pharm.* **2019**, *177*, 1409–1423. [CrossRef]
8. Lodi, A.; Saha, A.; Lu, X.; Wang, B.; Sentandreu, E.; Collins, M.; Kolonin, M.G.; DiGiovanni, J.; Tiziani, S. Combinatorial treatment with natural compounds in prostate cancer inhibits prostate tumor growth and leads to key modulations of cancer cell metabolism. *NPJ Precis. Oncol.* **2017**, *1*, 1–12. [CrossRef]
9. Minutolo, F.; Macchia, M.; Katzenellenbogen, B.S.; Katzenellenbogen, J.A. Estrogen receptor beta ligands: Recent advances and biomedical applications. *Med. Res. Rev.* **2011**, *31*, 364–442. [CrossRef]
10. Barbosa, A.M.; Martel, F. Targeting glucose transporters for breast cancer therapy: The effect of natural and synthetic compounds. *Cancers* **2020**, *12*, 154. [CrossRef]
11. Zhao, Z.; Jin, G.; Ge, Y.; Guo, Z. Naringenin inhibits migration of breast cancer cells via inflammatory and apoptosis cell signaling pathways. *Inflammopharmacology* **2019**, *27*, 1021–1036. [CrossRef] [PubMed]
12. Lim, W.; Park, S.; Bazer, F.W.; Song, G. Naringenin-induced apoptotic cell death in prostate cancer cells is mediated via the pi3k/akt and mapk signaling pathways. *J. Cell Biochem.* **2017**, *118*, 1118–1131. [CrossRef]
13. Nasr Bouzaiene, N.; Chaabane, F.; Sassi, A.; Chekir-Ghedira, L.; Ghedira, K. Effect of apigenin-7-glucoside, genkwanin and naringenin on tyrosinase activity and melanin synthesis in B16F10 melanoma cells. *Life Sci.* **2016**, *144*, 80–85. [CrossRef]
14. Arul, D.; Subramanian, P. Naringenin (citrus flavonone) induces growth inhibition, cell cycle arrest and apoptosis in human hepatocellular carcinoma cells. *Pathol. Oncol. Res.* **2013**, *19*, 763–770. [CrossRef] [PubMed]
15. Chandrika, B.B.; Steephan, M.; Kumar, T.R.S.; Sabu, A.; Haridas, M. Hesperetin and naringenin sensitize HER2 positive cancer cells to death by serving as HER2 tyrosine kinase inhibitors. *Life Sci.* **2016**, *160*, 47–56. [CrossRef] [PubMed]
16. Ke, J.Y.; Banh, T.; Hsiao, Y.H.; Cole, R.M.; Straka, S.R.; Yee, L.D.; Belury, M.A. Citrus flavonoid naringenin reduces mammary tumor cell viability, adipose mass, and adipose inflammation in obese ovariectomized mice. *Mol. Nutr. Food Res.* **2017**, *61*, 1600934. [CrossRef]

17. Camargo, C.A.; Gomes-Marcondes, M.C.; Wutzki, N.C.; Aoyama, H. Naringin inhibits tumor growth and reduces interleukin-6 and tumor necrosis factor alpha levels in rats with walker 256 carcinosarcoma. *Anticancer Res.* **2012**, *32*, 129–133.
18. Salehi, B.; Fokou, P.V.T.; Sharifi-Rad, M.; Zucca, P.; Pezzani, R.; Martins, N.; Sharifi-Rad, J. The therapeutic potential of naringenin: A review of clinical trials. *Pharmaceuticals* **2019**, *12*, 11. [CrossRef]
19. Rajamani, S.; Radhakrishnan, A.; Sengodan, T.; Thangavelu, S. Augmented anticancer activity of naringenin-loaded TPGS polymeric nanosuspension for drug resistive MCF-7 human breast cancer cells. *Drug Dev. Ind. Pharm.* **2018**, *44*, 1752–1761. [CrossRef]
20. Kwon, O.; Eck, P.; Chen, S.; Corpe, C.P.; Lee, J.H.; Kruhlak, M.; Levine, M. Inhibition of the intestinal glucose transporter GLUT2 by flavonoids. *FASEB J.* **2007**, *21*, 366–377. [CrossRef]
21. Akins, N.S.; Nielson, T.C.; Le, H.V. Inhibition of glycolysis and glutaminolysis: An emerging drug discovery approach to combat cancer. *Curr. Top. Med. Chem.* **2018**, *18*, 494–504. [CrossRef] [PubMed]
22. Stompor, M.; Broda, D.; Bajek-Bil, A. Dihydrochalcones: Methods of acquisition and pharmacological properties—A first systematic review. *Molecules* **2019**, *24*, 4468. [CrossRef] [PubMed]
23. Choi, B. Biochemical basis of anti-cancer-effects of phloretin—A natural dihydrochalcone. *Molecules* **2019**, *24*, 278. [CrossRef]
24. Hasan, S.; Taha, R.; Omri, H.E. Current opinions on chemoresistance: An overview. *Bioinformation* **2018**, *14*, 80–85. [CrossRef]
25. Shriwas, P.; Chen, X.; Kinghorn, A.D.; Ren, Y. Plant-derived glucose transport inhibitors with potential antitumor activity. *Phytother. Res.* **2020**, *34*, 1027–1040. [CrossRef] [PubMed]
26. Ma, L.; Wang, R.; Nan, Y.; Li, W.; Wang, Q.; Jin, F. Phloretin exhibits an anticancer effect and enhances the anticancer ability of cisplatin on non-small cell lung cancer cell lines by regulating expression of apoptotic pathways and matrix metalloproteinases. *Int. J. Oncol.* **2016**, *48*, 843–853. [CrossRef] [PubMed]
27. Abkin, S.V.; Ostroumova, O.S.; Komarova, E.Y.; Meshalkina, D.A.; Shevtsov, M.A.; Margulis, B.A.; Guzhova, I.V. Phloretin increases the anti-tumor efficacy of intratumorally delivered heat-shock protein 70 kDa (HSP70) in a murine model of melanoma. *Cancer Immunol. Immunother.* **2015**, *65*, 83–92. [CrossRef]
28. Qin, X.; Xing, Y.F.; Zhou, Z.; Yao, Y. Dihydrochalcone compounds isolated from crabapple leaves showed anticancer effects on human cancer cell lines. *Molecules* **2015**, *20*, 21193–21203. [CrossRef]
29. Xu, M.; Gu, W.; Shen, Z.; Wang, F. Anticancer activity of phloretin against human gastric cancer cell lines involves apoptosis, cell cycle arrest, and inhibition of cell invasion and JNK signalling pathway. *Med. Sci. Monit.* **2018**, *24*, 6551–6558. [CrossRef]
30. Duan, H.; Wang, R.; Yan, X.; Liu, H.; Zhang, Y.; Mu, D.; Han, J.; Li, X. Phloretin induces apoptosis of human esophageal cancer via a mitochondria-dependent pathway. *Oncol. Lett.* **2017**, *14*, 6763–6768. [CrossRef]
31. Wu, K.-H.; Ho, C.-T.; Chen, Z.-F.; Chen, L.-C.; Whang-Peng, J.; Lin, T.-N.; Ho, Y.-S. The apple polyphenol phloretin inhibits breast cancer cell migration and proliferation via inhibition of signals by type 2 glucose transporter. *J. Food Drug Anal.* **2017**. [CrossRef] [PubMed]
32. Szliszka, E.; Czuba, Z.P.; Mazur, B.; Paradysz, A.; Krol, W. Chalcones and dihydrochalcones augment TRAIL-mediated apoptosis in prostate cancer cells. *Molecules* **2010**, *15*, 5336–5353. [CrossRef] [PubMed]
33. Liu, Y.; Fan, C.; Pu, L.; Wei, C.; Jin, H.; Teng, Y.; Zhao, M.; Yu, A.C.; Jiang, F.; Shu, J.; et al. Phloretin induces cell cycle arrest and apoptosis of human glioblastoma cells through the generation of reactive oxygen species. *J. Neurooncol.* **2016**, *128*, 217–223. [CrossRef] [PubMed]
34. Zielinska, D.; Laparra-Llopis, J.M.; Zielinski, H.; Szawara-Nowak, D.; Giménez-Bastida, J.A. Role of apple phytochemicals, phloretin and phloridzin, in modulating processes related to intestinal inflammation. *Nutrients* **2019**, *11*, 1173. [CrossRef] [PubMed]
35. Yang, Y.C.; Lii, C.K.; Lin, A.H.; Yeh, Y.W.; Yao, H.T.; Li, C.C.; Liu, K.L.; Chen, H.W. Induction of glutathione synthesis and heme oxygenase 1 by the flavonoids butein and phloretin is mediated through the ERK/Nrf2 pathway and protects against oxidative stress. *Free Radic. Biol. Med.* **2011**, *51*, 2073–2081. [CrossRef]
36. Zhan, T.; Digel, M.; Kuch, E.M.; Stremmel, W.; Fullekrug, J. Silybin and dehydrosilybin decrease glucose uptake by inhibiting GLUT proteins. *J. Cell Biochem.* **2011**, *112*, 849–859. [CrossRef]
37. Delmas, D.; Xiao, J.; Vejux, A.; Aires, V. Silymarin and cancer: A dual strategy in both in chemoprevention and chemosensitivity. *Molecules* **2020**, *25*, 2009. [CrossRef]
38. Granchi, C.; Minutolo, F. Anticancer agents that counteract tumor glycolysis. *Chem. Med. Chem.* **2012**, *7*, 1318–1350. [CrossRef]

39. Bailon-Moscoso, N.; Cevallos-Solorzano, G.; Romero-Benavides, J.; Ramirez Orellana, M. Natural compounds as modulators of cell cycle arrest: Application for anticancer chemotherapies. *Curr. Genom.* **2017**, *18*, 106–131. [CrossRef]
40. Bijak, M.; Synowiec, E.; Sitarek, P.; Sliwiński, T.; Saluk-Bijak, J. Evaluation of the cytotoxicity and genotoxicity of flavonolignans in different cellular models. *Nutrients* **2017**, *9*, 1356. [CrossRef]
41. Luo, H.; Vong, C.T.; Chen, H.; Gao, Y.; Lyu, P.; Qiu, L.; Zhao, M.; Liu, Q.; Cheng, Z.; Zou, J.; et al. Naturally occurring anti-cancer compounds: Shining from Chinese herbal medicine. *Chin. Med.* **2019**, *14*, 48. [CrossRef] [PubMed]
42. Deep, G.; Agarwal, R. Chemopreventive efficacy of silymarin in skin and prostate cancer. *Integr. Cancer Ther.* **2007**, *6*, 130–145. [CrossRef]
43. Liao, H.; Wang, Z.; Deng, Z.; Ren, H.; Li, X. Curcumin inhibits lung cancer invasion and metastasis by attenuating GLUT1/MT1-MMP/MMP2 pathway. *Int. J. Clin. Exp. Med.* **2015**, *8*, 8948–8957.
44. Wang, K.; Fan, H.; Chen, Q.; Ma, G.; Zhu, M.; Zhang, X.; Zhang, Y.; Yu, J. Curcumin inhibits aerobic glycolysis and induces mitochondrial-mediated apoptosis through hexokinase II in human colorectal cancer cells in vitro. *Anticancer Drugs* **2015**, *26*, 15–24. [CrossRef] [PubMed]
45. Geng, C.; Li, J.; Ding, F.; Wu, G.; Yang, Q.; Sun, Y.; Zhang, Z.; Dong, T.; Tian, X. Curcumin suppresses 4-hydroxytamoxifen resistance in breast cancer cells by targeting SLUG/Hexokinase 2 pathway. *Biochem. Biophys. Res. Commun.* **2016**, *473*, 147–153. [CrossRef] [PubMed]
46. Fan, H.; Tian, W.; Ma, X. Curcumin induces apoptosis of HepG2 cells via inhibiting fatty acid synthase. *Target. Oncol.* **2014**, *9*, 279–286. [CrossRef]
47. Fan, H.; Liang, Y.; Jiang, B.; Li, X.; Xun, H.; Sun, J.; He, W.; Lau, H.T.; Ma, X. Curcumin inhibits intracellular fatty acid synthase and induces apoptosis in human breast cancer MDA-MB-231 cells. *Oncol. Rep.* **2016**, *35*, 2651–2656. [CrossRef]
48. Giordano, A.; Tommonaro, G. Curcumin and cancer. *Nutrients* **2019**, *11*, 2376. [CrossRef]
49. Tomeh, M.A.; Hadianamrei, R.; Zhao, X. A review of curcumin and its derivatives as anticancer agents. *Int. J. Mol. Sci.* **2019**, *20*, 1033. [CrossRef]
50. Zhang, Y.; Courtois, P.; Sener, A.; Malaisse, W.J. Dissimilar effects of D-mannoheptulose on the phosphorylation of alpha- versus beta-D-glucose by either hexokinase or glucokinase. *Int. J. Mol. Med.* **2004**, *14*, 107–112.
51. Jeon, Y.K.; Yoo, D.R.; Jang, Y.H.; Jang, S.Y.; Nam, M.J. Sulforaphane induces apoptosis in human hepatic cancer cells through inhibition of 6-phosphofructo-2-kinase/fructose-2,6-biphosphatase4, mediated by hypoxia inducible factor-1-dependent pathway. *Biochim. Biophys. Acta* **2011**, *1814*, 1340–1348. [CrossRef] [PubMed]
52. Liang, J.; Hansch, G.M.; Hubner, K.; Samstag, Y. Sulforaphane as anticancer agent: A double-edged sword? Tricky balance between effects on tumor cells and immune cells. *Adv. Biol. Regul.* **2019**, *71*, 79–87. [CrossRef] [PubMed]
53. Su, X.; Jiang, X.; Meng, L.; Dong, X.; Shen, Y.; Xin, Y. Anticancer activity of sulforaphane: The epigenetic mechanisms and the Nrf2 signaling pathway. *Oxid. Med. Cell. Longev.* **2018**, *2018*, 5438179. [CrossRef] [PubMed]
54. Alumkal, J.J.; Slottke, R.; Schwartzman, J.; Cherala, G.; Munar, M.; Graff, J.N.; Beer, T.M.; Ryan, C.W.; Koop, D.R.; Gibbs, A.; et al. A phase II study of sulforaphane-rich broccoli sprout extracts in men with recurrent prostate cancer. *Investig. New Drugs* **2015**, *33*, 480–489. [CrossRef] [PubMed]
55. Lozanovski, V.J.; Houben, P.; Hinz, U.; Hackert, T.; Herr, I.; Schemmer, P. Pilot study evaluating broccoli sprouts in advanced pancreatic cancer (POUDER trial)—Study protocol for a randomized controlled trial. *Trials* **2014**, *15*, 204. [CrossRef] [PubMed]
56. Nakazawa, M.; Uehara, T.; Nomura, Y. Koningic acid (a potent glyceraldehyde-3-phosphate dehydrogenase inhibitor)-induced fragmentation and condensation of DNA in NG108-15 cells. *J. Neurochem.* **1997**, *68*, 2493–2499. [CrossRef]
57. Rahier, N.J.; Molinier, N.; Long, C.; Deshmukh, S.K.; Kate, A.S.; Ranadive, P.; Verekar, S.A.; Jiotode, M.; Lavhale, R.R.; Tokdar, P.; et al. Anticancer activity of koningic acid and semisynthetic derivatives. *Bioorg. Med. Chem.* **2015**, *23*, 3712–3721. [CrossRef]
58. Ganapathy-Kanniappan, S. Evolution of GAPDH as a druggable target of tumor glycolysis? *Expert Opin. Ther. Targets* **2018**, *22*, 295–298. [CrossRef]

59. Chen, J.; Xie, J.; Jiang, Z.; Wang, B.; Wang, Y.; Hu, X. Shikonin and its analogs inhibit cancer cell glycolysis by targeting tumor pyruvate kinase-M2. *Oncogene* **2011**, *30*, 4297–4306. [CrossRef]
60. Sweeney, S.; Collins, M.; Pandey, R.; Chiou, J.; Lodi, A.; Tiziani, S. Identification of a synergistic combination of dimethylaminoparthenolide and shikonin alters metabolism and inhibits proliferation of pediatric precursor-B cell acute lymphoblastic leukemia. *Mol. Carcinogen.* **2020**, *59*, 399–411. [CrossRef]
61. Zhao, X.; Zhu, Y.; Hu, J.; Jiang, L.; Li, L.; Jia, S.; Zen, K. Shikonin inhibits tumor growth in mice by suppressing pyruvate kinase M2-mediated aerobic glycolysis. *Sci. Rep.* **2018**, *8*, 14517. [CrossRef] [PubMed]
62. Wang, Y.; Hao, F.; Nan, Y.; Qu, L.; Na, W.; Jia, C.; Chen, X. PKM2 inhibitor shikonin overcomes the cisplatin resistance in bladder cancer by inducing necroptosis. *Int. J. Biol. Sci.* **2018**, *14*, 1883–1891. [CrossRef] [PubMed]
63. Tang, J.C.; Zhao, J.; Long, F.; Chen, J.Y.; Mu, B.; Jiang, Z.; Ren, Y.; Yang, J. Efficacy of shikonin against esophageal cancer cells and its possible mechanisms in vitro and in vivo. *J. Cancer* **2018**, *9*, 32–40. [CrossRef] [PubMed]
64. Chen, J.; Jiang, Z.; Wang, B.; Wang, Y.; Hu, X. Vitamin K (3) and K (5) are inhibitors of tumor pyruvate kinase M2. *Cancer Lett.* **2012**, *316*, 204–210. [CrossRef] [PubMed]
65. Liu, J.; Wu, N.; Ma, L.; Liu, M.; Liu, G.; Zhang, Y.; Lin, X. Oleanolic acid suppresses aerobic glycolysis in cancer cells by switching pyruvate kinase type M isoforms. *PLoS ONE* **2014**, *9*, e91606. [CrossRef] [PubMed]
66. Gomez, M.S.; Piper, R.C.; Hunsaker, L.A.; Royer, R.E.; Deck, L.M.; Makler, M.T.; Vander Jagt, D.L. Substrate and cofactor specificity and selective inhibition of lactate dehydrogenase from the malarial parasite P. falciparum. *Mol. Biochem. Parasitol.* **1997**, *90*, 235–246. [CrossRef]
67. Feng, Y.; Xiong, Y.; Qiao, T.; Li, X.; Jia, L.; Han, Y. Lactate dehydrogenase: A key player in carcinogenesis and potential target in cancer therapy. *Cancer Med.* **2018**, *7*, 6124–6136. [CrossRef]
68. Kim, H.Y.; Lee, B.I.; Jeon, J.H.; Kim, D.K.; Kang, S.G.; Shim, J.K.; Kim, S.Y.; Kang, S.W.; Jang, H. Gossypol suppresses growth of temozolomide-resistant glioblastoma tumor spheres. *Biomolecules* **2019**, *9*, 595. [CrossRef]
69. Zhang, L.; Sun, S.; Wang, Y.; Mo, Y.; Xiong, F.; Zhang, S.; Zeng, Z.; Xiong, W.; Li, G.; Chen, H.; et al. Gossypol induces apoptosis of multiple myeloma cells through the JUN-JNK pathway. *Am. J. Cancer Res.* **2020**, *10*, 870–883.
70. Lu, M.D.; Li, L.Y.; Li, P.H.; You, T.; Wang, F.H.; Sun, W.J.; Zheng, Z.Q. Gossypol induces cell death by activating apoptosis and autophagy in HT-29 cells. *Mol. Med. Rep.* **2017**, *16*, 2128–2132. [CrossRef]
71. Lampson, B.L.; Davids, M.S. The development and current use of BCL-2 inhibitors for the treatment of chronic lymphocytic leukemia. *Curr. Hematol. Malig. Rep.* **2017**, *12*, 11–19. [CrossRef] [PubMed]
72. Volate, S.R.; Kawasaki, B.T.; Hurt, E.M.; Milner, J.A.; Kim, Y.S.; White, J.; Farrar, W.L. Gossypol induces apoptosis by activating p53 in prostate cancer cells and prostate tumor-initiating cells. *Mol. Cancer* **2010**, *9*, 461–470. [CrossRef] [PubMed]
73. Moon, D.O.; Choi, Y.H.; Moon, S.K.; Kim, W.J.; Kim, G.Y. Gossypol decreases tumor necrosis factor-alpha-induced intercellular adhesion molecule-1 expression via suppression of NF-kappaB activity. *Food Chem. Toxicol.* **2011**, *49*, 999–1005. [CrossRef] [PubMed]
74. Halestrap, A.P.; Denton, R.M. The specificity and metabolic implications of the inhibition of pyruvate transport in isolated mitochondria and intact tissue preparations by alpha-Cyano-4-hydroxycinnamate and related compounds. *Biochem. J.* **1975**, *148*, 97–106. [CrossRef]
75. Wilkins, L.R.; Brautigan, D.L.; Wu, H.; Yarmohammadi, H.; Kubicka, E.; Serbulea, V.; Leitinger, N.; Liu, W.; Haaga, J.R. Cinnamic acid derivatives enhance the efficacy of transarterial embolization in a rat model of hepatocellular carcinoma. *Cardiovasc. Interv. Radiol.* **2016**. [CrossRef]
76. Payen, V.L.; Mina, E.; Van Hée, V.F.; Porporato, P.E.; Sonveaux, P. Monocarboxylate transporters in cancer. *Mol. Metab.* **2020**, *33*, 48–66. [CrossRef]
77. Coss, R.A.; Storck, C.W.; Daskalakis, C.; Berd, D.; Wahl, M.L. Intracellular acidification abrogates the heat shock response and compromises survival of human melanoma cells. *Mol. Cancer Ther.* **2003**, *2*, 383–388.
78. Caruso, J.P.; Koch, B.J.; Benson, P.D.; Varughese, E.; Monterey, M.D.; Lee, A.E.; Dave, A.M.; Kiousis, S.; Sloan, A.E.; Mathupala, S.P. pH, lactate, and hypoxia: Reciprocity in regulating high-affinity monocarboxylate transporter expression in glioblastoma. *Neoplasia* **2017**, *19*, 121–134. [CrossRef]

79. Colen, C.B.; Shen, Y.; Ghoddoussi, F.; Yu, P.; Francis, T.B.; Koch, B.J.; Monterey, M.D.; Galloway, M.P.; Sloan, A.E.; Mathupala, S.P. Metabolic targeting of lactate efflux by malignant glioma inhibits invasiveness and induces necrosis: An in vivo study. *Neoplasia* **2011**, *13*, 620–632. [CrossRef]
80. Schonrogge, M.; Kerndl, H.; Zhang, X.; Kumstel, S.; Vollmar, B.; Zechner, D. Alpha-cyano-4-hydroxycinnamate impairs pancreatic cancer cells by stimulating the p38 signaling pathway. *Cell Signal.* **2018**, *47*, 101–108. [CrossRef]
81. Kumar, A.; Kant, S.; Singh, S.M. Alpha-Cyano-4-hydroxycinnamate induces apoptosis in Dalton's lymphoma cells: Role of altered cell survival-regulatory mechanisms. *Anticancer Drugs* **2013**, *24*, 158–171. [CrossRef] [PubMed]
82. Mele, L.; Paino, F.; Papaccio, F.; Regad, T.; Boocock, D.; Stiuso, P.; Lombardi, A.; Liccardo, D.; Aquino, G.; Barbieri, A.; et al. A new inhibitor of glucose-6-phosphate dehydrogenase blocks pentose phosphate pathway and suppresses malignant proliferation and metastasis in vivo. *Cell Death Dis.* **2018**, *9*, 572. [CrossRef] [PubMed]
83. Du, Q.H.; Peng, C.; Zhang, H. Polydatin: A review of pharmacology and pharmacokinetics. *Pharm. Biol.* **2013**, *51*, 1347–1354. [CrossRef] [PubMed]
84. Scalise, M.; Pochini, L.; Console, L.; Losso, M.A.; Indiveri, C. The human SLC1A5 (ASCT2) amino acid transporter: From function to structure and role in cell biology. *Front. Cell Dev. Biol.* **2018**, *6*, 96. [CrossRef]
85. Yin, R.; Li, T.; Tian, J.X.; Xi, P.; Liu, R.H. Ursolic acid, a potential anticancer compound for breast cancer therapy. *Crit. Rev. Food Sci. Nutr.* **2018**, *58*, 568–574. [CrossRef]
86. Leng, S.; Hao, Y.; Du, D.; Xie, S.; Hong, L.; Gu, H.; Zhu, X.; Zhang, J.; Fan, D.; Kung, H.F. Ursolic acid promotes cancer cell death by inducing Atg5-dependent autophagy. *Int. J. Cancer* **2013**, *133*, 2781–2790. [CrossRef]
87. Min, H.Y.; Jang, H.J.; Park, K.H.; Hyun, S.Y.; Park, S.J.; Kim, J.H.; Son, J.; Kang, S.S.; Lee, H.Y. The natural compound gracillin exerts potent antitumor activity by targeting mitochondrial complex II. *Cell Death Dis.* **2019**, *10*, 810. [CrossRef]
88. Hail, N., Jr.; Lotan, R. Examining the role of mitochondrial respiration in vanilloid-induced apoptosis. *J. Natl. Cancer Inst.* **2002**, *94*, 1281–1292. [CrossRef]
89. Yan, X.-J.; Yu, X.; Wang, X.-P.; Jiang, J.-F.; Yuan, Z.-Y.; Lu, X.; Lei, F.; Xing, D.-M. Mitochondria play an important role in the cell proliferation suppressing activity of berberine. *Sci. Rep.* **2017**, *7*, 41712. [CrossRef]
90. Zhang, J.S.; Lei, J.P.; Wei, G.Q.; Chen, H.; Ma, C.Y.; Jiang, H.Z. Natural fatty acid synthase inhibitors as potent therapeutic agents for cancers: A review. *Pharm. Biol.* **2016**, *54*, 1919–1925. [CrossRef]
91. Du, G.J.; Zhang, Z.; Wen, X.D.; Yu, C.; Calway, T.; Yuan, C.S.; Wang, C.Z. Epigallocatechin gallate (EGCG) is the most effective cancer chemopreventive polyphenol in green tea. *Nutrients* **2012**, *4*, 1679–1691. [CrossRef] [PubMed]
92. Yu, Y.; Deng, Y.; Lu, B.M.; Liu, Y.X.; Li, J.; Bao, J.K. Green tea catechins: A fresh flavor to anticancer therapy. *Apoptosis* **2014**, *19*, 1–18. [CrossRef] [PubMed]
93. Suganuma, M.; Saha, A.; Fujiki, H. New cancer treatment strategy using combination of green tea catechins and anticancer drugs. *Cancer Sci.* **2011**, *102*, 317–323. [CrossRef] [PubMed]
94. Wei, R.; Mao, L.; Xu, P.; Zheng, X.; Hackman, R.M.; Mackenzie, G.G.; Wang, Y. Suppressing glucose metabolism with epigallocatechin-3-gallate (EGCG) reduces breast cancer cell growth in preclinical models. *Food Funct.* **2018**, *9*, 5682–5696. [CrossRef] [PubMed]
95. Pournourmohammadi, S.; Grimaldi, M.; Stridh, M.H.; Lavallard, V.; Waagepetersen, H.S.; Wollheim, C.B.; Maechler, P. Epigallocatechin-3-gallate (EGCG) activates AMPK through the inhibition of glutamate dehydrogenase in muscle and pancreatic ß-cells: A potential beneficial effect in the pre-diabetic state? *Int. J. Biochem. Cell Biol.* **2017**, *88*, 220–225. [CrossRef] [PubMed]
96. Rauf, A.; Imran, M.; Butt, M.S.; Nadeem, M.; Peters, D.G.; Mubarak, M.S. Resveratrol as an anti-cancer agent: A review. *Crit. Rev. Food Sci. Nutr.* **2017**, *58*, 1428–1447. [CrossRef]
97. Pandey, P.R.; Okuda, H.; Watabe, M.; Pai, S.K.; Liu, W.; Kobayashi, A.; Xing, F.; Fukuda, K.; Hirota, S.; Sugai, T.; et al. Resveratrol suppresses growth of cancer stem-like cells by inhibiting fatty acid synthase. *Breast Cancer Res. Treat.* **2011**, *130*, 387–398. [CrossRef]
98. Rojas, C.; Pan-Castillo, B.; Valls, C.; Pujadas, G.; Garcia-Vallve, S.; Arola, L.; Mulero, M. Resveratrol enhances palmitate-induced ER stress and apoptosis in cancer cells. *PLoS ONE* **2014**, *9*, e113929. [CrossRef]

99. Kma, L. Synergistic effect of resveratrol and radiotherapy in control of cancers. *Asian Pac. J. Cancer Prev.* **2013**, *14*, 6197–6208. [CrossRef]
100. Zhu, W.; Lv, C.; Wang, J.; Gao, Q.; Zhu, H.; Wen, H. Patuletin induces apoptosis of human breast cancer SK-BR-3 cell line via inhibiting fatty acid synthase gene expression and activity. *Oncol. Lett.* **2017**, *14*, 7449–7454. [CrossRef]
101. Wang, Y.; Nie, F.; Ouyang, J.; Wang, X.; Ma, X. Inhibitory effects of sea buckthorn procyanidins on fatty acid synthase and MDA-MB-231 cells. *Tumor Biol.* **2014**, *35*, 9563–9569. [CrossRef] [PubMed]
102. Chiang, C.T.; Way, T.D.; Tsai, S.J.; Lin, J.K. Diosgenin, a naturally occurring steroid, suppresses fatty acid synthase expression in HER2-overexpressing breast cancer cells through modulating Akt, mTOR and JNK phosphorylation. *FEBS Lett.* **2007**, *581*, 5735–5742. [CrossRef] [PubMed]
103. Impheng, H.; Richert, L.; Pekthong, D.; Scholfield, C.N.; Pongcharoen, S.; Pungpetchara, I.; Srisawang, P. [6]-Gingerol inhibits de novo fatty acid synthesis and carnitine palmitoyltransferase-1 activity which triggers apoptosis in HepG2. *Am. J. Cancer Res.* **2015**, *5*, 1319–1336.
104. Lin, V.C.; Chou, C.H.; Lin, Y.C.; Lin, J.N.; Yu, C.C.; Tang, C.H.; Lin, H.Y.; Way, T.D. Osthole suppresses fatty acid synthase expression in HER2-overexpressing breast cancer cells through modulating Akt/mTOR pathway. *J. Agric. Food Chem.* **2010**, *58*, 4786–4793. [CrossRef] [PubMed]
105. Lee, J.S.; Sul, J.Y.; Park, J.B.; Lee, M.S.; Cha, E.Y.; Song, I.S.; Kim, J.R.; Chang, E.S. Fatty acid synthase inhibition by amentoflavone suppresses HER2/neu (erbB2) oncogene in SKBR3 human breast cancer cells. *Phytother. Res.* **2013**, *27*, 713–720. [CrossRef] [PubMed]
106. Liu, W.; Furuta, E.; Shindo, K.; Watabe, M.; Xing, F.; Pandey, P.R.; Okuda, H.; Pai, S.K.; Murphy, L.L.; Cao, D.; et al. Cacalol, a natural sesquiterpene, induces apoptosis in breast cancer cells by modulating Akt-SREBP-FAS signaling pathway. *Breast Cancer Res. Treat.* **2011**, *128*, 57–68. [CrossRef]
107. Murata, S.; Yanagisawa, K.; Fukunaga, K.; Oda, T.; Kobayashi, A.; Sasaki, R.; Ohkohchi, N. Fatty acid synthase inhibitor cerulenin suppresses liver metastasis of colon cancer in mice. *Cancer Sci.* **2010**, *101*, 1861–1865. [CrossRef]
108. Oh, J.; Hwang, I.H.; Hong, C.E.; Lyu, S.Y.; Na, M. Inhibition of fatty acid synthase by ginkgolic acids from the leaves of Ginkgo biloba and their cytotoxic activity. *J. Enzym. Inhib. Med. Chem.* **2012**, *28*, 565–568. [CrossRef]
109. Losada-Echeberría, M.; Herranz-López, M.; Micol, V.; Barrajón-Catalán, E. Polyphenols as promising drugs against main breast cancer signatures. *Antioxidants* **2017**, *6*, 88. [CrossRef] [PubMed]
110. Bruntz, R.C.; Lane, A.N.; Higashi, R.M.; Fan, T.W. Exploring cancer metabolism using stable isotope-resolved metabolomics (SIRM). *J. Biol. Chem.* **2017**, *292*, 11601–11609. [CrossRef] [PubMed]
111. Jang, C.; Chen, L.; Rabinowitz, J.D. Metabolomics and isotope tracing. *Cell* **2018**, *173*, 822–837. [CrossRef] [PubMed]
112. Gao, J.L.; Chen, Y.G. Natural compounds regulate glycolysis in hypoxic tumor microenvironment. *Biomed. Res. Int.* **2015**, *2015*, 354143. [CrossRef] [PubMed]
113. Marbaniang, C.; Kma, L. Dysregulation of glucose metabolism by oncogenes and tumor suppressors in cancer cells. *Asian Pac. J. Cancer Prev.* **2018**, *19*, 2377–2390. [PubMed]
114. Martinez-Outschoorn, U.E.; Peiris-Pages, M.; Pestell, R.G.; Sotgia, F.; Lisanti, M.P. Cancer metabolism: A therapeutic perspective. *Nat. Rev. Clin. Oncol.* **2017**, *14*, 113. [CrossRef]
115. De Alteriis, E.; Cartenì, F.; Parascandola, P.; Serpa, J.; Mazzoleni, S. Revisiting the crabtree/warburg effect in a dynamic perspective: A fitness advantage against sugar-induced cell death. *Cell Cycle* **2018**, *17*, 688–701. [CrossRef]
116. Adekola, K.; Rosen, S.T.; Shanmugam, M. Glucose transporters in cancer metabolism. *Curr. Opin. Oncol.* **2012**, *24*, 650–654. [CrossRef]
117. De Berardinis, R.J.; Mancuso, A.; Daikhin, E.; Nissim, I.; Yudkoff, M.; Wehrli, S.; Thompson, C.B. Beyond aerobic glycolysis: Transformed cells can engage in glutamine metabolism that exceeds the requirement for protein and nucleotide synthesis. *Proc. Natl. Acad. Sci. USA* **2007**, *104*, 19345–19350. [CrossRef]
118. Metallo, C.M.; Gameiro, P.A.; Bell, E.L.; Mattaini, K.R.; Yang, J.; Hiller, K.; Jewell, C.M.; Johnson, Z.R.; Irvine, D.J.; Guarente, L.; et al. Reductive glutamine metabolism by IDH1 mediates lipogenesis under hypoxia. *Nature* **2012**, *481*, 380–384. [CrossRef]
119. Jiang, L.; Shestov, A.A.; Swain, P.; Yang, C.; Parker, S.J.; Wang, Q.A.; Terada, L.S.; Adams, N.D.; McCabe, M.T.; Pietrak, B.; et al. Reductive carboxylation supports redox homeostasis during anchorage-independent growth. *Nature* **2016**, *532*, 255–258. [CrossRef]

120. Du, J.; Yanagida, A.; Knight, K.; Engel, A.L.; Vo, A.H.; Jankowski, C.; Sadilek, M.; Tran, V.T.; Manson, M.A.; Ramakrishnan, A.; et al. Reductive carboxylation is a major metabolic pathway in the retinal pigment epithelium. *Proc. Natl. Acad. Sci. USA* **2016**, *113*, 14710–14715. [CrossRef]
121. Mullen, A.R.; Wheaton, W.W.; Jin, E.S.; Chen, P.H.; Sullivan, L.B.; Cheng, T.; Yang, Y.; Linehan, W.M.; Chandel, N.S.; De Berardinis, R.J. Reductive carboxylation supports growth in tumour cells with defective mitochondria. *Nature* **2011**, *481*, 385–388. [CrossRef] [PubMed]
122. Kowalik, M.A.; Columbano, A.; Perra, A. Emerging role of the pentose phosphate pathway in hepatocellular carcinoma. *Front. Oncol.* **2017**, *7*, 87. [CrossRef] [PubMed]
123. Li, B.; Qiu, B.; Lee, D.S.; Walton, Z.E.; Ochocki, J.D.; Mathew, L.K.; Mancuso, A.; Gade, T.P.; Keith, B.; Nissim, I.; et al. Fructose-1,6-bisphosphatase opposes renal carcinoma progression. *Nature* **2014**, *513*, 251–255. [CrossRef] [PubMed]
124. Fan, J.; Ye, J.; Kamphorst, J.J.; Shlomi, T.; Thompson, C.B.; Rabinowitz, J.D. Quantitative flux analysis reveals folate-dependent NADPH production. *Nature* **2014**, *510*, 298–302. [CrossRef]
125. Lao-On, U.; Attwood, P.V.; Jitrapakdee, S. Roles of pyruvate carboxylase in human diseases: From diabetes to cancers and infection. *J. Mol. Med.* **2018**, *96*, 237–247. [CrossRef] [PubMed]
126. Forbes, N.S.; Meadows, A.L.; Clark, D.S.; Blanch, H.W. Estradiol stimulates the biosynthetic pathways of breast cancer cells: Detection by metabolic flux analysis. *Metab. Eng.* **2006**, *8*, 639–652. [CrossRef]
127. Gaude, E.; Schmidt, C.; Gammage, P.A.; Dugourd, A.; Blacker, T.; Chew, S.P.; Saez-Rodriguez, J.; O'Neill, J.S.; Szabadkai, G.; Minczuk, M.; et al. NADH shuttling couples cytosolic reductive carboxylation of glutamine with glycolysis in cells with mitochondrial dysfunction. *Mol. Cell* **2018**, *69*, 581–593. [CrossRef]
128. Lewis, C.A.; Parker, S.J.; Fiske, B.P.; McCloskey, D.; Gui, D.Y.; Green, C.R.; Vokes, N.I.; Feist, A.M.; Vander Heiden, M.G.; Metallo, C.M. Tracing compartmentalized NADPH metabolism in the cytosol and mitochondria of mammalian cells. *Mol. Cell* **2014**, *55*, 253–263. [CrossRef]
129. Pandey, R.; Riley, C.L.; Mills, E.M.; Tiziani, S. Highly sensitive and selective determination of redox states of coenzymes Q9 and Q10 in mice tissues: Application of orbitrap mass spectrometry. *Anal. Chim. Acta* **2018**, *1011*, 68–76. [CrossRef]
130. Stefely, J.A.; Pagliarini, D.J. Biochemistry of mitochondrial coenzyme q biosynthesis. *Trends Biochem. Sci.* **2017**, *42*, 824–843. [CrossRef]
131. Ducker, G.S.; Chen, L.; Morscher, R.J.; Ghergurovich, J.M.; Esposito, M.; Teng, X.; Kang, Y.; Rabinowitz, J.D. Reversal of cytosolic one-carbon flux compensates for loss of the mitochondrial folate pathway. *Cell Metab.* **2016**, *23*, 1140–1153. [CrossRef] [PubMed]

3

Bioactive Phenolic Compounds in the Modulation of Central and Peripheral Nervous System Cancers

Lorena Perrone [1,2], Simone Sampaolo [1] and Mariarosa Anna Beatrice Melone [1,3,*]

1 Department of Advanced Medical and Surgical Sciences, 2nd Division of Neurology, Center for Rare Diseases and InterUniversity Center for Research in Neurosciences, University of Campania "Luigi Vanvitelli", Via Sergio Pansini, 5 80131 Naples, Italy; perronelorena1@gmail.com (L.P.); simone.sampaolo@unicampania.it (S.S.)

2 Department of Chemistry and Biology, University Grenoble Alpes, 38400 Saint-Martin-d'Hères, France

3 Sbarro Institute for Cancer Research and Molecular Medicine, Department of Biology, Temple University, BioLife Building (015-00)1900 North 12th Street, Philadelphia, PA 19122-6078, USA

* Correspondence: marina.melone@unicampania.it

Abstract: Efficacious therapies are not available for the cure of both gliomas and glioneuronal tumors, which represent the most numerous and heterogeneous primary cancers of the central nervous system (CNS), and for neoplasms of the peripheral nervous system (PNS), which can be divided into benign tumors, mainly represented by schwannomas and neurofibromas, and malignant tumors of the peripheral nerve sheath (MPNST). Increased cellular oxidative stress and other metabolic aspects have been reported as potential etiologies in the nervous system tumors. Thus polyphenols have been tested as effective natural compounds likely useful for the prevention and therapy of this group of neoplasms, because of their antioxidant and anti-inflammatory activity. However, polyphenols show poor intestinal absorption due to individual intestinal microbiota content, poor bioavailability, and difficulty in passing the blood–brain barrier (BBB). Recently, polymeric nanoparticle-based polyphenol delivery improved their gastrointestinal absorption, their bioavailability, and entry into defined target organs. Herein, we summarize recent findings about the primary polyphenols employed for nervous system tumor prevention and treatment. We describe the limitations of their application in clinical practice and the new strategies aimed at enhancing their bioavailability and targeted delivery.

Keywords: brain cancer; gliomas; schwannomas; malignant tumors of the peripheral nerve sheath (MPNST); neurofibromas; polyphenols; bioavailability; nanoparticle-based delivery systems

---

1. Introduction

Primary tumors of the central nervous system (CNS) are a complex heterogeneous group of benign and malignant cancers, each with their unique biology, prognosis, and sensitivity to the proposed therapies. As a general rule, brain tumors are named according to the non-neoplastic cell types that they most closely resemble and/or to their location where they are located in the brain, as classified by the World Health Organization (WHO) [1].

Gliomas and glioneuronal tumors are the most frequent *heterogeneous group of* primary tumors of the CNS. Gliomas, representing about 30% of the whole CNS cancers and 80% of malignant brain tumors [2], develop from glial cells, so called because the ancients thought that these cells served as "glue" between neurons (glia = glue in Greek). It is actually a group of tumors, including astrocytomas, oligodendrogliomas, ependymomas, and mixed gliomas. *Gliomas* can be aggressive (high degree of malignancy) or have a more indolent behavior (low degree of malignancy). The highest-grade astrocytomas are known as glioblastoma. Non-glial tumors constitute the bulk of neoplasms encountered in the CNS. They include a wide variety of tumor types and a spectrum of behavior ranging from indolent *benign* to highly invasive.

Tumors of the peripheral nervous system (PNS) *can be divided into* benign *tumors, mainly represented by* schwannomas and neurofibromas, and malignant tumors of the peripheral nerve sheath (MPNST), which are a type of sarcoma with very low-frequency. Arising from the soft tissue that surrounds nerves, they develop sporadically or in a particular genetic context. Indeed, neurofibromas are part of the diagnostic criteria inclusion for neurofibromatosis type 1 (NF1), also named von Recklinghausen disease (Table 1) [3,4].

Table 1. Criteria for the clinical diagnosis of NF1 *(At least two are required)*.

Criterion	Features
Six or more café-au-lait macules	>5 mm before puberty >15 mm after puberty
Freckling	Axillary, inguinal
Neurofibromas	Two or more neurofibromas or one plexiform neurofibroma
Skeletal dysplasia	Sphenoid or tibial lesion
Lisch nodules	Two or more iris hamartomas
Optic glioma	Detected by neuroimaging (usually MRI)
First degree relative with NF1	Sibling or parent with NF1
Skeletal dysplasia	Sphenoid or tibial lesion

Similarly, the MPNST develop in 50% of cases in a context of NF1. On the other hand, schwannomas, especially tumors of acoustics, are a major diagnostic criterion for neurofibromatosis type 2 (NF2) (Table 2) [5].

Table 2. Diagnostic criteria for Neurofibromatosis type 2 (these include the National Institutes of Health (NIH) criteria with additional criteria).

Main Criteria	Additional Criteria
Bilateral vestibular schwannomas (VS) or family history of NF2 *plus* (1) Unilateral VS *or* (2) Any two of: meningioma, glioma, neurofibroma, schwannoma, posterior subcapsular lenticular opacities	Unilateral VS *plus* any two of: meningioma, glioma, neurofibroma, schwannoma, and posterior subcapsular opacities or Multiple meningioma (two or more) plus unilateral VS or any two of: glioma, neurofibroma, schwannoma, and cataract
NF2—Neurofibromatosis type 2; VS—vestibular schwannomas	

A recently published survey of the global incidence of brain cancer estimated that between 1990 and 2016 its worldwide incidence increased most in populations grouped in the low quintile of SDI, a socio demographic index indicator of income per capita, educational level, and total fertility rate. Moreover, it is proposed that significant differences in the incidence of CNS cancer between various geographical regions can be due not only to variations in diagnoses and reporting practices but also to genetic and environmental risk factors not yet identified [6].

Unfortunately, the sole accurate targeting of genetic lesions has been shown to be an incomplete strategy, unable to extend the survival of brain tumor patient [7,8]. In the past time, cancer has been considered as a set of diseases that are caused by the accumulation of genetic mutations, and that aberrant regulation of epigenetic mechanisms may lead to human diseases, including cancer. Contrary to genetic mutations, epigenetic modifications are reversible. For this reason, epigenetic alterations are considered more effective therapeutic targets. Indeed, recent studies confirm the relevance of diet and bioactive dietary compounds for the prevention of epigenetic alterations in cancer. In fact, while former epidemiological studies did not support any or very little association between consumption of vegetable and fruit and reduced risk of cancer, clinical studies based on case-control analysis as well as data produced by large clinical cohort studies indicate an inverse correlation between the incidence of certain types of cancer and the regular consumption of fruits and vegetables [9]. For this reason, it has been hypothesized that only certain types of fruits and vegetables, likely those containing polyphenols, can exert a protective effect against cancer [9]. Correspondingly, several studies investigating the effect of diet on cancer risk and cancer progression provided evidence that polyphenols derived from tea, red wine, cocoa, certain fruits, and olive oil have an impact on carcinogenesis and tumor progression [10]. Several polyphenols, in fact, exhibit potent anti-tumor activity through their capability to reverse epigenetic alterations leading to oncogene activation and down-regulation of tumor suppressor genes [11] by interacting with oxidative reactive intermediates [12] and mutagens [13], modulating the signaling molecules involved in cell-cycle regulation [14], regulating the expression of cancer-related genes [15], or inducing apoptosis [16,17].

Furthermore, the transition from normal to cancer cell is characterized by altered cellular energy metabolism [18,19]. Indeed, the energy metabolism drives the cascade of events which lead a cell to proliferate or to die.

It is known, for example, that tumors are characterized by enhanced glucose uptake and an increased glycolysis rate [9]. Indeed, polyphenols act as inhibitors of glucose absorption and metabolism in cancer [20,21].

Oxidative stress is a common alteration present in adult-onset brain tumors as well as in hereditary cancer of the nervous system, such as Neurofibromatosis type 1 (NF1) and Tuberous Sclerosis (TSC) [22,23]. Since polyphenols show a powerful antioxidant activity, several studies have analyzed their therapeutic potential to counteract tumor progression [23].

Taking into account recent studies, the present review aims to provide up-to-date data on the effect of polyphenols in preventing the progression of central and peripheral nervous system tumors, which helps to explore their therapeutic values for future clinical settings.

2. Polyphenols

Phenols are "molecules possessing at minimum one aromatic ring with one or more hydroxyl groups attached" [23]. They are subdivided into flavonoids and non-flavonoids [24] (Figure 1).

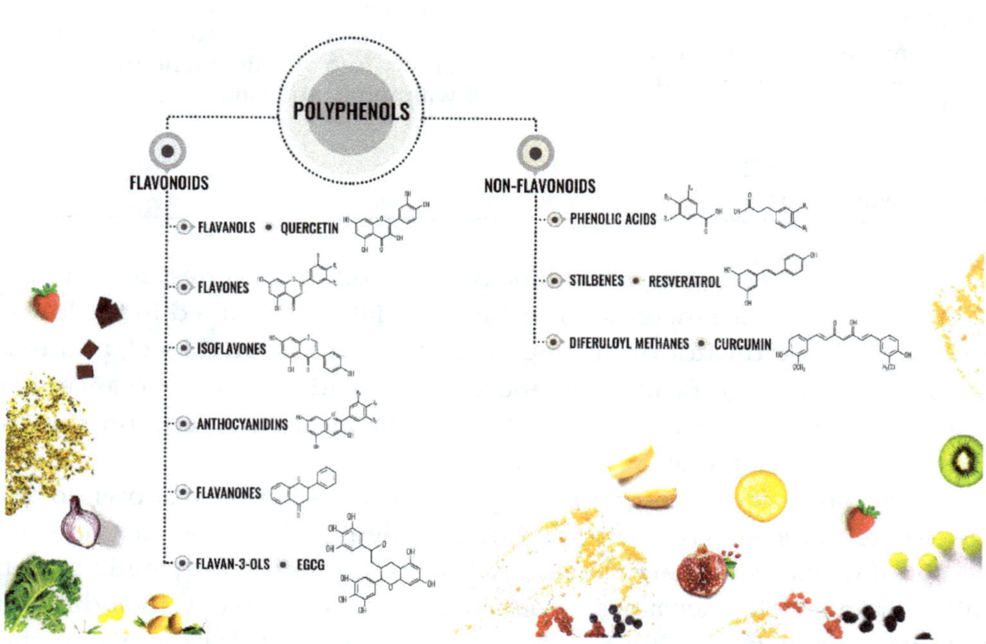

Figure 1. Chemical structures of different subtypes of polyphenols.

Flavonoids. They contain 15 carbons and two aromatic rings linked by a three-carbon bridge. This class includes: flavanols, flavones, isoflavones, flavanones, anthocyanidins, and flavan-3-ols [24].

a. Flavanols are represented in the whole plant kingdom excluding the algae. Flavonols include kaempferol, quercetin, isorhamnetin, and myricetin [24].
b. Flavones are contained in some herbs, such as Celery (*Apium graveolens*) and parsley (*Petrosilinum hortense*). They include apigenin, luteolin, wogonin, and baicalein [24].
c. Isoflavones are contained in leguminous plants. Soybeans (*Glycine max*) present a large amount of daidzein and genistein [24]. Chickpeas are enriched in biochanin A, while peanuts contain high levels of genistein. Since isoflavones show a structure similar to estrogens, they are also defined as phytoestrogens [24].
d. Flavanones are contained at elevated levels in the flavedo of citrus fruits. Hesperetin-7-O-rutinoside is also called hesperidin and is the most common member of this subclass and it is present also in apricots, plums, and bilberries [24].
e. Anthocyanidins are plant pigments, which react with organic acids and sugars, leading to the formation of molecules of different colors. The major components of this subclass are peonidin, pelargonidin, petunidin, cyanidin, delphinidin, and malvidin [24].
f. Flavan-3-ols. They can range from monomers (epicatechin and catechin) to oligomeric and polymeric proanthocyanidins (also called tannins). High concentrations of epicatechin-3-gallate (ECG) and epigallocatechin-3-gallate (EGCG) are present in green tea (*Camelia sinensis*) [24].

Non-flavonoids. They include the C_6-C_1 phenolic acids, which have a dietary relevance. The most common is the gallic acid, which is contained in numerous fruits and plants. Ellagitannins are contained in strawberries (*Fragaria ananassa*), raspberries (*Rubus idaeus*), blackberries (*Rubus spp*), persimmon (*Diospyros kaki*), pomegranates (*Punica granatum*), hazelnuts (*Corylus avellana*), and walnuts (*Juglans regia*) [24]. Belonging to this class are also: (i) secoiridoids and ligstroside, which are present in olive oil, (ii) stilbenes, whose major representing is resveratrol and is found in wine, and (iii) diferuloylmethanes that include curcumin, a curcuminoid of turmeric (Curcuma longa) [23].

3. Mechanisms of Cancer Modulation by Polyphenols

3.1. Regulation of Glucose Homeostasis

High proliferating tumor cells need to produce extra ATP to maintain their energy status, produce an increased biosynthesis of macromolecules, and maintain the cellular redox status [25]. For this reason, tumor cells need to reprogram the own metabolic flux with the aim of obtaining a surplus of ATP that is needed for an increased rate of proliferation [25]. Indeed, cancer cells are characterized by metabolic reprogramming involving an altered energy metabolism, called the Warburg effect, that shows elevated uptake and consumption of glucose and also enhanced creation of lactate buildup despite the presence of oxygen [26]. This metabolic change in tumor cells promotes cell proliferation and tumor progression by generating an increased level of glycolytic intermediates needed for the synthesis of new molecules. In addition, it augments the metabolism of glucose, which counteracts the excess metabolic formation of reactive oxygen species (ROS) in cancer cells [27]. Because of the necessity of extra ATP, glucose deprivation displays a higher cytotoxic effect on several cancer cells compared to normal cells. For this reason, inhibitors of glucose uptake and of oxidative metabolism (glycolysis inhibitors) are considered as therapeutic strategies against cancer [26]. Importantly, the Warburg effect, also defined as "aerobic lactatogenesis" [28], is considered an excellent target against cancer because therapeutic strategies directed against this metabolic shift will induce less negative side effects, leading to the reduction of treatment-associated morbidities. Indeed, several drugs targeting glucose metabolism are in trial or already approved compounds to treat cancer [29].

Several polyphenols exert an inhibitory effect on various steps of energy pathways in cancer cells, including inhibition of the uptake of glucose and block of enzymes involved in glucose metabolism.

Polyphenols interfere with the glucose transporters in various cell types, affecting glucose uptake. Gossypol decreases glucose uptake in various cell types by a competitive mechanism [30]. Naringenin inhibits basal as well insulin-induced uptake of glucose in tumoral cells by blocking PIP3/Akt and MAPK activity [31]. This inhibition of glucose uptake results in an anti-proliferative effect of naringenin treatment in cancer cells [31]. Genistein reduces glucose uptake in cancer cell lines [32]. Resveratrol inhibits glycolysis in cancer cells, where it also blocks glucose uptake by lowering the expression of the glucose transporter GLUT1 [33]. Resveratrol reduces cell viability in cancer cells. Such resveratrol-dependent reduction of GLUT1 depends on a reduction of ROS and subsequent down-regulation of the transcription factor HIF-1 -alpha [33]. Moreover, resveratrol reduces cell viability by directly inhibiting the 6-Phosphofructo-1-kinase-1 (PKF), an essential enzyme of the glycolytic pathway, leading to a decreased glucose utilization and reduced ATP levels in cancer cells [34]. The flavone hesperetin reduces basal glucose uptake in cancer cells by down-regulating GLUT1 [35]. It also impairs insulin-dependent glucose uptake in cancer cells by impairing GLUT4 translocation to the plasma membrane [35]. The flavonoids epigallocatechin-3-gallate (EGCG) and quercetin reduce glucose uptake and lactate production in tumoral cells [36]. The reduction of glucose uptake is independent from signaling pathways modulated by PKC, PKG, PKA, and calcium-calmodulin [36]. The reduction of glucose uptake and lactate production due to these flavonoids results in a cytotoxic and anti-proliferative effect [36]. Luteolin reduces the glycolytic flux in cancer cells but does not affect the glucose uptake [37]. 1,2,3,4,6-penta-O-galloyl-beta-d-glucose (PGG) down-regulates the genes encoding enzymes of the pyruvate metabolism, such as acylphosphatase, pyruvate carboxylase, and aldehyde dehydrogenase (ALDH3B1) in cancer cells [38].

3.2. Modulation of Advanced Glycation Endproducts (AGEs) and their Receptor (RAGE)

Aging, altered metabolism, and diet induce the formation of advanced glycation endproducts (AGEs), which participate in the progression of several diseases, including cancer [39–43]. Additionally, members of the AGEs family, such as N-carboxymethyllysine (CML) and argpyrimidine, are elevated in several tumors and are implicated in cancer progression [43]. Several polyphenols inhibit AGEs formation both in vitro and in vivo. Indeed, Tomato paste blocks the formation of AGEs [44], tea polyphenols interfere with AGEs formation in physiological conditions [45], and EGCG inhibits AGEs formation [46]. The receptor for AGEs (RAGE) is also involved in cancer cell invasion and metastasis [47]. Polyphenols interfere with RAGE activation and signaling. EGCG inhibits RAGE activation [48]. Quercetin reduces RAGE expression in cancer cells, inducing cell cycle arrest, autophagy, apoptosis, and chemo-sensitivity [49].

3.3. Modulation of Oxidative Stress and Related Signaling Pathways

Reactive oxygen species (ROS) induce tumor formation by producing genetic mutation, inducing oncogenes, and promoting oxidative stress. The last has an effect on cell proliferation, apoptosis, and survival. Tumor cells are characterized by enhanced ROS production, leading to redox unbalance. ROS induce the oxidation of protein cysteine residues, which may induce cellular proliferation [50]. ROS play a key function in tumor initiation, promotion, and progression [51]. ROS activate oncogenes, such as Ras and c-Myc, and promote p53-dependent DNA repair [52]. In addition, ROS promote cancer progression also by inducing the activation of several signaling pathways, such as the phosphoinositide-3-kinase (PI3K)/protein kinase B (AKT), mitogen-activated protein kinase (MAPK)/extracellular-signal-regulated kinase (ERK), the inhibitor of kappa B (IκB), kinase (IKK)/nuclear factor κB (NFκB), the protein kinase D (PKD), JNK, and PI3K, which in turn modulate the activity of several transcription factors that participate to cancer initiation/progression [52].

Polyphenols possess both anti-oxidant and pro-oxidant activity, which modulate cell proliferation and apoptotic pathways [53]. Quercetin scavenges superoxide anions, leading to the formation of H_2O_2, semiquinone, and quercetin radicals. The latter deplete the intracellular anti-oxidant systems [52]. Indeed, quercetin leads to ROS-dependent apoptosis, necrosis, and autophagy in cancer cells [52].

In addition, quercetin induces cell cycle arrest by modulating $p21^{WAF}$, cyclin B, and $p27^{KIP1}$ in cancer cells [52]. Notably, curcumin exerts opposite effects in cancer cells compared to its effects in normal cells, suggesting that curcumin can be beneficial in preventing cancer without affecting the homeostasis of normal cells. In normal cells, curcumin acts as an anti-oxidant by scavenging hydroxyl radicals, superoxide, nitric oxide, H2O2, and peroxynitrite [54]. In addition, curcumin regulates the expression of HO-1, GPX, and SOD in normal cells [54]. On the other hand, in cancer cells curcumin has a pro-oxidative effect that induces apoptosis [55]. Indeed, curcumin induces ROS formation in cancer cells [56,57]. Curcumin's pro-oxidative activity occurs in the mitochondrial membranes of cancer cells, leading to depolarization of mitochondrial and down-regulation of ATP synthesis, ultimately inducing apoptosis [58]. Curcumin-dependent ROS production in cancer cells induces Erk1/2 and p38 MAPK pathways that lead to autophagy [59]. Curcumin blocks the survival and proliferation of cancer stem cell through a ROS-mediated inhibition of NFκB and STAT3 in glioblastoma [60]. Capsaicin has been shown to exert beneficial effects against glioma. Indeed, in glioma, capsaicin (trans-8-methyl-N-vanillyl-6-nonenamide) affects the mitochondrial membrane potential, leading to ROS elevation and subsequent caspase 3 activation [61]. Capsaicin not only induces apoptosis but also cell cycle arrest [62]. EGCG possesses both anti-oxidant and pro-oxidant activity. It produces ROS by auto-oxidation [63]. EGCG induces apoptosis by inhibiting the PI3k/AKT pathway. In addition, it decreases the mitochondrial membrane potential, leading to apoptosis [52]. Phenethyl isothiocyanate (PEITC) decreases intracellular GSH, leading to enhanced ROS accumulation and mitochondrial dysfunction exclusively in cancer cells [64]. Benzyl isothiocyanate (BITC) induces oxidative stress in glioma cells by exhausting SOD and GSH levels, leading to caspase-mediated apoptosis [65]. Piperine blocks tumor growth by inducing oxidative stress, mitochondria dysfunction, and subsequent apoptosis [66]. Resveratrol inhibits tum initiation and progression by inducing apoptosis in neuroblastoma cells [67]. It promotes apoptosis by inducing the death receptors for TRAIL and FasL, ROS-dependent caspase activation, and p53 [68]. P-Coumaric acid (p-CoA) promotes apoptosis in cancer cells by enhancing ROS formation and inducing mitochondrial depolarization [69]. Naringenin promotes apoptosis in cancer cells through induction of ROS formation, which in turn leads to p38 MAPK-dependent caspase activation [70]. Gallic acid inhibits cancer cell growth by inducing ROS production [71]. Thus, we may conclude that several polyphenols counteract tumor progression by inducing cancer-specific ROS production.

3.4. Other Mechanisms

Polyphenols modify the metabolism of pro-carcinogens through mechanisms that alter the levels of cytochromes P450 (CYPs), which plays an essential role in cancer promotion [72]. Polyphenols produce epigenetic changes that have a preventive effect against cancer [73]. Polyphenols also show a preventive effect by inhibiting inflammation [74]. They also modulate the autophagy flux [75].

Polyphenols prevent metastasis formation by affecting the activity of urokinase and matrix metalloproteinases and by inhibiting angiogenesis through modulation of the vascular endothelial growth factor expression and receptor phosphorylation [76].

In addition, dietary polyphenols are employed together with conventional pharmacological therapy or cytotoxic agents used to treat drug-resistant cancer cells [74].

Several studies indicated herein tested the efficacy of polyphenols at concentrations equivalent to oral sub ministration of juices/extracts of natural substances containing polyphenols (range 100–800 mg/day), while other studies analyzed higher concentrations (range 10–75 μM). Notably, concentrations of polyphenols equivalent to diet intake show also beneficial effects.

4. Polyphenol Effects on Central Nervous System Cancers

Several risk factors are involved in the onset and progression of adult brain tumors: aging, diet, environmental exposure, head trauma, infections, and cigarette smoking [77]. Primary brain tumors are named gliomas and classified according to their putative original cell type. Glioblastoma multiform

(GBM) shows the highest aggressive phenotype (grade IV) representing the 60% of age-related brain tumors [78]. At present there is not definite cure for GBM; thus, researchers are looking at innovative therapeutic strategies [23].

Recent studies in vitro and in vivo have underlined the therapeutic efficacy against cancer of several polyphenols, such as quercetin, epigallocatechin-3-gallate (EGCG), resveratrol, and curcumin [79]. Moreover, it has been reported that the polyphenols' therapeutic potential is further enhanced when they are used in combination or added to pharmaceutical compounds [74,79].

4.1. *Curcumin Effects on Central Nervous System Cancers*

The effective anti-tumor activity of curcumin treatment in GBM has been shown by several studies [23,80]. Curcumin exerts a pro-differentiative effect in glioma-stem cells because of its activation of the autophagy flux [81]. In human glioblastoma T98G cells, this polyphenol induces the activation of both receptor-mediated and mitochondria-mediated proteolytic pathways, which in turn promote apoptosis [55]. Curcumin down-regulates the expression of cancer signaling pathways (i.e., Notch1 and pAKT), leading to blockade of cell growth, apoptosis, and inhibition of migration and invasion [82]. In human glioma cells, it lowers the protein levels of neuronal precursor cell-expressed developmentally down-regulated 4–1 (NEDD4) [82]. Delivery of curcumin into the brain of GBM mice produces the remission of tumor in 50% of the animals and modifies the phenotype of the microglia surrounding the tumor [83]. Curcumin exerts an efficient induction of autophagy [75], which can lead to apoptosis in cancer cells. Moreover, curcumin treatment in A172 human glioblastoma cells leads to cell death by inducing autophagy flux [84]. Another study confirmed that curcumin promotes autophagy in glioblastoma cells while it inhibits mitophagy [85]. Curcumin also blocks invasion and migration potential of glioblastoma U87 cells by decreasing the expression of fascin, an actin-binding protein involved in migration and invasion [86]. Noteworthy, curcumin exerts a radiosensitizing effect on GBM [87]. Moreover, curcumin acts as a photosensitizer in sNB-19 glioblastoma cells, showing that it can be used to improve the photodynamic therapy for GBM treatment [88].

4.2. *Resveratrol Effects on Central Nervous System Cancers*

Several studies demonstrate the efficacy of resveratrol in lowering tumorigenesis and preventing metastasis [23,89,90]. Resveratrol has a powerful capability of down-regulating the self-renewal and tumor-initiating capability of glioma stem cells obtained from GBM patients by inducing the p53/ p21 pathway [91]. Resveratrol possesses a potent effect in inhibiting the invasion and migration capability of glioblastoma cells by activating the RhoA/ROCK pathway [92]. Resveratrol decreases cell growth and motility, enhances cell death, and interferes with the epithelial-mesenchymal transition modulating the Wnt signaling pathway [93]. Resveratrol lowers tumorigenic potential and improves the effects of radiotherapy in vitro and in vivo against GBM-derived tumor stem cells to by inhibiting the signal transducer and activator of transcription 3 (STAT3) [94]. Resveratrol blocks the growth of U-87MG glioblastoma cells and lowers the expression of human telomerase reverse transcriptase (hTERT) as well as the catalytic subunit of the telomerase and a biomarker of cell immortalization, confirming that resveratrol can be used as a therapeutic agent for GBM [95]. The postoperative administration of resveratrol results in a significant prognosis amelioration of rat-advanced orthotopic glioblastoma by reducing growth, inducting apoptosis, and suppressing STAT3 signaling [96]. In addition, resveratrol blocks epithelial-mesenchymal transition in GBM by modulating Smad signaling [97].

In combination with Paclitaxel, resveratrol enhances the oxidant and apoptotic effect of the pharmacological compound by activating the TRPM2 channel in glioblastoma cells [98].

4.3. *EGCG Effects on Central Nervous System Cancers*

Several studies show the beneficial effect of EGCG as a therapeutic agent for brain tumors [23]. EGCG exerts an inhibitory effect in three glioma cell lines by modulating the epidermal growth factor-1 (EGF-1) [99]. EGCG potentiates the effects of ionizing radiation (IR) in GBM by modulating the activity of Ras homolog gene family member A (RhoA) and survivin, with the last being involved in the regulation of apoptosis. Treatment with EGCG combined with radiotherapy ameliorates the efficacy of IR treatments [100]. EGCG also enhances the anti-cancer activity of cytotoxic agents [101]. Indeed, in a mouse model of glioblastoma, EGCG enhances the anti-cancer potential of temozolomide, which promotes DNA damage [101]. Treatment with EGCG alone or in combination with temozolomide affects glioma stem cell survival and migration capability, as well as inhibits neurosphere formation [102]. In addition, such treatments induce apoptosis by down-regulating p-Akt and Bcl-2 [102]. In human glioblastoma U251 cells, EGCG promotes apoptosis and blocks cell-growth because of inhibiting the JAK2/STAT3 signaling pathway [103]. EGCG suppresses the invasion properties of human glioblastoma T-98G cells by down-regulating MMP-2 and MMP-9 expression [104]. Interestingly, EGCG inhibits the effects of the glucose-regulated protein 78 (GRP78), which is up-regulated in GBM by direct protein–protein interaction that results in a conformational change in GRP78, probably leading to its inactivation [105]. At the low concentration of 100 nM, EGCG activates endogenous repair pathways while at higher concentrations, EGCG induces ROS production and autophagy [106]. These data suggest that drinking green tea containing low concentrations of EGCG may exert a chemo-preventive effect against GBM, while higher concentrations (500 μM) show a therapeutic effect [106]. Importantly, EGCG inhibits the expression of O^6-Methylguanine DNA-Methyltransferase (MGMT) in GBM-derived cells only, which is an essential regulator of the resistance to temozolomide (TMZ) in glioblastomas. EGCG treatment in two GBM cell lines (GBM-XD and T98G) results in suppression of MGMT expression, abolishes TMZ resistance, and prevents β catenin translocation into the nucleus [107]. On the contrary, the addition of EGCG to non-tumor glial cell culture (GliaX) enhances MGMT expression by inhibiting the methylation of the MGMT promoter [107]. Recently, it has been shown that EGCG induces telomere shortening in U251 glioblastoma, leading to senescence [108]. In addition, it also promotes telomere-independent genotoxicity [108].

4.4. *Quercetin Effects on Central Nervous System Cancers*

The therapeutic potential of quercetin for the cure of GBM has been extensively analyzed [23]. The glycoside form of quercetin called Rutin exerts an anti-proliferative effect on human GBM cells [109]. Rutin reduces the survival and proliferation of GL-15 cell lines, resulting in a decrement of phosphorylated extracellular signal-regulated protein kinases 1 and 2 (ERK1/2), which exert an essential role in cell proliferation and apoptosis modulation [109]. In GBM cell cultures, rutin induces astroglial differentiation and apoptosis [109]. In GBM cultures, treatment with quercetin alone or together with temozolomide, induces apoptosis, whereas it does not affect autophagy [110]. Treatment with quercetin or its addition during with irradiation promotes apoptosis. This anti-cancer effect is due to activation of caspase-3 and poly [ADP-ribose] polymerase 1 (PARP-1), which are concomitant to the inhibition of the Akt pathway [111]. In GBM cells, co-treatment with rutin and temozolomide results in enhanced cytotoxicity because of inhibition of the autophagy flux [112]. Studies in subcutaneous and orthotopic xenograft using concomitant treatment with temozolomide and rutin show a decreased tumor volumes, while treatment with temozolomide or rutin alone is less effective [112]. In U251 glioblastoma human cells, quercetin inhibits cell proliferation and viability as well as invasion and migration properties [113,114].

Quercetin shows a pro-apoptotic effect also because it regulates the expression of apoptotic genes and because it induces the cell cycle arrest [113]. Using U87MG, C6, and U138 glioblastoma cultures, we demonstrated that the water extract of *Ruta graveolens* L. promotes cell death. We also found that rue activates ERK1/2 and AKT, resulting in an inhibition of cell growth. We also show that rutin, the major component of the *Ruta graveolens* water extract, is unable to induce cell death [115]. Quercetin in combination with sodium butyrate promotes apoptosis in rat C6 and human T98G GBM cells by inhibiting autophagy [116].

5. Polyphenol Effects on Tumors of the Peripheral Nervous System

Neurofibromatosis type 1 (NF1) is an autosomal dominant disorder showing complex phenotypes and it is caused by inherited mutations in the NF1 gene, which is a tumor suppressor. Almost all NF1 patients develop pigmentary lesions (café-au-lait macules, skinfold freckling, and Lisch nodules) and dermal neurofibromas (Table 1). In some patients are also present brain tumors (glioblastoma and optic pathway gliomas), peripheral nerve tumors (plexiform neurofibromas, spinal neurofibromas, and malignant peripheral nerve sheath tumors), skeletal abnormalities (tibial pseudarthrosis, orbital dysplasia, and scoliosis), attention deficits, learning disabilities, and social and behavioral problems, which impair the quality of life [117].

Neurofibromatosis type 2 (NF2) is a genetic disorder characterized by the presence of multiple benign tumors of the peripheral and central nervous system (including meningiomas, schwannomas, and ependymomas) (Table 2).

NF2 patients are almost always diagnosed late in life, around the second or third decade of life [118,119]. NF2 is characterized by the presence of benign tumors. However, such tumors can induce mortality that is associated to the location of the tumors as well as can be promoted by the treatments. Currently, the only therapy available consists in a local treatment of the tumors and is not effective. Thus, there is a need to develop systemic therapies aimed to improve the outcome of NF2 [23,119].

It is well documented that a healthy diet including a high consumption of fruit and vegetables has a preventive effect against cancer and results in a lower incidence of tumor development and tumor-induced mortality [120].

Recently, researchers started to investigate the chemopreventive and/or chemotherapeutic potential of polyphenolic compounds [120]. Since polyphenols possess anti-oxidant proprieties, their consumption has a beneficial effect against the high levels of oxidative stress produced by cancer cells [51].

5.1. Curcumin Effects on Tumors of the Peripheral Nervous System

Curcumin reduces proliferation and enhances the apoptosis rate in HEI-193 human schwannoma cells [118]. These results indicate that administration of curcumin to patients with NF2 schwannomas may exert a beneficial effect. We describe the first experience with curcumin supplementation in NF1 patients. We show that a therapeutic strategy involving a high adherence to the Mediterranean diet together with the administration of 1200 mg/day of curcumin results in a significant reduction of the number and volume of cutaneous neurofibromas in NF1 patients [121]. Notably, we demonstrate by Magnetic Resonance Imaging that in one patient this therapeutic strategy results in a sensible reduction in volume (28%) of a large cranial plexiform neurofibroma. On the contrary, administration of curcumin in association with a Western diet has not effect on NF1 tumors, suggesting that some components in the Mediterranean diet may improve curcumin bioavailability and activity [121]. A recent study revealed that calebin-A, derived from turmeric *Curcuma longa*, (a) inhibits the cell growth in the malignant peripheral nerve sheath tumor (MPNST) transformed from NF1-related plexiform neurofibroma, and (b) blocks cell growth in primary neurofibroma cells [122]. Calebin-A induces the cell cycle arrest and decreases hTERT, phosphorylated- ERK1/2, -AKT, and surviving [122].

5.2. EGCG Effects on Tumors of the Peripheral Nervous System

Only one study reported that EGCG reduces the proliferation of an MPNST transformed from NF1-related plexiform neurofibroma [122].

6. Bioavailability of Dietary Polyphenols

Several studies have indicated that dietary polyphenols exert neuroprotective functions. However, their clinical application is still limited. In fact, polyphenols exert poor effect in vivo when compared to their activity in vitro [123,124]. The difference between in vitro and in vivo effects of polyphenols is mainly associated to their poor absorption, rapid metabolism, and massive system elimination, which represent a limitation regarding their therapeutic action and clinical application [125]. Several studies underline that the chemical structure of polyphenols plays a key role in modulating the rate and extent of their absorption upon ingestion [74]. Noteworthy, the individual variability in drug absorption and metabolism has a key role in modulating the effects of polyphenols in vivo. Indeed, the absorption is regulated by the local microflora, by the metabolic activity and by the hepatic function [126]. In addition, the CNS is protected by the blood brain barrier (BBB), which regulates the transport of molecules into the CNS. Thus, the transport across the BBB further limits the therapeutic potential of dietary polyphenols. For this reason, several ongoing research projects are studying how to improve the bioavailability of polyphenols [125]. These studies aim at ameliorating the biochemical stability and transport across the BBB of the polyphenols as well as decreasing their degradation [125]. Another study investigated the transport across the BBB of bioavailable phenolic sulfates derived from the colonic metabolism of berries [127]. They found that these compounds show a differential transport across the BBB, which was related to their chemical structure. In addition, they discovered that these compounds were further metabolized by the endothelial cells, leading to the production of novel molecules with potential bioactivity [127]. This study also demonstrated that pre-treatment with these compounds (a) ameliorated the response to oxidative stress and toxicity and (b) reduced the inflammatory response by modulating NF-kB activity [127]. Thus, this study demonstrated that these polyphenols cross the BBB and exert a neuroprotective and anti-inflammatory function. Furthermore, it has been shown that the gut microbiota metabolize the dietary polyphenols, promoting the production of bioactive molecules that cross the BBB and modulate the neuronal function by acting as neurotransmitters [128]. Interestingly, dietary polyphenols modulate the bacterial composition of the gut microbiota, acting on the microbiota-gut-brain axis, which is considered as a neuroendocrine system [128]. These studies support the hypothesis that dietary polyphenols exert a beneficial effect by modulating the gut microbiota, leading to a neuroprotective effect via the gut-brain axis. Thus, they may have a therapeutic role in the prevention of diseases affecting the nervous system [128].

However, several challenges remain. These include (a) the exploration of the therapeutic interplay between polyphenols or other natural substances contained in the Mediterranean diet [121,129], (b) their molecular characterization, and (c) the definition of optimal absorption levels and bioavailability improvement. This is necessary to ensure therapeutic efficacy, that these substances cross the intestinal and blood–brain barriers, and that matrices can be developed for the release of product formulations. Indeed, nanotechnology can provide new materials for the delivery of polyphenols, improving their absorption and efficacy [130]. These technologies can provide food-based nanodelivery vehicles with different surface properties. To date, several nanovehicles, such as nanoemulsions, protein-polysaccharide coacervas, liposomes, and small cochlear structures, are produced only on a laboratory scale. In the future these systems will have applications in the development of functional foods at an industry scale [131].

7. Clinical Trials

To date, the US National Institute of Health database shows only two completed clinical trials using curcumin and polyphenols for the treatment of GBM (http://www.clinicaltrial.gov/; searching for: "Glioblastoma multiforme" and "Curcumin" and "polyphenols"; and http://www.clinicaltrial.gov/; searching for: "Glioblastoma multiforme" and "Curcumin"). There are no any curcumin-based clinical trials for NF2 or NF1 treatments (http://www.clinicaltrial.gov/; searching for: "Neurofibromatosis type 2" and "Curcumin").

8. Conclusions

The incidence of brain tumors has been increasing recently. Despite considerable efforts to find an effective therapy, the treatment of some cancers of the nervous system still remains a challenge in a war in which, thus far, few battles have been won. The numerous metabolic aspects underlying the tumors of the CNS and PNS have opened the way to new therapeutic approaches that see an interesting therapeutic strategy in diet and, in particular, foods with anti-oxidant activity. In particular, several studies have underlined the beneficial effect of dietary polyphenols for the prevention of tumors of the CNS and PNS.

Furthermore, recent studies have revealed the positive effect of polyphenols on the microbioma-intestine-brain axis, demonstrating the therapeutic potential of dietary polyphenols in the prevention of diseases affecting the nervous system.

However, the low bioavailability of dietary polyphenols is still a limitation for their introduction into clinical practice. A promising solution lies in polymeric nanoparticle-based polyphenol delivery systems that prevent the degradation of bioactive compounds and enhance their absorption and bioavailability.

Author Contributions: L.P., S.S., and M.A.B.M. wrote the manuscript. All the authors reviewed the final version and agree to publication. All authors have read and agreed to the published version of the manuscript.

Acknowledgments: We are grateful to Antonia Auletta for preparing the figures.

References

1. Louis, D.N.; Perry, A.; Reifenberger, G.; von Deimling, A.; Figarella-Branger, D.; Cavenee, W.K.; Ohgaki, H.; Wiestler, O.D.; Kleihues, P.; Ellison, D.W. The 2016 World Health Organization Classification of Tumors of the Central Nervous System: A summary. *Acta Neuropathol.* **2016**, *131*, 803–820. [CrossRef] [PubMed]
2. Goodenberger, M.L.; Jenkins, R.B. Genetics of adult glioma. *Cancer Genet.* **2012**, *205*, 613–621. [CrossRef] [PubMed]
3. National Institutes of Health. Consensus Development Conference Statement: Neurofibromatosis. Bethesda, Md., USA, July 13–15, 1987. *Neurofibromatosis* **1988**, *1*, 172–178.
4. Giugliano, T.; Santoro, C.; Torella, A.; Del Vecchio Blanco, F.; Grandone, A.; Onore, M.E.; Melone, M.A.B.; Straccia, G.; Melis, D.; Piccolo, V.; et al. Clinical and Genetic Findings in Children with Neurofibromatosis Type 1, Legius Syndrome, and Other Related Neurocutaneous Disorders. *Genes* **2019**, *10*, 580. [CrossRef]
5. Evans, D.G. Neurofibromatosis type 2 (NF2): A clinical and molecular review. *Orphanet. J. Rare Dis.* **2009**, *4*, 16. [CrossRef]
6. GBD 2016 Brain and Other CNS Cancer Collaborators. Global, regional, and national burden of brain and other CNS cancer, 1990–2016: A systematic analysis for the Global Burden of Disease Study 2016. *Lancet Neurol.* **2019**, *18*, 376–393. [CrossRef]
7. Dhez, A.C.; Benedetti, E.; Antonosante, A.; Panella, G.; Ranieri, B.; Florio, T.M.; Cristiano, L.; Angelucci, F.; Giansanti, F.; Di Leandro, L.; et al. Targeted therapy of human glioblastoma via delivery of a toxin through a peptide directed to cell surface nucleolin. *J. Cell Physiol.* **2018**, *233*, 4091–4105. [CrossRef]
8. Mack, S.C.; Hubert, C.G.; Miller, T.E.; Taylor, M.D.; Rich, J.N. An epigenetic gateway to brain tumor cell identity. *Nat. Neurosci.* **2016**, *19*, 10–19. [CrossRef]
9. Vauzour, D.; Rodriguez-Mateos, A.; Corona, G.; Oruna-Concha, M.J.; Spencer, J.P. Polyphenols and human health: Prevention of disease and mechanisms of action. *Nutrients* **2010**, *2*, 1106–1131. [CrossRef]
10. Middleton, E., Jr.; Kandaswami, C.; Theoharides, T.C. The effects of plant flavonoids on mammalian cells: Implications for inflammation, heart disease, and cancer. *Pharm. Res.* **2000**, *52*, 673–751.
11. Carlos-Reyes, Á.; López-González, J.S.; Meneses-Flores, M.; Gallardo-Rincón, D.; Ruíz-García, E.; Marchat, L.A.; Astudillo-de la Vega, H.; Hernández de la Cruz, O.N.; López-Camarillo, C. Dietary Compounds as Epigenetic Modulating Agents in Cancer. *Front. Genet.* **2019**, *10*, 79. [CrossRef] [PubMed]
12. Duthie, S.J.; Dobson, V.L. Dietary flavonoids protect human colonocyte DNA from oxidative attack in vitro. *Eur. J. Nutr.* **1999**, *38*, 28–34. [CrossRef] [PubMed]
13. Calomme, M.; Pieters, L.; Vlietinck, A.; Vanden Berghe, D. Inhibition of bacterial mutagenesis by Citrus flavonoids. *Planta Med.* **1996**, *62*, 222–226. [CrossRef] [PubMed]

14. Plaumann, B.; Fritsche, M.; Rimpler, H.; Brandner, G.; Hess, R.D. Flavonoids activate wild-type p53. *Oncogene* **1996**, *13*, 1605–1614.

15. van Erk, M.J.; Roepman, P.; van der Lende, T.R.; Stierum, R.H.; Aarts, J.M.; van Bladeren, P.J.; van Ommen, B. Integrated assessment by multiple gene expression analysis of quercetin bioactivity on anticancer-related mechanisms in colon cancer cells in vitro. *Eur. J. Nutr.* **2005**, *44*, 143–156. [CrossRef]

16. Fabiani, R.; De Bartolomeo, A.; Rosignoli, P.; Servili, M.; Montedoro, G.F.; Morozzi, G. Cancer chemoprevention by hydroxytyrosol isolated from virgin olive oil through G1 cell cycle arrest and apoptosis. *Eur. J. Cancer Prev.* **2002**, *11*, 351–358. [CrossRef]

17. Mantena, S.K.; Baliga, M.S.; Katiyar, S.K. Grape seed proanthocyanidins induce apoptosis and inhibit metastasis of highly metastatic breast carcinoma cells. *Carcinogenesis* **2006**, *27*, 1682–1691. [CrossRef]

18. Cirillo, A.; Di Salle, A.; Petillo, O.; Melone, M.A.; Grimaldi, G.; Bellotti, A.; Torelli, G.; De'Santi, M.S.; Cantatore, G.; Marinelli, A.; et al. High grade glioblastoma is associated with aberrant expression of ZFP57, a protein involved in gene imprinting, and of CPT1A and CPT1C that regulate fatty acid metabolism. *Cancer Biol. Ther.* **2014**, *15*, 735–741. [CrossRef]

19. Melone, M.A.B.; Valentino, A.; Margarucci, S.; Galderisi, U.; Giordano, A.; Peluso, G. The carnitine system and cancer metabolic plasticity. *Cell Death Dis.* **2018**, *9*, 228. [CrossRef]

20. León, D.; Uribe, E.; Zambrano, A.; Salas, M. Implications of Resveratrol on Glucose Uptake and Metabolism. *Molecules* **2017**, *22*, 398. [CrossRef]

21. Siddiqui, F.A.; Prakasam, G.; Chattopadhyay, S.; Rehman, A.U.; Padder, R.A.; Ansari, M.A.; Irshad, R.; Mangalhara, K.; Bamezai, R.; Husain, M.; et al. Curcumin decreases Warburg effect in cancer cells by down-regulating pyruvate kinase M2 via mTOR-HIF1α inhibition. *Sci. Rep.* **2018**, *8*, 8323. [CrossRef] [PubMed]

22. Incecik, F.; Avcıoğlu, G.; Erel, Ö.; Neşelioğlu, S.; Besen, S.; Altunbaşak, S. Dynamic thiol/disulphide homeostasis in children with neurofibromatosis type 1 and tuberous sclerosis. *Acta Neurol. Belg.* **2019**, *119*, 419–422. [CrossRef] [PubMed]

23. Squillaro, T.; Schettino, C.; Sampaolo, S.; Galderis, U.; Di Iorio, G.; Giordano, A.; Melone, M.A.B. Adult-onset brain tumors and neurodegeneration: Are polyphenols protective? *J. Cell Physiol.* **2017**, *233*, 3955–3967. [CrossRef] [PubMed]

24. Del Rio, D.; Rodriguez-Mateos, A.; Spencer, J.P.; Tognolini, M.; Borges, G.; Crozier, A. Dietary (poly)phenolics in human health: Structures, bioavailability, and evidence of protective effects against chronic diseases. *Antioxid. Redox Signal.* **2013**, *18*, 1818–1892. [CrossRef]

25. Cairns, R.A.; Harris, I.S.; Mak, T.W. Regulation of cancer cell metabolism. *Nat. Rev. Cancer* **2011**, *11*, 85–95. [CrossRef]

26. Hanahan, D.; Weinberg, R.A. Hallmarks of cancer: The next generation. *Cell* **2011**, *144*, 646–674. [CrossRef]

27. Aykin-Burns, N.; Ahmad, I.M.; Zhu, Y.; Oberley, L.W.; Spitz, D.R. Increased levels of superoxide and H2O2 mediate the differential susceptibility of cancer cells versus normal cells to glucose deprivation. *Biochem. J.* **2009**, *418*, 29–37. [CrossRef]

28. Martel, F.; Guedes, M.; Keating, E. Effect of polyphenols on glucose and lactate transport by breast cancer cells. *Breast Cancer Res. Treat.* **2016**, *157*, 1–11. [CrossRef]

29. Luengo, A.; Gui, D.Y.; Vander-Heiden, M.G. Targeting metabolism for cancer therapy. *Cell Chem. Biol.* **2017**, *24*, 1161–1180. [CrossRef]

30. Pérez, A.; Ojeda, P.; Valenzuela, X.; Ortega, M.; Sánchez, C.; Ojeda, L.; Castro, M.; Cárcamo, J.G.; Rauch, M.C.; Concha, I.I.; et al. Endofacial competitive inhibition of the glucose transporter 1 activity by gossypol. *Am. J. Physiol. Cell Physiol.* **2009**, *297*, C86–C93. [CrossRef]

31. Harmon, A.W.; Patel, Y.M. Naringenin inhibits glucose uptake in MCF-7 breast cancer cells: A mechanism for impaired cellular proliferation. *Breast Cancer Res. Treat.* **2004**, *85*, 103–110. [CrossRef] [PubMed]

32. Lim, H.A.; Kim, J.H.; Kim, J.H.; Sung, M.K.; Kim, M.K.; Park, J.H.; Kim, J.S. Genistein induces glucose-regulated protein 78 in mammary tumor cells. *J. Med. Food* **2006**, *9*, 28–32. [CrossRef]

33. Jung, K.H.; Lee, J.H.; Thien-Quach, C.H.; Paik, J.Y.; Oh, H.; Park, J.W.; Lee, E.J.; Moon, S.H.; Lee, K.H. Resveratrol suppresses cancer cell glucose uptake by targeting reactive oxygen species-mediated hypoxia-inducible factor-1α activation. *J. Nucl. Med.* **2013**, *54*, 2161–2167. [CrossRef] [PubMed]

34. Gomez, L.S.; Zancan, P.; Marcondes, M.C.; Ramos-Santos, L.; Meyer-Fernandes, J.R.; Sola-Penna, M.; Da Silva, D. Resveratrol decreases breast cancer cell viability and glucose metabolism by inhibiting 6-phosphofructo-1-kinase. *Biochimie* **2013**, *98*, 1336–1343. [CrossRef] [PubMed]

35. Yang, Y.; Wolfram, J.; Boom, K.; Fang, X.; Shen, H.; Ferrari, M. Hesperetin impairs glucose uptake and inhibits proliferation of breast cancer cells. *Cell Biochem. Funct.* **2013**, *31*, 374–379. [CrossRef]
36. Moreira, L.; Araújo, I.; Costa, T.; Correia-Branco, A.; Faria, A.; Martel, F.; Keating, E. Quercetin and epigallocatechin gallate inhibit glucose uptake and metabolism by breast cancer cells by an estrogen receptor-independent mechanism. *Exp. Cell Res.* **2013**, *319*, 1784–1795. [CrossRef]
37. Du, G.J.; Song, Z.H.; Lin, H.H.; Han, X.F.; Zhang, S.; Yang, Y.M. Luteolin as a gly-colysis inhibitor offers superior efficacy and lesser toxicity of doxorubicin in breast cancer cells. *Biochem. Biophys. Res. Commun.* **2008**, *372*, 497–502. [CrossRef]
38. Yu, W.S.; Jeong, S.J.; Kim, J.H.; Lee, H.J.; Song, H.S.; Kim, M.S.; Ko, E.; Lee, H.J.; Khil, J.H.; Jang, H.J.; et al. The genome-wide expression profile of 1,2,3,4,6-penta-O-galloyl-β-D-glucose-treated MDA-MB-231 breast cancer cells: Molecular target on cancer metabolism. *Mol. Cells* **2011**, *32*, 123–132. [CrossRef]
39. Anzilotti, S.; Giampà, C.; Laurenti, D.; Perrone, L.; Bernardi, G.; Melone, M.A.; Fusco, F.R. Immunohistochemical localization of receptor for advanced glycation end (RAGE) products in the R6/2 mouse model of Huntington's disease. *Brain Res. Bull.* **2012**, *87*, 350–358. [CrossRef]
40. Aragno, M.; Mastrocola, R. Dietary Sugars and Endogenous Formation of Advanced Glycation Endproducts: Emerging Mechanisms of Disease. *Nutrients* **2017**, *9*, 385. [CrossRef]
41. Perrone, L.; Grant, W.B. Observational and ecological studies of dietary advanced glycation end products in national diets and Alzheimer's disease incidence and prevalence. *J. Alzheimers Dis.* **2015**, *45*, 965–979. [CrossRef] [PubMed]
42. Perrone, L.; Sbai, O.; Nawroth, P.P.; Bierhaus, A. The Complexity of Sporadic Alzheimer's Disease Pathogenesis: The Role of RAGE as Therapeutic Target to Promote Neuroprotection by Inhibiting Neurovascular Dysfunction. *Int. J. Alzheimers Dis.* **2012**, *2012*, 734956. [CrossRef] [PubMed]
43. van Heist, J.; Niessen, H.; Hoekman, K.; Schalkwij, C. Advanced glycation end products in human cancer tissues: Detection of Nepsilon-(carboxymethyl)lysine and argpryrimidine. *Ann. N. Y. Acad. Sci.* **2005**, *1043*, 725–733. [CrossRef] [PubMed]
44. Kiho, T.; Usui, S.; Hirano, K.; Aizawa, K.; Inakuma, T. Tomato paste fraction inhibiting the formation of advance glycation end-products. *Biosci. Biotechnol. Biochem.* **2004**, *1*, 200–205. [CrossRef]
45. Lo, C.-Y.; Li, S.; Tan, D.; Pan, M.-H.; Sang, S.; Ho, C.-T. Trapping reactions of reactive carbonyl species with tea polyphenols in simulated physiological conditions. *Mol. Nutr. Food Res.* **2006**, *50*, 1118–1128. [CrossRef]
46. Sang, S.; Shao, X.; Bai, N.; Lo, C.-Y.; Yang, C.; Ho, C.-T. Tea polyphenol (−)-Epigallocatechin-3-Gallate: A new trapping agent of reactive dicarbonyl species. *Chem. Res. Toxicol.* **2007**, *20*, 1862–1870. [CrossRef]
47. Palanissami, G.; Paul, S.F.D. RAGE and Its Ligands: Molecular Interplay Between Glycation, Inflammation, and Hallmarks of Cancer-a Review. *Horm. Cancer* **2018**, *9*, 295–325. [CrossRef]
48. Takada, M.; Ku, Y.; Toyama, H.; Suzuki, Y.; Kuroda, Y. Suppressive effects of tea polyphenol and conformational changes with receptor for advanced glycation en products (RAGE) expression in human hepatoma cells. *Hepatogastroenterology* **2002**, *49*, 928–931.
49. Lan, C.Y.; Chen, S.Y.; Kuo, C.W.; Lu, C.C.; Yen, G.C. Quercetin facilitates cell death and chemosensitivity through RAGE/PI3K/AKT/mTOR axis in human pancreatic cancer cells. *J. Food Drug Anal.* **2019**, *27*, 887–896. [CrossRef]
50. Schieber, M.; Chandel, N.S. ROS function in redox signaling and oxidative stress. *Curr. Biol.* **2014**, *24*, R453–R462. [CrossRef]
51. Liou, G.Y.; Storz, P. Reactive oxygen species in cancer. *Free Radic. Res.* **2010**, *44*, 479–496. [CrossRef] [PubMed]
52. NavaneethaKrishnan, S.; Rosales, J.L.; Lee, K.Y. ROS-Mediated Cancer Cell Killing through Dietary Phytochemicals. *Oxid. Med. Cell Longev.* **2019**, *2019*, 905154. [CrossRef] [PubMed]
53. Gibellini, L.; Pinti, M.; Nasi, M.; De Biasi, S.; Roat, E.; Bertoncelli, L.; Cossarizza, A. Interfering with ROS Metabolism in Cancer Cells: The Potential Role of Quercetin. *Cancers* **2010**, *2*, 1288–1311. [CrossRef] [PubMed]
54. Gibellini, L.; Bianchini, E.; De Biasi, S.; Nasi, M.; Cossarizza, A.; Pinti, M. Natural compounds modulating mitochon-drial functions. *Evid. Based Complement. Altern. Med.* **2015**, *2015*, 527209. [CrossRef]
55. Karmakar, S.; Banik, N.L.; Patel, S.J.; Ray, S.K. Curcumin activated both receptor-mediated and mitochondria-mediated proteolytic pathways for apoptosis in human glioblastoma T98G cells. *Neurosci. Lett.* **2006**, *407*, 53–58. [CrossRef]

56. Bhaumik, S.; Anjum, R.; Rangaraj, N.; Pardhasaradhi, B.V.V.; Khar, A. Curcumin mediated apoptosis in AK-5 tumor cells involves the production of reactive oxygen intermediates. *FEBS Lett.* **1999**, *456*, 311–314. [CrossRef]
57. Thayyullathil, F.; Chathoth, S.; Hago, A.; Patel, M.; Galadari, S. Rapid reactive oxygen species (ROS) generation induced by curcumin leads to caspase-dependent and -independent apoptosis in L929 cells. *Free Radic. Biol. Med.* **2008**, *45*, 1403–1412. [CrossRef]
58. Morin, D.; Barthelemy, S.; Zini, R.; Labidalle, S.; Tillement, J.P. Curcumin induces the mitochondrial permeability transition pore mediated by membrane protein thiol oxidation. *FEBS Lett.* **2001**, *495*, 131–136. [CrossRef]
59. Lee, Y.J.; Kim, N.Y.; Suh, Y.A.; Lee, C. Involvement of ROS in curcumin-induced autophagic cell death. *Korean J. Physiol. Pharmacol.* **2011**, *15*, 1–7. [CrossRef]
60. Gersey, Z.C.; Rodriguez, G.A.; Barbarite, E.; Sanchez, A.; Walters, W.M.; Ohaeto, K.C.; Komotar, R.J.; Graham, R.M. Curcumin decreases malignant characteristics of glioblastoma stem cells via induction of reactive oxygen species. *BMC Cancer* **2017**, *17*, 99. [CrossRef]
61. Xie, L.; Xiang, G.H.; Tang, T.; Tang, Y.; Zhao, L.Y.; Liu, D.; Zhang, Y.R.; Tang, J.T.; Zhou, S.; Wu, D.H. Capsaicin and dihydrocapsaicin induce apoptosis in human glioma cells via ROS and Ca2+-mediated mitochondrial pathway. *Mol. Med. Rep.* **2016**, *14*, 4198–4208. [CrossRef]
62. Lin, C.H.; Lu, W.C.; Wang, C.W.; Chan, Y.C.; Chen, M.K. Capsaicin induces cell cycle arrest and apoptosis in human KB cancer cells. *BMC Complement. Altern. Med.* **2013**, *13*, 46. [CrossRef]
63. Min, K.J.; Kwon, T.K. Anticancer effects and molecular mechanisms of epigallocatechin-3-gallate. *Integr. Med. Res.* **2014**, *3*, 16–24. [CrossRef]
64. Trachootham, D.; Zhou, Y.; Zhang, H.; Demizu, Y.; Chen, Z.; Pelicano, H.; Chiao, P.J.; Achanta, G.; Arlinghaus, R.B.; Liu, J.; et al. Selective killing of oncogenically transformed cells through a ROS-mediated mechanism by beta-phenylethyl isothiocyanate. *Cancer Cell* **2006**, *10*, 241–252. [CrossRef]
65. Zhu, Y.; Zhuang, J.X.; Wang, Q.; Zhang, H.Y.; Yang, P. Inhibitory effect of benzyl isothiocyanate on proliferation in vitro of human glioma cells. *Asian Pac. J. Cancer Prev.* **2013**, *14*, 2607–2610. [CrossRef]
66. Rather, R.A.; Bhagat, M. Cancer chemoprevention and piperine: Molecular mechanisms and therapeutic opportunities. *Front. Cell Dev. Biol.* **2018**, *6*, 10. [CrossRef]
67. Chen, Y.; Tseng, S.H.; Lai, H.S.; Chen, W.J. Resveratrol-induced cellular apoptosis and cell cycle arrest in neuroblas-toma cells and antitumor effects on neuroblastoma in mice. *Surgery* **2004**, *136*, 57–66. [CrossRef]
68. Shankar, S.; Chen, Q.; Siddiqui, I.; Sarva, K.; Srivastava, R.K. Sensitization of TRAIL-resistant LNCaP cells by resveratrol (3, 4′, 5 tri-hydroxystilbene): Molecular mechanisms and therapeutic potential. *J. Mol. Signal.* **2007**, *2*, 7. [CrossRef]
69. Rosa, L.D.S.; Jordão, N.A.; Soares, N.D.; DeMesquita, J.F.; Monteiro, M.; Teodoro, A.J. Pharmacokinetic, Antipro-liferative and Apoptotic Effects of Phenolic Acids in Human Colon Adenocarcinoma Cells Using In Vitro and In Silico Approaches. *Molecules* **2018**, *23*, 2569. [CrossRef]
70. Totta, P.; Acconcia, F.; Leone, S.; Cardillo, I.; Marino, M. Mechanisms of Naringenin-induced Apoptotic Cascade in Cancer Cells: Involvement of Estrogen Receptor α and β Signalling. *IUBMB Life* **2004**, *56*, 491–499. [CrossRef]
71. You, B.R.; Kim, S.Z.; Kim, S.H.; Park, W.H. Gallic acid-induced lung cancer cell death is accompanied by ROS increase and glutathione depletion. *Mol. Cell. Biochem.* **2011**, *357*, 295–303. [CrossRef]
72. Scalbert, A.; Manach, C.; Morand, C.; Remesy, C.; Jimenez, L. Dietary polyphenols and the prevention of diseases. *Crit. Rev. Food Sci. Nutr.* **2005**, *45*, 287–306. [CrossRef]
73. Thakur, V.S.; Gupta, K.; Gupta, S. The chemopreventive and chemotherapeutic potentials of tea polyphenols. *Curr. Pharm. Biotechnol.* **2012**, *13*, 191–199. [CrossRef]
74. Pandey, K.B.; Rizvi, S.I. Plant polyphenols as dietary antioxidants in human health and disease. *Oxidative Med. Cell. Longev.* **2009**, *2*, 270–278. [CrossRef]
75. Perrone, L.; Squillaro, T.; Napolitano, F.; Terracciano, C.; Sampaolo, S.; Melone, M.A.B. The Autophagy Signaling Pathway: A Potential Multifunctional Therapeutic Target of Curcumin in Neurological and Neuromuscular Diseases. *Nutrients* **2019**, *11*, 1881. [CrossRef]
76. Beltz, L.A.; Bayer, D.K.; Moss, A.L.; Simet, I.M. Mechanisms of cancer prevention by green and black tea polyphenols. *Anti-Cancer Agents Med. Chem.* **2006**, *6*, 389–406. [CrossRef]
77. Anand, P.; Kunnumakkara, A.B.; Sundaram, C.; Harikumar, K.B.; Tharakan, S.T.; Lai, O.S.; Sung, B.; Aggarwal, B.B. Cancer is a preventable disease that requires major lifestyle changes. *Pharm. Res.* **2008**, *25*, 2200. [CrossRef]

78. Stoll, E.A.; Horner, P.J.; Rostomily, R.C. The impact of age on oncogenic potential: Tumor-initiating cells and the brain microenvironment. *Aging Cell* **2013**, *12*, 733–741. [CrossRef]
79. Niedzwiecki, A.; Roomi, M.W.; Kalinovsky, T.; Rath, M. Anticancer efficacy of polyphenols and their combinations. *Nutrients* **2016**, *8*, 552. [CrossRef]
80. Shahcheraghi, S.H.; Zangui, M.; Lotfi, M.; Ghayour-Mobarhan, M.; Ghorbani, A.; Jaliani, H.Z.; Sadeghnia, H.R.; Sahebkar, A. Therapeutic Potential of Curcumin in the Treatment of Glioblastoma Multiforme. *Curr. Pharm. Des.* **2019**, *25*, 333–342. [CrossRef]
81. Zhuang, W.; Long, L.; Zheng, B.; Ji, W.; Yang, N.; Zhang, Q.; Liang, Z. Curcumin promotes differentiation of glioma-initiating cells by inducing autophagy. *Cancer Sci.* **2012**, *103*, 684–690. [CrossRef]
82. Wang, X.; Deng, J.; Yuan, J.; Tang, X.; Wang, Y.; Chen, H.; Liu, Y.; Zhou, L. Curcumin exerts its tumor suppressive function via inhibition of NEDD4 oncoprotein in glioma cancer cells. *Int. J. Oncol.* **2017**, *51*, 467–477. [CrossRef]
83. Mukherjee, S.; Baidoo, J.; Fried, A.; Atwi, D.; Dolai, S.; Boockvar, J.; Symons, M.; Ruggieri, R.; Raja, K.; Banerjee, P. Curcumin changes the polarity of tumor-associated microglia and eliminates glioblastoma. *Int. J. Cancer* **2016**, *139*, 2838–2849. [CrossRef]
84. Lee, J.E.; Yoon, S.S.; Moon, E.Y. Curcumin-Induced Autophagy Augments Its Antitumor Effect against A172 Human Glioblastoma Cells. *Biomol. Ther.* **2019**, *27*, 484–491. [CrossRef]
85. Maiti, P.; Scott, J.; Sengupta, D.; Al-Gharaibeh, A.; Dunbar, G.L. Curcumin and Solid Lipid Curcumin Particles Induce Autophagy, but Inhibit Mitophagy and the PI3K-Akt/mTOR Pathway in Cultured Glioblastoma Cells. *Int. J. Mol. Sci.* **2019**, *20*, 399. [CrossRef]
86. Park, K.S.; Yoon, S.Y.; Park, S.H.; Hwang, J.H. Anti-Migration and Anti-Invasion Effects of Curcumin via Suppression of Fascin Expression in Glioblastoma Cells. *Brain Tumor. Res. Treat.* **2019**, *7*, 16–24. [CrossRef]
87. Sak, K. Radiosensitizing Potential of Curcumin in Different Cancer Models. *Nutr. Cancer* **2019**, *24*, 1–14. [CrossRef]
88. Kielbik, A.; Wawryka, P.; Przystupski, D.; Rossowska, J.; Szewczyk, A.; Saczko, J.; Kulbacka, J.; Chwiłkowska, A. Effects of Photosensitization of Curcumin in Human Glioblastoma Multiforme Cells. *In Vivo* **2019**, *33*, 1857–1864. [CrossRef]
89. Pawlowska, E.; Szczepanska, J.; Szatkowska, M.; Blasiak, J. An Interplay between Senescence, Apoptosis and Autophagy in Glioblastoma Multiforme-Role in Pathogenesis and Therapeutic Perspective. *Int. J. Mol. Sci.* **2018**, *19*, 889. [CrossRef]
90. Pistollato, F.; Bremer-Hoffmann, S.; Basso, G.; Cano, S.S.; Elio, I.; Vergara, M.M.; Giampieri, F.; Battino, M. Targeting Glioblastoma with the Use of Phytocompounds and Nanoparticles. *Target Oncol.* **2016**, *11*, 1–16. [CrossRef]
91. Sato, A.; Okada, M.; Shibuya, K.; Watanabe, E.; Seino, S.; Suzuki, K.; Narita, Y.; Shibui, S.; Kayama, T.; Kitanaka, C. Resveratrol promotes proteasome-dependent degradation of Nanog via p53 activation and induces differentiation of glioma stem cells. *Stem. Cell Res.* **2013**, *11*, 601–610. [CrossRef]
92. Xiong, W.; Yin, A.; Mao, X.; Zhang, W.; Huang, H.; Zhang, X. Resveratrol suppresses human glioblastoma cell migration and invasion via activation of RhoA/ROCK signaling pathway. *Oncol. Lett.* **2016**, *11*, 484–490. [CrossRef]
93. Cilibrasi, C.; Riva, G.; Romano, G.; Cadamuro, M.; Bazzoni, R.; Butta, V.; Paoletta, L.; Dalprà, L.; Strazzabosco, M.; Lavitrano, M.; et al. Resveratrol Impairs Glioma Stem Cells Proliferation and Motility by Modulating the Wnt Signaling Pathway. *PLoS ONE* **2017**, *12*, e0169854. [CrossRef]
94. Yang, Y.P.; Chang, Y.L.; Huang, P.I.; Chiou, G.Y.; Tseng, L.M.; Chiou, S.H.; Chen, M.H.; Chen, M.T.; Shih, Y.H.; Chang, C.; et al. Resveratrol suppresses tumorigenicity and enhances radiosensitivity in primary glioblastoma tumor initiating cells by inhibiting the STAT3 axis. *J. Cell Physiol.* **2012**, *227*, 976–993. [CrossRef]
95. Mirzazadeh, A.; Kheirollahi, M.; Farashahi, E.; Sadeghian-Nodoushan, F.; Sheikhha, M.H.; Aflatoonian, B. Assessment Effects of Resveratrol on Human Telomerase Reverse Transcriptase Messenger Ribonucleic Acid Transcript in Human Glioblastoma. *Adv. Biomed. Res.* **2017**, *6*, 73.
96. Song, X.; Shu, X.H.; Wu, M.L.; Zheng, X.; Jia, B.; Kong, Q.Y.; Liu, J.; Li, H. Postoperative resveratrol administration improves prognosis of rat orthotopic glioblastomas. *BMC Cancer* **2018**, *18*, 871. [CrossRef]
97. Song, Y.; Chen, Y.; Li, Y.; Lyu, X.; Cui, J.; Cheng, Y.; Zheng, T.; Zhao, L.; Zhao, G. Resveratrol Suppresses Epithelial-Mesenchymal Transition in GBM by Regulating Smad-Dependent Signaling. *Biomed. Res. Int.* **2019**, *2019*, 1321973. [CrossRef]
98. Öztürk, Y.; Günaydın, C.; Yalçın, F.; Nazıroğlu, M.; Braidy, N. Resveratrol Enhances Apoptotic and Oxidant Effects of Paclitaxel through TRPM2 Channel Activation in DBTRG Glioblastoma Cells. *Oxid. Med. Cell Longev.* **2019**, *2019*, 4619865. [CrossRef]

99. Yokoyama, S.; Hirano, H.; Wakimaru, N.; Sarker, K.P.; Kuratsu, J. Inhibitory effect of epigallocatechin-gallate on brain tumor cell lines in vitro. *Neuro-Oncology* **2001**, *3*, 22–28. [CrossRef]
100. McLaughlin, N.; Annabi, B.; Bouzeghrane, M.; Temme, A.; Bahary, J.P.; Moumdjian, R.; Beliveau, R. The Survivin-mediated radio-resistant phenotype of glioblastomas is regulated by RhoA and inhibited by the green tea polyphenol (−)-epigallocatechin-3-gallate. *Brain Res.* **2006**, *1071*, 1–9. [CrossRef]
101. Chen, T.C.; Wang, W.; Golden, E.B.; Thomas, S.; Sivakumar, W.; Hofman, F.M.; Louie, S.G.; Schönthal, A.H. Green tea epigallocatechin gallate enhances therapeutic efficacy of temozolomide in orthotopic mouse glioblastoma models. *Cancer Lett.* **2011**, *302*, 100–108. [CrossRef]
102. Zhang, Y.; Wang, S.X.; Ma, J.W.; Li, H.Y.; Ye, J.C.; Xie, S.M.; Du, B.; Zhong, X.Y. EGCG inhibits properties of glioma stem-like cells and synergizes with temozolomide through downregulation of P-glycoprotein inhibition. *J. Neurooncol.* **2015**, *121*, 41–52. [CrossRef]
103. Sui, X.M.; Wang, J.X.; Zhu, Q.W.; Zhang, Q.F. Epigallocatechin-3-gallate induces apoptosis and proliferation inhibition of glioma cell through suppressing JAK2/STAT3 signaling pathway. *Int. J. Clin. Exp. Med.* **2016**, *9*, 10995–11001.
104. Roomi, M.W.; Kalinovsky, T.; Rath, M.; Niedzwiecki, A. Modulation of MMP-2 and MMP-9 secretion by cytokines, inducers and inhibitors in human glioblastoma T-98G cells. *Oncol. Rep.* **2017**, *37*, 1907–1913. [CrossRef]
105. Gurusinghe, K.R.D.S.N.S.; Mishra, A.; Mishra, S. Glucose-regulated protein 78 substrate-binding domain alters its conformation upon EGCG inhibitor binding to nucleotide-binding domain: Molecular dynamics studies. *Sci. Rep.* **2018**, *8*, 5487. [CrossRef]
106. Grube, S.; Ewald, C.; Kögler, C.; Lawson-McLean, A.; Kalff, R.; Walter, J. Achievable Central Nervous System Concentrations of the Green Tea Catechin EGCG Induce Stress in Glioblastoma Cells in Vitro. *Nutr. Cancer* **2018**, *70*, 1145–1158. [CrossRef]
107. Xie, C.R.; You, C.G.; Zhang, N.; Sheng, H.S.; Zheng, X.S. Epigallocatechin Gallate Preferentially Inhibits O6-Methylguanine DNA-Methyltransferase Expression in Glioblastoma Cells Rather than in Nontumor Glial Cells. *Nutr. Cancer* **2018**, *70*, 1339–1347. [CrossRef]
108. Udroiu, I.; Marinaccio, J.; Sgura, A. Epigallocatechin-3-gallate induces telomere shortening and clastogenic damage in glioblastoma cells. *Environ. Mol. Mutagen.* **2019**, *60*, 683–692. [CrossRef]
109. Santos, B.L.; Silva, A.R.; Pitanga, B.P.; Sousa, C.S.; Grangeiro, M.S.; Fragomeni, B.O.; Coelho, P.L.; Oliveira, M.N.; Menezes-Filho, N.J.; Costa, M.F.; et al. Antiproliferative, proapoptotic and morphogenic effects of the flavonoid rutin on human glioblastoma cells. *Food Chem.* **2011**, *127*, 404–411. [CrossRef]
110. Jakubowicz-Gil, J.; Langner, E.; Badziul, D.; Wertel, I.; Rzeski, W. Apoptosis induction in human glioblastoma multiforme T98G cells upon temozolomide and quercetin treatment. *Tumour Biol. J. Int. Soc. Oncodev. Biol. Med.* **2013**, *34*, 2367–2378. [CrossRef]
111. Pozsgai, E.; Bellyei, S.; Cseh, A.; Boronkai, A.; Racz, B.; Szabo, A.; Sumegi, B.; Hocsak, E. Quercetin increases the efficacy of glioblastoma treatment compared to standard chemoradiotherapy by the suppression of PI-3-kinase-Akt pathway. *Nutr. Cancer* **2013**, *65*, 1059–1066. [CrossRef]
112. Zhang, P.; Sun, S.; Li, N.; Ho, A.S.W.; Kiang, K.M.Y.; Zhang, X.; Cheng, Y.S.; Poon, M.W.; Lee, D.; Pu, J.K.S.; et al. Rutin increases the cytotoxicity of temozolomide in glioblastoma via autophagy inhibition. *J. Neurooncol.* **2017**, *132*, 393–400. [CrossRef]
113. Liu, Y.; Tang, Z.G.; Lin, Y.; Qu, X.G.; Lv, W.; Wang, G.B.; Li, C.L. Effects of quercetin on proliferation and migration of human glioblastoma U251 cells. *Biomed. Pharm.* **2017**, *92*, 33–38. [CrossRef]
114. Liu, Y.; Tang, Z.G.; Yang, J.Q.; Zhou, Y.; Meng, L.H.; Wang, H.; Li, C.L. Low concentration of quercetin antagonizes the invasion and angiogenesis of human glioblastoma U251 cells. *Onco Targets Ther.* **2017**, *10*, 4023–4028. [CrossRef]
115. Gentile, M.T.; Ciniglia, C.; Reccia, M.G.; Volpicelli, F.; Gatti, M.; Thellung, S.; Florio, T.; Melone, M.A.; Colucci-D'Amato, L. Ruta graveolens L. induces death of glioblastoma cells and neural progenitors, but not of neurons, via ERK 1/2 and AKT activation. *PLoS ONE* **2015**, *10*, e0118864. [CrossRef]
116. Taylor, M.A.; Khathayer, F.; Ray, S.K. Quercetin and Sodium Butyrate Synergistically Increase Apoptosis in Rat C6 and Human T98G Glioblastoma Cells Through Inhibition of Autophagy. *Neurochem. Res.* **2019**, *44*, 1715–1725. [CrossRef]
117. Tora, M.S.; Xenos, D.; Texakalidis, P.; Boulis, N.M. Treatment of neurofibromatosis 1-associated malignant peripheral nerve sheath tumors: A systematic review. *Neurosurg. Rev.* **2019**, 1–8. [CrossRef]

118. Angelo, L.S.; Wu, J.Y.; Meng, F.; Sun, M.; Kopetz, S.; McCutcheon, I.E.; Slopis, J.M.; Kurzrock, R. Combining curcumin (diferuloylmethane) and heat shock protein inhibition for neurofibromatosis 2 treatment: Analysis of response and resistance pathways. *Mol. Cancer* **2011**, *10*, 2094–2103. [CrossRef]
119. Blakeley, J. Development of drug treatments for neurofibromatosis type 2-associated vestibular schwannoma. *Curr. Opin. Otolaryngol. Head Neck Surg.* **2012**, *20*, 372–379. [CrossRef]
120. Turrini, E.; Ferruzzi, L.; Fimognari, C. Potential effects of pomegranate polyphenols in cancer prevention and therapy. *Oxidative Med. Cell. Longev.* **2015**, *2015*, 938475. [CrossRef]
121. Esposito, T.; Schettino, C.; Polverino, P.; Allocca, S.; Adelfi, L.; D'Amico, A.; Capaldo, G.; Varriale, B.; Di Salle, A.; Peluso, G.; et al. Synergistic Interplay between Curcumin and Polyphenol-Rich Foods in the Mediterranean Diet: Therapeutic Prospects for Neurofibromatosis 1 Patients. *Nutrients* **2017**, *9*, 783. [CrossRef] [PubMed]
122. Lee, M.J.; Tsai, Y.J.; Lin, M.Y.; You, H.L.; Kalyanam, N.; Ho, C.T.; Pan, M.H. Calebin-A induced death of malignant peripheral nerve sheath tumor cells by activation of histone acetyltransferase. *Phytomedicine* **2019**, *57*, 377–384. [CrossRef] [PubMed]
123. Hu, M.; Wu, B.; Liu, Z. Bioavailability of polyphenols and flavonoids in the era of precision medicine. *Mol Pharm* **2017**, *14*, 2861–2863. [CrossRef] [PubMed]
124. Teng, H.; Chen, L. Polyphenols and bioavailability: An update. *Crit. Rev. Food Sci. Nutr.* **2019**, *59*, 2040–2051. [CrossRef]
125. Pandareesh, M.D.; Mythri, R.B.; Srinivas Bharath, M.M. Bioavailability of dietary polyphenols: Factors contributing to their clinical application in CNS diseases. *Neurochem. Int.* **2015**, *89*, 198–208. [CrossRef]
126. Squillaro, T.; Peluso, G.; Melone, M.A.B. Nanotechnology-based polyphenol delivery: A novel therapeutic strategy for the treatment of age-related neurodegenerative disorder. *Austin Aging Res.* **2017**, *1*, 1004–1009.
127. Figueira, I.; Garcia, G.; Pimpão, R.C.; Terrasso, A.P.; Costa, I.; Almeida, A.F.; Tavares, L.; Pais, T.F.; Pinto, P.; Ventura, M.R.; et al. Polyphenols journey through blood-brain barrier towards neuronal protection. *Sci. Rep.* **2017**, *7*, 11456. [CrossRef]
128. Filosa, S.; Di Meo, F.; Crispi, S. Polyphenols-gut microbiota interplay and brain neuromodulation. *Neural. Regen. Res.* **2018**, *13*, 2055–2059.
129. Finicelli, M.; Squillaro, T.; Di Cristo, F.; Di Salle, A.; Melone, M.A.B.; Galderisi, U.; Peluso, G. Metabolic syndrome, Mediterranean diet, and polyphenols: Evidence and perspectives. *J. Cell Physiol.* **2019**, *234*, 5807–5826. [CrossRef]
130. Squillaro, T.; Cimini, A.; Peluso, G.; Giordano, A.; Melone, M.A.B. Nano-delivery systems for encapsulation of dietary polyphenols: An experimental approach for neurodegenerative diseases and brain tumors. *Biochem. Pharm.* **2018**, *154*, 303–317. [CrossRef]
131. Singh, H. Nanotechnology Applications in Functional Foods; Opportunities and Challenges. *Prev. Nutr. Food Sci.* **2016**, *21*, 1–8. [CrossRef]

4

EGCG Mediated Targeting of Deregulated Signaling Pathways and Non-Coding RNAs in Different Cancers: Focus on JAK/STAT, Wnt/β-Catenin, TGF/SMAD, NOTCH, SHH/GLI and TRAIL Mediated Signaling Pathways

Ammad Ahmad Farooqi [1], Marina Pinheiro [2,*], Andreia Granja [2], Fulvia Farabegoli [3], Salette Reis [2], Rukset Attar [4], Uteuliyev Yerzhan Sabitaliyevich [5], Baojun Xu [6] and Aamir Ahmad [7]

1. Institute of Biomedical and Genetic Engineering (IBGE), Islamabad 54000, Pakistan; ammadfarooqi@rlmclahore.com
2. LAQV, REQUIMTE, Departamento de Ciências Químicas, Faculdade de Farmácia, Universidade do Porto, 4050-313 Porto, Portugal; andreia26293@gmail.com (A.G.); shreis@ff.up.pt (S.R.)
3. Department of Pharmacy and Biotechnology (FaBiT), University of Bologna, 40126 Bologna, Italy; fulvia.farabegoli@unibo.it
4. Department of Obstetrics and Gynecology, Yeditepe University, Ataşehir/İstanbul 34755, Turkey; ruksetattar@hotmail.com
5. Department of Health Policy and Health Care Development, Kazakh Medical University of Continuing Education, Almaty 050004, Kazakhstan; e.uteuliyev@ksph.kz
6. Food Science and Technology Program, Beijing Normal University-Hong Kong Baptist University United International College, Zhuhai 519087, China; baojunxu@uic.edu.hk
7. Department of Medicine, University of Alabama at Birmingham, Birmingham, AL 35205, USA; aamirahmad100@gmail.com

* Correspondence: mpinheiro@ff.up.pt

Abstract: Decades of research have enabled us to develop a better and sharper understanding of multifaceted nature of cancer. Next-generation sequencing technologies have leveraged our existing knowledge related to intra- and inter-tumor heterogeneity to the next level. Functional genomics have opened new horizons to explore deregulated signaling pathways in different cancers. Therapeutic targeting of deregulated oncogenic signaling cascades by products obtained from natural sources has shown promising results. Epigallocatechin-3-gallate (EGCG) has emerged as a distinguished chemopreventive product because of its ability to regulate a myriad of oncogenic signaling pathways. Based on its scientifically approved anticancer activity and encouraging results obtained from preclinical trials, it is also being tested in various phases of clinical trials. A series of clinical trials associated with green tea extracts and EGCG are providing clues about significant potential of EGCG to mechanistically modulate wide ranging signal transduction cascades. In this review, we comprehensively analyzed regulation of JAK/STAT, Wnt/β-catenin, TGF/SMAD, SHH/GLI, NOTCH pathways by EGCG. We also discussed most recent evidence related to the ability of EGCG to modulate non-coding RNAs in different cancers. Methylation of the genome is also a widely studied mechanism and EGCG has been shown to modulate DNA methyltransferases (DNMTs) and protein enhancer of zeste-2 (EZH2) in multiple cancers. Moreover, the use of nanoformulations to increase the bioavailability and thus efficacy of EGCG will be also addressed. Better understanding of the pleiotropic abilities of EGCG to modulate intracellular pathways along with the development of effective EGCG delivery vehicles will be helpful in getting a step closer to individualized medicines.

Keywords: EGCG; signaling pathways; non-coding RNAs; anti-cancer drug

---

1. Introduction

Genomic approaches such as whole genome sequencing and genetic mapping have helped considerably in the identification of many genetic variants in multiple components of cell signaling pathways. Moreover, advancements in functional genomics have marked a new frontier in molecular oncology. Epigallocatechin-3-gallate (EGCG) is a phenolic compound present in tea and has captivated tremendous attention in the past two decades because of its premium pharmacological properties. There is a wide variety of reviews published with reference to EGCG mediated anticancer effects [1–4]. However, in this review we focused on EGCG mediated modulation of deregulation cell signaling pathways in different cancers. We partitioned this multi-component review into different sections. We will open the review by critical analysis of layered regulation of the JAK-STAT pathway by EGCG.

2. Targeting of JAK/STAT Signaling

The JAK-STAT pathway constitutes a rapid membrane-to-nucleus signaling module that has been shown to play fundamental role in cancer development and progression (shown in Figure 1). In this section, we will discuss in detail how EGCG modulated JAK/STAT signaling. EGCG has been shown to interfere with the JAK/STAT pathway at different steps, which includes inhibition of STAT phosphorylation and restriction of nuclear transportation of STAT proteins.

EGCG remarkably reduced tyrosine and serine phosphorylation of signal transducer and activator of transcription 1 (STAT1) [5]. Moreover, phosphorylation of protein kinase C delta PKC-delta, Janus kinase 1 (JAK1), and Janus kinase 2 (JAK2), which are the upstream activators of STAT1 are also inhibited by EGCG in interferon gamma (IFNγ)-stimulated oral cancer cells (shown in Figure 1) [5]. EGCG-mono-palmitate (EGCG-MP), a highly active derivative of EGCG effectively activated Src homology 2 domain-containing tyrosine phosphatase-1 (SHP-1) which consequentially resulted in reduction of phosphorylated levels of BCR-ABL and signal transducer and activator of transcription 3 (STAT3) in human chronic myeloid leukemia (CML) cells (shown in Figure 1) [6]. EGCG-MP treatment more efficiently induced regression of tumor growth in BALB/c athymic nude mice [6]. EGCG potently inhibited BCR/ABL oncoprotein and the JAK2/STAT3/AKT pathway in BCR/ABL+ CML cell lines [7]. Curcumin worked synchronously with EGCG and considerably interfered with tumor conditioned media-induced transition of normal endothelial cells toward tumor endothelial cells by inhibition of the JAK/STAT3 signaling pathway [8].

EGCG significantly reduced phosphorylation of STAT3 on the 705th tyrosine residue and improved sensitivity of cisplatin-resistant oral cancer cells [9]. Fundamental role-play of STAT signaling had previously been studied in invasive breast cancers and matched lymph nodes using quantitative immunofluorescence [10]. STAT proteins were analyzed in lymph nodes and paired primary breast cancer tissues. There was higher expression of cytoplasmic STAT1, p-STAT3 (Ser727), STAT5, and nuclear p-STAT3 (Ser727) in the nodes [10]. c-Myb overexpression induced activation of NF-κB and STAT3 signaling to enhance proliferation, invasion, and resistance against cisplatin [11]. However, c-Myb silencing inhibited proliferation, invasive potential, and sensitized ovarian cancer cells to cisplatin. EGCG completely inhibited c-Myb-mediated proliferative and invasive abilities of ovarian cancer cells [11].

EGCG dose-dependently reduced phosphorylated levels of STAT1 and STAT3 [12]. Quercetin and EGCG worked synergistically and exerted inhibitory effects on cytokine-mediated upregulation of iNOS (inducible nitric oxide synthase) and ICAM-1 (intercellular adhesion molecule-1) via JAK/STAT cascade in cholangiocarcinoma cells (Figure 1) [12].

Indoleamine 2,3-dioxygenase (IDO) is a tryptophan catabolic enzyme. IDO mechanistically regulates immunological response and enables tumor cells to evade the immune system [13].

IFN-γ increased mRNA and protein levels of IDO in HT29 and SW837 colorectal cancer cells. EGCG dose-dependently decreased IFN-γ-induced expression of IDO in SW837 cells. Increase in p-STAT1 level induced by IFN-γ was also found to be markedly repressed by EGCG. Data obtained from reporter assays clearly revealed that EGCG inhibited the transcriptional activity of IDO promoter and blocked binding of p-STAT1 to gamma-activated sequence (GAS) sites on the promoters of target genes (Figure 1) [13].

Toxicological analysis of EGCG highlighted its efficacy and minimum off-target effects. Orally administered EGCG mitigated cisplatin-induced hearing loss along with a marked reduction in the loss of outer hair cells in the basal cochlear region. Importantly, chemotherapeutic drug-induced toxicity was also reduced mainly though suppression of apoptotic markers and oxidative stress [14].

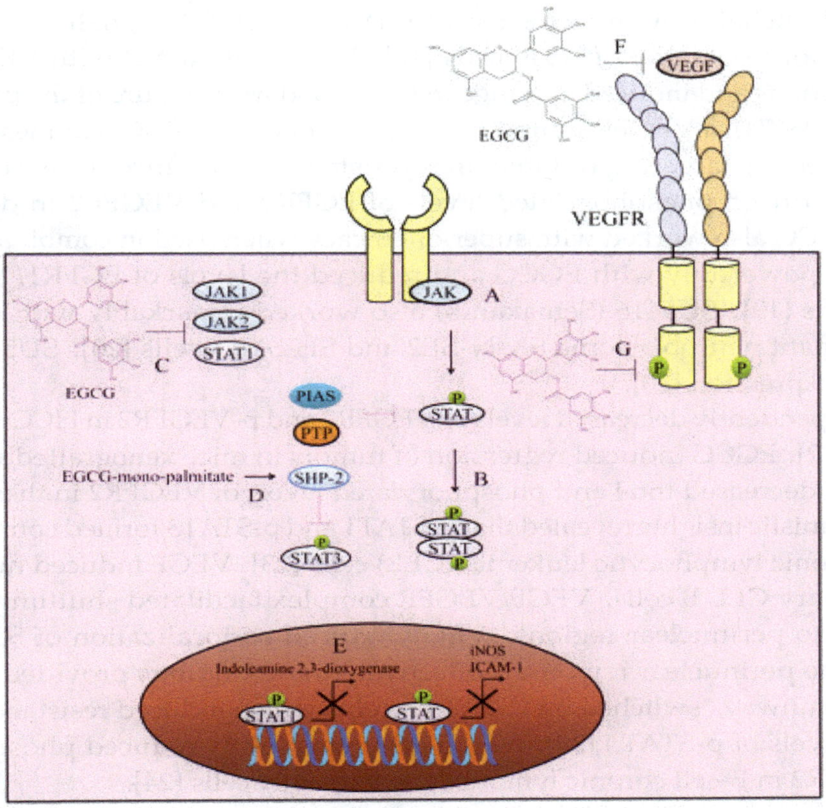

Figure 1. Regulation of the JAK/STAT pathway by epigallocatechin-3-gallate (EGCG). (**A**,**B**) Janus kinase (JAK) mediated phosphorylation of STAT proteins promoted their accumulation in nucleus to regulate expression of a plethora of genes. (**C–E**) EGCG showcased remarkable ability to shut down the JAK/STAT pathway by inhibition of Janus kinase 1 (JAK1), Janus kinase 2 (JAK2), signal transducer and activator of transcription 1 (STAT1), signal transducer and activator of transcription 3 (STAT3). EGCG also activated negative regulators of STAT-driven signaling. Activation of Src homology 2 domain-containing tyrosine phosphatase-1 (SHP-2) was effective in inhibition of JAK/STAT signaling. Different oncogenes particularly, inducible nitric oxide synthase (iNOS), intercellular adhesion molecule-1 (ICAM-1), and indoleamine 2,3-dioxygenase have been shown to be under direct control of STAT signaling. (**F**,**G**) Vascular endothelial growth factor vascular endothelial growth factor receptor (VEGF/VEGFR) signaling is also regulated by EGCG. EGCG interacted with VEGF. Additionally, EGCG inhibited phosphorylation of VEGFR.

It has recently been reported that IFNγ-mediated PD-L1 levels were noted to be downregulated after treatment with green tea extracts and EGCG mainly through inhibition of JAK2/STAT1 signaling in A549 cells [15]. Likewise, EGF-stimulated PD-L1 upregulation was reduced in EGCG-treated Lu99 cells by inactivation of EGFR/AKT transduction cascade. Additionally, green tea extracts notably reduced average number of tumors and percentage of PD-L1$^+$ cells in lungs of A/J mice intraperitoneally injected with a cigarette smoke toxin. EGCG reduced mRNA levels of PD-L1 in F10-OVA cells and enhanced expression of interleukin-2 in tumor-specific CD3$^+$ T cells [15]. Collectively these findings suggested that green tea catechin acted as a useful immunological checkpoint inhibitor.

Confluence of information suggested central role of JAK/STAT signaling in different cancers. EGCG mediated inhibition of JAK/STAT signaling via activation of negative regulators (SHP-2) and inactivation of positive regulators (JAK1, JAK2) has gradually gained appreciation. Additionally, different fusion oncoproteins (BCR-ABL) are also exclusively targeted by EGCG.

3. VEGF/VEGFR Signaling

EGCG and silibinin worked synergistically and inhibited vascular endothelial growth factor/vascular endothelial growth factor receptor (VEGF/VEGFR) signaling. EGCG and Silibinin also reduced migratory potential of A549 cells [16]. EGCG interacted with VEGF mainly through hydrophobic interactions and induced a change in the secondary structure of the protein (Figure 1) [17].

Vandetanib (ZD6474), a VEGFR inhibitor was co-loaded with EGCG in mesoporous Silica-Gold nanoclusters for effective targeting of tamoxifen-resistant breast cancer cells [18]. Vandetanib and EGCG effectively reduced phosphorylated levels of EGFR2 and VEGFR2 in drug-resistant breast cancer cells [18]. EGCG also worked with superior efficacy when used in combination with tamoxifen. Tamoxifen worked powerfully with EGCG and reduced the levels of EGFR1, VEGF, and VEGFR1 in breast cancer cells [19]. SU5416 (Semaxanib) also worked remarkably with EGCG and induced apoptosis in malignant neuroblastoma SK-N-BE2 and SH-SY5Y cells [20]. SU5416 and EGCG also inhibited VEGFR2 expression [20].

EGCG dose-dependently decreased levels of VEGFR2 and p-VEGFR2 in HCC and colorectal cancer cells (Figure 1) [21,22]. EGCG induced regression of tumors in mice xenografted with either HuH7 or SW837 cells. EGCG decreased total and phosphorylated levels of VEGFR2 in these xnografts [21,22].

Detailed mechanistic insights revealed that p-STAT1 and p-STAT3 formed complexes with VEGFR1 and VEGFR2 in chronic lymphocytic leukemia (CLL) cells [23]. VEGF induced nuclear accumulation of p-STAT3 in primary CLL B cells. VEGF/VEGFR complex facilitated shuttling of STAT3 from the plasma membrane to perinuclear regions. VEGF induced co-localization of STAT3, VEGFR1 and VEGFR2 to the same perinuclear regions. Collectively these findings provided clear evidence that the VEGF/VEGFR pathway "switched on" STAT proteins which induced resistance against apoptosis. EGCG decreased levels of p-STAT3 [23]. EGCG also remarkably reduced phosphorylated levels of VEGFR1 and VEGFR2 in B-cell chronic lymphocytic leukemia cells [24].

4. Regulation of Methylation-Associated Machinery

PRC2 (Polycomb repressive complex-2) is a transcriptional repressive complex that consists of three essential proteins: EZH2 (enhancer of zeste-2), EED (embryonic ectoderm development), and SUZ12 (suppressor of zeste 12). A series of structural studies have shown that EZH2 context-dependent trimethylates lysine 27 on histone 3 (H3K27) to promote transcriptional inactivation of target genes (shown in Figure 2).

EZH2-mediated trimethylation of H3K27 induced transcriptional repression of TIMP3 (tissue inhibitor of metalloproteinases-3). However, EGCG demonstrated remarkable ability to inhibit EZH2-mediated trimethylation. There was a considerable reduction in the levels of enhancers of zeste homolog 2 (EZH2) and H3K27me3 repressive marks at the promoter region of TIMP-3. Additionally, there was an evident increase in histone H3K9/18 acetylation [25]. Essentially, green tea polyphenols and EGCG treatment significantly reduced class I histone deacetylases (HDAC) activity/expression in prostate cancer cells. Furthermore, levels of EZH2 and H3K27me3 were also found to be reduced in prostate cancer cells [25]. Data clearly suggested that EGCG efficiently demonstrated multi-layered regulation of HDACs and EZH2.

Due to the fundamental role of EZH2 in cancer progression, different inhibitors of EZH2 have been designed and tested for evaluation of efficacy. EGCG and GSK343 (EZH2 inhibitor) exerted inhibitory effects on the proliferation, invasive and migratory potential of the cells, and suppressed EZH2-mediated trimethylation of H3K27 [26].

Recent advancements in the biochemical characterization of polycomb-group (PcG) complexes have revealed a broad range of new proteins, which assemble to form multi-protein complexes. All PRC1 complexes contain Ring1B, which has the E3 ubiquitin ligase activity of the complex. Complexes also include PCGF4/BMI-1 in association with Ring1B to regulate epigenetic modifications [27]. EGCG reduced BMI-1 and EZH2 levels in SCC-13 cells [28].

PML–RARα homodimers worked synchronously with co-repressors and histone deacetylases (HDACs) and consequentially enhanced DNA methylation [29]. EGCG reduced the levels of HDAC1 and PML/RARα in leukemic cells (Figure 2) [30].

Groundbreaking discoveries in biology of epigenome have enabled us to develop a sharp comprehension of highly intricate and well-coordinated interplay of HDACs, histone methyltransferases, and DNA methyltransferases. EGCG has emerged as a master-regulator of epigenetic-associated machinery.

Chromatin immunoprecipitation (ChIP) analyses revealed that EGCG enhanced hyperacetylated H4 and acetylated H3K14 histones within promoter regions of p27, PCAF, C/EBP and reduced binding of PRC2 core component genes EZH2, SUZ12, and EED [31].

EGCG significantly reduced enzymatic activities of DNA methyltransferase (DNMT) and HDAC in HeLa cells [32]. Moreover, EGCG also reduced expression level of DNMT3B whereas expression levels of HDAC1 remained unchanged [32]. GTP/EGCG-promoted acetylation of p53 and enhanced its binding to the promoters of Bax and p21/waf1. Treatment of cells with GTPs and EGCG dose- and time-dependently inhibited class I HDACs [33].

Am80 is a structurally different synthetic retinoid from all-trans-retinoic acid. EGCG and Am80 increased acetylated-p53 and acetylated-α-tubulin through suppression of HDAC activity. Use of specific inhibitors against HDAC4 and HDAC5 strongly induced p21waf1 gene expression. Additionally, HDAC6 inhibition induced upregulation of GADD153 and p21waf1 [34].

UHRF1 (ubiquitin-like containing PHD and Ring finger 1) contributed to inactivation of tumor suppressor genes by directing the binding of DNA methyltransferase 1 (DNMT1) to hemi-methylated promoters [35]. EGCG downregulated DNMT1 and UHRF1 expression and consequently upregulated p73 and p16 (INK4A) in Jurkat cells. UHRF1 downregulation was dependent upon the generation of ROS by EGCG. Upregulation of p16 (INK4A) correlated strongly with reduction in the binding of UHRF1 to the promoter region. UHRF1 overexpression counteracted EGCG-induced apoptosis and upregulation of p73 and p16 (INK4A) [35].

EGCG effectively reduced 5-methylcytosine, DNMT activity, mRNA and protein levels of DNMT1, DNMT3a, and DNMT3b [36]. EGCG decreased HDAC activity and increased levels of acetylated H3K9 and H3K14, H4K5, H4K12, and H4K16 but decreased levels of methylated H3-Lys 9. Collectively, because of inhibition of DNMTs and HDACs, EGCG induced re-expression of p16INK4a and Cip1/p21 [36].

Gazing through a molecular lens clearly highlighted contextual push and pull between various versatile regulators associated with methylation. Substantial fraction of information gathered through high-quality research has unraveled that a broad range of tumor suppressors are epigenetically silenced during cancer progression. Selective targeting of DNMTs and HDACs specifically in cancer cells is very challenging and needs to be comprehensively investigated in EGCG-treated preclinical models. In the upcoming section we will analyze how EGCG modulated deregulated TGF/SMAD signaling.

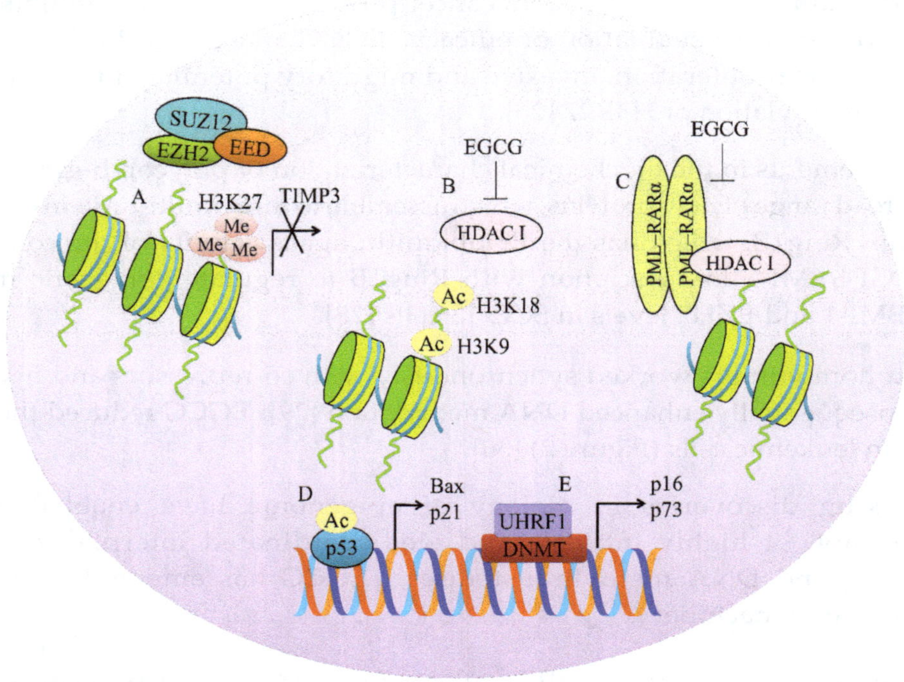

Figure 2. Interconnected and orchestrated interplay among various regulators of epigenetic modifying machinery. (**A**) Protein enhancer of zeste-2 (EZH2), embryonic ectoderm development (EED), and suppressor of zeste 12 (SUZ12) worked synchronously to trimethylate H3K27 and transcriptionally repressed tissue inhibitor of metalloproteinases-3 (TIMP-3). (**B**) Class 1 histone deacetylases (HDACs) were inhibited by EGCG to increase acetylation at H3K9 and H3K18. (**C**) PML–RARα homodimers worked collaboratively with HDAC to regulate expression of target genes. However, EGCG effectively inhibited PML–RARα and HDAC. (**D**) Acetylation of proteins has also been investigated. Acetylated p53 stimulated expression of Bax and p21. (**E**) Ubiquitin-like containing PHD and Ring finger 1 (UHRF1) and DNA methyltransferase (DNMT) also notably downregulated p16 and p73.

5. TGF/SMAD Signaling

Binding of TGFβ superfamily ligands to a type II receptor facilitated closer positioning of type I receptor and phosphorylated it [37]. More importantly, type-I receptor mediated phosphorylation of receptor-regulated SMADs (R-SMADs), which promoted formation of a complex with common mediator SMAD (co-SMAD) (shown in Figure 3). Structural studies had shown that the R-SMAD/co-SMAD complex accumulated in the nucleus to transcriptionally modulate the expression of target genes [38]. Epithelial to mesenchymal transition (EMT) is a highly complex mechanism induced by TGF/SMAD signaling. SMAD2/3 proteins have been shown to stimulate the expression of Snail and Slug in different cancers [39].

In this section, we will provide an overview of multi-layered regulation of TGF/SMAD signaling by EGCG in different cancers. Inhibition of phosphorylation of R-SMADs will inhibit TGF/SMAD signaling. Consequentially, TGF/SMAD signaling inhibition will result in repression of EMT-associated markers.

EGCG effectively reduced p-SMAD3, Snail, and Slug levels in ovarian cancer cells [40]. EGCG considerably suppressed EMT, invasive and migratory capacity of anaplastic thyroid carcinoma (ATC) 8505C cells by regulation of the TGFβ/SMAD pathway [41]. EGCG exerted inhibitory effects on TGFβ1-induced expression of EMT markers (vimentin) in 8505C cells. EGCG was noted to completely block the phosphorylation of SMAD2/3 and nuclear accumulation of SMAD4 [41].

Apart from phosphorylation, acetylation of SMAD proteins is also an intricate mechanism. p300/CBP, a histone acetyltransferase, has been shown to post-translationally modify SMAD proteins. TGFβ1-driven activation of p300/CBP mediated EMT mainly through acetylation of SMAD2 and SMAD3 [42]. EGCG inhibited p300/CBP activity in lung cancer cells. EGCG strongly repressed

TGFβ1-induced EMT and reversed the upregulation of different target genes associated with EMT. EGCG inhibited TGFβ1-mediated activation of p300/CBP. EGCG inhibited TGFβ1-mediated EMT by interfering with the acetylated state of SMAD2 and SMAD3 in lung cancer cells [42].

TGFβ potently induced epithelial–mesenchymal transition (EMT) in NSCLC cells but EGCG reversed TGFβ-induced morphological alterations [43]. EGCG upregulated the expression of E-cadherin and downregulated the expression of vimentin. Data obtained through immunofluorescence also provided clear clues that E-cadherin was upregulated, and vimentin was downregulated by EGCG [43]. Moreover, EGCG effectively inhibited TGFβ-induced migratory and invasive potential of NSCLC cells. EGCG inhibited TGFβ-induced EMT at the transcriptional level. Expectedly, EGCG reduced phosphorylated levels of ERK1/2 (extracellular signal-regulated protein kinases 1/2) and SMAD2 and also inhibited the accumulation of SMAD2 in the nucleus. EGCG repressed the expression of transcriptional factors Slug, Snail, Twist, and ZEB1 and upregulated E-cadherin expression (Figure 3) [43].

Interestingly, different peptide aptamers have been designed to effectively inhibit interaction of SMAD2 and SMAD3 with SMAD4. Therefore, it might be advantageous to combine EGCG with different TGFβ signaling inhibitors to inhibit tumor growth in xenografted mice. More importantly, it will also be exciting to evaluate EGCG-mediated regulation of negative regulators (SMURFs and NEDDs) of the TGF/SMAD pathway.

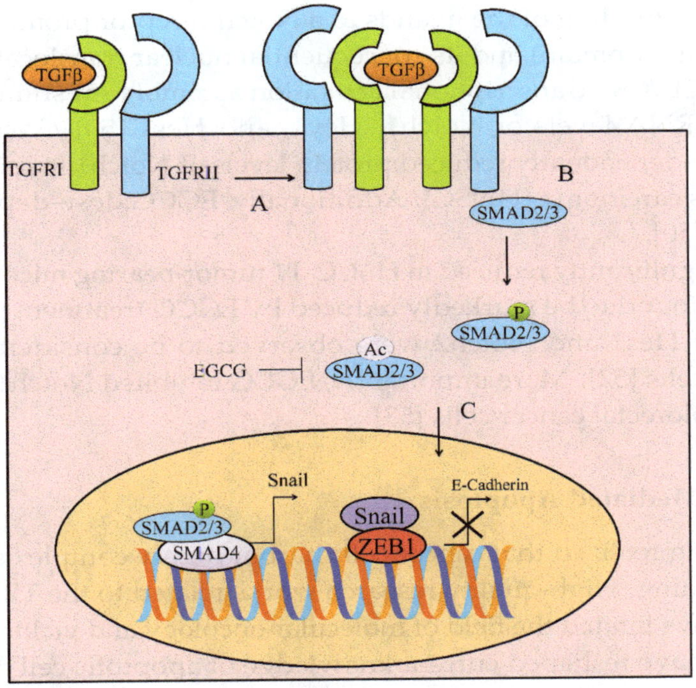

Figure 3. (**A**,**B**) Binding of TGFβ superfamily ligands to a type II receptor induced juxtapositioning of type I receptor. Phosphorylation of SMAD2/3 promoted its accumulation in the nucleus. SMAD2/3 have been shown to stimulate expression of Snail and Slug. Apart from phosphorylation, additional post-translational modifications, particularly acetylation, have also been observed in TGF/SMAD signaling. EGCG inhibited acetylation of SMAD proteins.

6. Regulation of Wnt/β-Catenin Pathway

Detailed mechanistic insights revealed that in the absence of Wnt signal, β-catenin was phosphorylated by APC (adenomatous polyposis coli)/Axin/GSK3β complex and degraded by proteasome [44]. However, activation of the membrane receptors by Wnt signal resulted in the phosphorylation and degradation of GSK3β. EGCG inhibited phosphorylation of GSK3β, upregulated GSK3β expression, and decreased the levels of β-catenin in colorectal cancer cells [44].

O^6-methylguanine (O6-meG) DNA-methyltransferase (MGMT) is a versatile mediator of temozolomide resistance in glioblastomas. TCF/LEF-binding sites within the promoter region of the MGMT gene have previously been identified [45]. Intriguingly, there is evidence of regulation of MGMT by WNT/β-catenin signaling. EGCG not only prevented translocation of β-catenin into the nucleus but also reduced the levels of transcriptional factors TCF1 and LEF1 [46]. Overall these findings clearly suggested that EGCG repressed MGMT expression via inhibition of the β-catenin-driven pathway.

EGCG not only reduced mRNA levels and transcriptional activities of β-catenin in p53 wild-type-expressing KB cells but also promoted ubiquitylation and degradation of β-catenin [47]. EGCG dose-dependently suppressed β-catenin expression in MDA-MB-231 cells [48]. EGCG worked synergistically with gemcitabine and exerted stronger inhibitory effects on β-catenin and N-cadherin in pancreatic cancer cells [49].

Clinical trials of CWP232291 (NCT01398462) and PRI-724 (NCT01302405; NCT01764477) are providing important clinically relevant information and it will be interesting to combine these agents with EGCG for evaluation of robust inhibition of β-catenin-driven signaling and tumor growth inhibitory effects in xenografted mice.

7. Regulation of Notch Pathway

The Notch signaling pathway consists of the Notch receptor, Notch ligand, DNA-binding protein, and Notch regulatory molecules. Notch is a transmembrane protein that mediates communication between neighboring cells. Binding of the ligands to a Notch receptor promoted proteolytic cleavage of NICD (Notch intracellular domain) and its consequential nuclear translocation where it complexed with CSL and formed NICD/CSL transcriptional activation assembly for stimulation of HES and HEY.

EGCG decreased mRNA levels of Notch1, Hey1, and Hes1 [50]. Western blot assay clearly indicated that EGCG dose-dependently reduced protein levels of Notch1 in cancer stem cells (CSCs) of head and neck squamous carcinoma (HNSC). Additionally, EGCG dose-dependently decreased the Notch promoter activity [50].

Tumor growth was significantly reduced in HuCC-T1 tumor-bearing mice subcutaneously injected with EGCG. Notch1 was found to be markedly reduced by EGCG treatment [51].

Expression levels of Hes1 and Notch2 were observed to be considerably reduced in EGCG treated colorectal cancer cells [52]. More importantly, EGCG inhibited Notch1 and cleaved-Notch1 in 5-fluorouracil-resistant colorectal cancer cells [53].

8. Regulation of TRAIL Mediated Apoptosis

Increasingly it is being realized that cancer cells harbor highly complex signaling networks that resist apoptotic programming. High-quality research works related to the TRAIL-mediated pathway in the past two decades have ignited the field of molecular oncology and yielded a stream of preclinical and clinical insights that have reshaped current knowledge of apoptotic cell death.

GCG and TRAIL synergistically reduced Bcl-XL, Bcl-2, and FLIP. Whereas, combinatorial treatment activated capase-8, -9, and -3 in nasopharyngeal carcinoma cells [54].

EGCG and TRAIL also worked effectively against renal cell carcinoma and pancreatic cancer cells [55,56].

EGCG restored sensitivity of HCC cells to TRAIL-induced apoptosis [57]. EGCG upregulated caspase-3 activity and simultaneously downregulated Bcl-2 levels. EGCG also induced upregulation of DR4 and DR5 [57]. EGCG and TRAIL robustly enhanced DR4 levels. Furthermore, FLIP levels were reduced in prostate cancer cells treated in combination with EGCG and TRAIL [58]. Collectively these findings suggested that EGCG might be helpful in increasing the protein levels as well as cell surface expression of death receptors. There is sufficient experimental evidence related to reduction in the cell surface levels of death receptors. Death receptors are internalized and degraded in various cancers. Therefore, EGCG might play its role in stabilizing the levels of death receptors.

PEA15 (phosphoprotein-enriched in astrocytes) is an oncoprotein [59]. It has previously been reported that AKT-induced PEA15 phosphorylation and increased its stability. EGCG downregulated PEA levels mainly through inactivation of AKT. However, overexpression of PEA15 severely impaired apoptotic cell death induced by EGCG and TRAIL [59].

Certain hints had emerged which highlighted that EGCG inhibited TRAIL-induced apoptosis and activated autophagic flux in colon cancer cells. Inhibition of autophagic flux induced death receptor-driven apoptosis in colon cancer cells [60].

These scientific findings are intriguing and future research must converge on identification of additional protein targets in the TRAIL-driven pathway. Essentially, the TRAIL mediated pathway is regulated by long non-coding RNAs as well. Therefore, it will be paramount to unravel underlying mechanisms of TRAIL resistance and identification of proteins, which can be targeted to restore apoptosis in TRAIL-resistant cancers. Keeping in view the fact that TRAIL-based therapeutics and death receptor-targeting agonistic antibodies have entered into various phases of clinical trials, any progress in improving the efficacy of TRAIL-based therapeutics will be advantageous.

9. Regulation of Non-Coding RNAs by EGCG in Different Cancers

Discovery of non-coding RNAs has revolutionized our current understanding of the mechanisms that regulate post-transcriptional processes. The field of non-coding RNA has been extensively explored and researchers have witnessed groundbreaking advancements in disentangling the complicated web ranging from biogenesis of non-coding RNAs to post-transcriptional regulation of a myriad of target mRNAs.

A wealth of information has unveiled a fundamental role of non-coding RNAs in different cancers and researchers have experimentally verified the effects of natural and synthetic products on wide-ranging microRNAs and long non-coding RNAs in different cancers.

9.1. Tumor Suppressor miRNAs

miR-485, a tumor suppressor microRNA, has been found to be frequently downregulated in various cancers. CD44 was directly targeted by miR-485 in A549-cisplatin resistant lung cancer cells. CD44 was overexpressed in A549-cisplatin resistant lung cancer cells but EGCG treatment exerted repressive effects on CD44 levels by enhancing miR-485-mediated targeting of CD44 [61]. EGCG also induced regression of tumors in mice xenografted with A549-cisplatin resistant lung cancer cells.

miR-485-5p directly targeted RXRα in drug-resistant lung cancer cells. EGCG repressed CSC-like properties via modulation of the miR-485-5p/RXRα axis [62]. miR-155 is a tumor suppressor miRNA reportedly involved in enhancing drug sensitivity of cancer cells [63]. EGCG promoted NF-κB mediated upregulation of miR-155. Resultantly, miR-155 enhanced drug sensitivity of colorectal cancer cells by directly targeting MDR1 [63]. IGF2BP1 and IGF2BP3 are direct targets of miR-1275 in different cancers [64]. EGCG stimulated the expression of miR-1275 and potentiated targeting of IGF2BP1 and IGF2BP3 by miR-1275 in HCC cells [65].

9.2. Oncogenic miRNAs

miR-221/222 played a central role in drug resistance. Knockdown of miR-221/222 inhibited proliferation of drug-resistant breast cancer cells [66]

Suberoylanilide hydroxamic acid (SAHA), an HDAC inhibitor worked effectively with EGCG and markedly reduced expression of miR-221/222 in triple-negative breast cancer cells [67].

9.3. Targeting of Oncogenic LncRNAs

SOX2OT variant 7 effectively promoted Notch3/DLL3 signaling in osteosarcoma stem cells (OSCs) [68]. NOTCH target genes HEY1 and HES1 were found to be notably enhanced in variant 7-expressing OSCs. EGCG efficiently inhibited the levels of HEY1 and HES1 in OSCs. However, EGCG mediated inhibitory effects were noted to be impaired in variant 7-expressing cells [68]. EGCG mediated tumor regression was not observed in mice xenografted with variant 7-expressing OSCs. However, EGCG treatment and NOTCH3 knockdown induced reduction in tumor growth in mice inoculated with variant 7-expressing OSCs [68].

EGCG also downregulated lncRNA-AF085935 in HCC cells. It was suggested that lncRNA-AF085935 promoted proliferation of HCC cells [69]. However, the study did not clearly provide a link between lncRNA-AF085935 and its targets and how lncRNA-AF085935 regulated apoptosis and proliferation in HCC cells.

9.4. Tumor Suppressor LncRNAs

EGCG had been shown to induce the expression of cisplatin transporter CTR1 (copper transporter 1) in cancer cells [70]. EGCG upregulated CTR1 and enhanced accumulation of intracellular platinum in NSCLC cells. hsa-miR-98-5p suppressed CTR1, whereas NEAT1 (nuclear enriched abundant transcript 1) enhanced its expression. hsa-miR-98-5p had specific complementary binding sites for NEAT1. Essentially, NEAT1 acted as a competitive endogenous RNA and upregulated EGCG-triggered CTR1 by sponging away hsa-miR-98-5p in NSCLC cells [70].

It seems surprising to note that available scientific proof related to regulation of non-coding RNAs by EGCG is limited. Keeping in view the wealth of information about remarkable pharmacological properties of EGCG, it is paramount to uncover how EGCG modulated different miRNAs, lncRNA, and circular RNAs in different cancers. Identification of the list of tumor suppressor and oncogenic non-coding RNAs regulated by EGCG in different cancers will be highly valuable in combinatorial treatments.

10. Nanotechnological Approaches for Effective Delivery of EGCG to the Target Sites

Despite the ability of EGCG to modulate several cancer-related mechanisms there are still major hurdles for the establishment of EGCG in clinical settings. The therapeutic concentrations of EGCG (between 1 and 10 μM) in the majority of the studies are much higher than the concentrations monitored in the plasma or tissues of animals or in human plasma (usually lower than 1 μM) after tea ingestion. In fact, even after the consumption of 7–9 cups of tea the EGCG concentration in plasma was still lower than 1 μM [71] and for that reason the use of nanotechnology, particularly the development of nanoparticles (NPs) as drug delivery systems, represent a promising approach to increase the bioavailability of EGCG. Nanotechnology corresponds to the science that studies and creates materials with dimensions between 1 and 1000 nm. NPs have at least one of the dimensions in the nanoscale range [72]. There are several types of NPs and for more comprehensive and detailed information the reader can consult the following revisions [73–76]. The different properties of the NPs can be used for medical purposes. Due to their small scale, NPs are excellent drug carriers, and since they can be modified in various factors such as size, chemical composition, outer layer, and others they are very versatile [77]. Furthermore, NPs can modify the pharmacokinetics and the stability of the carrier compound, being, for that reason, a promising strategy to improve EGCG bioavailability profile [78]. Another interesting characteristic of NPs is the possibility to enhance the cellular uptake or even the cellular targeting by modifying the outer layer with different ligands expressed in the target cells to assign particular characteristics in a strategy known by active targeting [79]. This is a useful strategy to improve the bioavailability and stability of EGCG even further, enhancing the utilization options and ultimately enhancing the anti-cancer properties of EGCG. The main types of NPs used for the delivery of EGCG reported in the literature are gold, polymeric, lipid-based, and inorganic NPs (shown in Figure 4). The majority of the NPs are designed to be at the range of approximately 200 nm since this size allows the administration of the NPs by the oral and intravenous routes. Other types of NPs were also used for the encapsulation of EGCG for the purpose of cancer therapy, including carbohydrates, transition metals, and inorganic materials [80–82]. The use of targeting ligands further increased cancer cell specificity and improved the anti-tumor effects of EGCG and, for that reason, folic acid has been used frequently to functionalize the NPs, since the folic acid receptor is overexpressed in tumor cells.

However, other ligands can also be used, including antibodies, carbohydrates, or polysaccharides and other molecules [83]. A summary of the studies using different EGCG nanocarriers for cancer management and carried out in cell lines and in animals is depicted in Table 1.

Table 1. Different types of EGCG nanocarriers for cancer management.

Type of Nanoparticles	Route of Administration	Target Organ	Outcome	Ref.
Gold	Oral, intra-tumoral and intra-peritoneal	Bladder	Tumor volume reduction in a bladder xenograft model	[84]
Gold	Intra-tumoral	Skin	Tumor volume reduction in a melanoma cells in a mouse model	[85]
Gold	N/A	Autonomic nervous system	Induction of apoptosis in neuroblastoma cells	[86]
Gold	N/A	Liver	Toxicity in tumor cells and protection of normal mouse hepatocytes	[87]
Polymeric	N/A	Prostate	Toxicity in prostate cancer cell line	[88]
Polymeric	N/A	Colon and rectum	DNA damage levels in samples of lymphocytes from colorectal cancer patients	[89]
Polymeric	N/A	Breast	Toxicity in breast cancer cell line and patient-derived cells	[90]
Polymeric	Intra-tumoral	Prostate	Tumor size reduction in mice model of prostate cancer	[91]
Polymeric	Oral	Prostate	Tumor size reduction in mice model of prostate cancer	[92]
Polymeric	Oral	Skin	Toxicity in human melanoma cells	[93]
Polymeric	N/A	Stomach and intestine	Anti-tumoral activity in gastrointestinal cancer cell line	[94]
Polymeric	N/A	Breast	Inhibition of breast cancer cell line viability	[95]
Lipid-based	Topic and intra-tumoral	Skin	Accumulation of EGCG in the tissues in a mice model of basal cell carcinoma	[96]
Lipid-based	Intra-tumoral	Skin	Apoptosis in a mice model of basal cell carcinoma	[97]
Lipid-based	N/A	Breast	Anti-proliferative and pro-apoptotic effect in a breast cancer cell line	[98]
Lipid-based	N/A	Breast	Cell apoptosis and cell invasion inhibition in a breast cancer cell line	[99]
Sugar-based	N/A	Prostate	Cell viability inhibition in a prostate cancer cell line	[80]
Inorganic	Intra-tumoral	Liver	Tumor growth reduction in a mouse model of liver cancer	[81]
Inorganic	N/A	Prostate	Anti-tumoral activity in prostate cell line	[82]

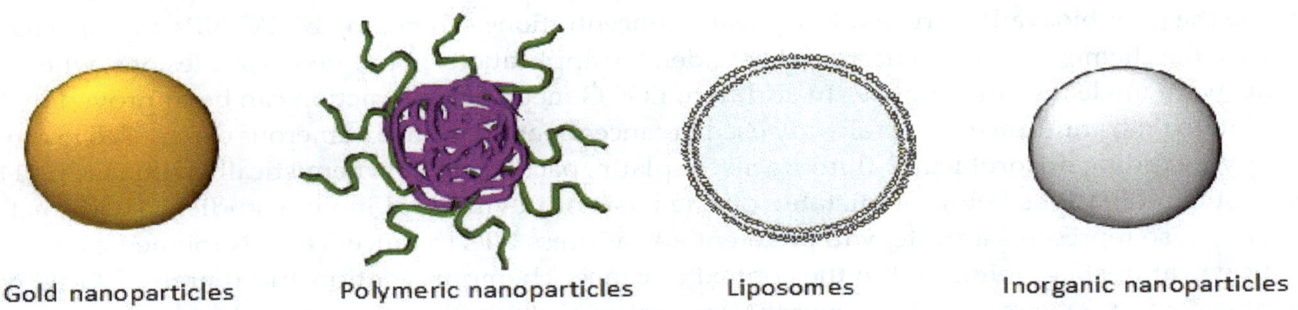

Figure 4. Main types of nanoparticles (NPs) used for the delivery of EGCG.

Gold NPs as EGCG delivery systems have been exploited in several types of cancer since gold has anti-cancer properties per se [85,100]. Several reports have described the in vitro and in vivo efficacy of gold NPs in conjugation with EGCG for cancer treatment, including for the bladder, melanoma, neuroblastoma, and hepatocarcinoma [84–87]. These nanocarriers also demonstrated a high biocompatibility, inducing low damage to human red blood cells and therefore no toxicity for the dose tested was observed. The NPs made of polymers approved and recognized as safe by the US Food and Drug Administration (FDA) are also suitable for cancer applications [89,101]. Several groups have already encapsulated EGCG into different polymeric NPs for cancer therapy, including for the treatment of prostate cancer, colorectal, breast cancer, melanoma, and gastrointestinal cancer [88–95]. Despite the high toxicity towards cancer cells these NPs demonstrated absence of toxicity for normal cells. Liposomes and lipid NPs are lipid-based NPs in composition and for that reason are biodegradable and present minimal levels of toxicity [97]. There are some studies reporting the use of lipid-nanocarriers for the delivery of EGCG to cancer cells [96–99]. All of the studies were used for the treatment of breast cancer with results that demonstrated efficacy and security in vitro and in vivo, including in the MDA-MB-231 cell line, which is a model of the triple-negative cancer and considered more aggressive and associated with poorer outcome than other types of breast cancer.

11. Potential Clinical Applications

EGCG drug delivery systems based in NPs might represent an extraordinary resource to improve the application of EGCG in chemoprevention or to introduce the use of EGCG in the therapy of cancer. The idea of using drug delivery systems, such as NPs for loading EGCG, preserving its structure, and allowing to circumvent the limitations of the low bioavailability associated with the oral administration of free EGCG has a tremendous potentiality since increasing the amount of EGCG inside the cells will potentialize the effect of EGCG in the molecular targets and the effect of deregulated oncogenic signaling cascades and, therefore, determine better cancer outcomes in comparison with free EGCG. For instance, EGCG loaded in polylactic acid–polyethylene glycol NPs preserved the biological activity and efficacy on molecular targets in vitro and in xenograft tumors with over 10-fold dose advantage in comparison with EGCG alone [91]. Indeed, in vitro and in vivo studies are mandatory to verify whether EGCG loaded in NPs maintain EGCG mechanism of action and to understand if the efficacy on molecular targets is at least retained or increased. In view of a safe application, the toxicity of engineered NPs associated with EGCG needs to be fully investigated. For instance, transition metal oxide NPs have been found to increase oxidative stress, disturb calcium homeostasis, and deregulate cell cycle [102]. The activation of the immune system, specifically macrophage activation and cytokine release has been also reported [103]. Thus, lipid-based NPs show higher level of biocompatibility and bioavailability, emerging as the best candidates for pharmaceutical and clinical applications. In this context, EGCG loaded solid lipid NPs as an oral delivery system did not show any toxicity in rats [104]. Different nanoformulations, including EGCG, also showed great biocompatibility with no or very modest toxicity in animal models [105,106]. All these findings encourage the efforts to invest in biocompatible EGCG NPs to be used on humans, as interventional studies in pre-cancerous lesions, including prostate, breast, colon, and Barret's Esophagus [107–110] demonstrated EGCG efficacy despite the poor bioavailability and low plasma concentrations. Therefore, EGCG NPs are expected to improve the chemopreventive effects and to widen the applications in pre-neoplastic lesions, where the results were unclear or incomplete. In addition, EGCG mechanism of action can be improved by the association with anti-cancer drugs already used in cancer treatment since numerous drugs used in cancer therapy, including doxorubicin, 5-flurouracile, cisplatin, paclitaxel, act synergistically with EGCG [111], the best combinations being predictable on the basis of in vitro and in vivo studies. Lastly, active targeting also represents a strategy to preferentially address NPs to cancer cells. Nanomedicine-based therapy is at the beginning, but in the context of cancer chemoprevention and therapy, EGCG NPs might become a powerful strategy over the conventional chemotherapy approach.

Clinical Trials Evaluating EGCG

Given the promising reports from preclinical studies, EGCG has been tested in various clinical studies. Postmenopausal women are at high risk of developing breast cancer and, therefore, EGCG safety clinical trials have been conducted targeting this population. EGCG can afford benefit in terms of regulating LDL-cholesterol as well as glucose and insulin, as reported by a double-blind, randomized, placebo-controlled intervention study in healthy postmenopausal women [112]. A subsequent ancillary study of a double-blind, randomized, placebo-controlled, parallel-arm trial further confirmed the benefit of EGCG but reported the total cholesterol levels reductions only in women with elevated baseline levels [113]. In postmenopausal women, a daily dose of 843 mg EGCG has been reported to be generally well-tolerated with only a small fraction (6.7%) of women reporting adverse events [114]. This dose of 843 mg EGCG, when administered for a year, can reduce mammographic density in relatively younger women (50–55 years) but not in postmenopausal women, as suggested by phase II trial [115]. Not only in breast cancer patients or women at high breast cancer risk, EGCG is well-tolerated by chronic lymphocytic leukemia (CLL) patients as well [116]. Further, EGCG, at a daily dose as low as 44.9 mg for 4 weeks prior to surgery, has been reported to result in increased bioavailability, including accumulations in breast tumor tissue, in early stage breast cancer patients [108].

A randomized trial reported no reduction in likelihood of prostate cancer in men with high-grade prostatic intraepithelial neoplasia, compared to placebo, after a year on 400 mg EGCG dose per day [117]. It is possible that this might be related to the dose tested in this study as a previous study which tested the effects of 800 mg EGCG administered to 26 patients with positive prostate biopsies reported significant reductions in PSA, HGF, and VEGF, with no associated liver toxicity [118]. Similarly, a phase II pharmacodynamic prevention trial in bladder cancer patients indicated a possible reduction in PCNA and clusterin levels upon 2–4 weeks administration of EGCG prior to transurethral resection of bladder tumor or cystectomy [119].

EGCG has been tested in cancer clinical trials not just for the direct anticancer effects, but also for possible effects on co-morbidities. In lung cancer patients with an unresectable stage III disease, a phase I study was conducted to evaluate the efficacy of EGCG against chemotherapy related esophagitis [120]. Patients, divided in six cohorts receiving six different doses of EGCG, were administered EGCG once grade 2 esophagitis occurred. The study reported dramatic regression of esophagitis to grade 0/1 in 22 of 24 patients (91.7% cases), thus underlying the effectiveness of EGCG. On similar lines, a prospective phase II trial confirmed that EGCG can be effective against acute radiation-induced esophagitis as well [121]. Topical administration of EGCG to the radiation field, post-mastectomy and radiotherapy, can resolve radiation dermatitis, as revealed in a phase I study [122].

12. Concluding Remarks

Recent breakthroughs in novel single-cell profiling and spatial transcriptomics have leveraged our understanding to a new level and helped us to find new answers to a critical question of how cancers move through space and time. Importantly, with rapidly increasing sensitivity of detection methods, we also require novel approaches to conceptually analyze single-cell data with observations at the tissue and organ level.

We have developed a near to complete understanding of VEGF/VEGFR signaling pathways. Studies have shown that relative abundance of the cell surface expression of various VEGFRs and their affiliations for specific VEGF ligands play a fundamental role in the initial set of dimeric constellations. Deeper knowledge of this multifaceted signaling web is key to result-oriented therapeutic targeting. Likewise, EGCG mediated targeting of Wnt/β-catenin has been explored and it needs to be tested comprehensively in different types of cancers. Henceforth xenografted mice bearing β-catenin-overexpressing cancer cells will be helpful in uncovering the true potential of EGCG. Likewise, there is a need to unveil if EGCG inhibited β-catenin activation by functionalization of negative regulators of Wnt signaling. Accordingly, TGF/SMAD signaling regulation by EGCG needs to be addressed more conceptually. Inhibition of SMAD phosphorylation by EGCG is a single dimension of this highly intricate mechanism. Available evidence enlightens involvement of SMURFs and NEDDs in inhibition of TGF/SMAD signaling. Therefore, additional key players of TGF/SMAD signaling also need in-depth research. Regulation of Notch signaling by EGCG seems to be sparsely studied. Therefore, we still have incomplete information about targeting of proteolytically cleaved segment of Notch-intracellular domain (NICD) in regulation of the target gene network. Does EGCG inhibit NICD nuclear accumulation or whether it also interferes with repressor/co-repressor and activator/co-activator machinery needs more answers. On a similar note, SHH/Gli pathway regulation by EGCG requires initial cellular studies. Furthermore, Gli-overexpressing cancers have to be treated with EGCG and combinatorial treatments.

Despite the absence of clinical trials, the NPs loaded with EGCG might be an efficient and safe strategy for the treatment of several cancers, especially breast and prostate cancer. Thus, clinical trials should be conducted to establish the clinical potential of the NPs loaded with EGCG alone or in addition with the conventional anti-cancer drugs.

Author Contributions: Conceptualization, A.A.F. and M.P.; Writing Original Draft Preparation, A.A.F., M.P., A.G., F.F., S.R., R.A., U.Y.S., B.X., A.A.; Writing Review & Editing, A.A.F., M.P., A.G., F.F., S.R., R.A., U.Y.S., B.X., A.A.; Visualization, A.A.F., M.P., A.G., F.F., S.R., R.A., U.Y.S., B.X., A.A.; Supervision, A.A.F. and M.P.; Funding and Acquisition. M.P. and S.R. All authors have read and agreed to the published version of the manuscript.

Acknowledgments: This work received financial support from the European Union (FEDER funds through COMPETE POCI-01-0145-FEDER-30624) and National Funds (FCT, Fundação para a Ciência e Tecnologia) through project PTDC/BTM-MAT/30624/2017. Marina Pinheiro thanks FCT for funding through program DL 57/2016—Norma transitória. Andreia Granja thanks FCT and POPH (Programa Operacional Potencial Humano) for the PhD grant (SFRH/BD/130147/2017). This work was also supported by FCT through the FCT PhD Programs, specifically by the BiotechHealth Program (Doctoral Program on Cellular and Molecular Biotechnology Applied to Health Sciences).

References

1. Yang, C.S.; Wang, X.; Lu, G.; Picinich, S.C. Cancer prevention by tea: Animal studies, molecular mechanisms and human relevance. *Nat. Rev. Cancer* **2009**, *9*, 429–439. [CrossRef] [PubMed]
2. Tauber, A.L.; Schweiker, S.S.; Levonis, S.M. From tea to treatment; epigallocatechin gallate and its potential involvement in minimizing the metabolic changes in cancer. *Nutr. Res.* **2020**, *74*, 23–36. [CrossRef] [PubMed]
3. Saeki, K.; Hayakawa, S.; Nakano, S.; Ito, S.; Oishi, Y.; Suzuki, Y.; Isemura, M. In Vitro and In Silico Studies of the Molecular Interactions of Epigallocatechin-3-O-gallate (EGCG) with Proteins That Explain the Health Benefits of Green Tea. *Molecules* **2018**, *23*, 1295. [CrossRef] [PubMed]
4. Negri, A.; Naponelli, V.; Rizzi, F.; Bettuzzi, S. Molecular Targets of Epigallocatechin-Gallate (EGCG): A Special Focus on Signal Transduction and Cancer. *Nutrients* **2018**, *10*, 1936. [CrossRef] [PubMed]
5. Cheng, C.W.; Shieh, P.C.; Lin, Y.C.; Chen, Y.J.; Lin, Y.H.; Kuo, D.H.; Liu, J.Y.; Kao, J.Y.; Kao, M.C.; Way, T.D. Indoleamine 2,3-dioxygenase, an immunomodulatory protein, is suppressed by (-)-epigallocatechin-3-gallate via blocking of gamma-interferon-induced JAK-PKC-delta-STAT1 signaling in human oral cancer cells. *J. Agric. Food Chem.* **2010**, *58*, 887–894. [CrossRef]
6. Jung, J.H.; Yun, M.; Choo, E.J.; Kim, S.H.; Jeong, M.S.; Jung, D.B.; Lee, H.; Kim, E.O.; Kato, N.; Kim, B.; et al. A derivative of epigallocatechin-3-gallate induces apoptosis via SHP-1-mediated suppression of BCR-ABL and STAT3 signalling in chronic myelogenous leukaemia. *Br. J. Pharmacol.* **2015**, *172*, 3565–3578. [CrossRef]
7. Xiao, X.; Jiang, K.; Xu, Y.; Peng, H.; Wang, Z.; Liu, S.; Zhang, G. (-)-Epigallocatechin-3-gallate induces cell apoptosis in chronic myeloid leukaemia by regulating Bcr/Abl-mediated p38-MAPK/JNK and JAK2/STAT3/AKT signalling pathways. *Clin. Exp. Pharmacol. Physiol.* **2019**, *46*, 126–136. [CrossRef]
8. Jin, G.; Yang, Y.; Liu, K.; Zhao, J.; Chen, X.; Liu, H.; Bai, R.; Li, X.; Jiang, Y.; Zhang, X.; et al. Combination curcumin and (-)-epigallocatechin-3-gallate inhibits colorectal carcinoma microenvironment-induced angiogenesis by JAK/STAT3/IL-8 pathway. *Oncogenesis* **2017**, *6*, e384. [CrossRef]

9. Yuan, C.H.; Horng, C.T.; Lee, C.F.; Chiang, N.N.; Tsai, F.J.; Lu, C.C.; Chiang, J.H.; Hsu, Y.M.; Yang, J.S.; Chen, F.A. Epigallocatechin gallate sensitizes cisplatin-resistant oral cancer CAR cell apoptosis and autophagy through stimulating AKT/STAT3 pathway and suppressing multidrug resistance 1 signaling. *Environ. Toxicol.* **2017**, *32*, 845–855. [CrossRef]
10. Huang, R.; Faratian, D.; Sims, A.H.; Wilson, D.; Thomas, J.S.; Harrison, D.J.; Langdon, S.P. Increased STAT1 signaling in endocrine-resistant breast cancer. *PLoS ONE* **2014**, *9*, e94226. [CrossRef]
11. Tian, M.; Tian, D.; Qiao, X.; Li, J.; Zhang, L. Modulation of Myb-induced NF-kB-STAT3 signaling and resulting cisplatin resistance in ovarian cancer by dietary factors. *J. Cell. Physiol.* **2019**, *234*, 21126–21134. [CrossRef] [PubMed]
12. Senggunprai, L.; Kukongviriyapan, V.; Prawan, A.; Kukongviriyapan, U. Quercetin and EGCG exhibit chemopreventive effects in cholangiocarcinoma cells via suppression of JAK/STAT signaling pathway. *Phytother. Res. PTR* **2014**, *28*, 841–848. [CrossRef] [PubMed]
13. Ogawa, K.; Hara, T.; Shimizu, M.; Nagano, J.; Ohno, T.; Hoshi, M.; Ito, H.; Tsurumi, H.; Saito, K.; Seishima, M.; et al. (-)-Epigallocatechin gallate inhibits the expression of indoleamine 2,3-dioxygenase in human colorectal cancer cells. *Oncol. Lett.* **2012**, *4*, 546–550. [CrossRef] [PubMed]
14. Borse, V.; Al Aameri, R.F.H.; Sheehan, K.; Sheth, S.; Kaur, T.; Mukherjea, D.; Tupal, S.; Lowy, M.; Ghosh, S.; Dhukhwa, A.; et al. Epigallocatechin-3-gallate, a prototypic chemopreventative agent for protection against cisplatin-based ototoxicity. *Cell Death Dis.* **2017**, *8*, e2921. [CrossRef] [PubMed]
15. Rawangkan, A.; Wongsirisin, P.; Namiki, K.; Iida, K.; Kobayashi, Y.; Shimizu, Y.; Fujiki, H.; Suganuma, M. Green Tea Catechin Is an Alternative Immune Checkpoint Inhibitor that Inhibits PD-L1 Expression and Lung Tumor Growth. *Molecules* **2018**, *23*, 2071. [CrossRef] [PubMed]
16. Mirzaaghaei, S.; Foroughmand, A.M.; Saki, G.; Shafiei, M. Combination of Epigallocatechin-3-gallate and Silibinin: A Novel Approach for Targeting Both Tumor and Endothelial Cells. *ACS Omega* **2019**, *4*, 8421–8430. [CrossRef]
17. Perez-Moral, N.; Needs, P.W.; Moyle, C.W.A.; Kroon, P.A. Hydrophobic Interactions Drive Binding between Vascular Endothelial Growth Factor-A (VEGFA) and Polypheolic Inhibitors. *Molecules* **2019**, *24*, 2785. [CrossRef]
18. Kumar, B.N.P.; Puvvada, N.; Rajput, S.; Sarkar, S.; Mahto, M.K.; Yallapu, M.M.; Pathak, A.; Emdad, L.; Das, S.K.; Reis, R.L.; et al. Targeting of EGFR, VEGFR2, and Akt by Engineered Dual Drug Encapsulated Mesoporous Silica-Gold Nanoclusters Sensitizes Tamoxifen-Resistant Breast Cancer. *Mol. Pharm.* **2018**, *15*, 2698–2713. [CrossRef]
19. Scandlyn, M.; Stuart, E.; Somers-Edgar, T.; Menzies, A.; Rosengren, R. A new role for tamoxifen in oestrogen receptor-negative breast cancer when it is combined with epigallocatechin gallate. *Brit. J. Cancer* **2008**, *99*, 1056–1063. [CrossRef]
20. Mohan, N.; Karmakar, S.; Banik, N.L.; Ray, S.K. SU5416 and EGCG work synergistically and inhibit angiogenic and survival factors and induce cell cycle arrest to promote apoptosis in human malignant neuroblastoma SH-SY5Y and SK-N-BE2 cells. *Neurochem. Res.* **2011**, *36*, 1383–1396. [CrossRef]
21. Shirakami, Y.; Shimizu, M.; Adachi, S.; Sakai, H.; Nakagawa, T.; Yasuda, Y.; Tsurumi, H.; Hara, Y.; Moriwaki, H. (-)-Epigallocatechin gallate suppresses the growth of human hepatocellular carcinoma cells by inhibiting activation of the vascular endothelial growth factor-vascular endothelial growth factor receptor axis. *Cancer Sci.* **2009**, *100*, 1957–1962. [CrossRef] [PubMed]
22. Shimizu, M.; Shirakami, Y.; Sakai, H.; Yasuda, Y.; Kubota, M.; Adachi, S.; Tsurumi, H.; Hara, Y.; Moriwaki, H. (-)-Epigallocatechin gallate inhibits growth and activation of the VEGF/VEGFR axis in human colorectal cancer cells. *Chem. Biol. Interact.* **2010**, *185*, 247–252. [CrossRef] [PubMed]
23. Lee, Y.K.; Shanafelt, T.D.; Bone, N.D.; Strege, A.K.; Jelinek, D.F.; Kay, N.E. VEGF receptors on chronic lymphocytic leukemia (CLL) B cells interact with STAT 1 and 3: Implication for apoptosis resistance. *Leukemia* **2005**, *19*, 513–523. [CrossRef] [PubMed]
24. Lee, Y.K.; Bone, N.D.; Strege, A.K.; Shanafelt, T.D.; Jelinek, D.F.; Kay, N.E. VEGF receptor phosphorylation status and apoptosis is modulated by a green tea component, epigallocatechin-3-gallate (EGCG), in B-cell chronic lymphocytic leukemia. *Blood* **2004**, *104*, 788–794. [CrossRef]
25. Deb, G.; Shankar, E.; Thakur, V.S.; Ponsky, L.E.; Bodner, D.R.; Fu, P.; Gupta, S. Green tea-induced epigenetic reactivation of tissue inhibitor of matrix metalloproteinase-3 suppresses prostate cancer progression through histone-modifying enzymes. *Mol. Carcinog.* **2019**, *58*, 1194–1207. [CrossRef]

26. Ying, L.; Yan, F.; Williams, B.R.; Xu, P.; Li, X.; Zhao, Y.; Hu, Y.; Wang, Y.; Xu, D.; Dai, J. (-)-Epigallocatechin-3-gallate and EZH2 inhibitor GSK343 have similar inhibitory effects and mechanisms of action on colorectal cancer cells. *Clin. Exp. Pharmacol. Physiol.* **2018**, *45*, 58–67. [CrossRef]
27. Schwartz, Y.B.; Pirrotta, V. A new world of Polycombs: Unexpected partnerships and emerging functions. *Nat. Rev. Genet.* **2013**, *14*, 853–864. [CrossRef]
28. Balasubramanian, S.; Adhikary, G.; Eckert, R.L. The Bmi-1 polycomb protein antagonizes the (-)-epigallocatechin-3-gallate-dependent suppression of skin cancer cell survival. *Carcinogenesis* **2010**, *31*, 496–503. [CrossRef]
29. De The, H.; Chen, Z. Acute promyelocytic leukaemia: Novel insights into the mechanisms of cure. *Nat. Rev. Cancer* **2010**, *10*, 775–783. [CrossRef]
30. Moradzadeh, M.; Roustazadeh, A.; Tabarraei, A.; Erfanian, S.; Sahebkar, A. Epigallocatechin-3-gallate enhances differentiation of acute promyelocytic leukemia cells via inhibition of PML-RARalpha and HDAC1. *Phytother. Res. PTR* **2018**, *32*, 471–479. [CrossRef]
31. Borutinskaite, V.; Virksaite, A.; Gudelyte, G.; Navakauskiene, R. Green tea polyphenol EGCG causes anti-cancerous epigenetic modulations in acute promyelocytic leukemia cells. *Leuk. Lymphoma* **2018**, *59*, 469–478. [CrossRef] [PubMed]
32. Khan, M.A.; Hussain, A.; Sundaram, M.K.; Alalami, U.; Gunasekera, D.; Ramesh, L.; Hamza, A.; Quraishi, U. (-)-Epigallocatechin-3-gallate reverses the expression of various tumor-suppressor genes by inhibiting DNA methyltransferases and histone deacetylases in human cervical cancer cells. *Oncol. Rep.* **2015**, *33*, 1976–1984. [CrossRef] [PubMed]
33. Thakur, V.S.; Gupta, K.; Gupta, S. Green tea polyphenols increase p53 transcriptional activity and acetylation by suppressing class I histone deacetylases. *Int. J. Oncol.* **2012**, *41*, 353–361. [CrossRef] [PubMed]
34. Oya, Y.; Mondal, A.; Rawangkan, A.; Umsumarng, S.; Iida, K.; Watanabe, T.; Kanno, M.; Suzuki, K.; Li, Z.; Kagechika, H.; et al. Down-regulation of histone deacetylase 4, -5 and -6 as a mechanism of synergistic enhancement of apoptosis in human lung cancer cells treated with the combination of a synthetic retinoid, Am80 and green tea catechin. *J. Nutr. Biochem.* **2017**, *42*, 7–16. [CrossRef]
35. Achour, M.; Mousli, M.; Alhosin, M.; Ibrahim, A.; Peluso, J.; Muller, C.D.; Schini-Kerth, V.B.; Hamiche, A.; Dhe-Paganon, S.; Bronner, C. Epigallocatechin-3-gallate up-regulates tumor suppressor gene expression via a reactive oxygen species-dependent down-regulation of UHRF1. *Biochem. Biophys. Res. Commun.* **2013**, *430*, 208–212. [CrossRef]
36. Nandakumar, V.; Vaid, M.; Katiyar, S.K. (-)-Epigallocatechin-3-gallate reactivates silenced tumor suppressor genes, Cip1/p21 and p16INK4a, by reducing DNA methylation and increasing histones acetylation in human skin cancer cells. *Carcinogenesis* **2011**, *32*, 537–544. [CrossRef]
37. Massague, J. How cells read TGF-beta signals. *Nat. Rev. Mol. Cell Biol.* **2000**, *1*, 169–178. [CrossRef]
38. Ikushima, H.; Miyazono, K. TGFbeta signalling: A complex web in cancer progression. *Nat. Rev. Cancer* **2010**, *10*, 415–424. [CrossRef]
39. Brandl, M.; Seidler, B.; Haller, F.; Adamski, J.; Schmid, R.M.; Saur, D.; Schneider, G. IKK(alpha) controls canonical TGF(ss)-SMAD signaling to regulate genes expressing SNAIL and SLUG during EMT in panc1 cells. *J. Cell Sci.* **2010**, *123*, 4231–4239. [CrossRef]
40. Sicard, A.A.; Dao, T.; Suarez, N.G.; Annabi, B. Diet-Derived Gallated Catechins Prevent TGF-beta-Mediated Epithelial-Mesenchymal Transition, Cell Migration and Vasculogenic Mimicry in Chemosensitive ES-2 Ovarian Cancer Cells. *Nutr. Cancer* **2020**, 1–12. [CrossRef]
41. Li, T.; Zhao, N.; Lu, J.; Zhu, Q.; Liu, X.; Hao, F.; Jiao, X. Epigallocatechin gallate (EGCG) suppresses epithelial-Mesenchymal transition (EMT) and invasion in anaplastic thyroid carcinoma cells through blocking of TGF-beta1/Smad signaling pathways. *Bioengineered* **2019**, *10*, 282–291. [CrossRef] [PubMed]
42. Ko, H.; So, Y.; Jeon, H.; Jeong, M.H.; Choi, H.K.; Ryu, S.H.; Lee, S.W.; Yoon, H.G.; Choi, K.C. TGF-beta1-induced epithelial-mesenchymal transition and acetylation of Smad2 and Smad3 are negatively regulated by EGCG in human A549 lung cancer cells. *Cancer Lett.* **2013**, *335*, 205–213. [CrossRef] [PubMed]
43. Liu, L.C.; Tsao, T.C.; Hsu, S.R.; Wang, H.C.; Tsai, T.C.; Kao, J.Y.; Way, T.D. EGCG inhibits transforming growth factor-beta-mediated epithelial-to-mesenchymal transition via the inhibition of Smad2 and Erk1/2 signaling pathways in nonsmall cell lung cancer cells. *J. Agric. Food Chem.* **2012**, *60*, 9863–9873. [CrossRef] [PubMed]

44. Chen, Y.; Wang, X.Q.; Zhang, Q.; Zhu, J.Y.; Li, Y.; Xie, C.F.; Li, X.T.; Wu, J.S.; Geng, S.S.; Zhong, C.Y.; et al. (-)-Epigallocatechin-3-Gallate Inhibits Colorectal Cancer Stem Cells by Suppressing Wnt/beta-Catenin Pathway. *Nutrients* **2017**, *9*, 572. [CrossRef]
45. Wickstrom, M.; Dyberg, C.; Milosevic, J.; Einvik, C.; Calero, R.; Sveinbjornsson, B.; Sanden, E.; Darabi, A.; Siesjo, P.; Kool, M.; et al. Wnt/beta-catenin pathway regulates MGMT gene expression in cancer and inhibition of Wnt signalling prevents chemoresistance. *Nat. Commun.* **2015**, *6*, 8904. [CrossRef]
46. Xie, C.R.; You, C.G.; Zhang, N.; Sheng, H.S.; Zheng, X.S. Epigallocatechin Gallate Preferentially Inhibits O(6)-Methylguanine DNA-Methyltransferase Expression in Glioblastoma Cells Rather than in Nontumor Glial Cells. *Nutr. Cancer* **2018**, *70*, 1339–1347. [CrossRef]
47. Shin, Y.S.; Kang, S.U.; Park, J.K.; Kim, Y.E.; Kim, Y.S.; Baek, S.J.; Lee, S.H.; Kim, C.H. Anti-cancer effect of (-)-epigallocatechin-3-gallate (EGCG) in head and neck cancer through repression of transactivation and enhanced degradation of beta-catenin. *Phytomedicine* **2016**, *23*, 1344–1355. [CrossRef]
48. Hong, O.-Y.; Noh, E.-M.; Jang, H.-Y.; Lee, Y.-R.; Lee, B.K.; Jung, S.H.; Kim, J.-S.; Youn, H.J. Epigallocatechin gallate inhibits the growth of MDA-MB-231 breast cancer cells via inactivation of the β-catenin signaling pathway. *Oncol. Lett.* **2017**, *14*, 441–446. [CrossRef]
49. Wei, R.; Penso, N.E.C.; Hackman, R.M.; Wang, Y.; Mackenzie, G.G. Epigallocatechin-3-Gallate (EGCG) Suppresses Pancreatic Cancer Cell Growth, Invasion, and Migration partly through the Inhibition of Akt Pathway and Epithelial-Mesenchymal Transition: Enhanced Efficacy when Combined with Gemcitabine. *Nutrients* **2019**, *11*, 1856. [CrossRef]
50. Lee, S.H.; Nam, H.J.; Kang, H.J.; Kwon, H.W.; Lim, Y.C. Epigallocatechin-3-gallate attenuates head and neck cancer stem cell traits through suppression of Notch pathway. *Eur. J. Cancer* **2013**, *49*, 3210–3218. [CrossRef]
51. Kwak, T.W.; Park, S.B.; Kim, H.-J.; Jeong, Y.-I.; Kang, D.H. Anticancer activities of epigallocatechin-3-gallate against cholangiocarcinoma cells. *Oncol. Targets Ther.* **2016**, *10*, 137–144. [CrossRef] [PubMed]
52. Jin, H.; Gong, W.; Zhang, C.; Wang, S. Epigallocatechin gallate inhibits the proliferation of colorectal cancer cells by regulating Notch signaling. *Oncol. Targets Ther.* **2013**, *6*, 145–153. [CrossRef] [PubMed]
53. Toden, S.; Tran, H.M.; Tovar-Camargo, O.A.; Okugawa, Y.; Goel, A. Epigallocatechin-3-gallate targets cancer stem-like cells and enhances 5-fluorouracil chemosensitivity in colorectal cancer. *Oncotarget* **2016**. [CrossRef] [PubMed]
54. Li, P.; Li, S.; Yin, D.; Li, J.; Wang, L.; Huang, C.; Yang, X. EGCG sensitizes human nasopharyngeal carcinoma cells to TRAIL-mediated apoptosis by activation NF-kappaB. *Neoplasma* **2017**, *64*, 74–80. [CrossRef]
55. Wei, R.; Zhu, G.; Jia, N.; Yang, W. Epigallocatechin-3-gallate Sensitizes Human 786-O Renal Cell Carcinoma Cells to TRAIL-Induced Apoptosis. *Cell Biochem. Biophys.* **2015**, *72*, 157–164. [CrossRef]
56. Basu, A.; Haldar, S. Combinatorial effect of epigallocatechin-3-gallate and TRAIL on pancreatic cancer cell death. *Int. J. Oncol.* **2009**, *34*, 281–286. [CrossRef]
57. Abou El Naga, R.N.; Azab, S.S.; El-Demerdash, E.; Shaarawy, S.; El-Merzabani, M.; Ammar el, S.M. Sensitization of TRAIL-induced apoptosis in human hepatocellular carcinoma HepG2 cells by phytochemicals. *Life Sci.* **2013**, *92*, 555–561. [CrossRef]
58. Siddiqui, I.A.; Malik, A.; Adhami, V.M.; Asim, M.; Hafeez, B.B.; Sarfaraz, S.; Mukhtar, H. Green tea polyphenol EGCG sensitizes human prostate carcinoma LNCaP cells to TRAIL-mediated apoptosis and synergistically inhibits biomarkers associated with angiogenesis and metastasis. *Oncogene* **2008**, *27*, 2055–2063. [CrossRef]
59. Siegelin, M.D.; Habel, A.; Gaiser, T. Epigalocatechin-3-gallate (EGCG) downregulates PEA15 and thereby augments TRAIL-mediated apoptosis in malignant glioma. *Neurosci. Lett.* **2008**, *448*, 161–165. [CrossRef]
60. Kim, S.W.; Moon, J.H.; Park, S.Y. Activation of autophagic flux by epigallocatechin gallate mitigates TRAIL-induced tumor cell apoptosis via down-regulation of death receptors. *Oncotarget* **2016**, *7*, 65660–65668. [CrossRef]
61. Jiang, P.; Xu, C.; Chen, L.; Chen, A.; Wu, X.; Zhou, M.; Haq, I.U.; Mariyam, Z.; Feng, Q. EGCG inhibits CSC-like properties through targeting miR-485/CD44 axis in A549-cisplatin resistant cells. *Mol. Carcinog.* **2018**, *57*, 1835–1844. [CrossRef] [PubMed]
62. Jiang, P.; Xu, C.; Chen, L.; Chen, A.; Wu, X.; Zhou, M.; Haq, I.U.; Mariyam, Z.; Feng, Q. Epigallocatechin-3-gallate inhibited cancer stem cell-like properties by targeting hsa-mir-485-5p/RXRalpha in lung cancer. *J. Cell Biochem.* **2018**, *119*, 8623–8635. [CrossRef] [PubMed]

63. La, X.; Zhang, L.; Li, Z.; Li, H.; Yang, Y. (-)-Epigallocatechin Gallate (EGCG) Enhances the Sensitivity of Colorectal Cancer Cells to 5-FU by Inhibiting GRP78/NF-kappaB/miR-155-5p/MDR1 Pathway. *J. Agric. Food Chem.* **2019**, *67*, 2510–2518. [CrossRef] [PubMed]
64. Fawzy, I.O.; Hamza, M.T.; Hosny, K.A.; Esmat, G.; El Tayebi, H.M.; Abdelaziz, A.I. miR-1275: A single microRNA that targets the three IGF2-mRNA-binding proteins hindering tumor growth in hepatocellular carcinoma. *FEBS Lett.* **2015**, *589*, 2257–2265. [CrossRef]
65. Shaalan, Y.M.; Handoussa, H.; Youness, R.A.; Assal, R.A.; El-Khatib, A.H.; Linscheid, M.W.; El Tayebi, H.M.; Abdelaziz, A.I. Destabilizing the interplay between miR-1275 and IGF2BPs by Tamarix articulata and quercetin in hepatocellular carcinoma. *Nat. Prod. Res.* **2018**, *32*, 2217–2220. [CrossRef]
66. Rao, X.; Di Leva, G.; Li, M.; Fang, F.; Devlin, C.; Hartman-Frey, C.; Burow, M.E.; Ivan, M.; Croce, C.M.; Nephew, K.P. MicroRNA-221/222 confers breast cancer fulvestrant resistance by regulating multiple signaling pathways. *Oncogene* **2011**, *30*, 1082–1097. [CrossRef]
67. Lewis, K.A.; Jordan, H.R.; Tollefsbol, T.O. Effects of SAHA and EGCG on Growth Potentiation of Triple-Negative Breast Cancer Cells. *Cancers* **2018**, *11*, 23. [CrossRef]
68. Wang, W.; Chen, D.; Zhu, K. SOX2OT variant 7 contributes to the synergistic interaction between EGCG and Doxorubicin to kill osteosarcoma via autophagy and stemness inhibition. *J. Exp. Clin. Cancer Res.* **2018**, *37*, 37. [CrossRef]
69. Sabry, D.; Abdelaleem, O.O.; El Amin Ali, A.M.; Mohammed, R.A.; Abdel-Hameed, N.D.; Hassouna, A.; Khalifa, W.A. Anti-proliferative and anti-apoptotic potential effects of epigallocatechin-3-gallate and/or metformin on hepatocellular carcinoma cells: In vitro study. *Mol. Biol. Rep.* **2019**, *46*, 2039–2047. [CrossRef]
70. Jiang, P.; Wu, X.; Wang, X.; Huang, W.; Feng, Q. NEAT1 upregulates EGCG-induced CTR1 to enhance cisplatin sensitivity in lung cancer cells. *Oncotarget* **2016**, *7*, 43337–43351. [CrossRef]
71. Peter, B.; Bosze, S.; Horvath, R. Biophysical characteristics of proteins and living cells exposed to the green tea polyphenol epigallocatechin-3-gallate (EGCg): Review of recent advances from molecular mechanisms to nanomedicine and clinical trials. *Eur. Biophys. J. EBJ* **2017**, *46*, 1–24. [CrossRef] [PubMed]
72. Nikalje, A.P. Nanotechnology and its applications in medicine. *Med. Chem.* **2015**, *5*, 081–089. [CrossRef]
73. Bhatia, S. Nanoparticles types, classification, characterization, fabrication methods and drug delivery applications. In *Natural Polymer Drug Delivery Systems*; Springer: Cham, Switzerland, 2016; pp. 33–93.
74. Senapati, S.; Mahanta, A.K.; Kumar, S.; Maiti, P. Controlled drug delivery vehicles for cancer treatment and their performance. *Signal. Transduct. Target. Ther.* **2018**, *3*, 7. [CrossRef] [PubMed]
75. Liu, W.T. Nanoparticles and their biological and environmental applications. *J. Biosci. Bioeng.* **2006**, *102*, 1–7. [CrossRef] [PubMed]
76. Yih, T.C.; Al-Fandi, M. Engineered nanoparticles as precise drug delivery systems. *J. Cell Biochem.* **2006**, *97*, 1184–1190. [CrossRef] [PubMed]
77. Sanvicens, N.; Marco, M.P. Multifunctional nanoparticles—Properties and prospects for their use in human medicine. *Trends Biotechnol.* **2008**, *26*, 425–433. [CrossRef]
78. Granja, A.; Frias, I.; Neves, A.R.; Pinheiro, M.; Reis, S. Therapeutic Potential of Epigallocatechin Gallate Nanodelivery Systems. *BioMed Res. Int.* **2017**, *2017*, 5813793. [CrossRef]
79. Cho, K.; Wang, X.U.; Nie, S.; Shin, D.M. Therapeutic nanoparticles for drug delivery in cancer. *Clin. Cancer Res.* **2008**, *14*, 1310–1316. [CrossRef]
80. Rocha, S.; Generalov, R.; Peres, I.; Juzenas, P. Epigallocatechin gallate-loaded polysaccharide nanoparticles for prostate cancer chemoprevention. *Nanomedicine* **2011**, *6*, 79–87. [CrossRef]
81. Zhou, Y.; Yu, Q.; Qin, X.; Bhavsar, D.; Yang, L.; Chen, Q.; Zheng, W.; Chen, L.; Liu, J. Improving the anticancer efficacy of laminin receptor-specific therapeutic ruthenium nanoparticles (RuBB-loaded EGCG-RuNPs) via ROS-dependent apoptosis in SMMC-7721 cells. *ACS Appl. Mater. Interf.* **2016**, *8*, 15000–15012. [CrossRef]
82. Shafiei, S.S.; Solati-Hashjin, M.; Samadikuchaksaraei, A.; Kalantarinejad, R.; Asadi-Eydivand, M.; Abu Osman, N.A. Epigallocatechin Gallate/Layered Double Hydroxide Nanohybrids: Preparation, Characterization, and In Vitro Anti-Tumor Study. *PLoS ONE* **2015**, *10*, e0136530. [CrossRef] [PubMed]
83. Muhamad, N.; Plengsuriyakarn, T.; Na-Bangchang, K. Application of active targeting nanoparticle delivery system for chemotherapeutic drugs and traditional/herbal medicines in cancer therapy: A systematic review. *Int. J. Nanomed.* **2018**, *13*, 3921–3935. [CrossRef] [PubMed]

84. Hsieh, D.-S.; Wang, H.; Tan, S.-W.; Huang, Y.-H.; Tsai, C.-Y.; Yeh, M.-K.; Wu, C.-J. The treatment of bladder cancer in a mouse model by epigallocatechin-3-gallate-gold nanoparticles. *Biomaterials* **2011**, *32*, 7633–7640. [CrossRef] [PubMed]
85. Chen, C.C.; Hsieh, D.S.; Huang, K.J.; Chan, Y.L.; Hong, P.D.; Yeh, M.K.; Wu, C.J. Improving anticancer efficacy of (-)-epigallocatechin-3-gallate gold nanoparticles in murine B16F10 melanoma cells. *Drug Des. Dev. Ther.* **2014**, *8*, 459–473. [CrossRef]
86. Sanna, V.; Pala, N.; Dessi, G.; Manconi, P.; Mariani, A.; Dedola, S.; Rassu, M.; Crosio, C.; Iaccarino, C.; Sechi, M. Single-step green synthesis and characterization of gold-conjugated polyphenol nanoparticles with antioxidant and biological activities. *Int. J. Nanomed.* **2014**, *9*, 4935–4951. [CrossRef]
87. Mukherjee, S.; Ghosh, S.; Das, D.K.; Chakraborty, P.; Choudhury, S.; Gupta, P.; Adhikary, A.; Dey, S.; Chattopadhyay, S. Gold-conjugated green tea nanoparticles for enhanced anti-tumor activities and hepatoprotection—Synthesis, characterization and in vitro evaluation. *J. Nutr. Biochem.* **2015**. [CrossRef]
88. Sanna, V.; Pintus, G.; Roggio, A.M.; Punzoni, S.; Posadino, A.M.; Arca, A.; Marceddu, S.; Bandiera, P.; Uzzau, S.; Sechi, M. Targeted biocompatible nanoparticles for the delivery of (-)-epigallocatechin 3-gallate to prostate cancer cells. *J. Med. Chem.* **2011**, *54*, 1321–1332. [CrossRef]
89. Alotaibi, A.; Bhatnagar, P.; Najafzadeh, M.; Gupta, K.C.; Anderson, D. Tea phenols in bulk and nanoparticle form modify DNA damage in human lymphocytes from colon cancer patients and healthy individuals treated in vitro with platinum based-chemotherapeutic drugs. *Nanomedicine* **2012**, *4*, 2012. [CrossRef]
90. Narayanan, S.; Mony, U.; Vijaykumar, D.K.; Koyakutty, M.; Paul-Prasanth, B.; Menon, D. Sequential release of epigallocatechin gallate and paclitaxel from PLGA-casein core/shell nanoparticles sensitizes drug-resistant breast cancer cells. *Nanomed. Nanotechnol. Biol. Med.* **2015**, *11*, 1399–1406. [CrossRef]
91. Siddiqui, I.A.; Adhami, V.M.; Bharali, D.J.; Hafeez, B.B.; Asim, M.; Khwaja, S.I.; Ahmad, N.; Cui, H.; Mousa, S.A.; Mukhtar, H. Introducing Nanochemoprevention as a Novel Approach for Cancer Control: Proof of Principle with Green Tea Polyphenol Epigallocatechin-3-Gallate. *Cancer Res.* **2009**, *69*, 1712–1716. [CrossRef]
92. Khan, N.; Bharali, D.J.; Adhami, V.M.; Siddiqui, I.A.; Cui, H.; Shabana, S.M.; Mousa, S.A.; Mukhtar, H. Oral administration of naturally occurring chitosan-based nanoformulated green tea polyphenol EGCG effectively inhibits prostate cancer cell growth in a xenograft model. *Carcinogenesis* **2014**, *35*, 415–423. [CrossRef] [PubMed]
93. Siddiqui, I.A.; Bharali, D.J.; Nihal, M.; Adhami, V.M.; Khan, N.; Chamcheu, J.C.; Khan, M.I.; Shabana, S.; Mousa, S.A.; Mukhtar, H. Excellent anti-proliferative and pro-apoptotic effects of (-)-epigallocatechin-3-gallate encapsulated in chitosan nanoparticles on human melanoma cell growth both in vitro and in vivo. *Nanomed. Nanotechnol. Biol. Med.* **2014**, *10*, 1619–1626. [CrossRef] [PubMed]
94. Hu, B.; Xie, M.; Zhang, C.; Zeng, X. Genipin-structured peptide-polysaccharide nanoparticles with significantly improved resistance to harsh gastrointestinal environments and their potential for oral delivery of polyphenols. *J. Agric. Food Chem.* **2014**, *62*, 12443–12452. [CrossRef] [PubMed]
95. Shutava, T.G.; Balkundi, S.S.; Vangala, P.; Steffan, J.J.; Bigelow, R.L.; Cardelli, J.a.; O'Neal, D.P.; Lvov, Y.M. Layer-by-layer-coated gelatin nanoparticles as a vehicle for delivery of natural polyphenols. *ACS Nano* **2009**, *3*, 1877–1885. [CrossRef]
96. Fang, J.-Y.; Hung, C.-F.; Hwang, T.-L.; Huang, Y.-L. Physicochemical characteristics and in vivo deposition of liposome-encapsulated tea catechins by topical and intratumor administrations. *J. Drug Target.* **2005**, *13*, 19–27. [CrossRef]
97. Fang, J.-Y.; Lee, W.-R.; Shen, S.-C.; Huang, Y.-L. Effect of liposome encapsulation of tea catechins on their accumulation in basal cell carcinomas. *J. Dermatol. Sci.* **2006**, *42*, 101–109. [CrossRef]
98. De Pace, R.C.C.; Liu, X.; Sun, M.; Nie, S.; Zhang, J.; Cai, Q.; Gao, W.; Pan, X.; Fan, Z.; Wang, S. Anticancer activities of (−)-epigallocatechin-3-gallate encapsulated nanoliposomes in MCF7 breast cancer cells. *J. Liposome Res.* **2013**, *23*, 187–196. [CrossRef]
99. Ramadass, S.K.; Anantharaman, N.V.; Subramanian, S.; Sivasubramanian, S.; Madhan, B. Paclitaxel/epigallocatechin gallate coloaded liposome: A synergistic delivery to control the invasiveness of MDA-MB-231 breast cancer cells. *Coll. Surf. B Biointerfaces* **2015**, *125*, 65–72. [CrossRef]
100. Jain, S.; Hirst, D.G.; O'Sullivan, J.M. Gold nanoparticles as novel agents for cancer therapy. *Brit. J. Radiol.* **2012**, *85*, 101–113. [CrossRef]

101. Elsabahy, M.; Wooley, K.L. Design of polymeric nanoparticles for biomedical delivery applications. *Chem. Soc. Rev.* **2012**, *41*, 2545–2561. [CrossRef]
102. Huang, Y.-W.; Cambre, M.; Lee, H.-J. The Toxicity of Nanoparticles Depends on Multiple Molecular and Physicochemical Mechanisms. *Int. J. Mol. Sci.* **2017**, *18*, 2702. [CrossRef] [PubMed]
103. Halamoda-Kenzaoui, B.; Bremer-Hoffmann, S. Main trends of immune effects triggered by nanomedicines in preclinical studies. *Int. J. Nanomed.* **2018**, *13*, 5419–5431. [CrossRef] [PubMed]
104. Ramesh, N.; Mandal, A.K.A. Pharmacokinetic, toxicokinetic, and bioavailability studies of epigallocatechin-3-gallate loaded solid lipid nanoparticle in rat model. *Drug Dev. Ind. Pharm.* **2019**, *45*, 1506–1514. [CrossRef] [PubMed]
105. Sanna, V.; Singh, C.K.; Jashari, R.; Adhami, V.M.; Chamcheu, J.C.; Rady, I.; Sechi, M.; Mukhtar, H.; Siddiqui, I.A. Targeted nanoparticles encapsulating (−)-epigallocatechin-3-gallate for prostate cancer prevention and therapy. *Sci. Rep.* **2017**, *7*. [CrossRef] [PubMed]
106. Ding, J.; Liang, T.; Min, Q.; Jiang, L.; Zhu, J.J. "Stealth and Fully-Laden" Drug Carriers: Self-Assembled Nanogels Encapsulated with Epigallocatechin Gallate and siRNA for Drug-Resistant Breast Cancer Therapy. *ACS Appl. Mater. Interfaces* **2018**, *10*, 9938–9948. [CrossRef]
107. Bettuzzi, S.; Brausi, M.; Rizzi, F.; Castagnetti, G.; Peracchia, G.; Corti, A. Chemoprevention of human prostate cancer by oral administration of green tea catechins in volunteers with high-grade prostate intraepithelial neoplasia: A preliminary report from a one-year proof-of-principle study. *Cancer Res.* **2006**, *66*, 1234–1240. [CrossRef]
108. Lazzeroni, M.; Guerrieri-Gonzaga, A.; Gandini, S.; Johansson, H.; Serrano, D.; Cazzaniga, M.; Aristarco, V.; Macis, D.; Mora, S.; Caldarella, P.; et al. A Presurgical Study of Lecithin Formulation of Green Tea Extract in Women with Early Breast Cancer. *Cancer Prev. Res.* **2017**, *10*, 363–370. [CrossRef]
109. Shin, C.M.; Lee, D.H.; Seo, A.Y.; Lee, H.J.; Kim, S.B.; Son, W.C.; Kim, Y.K.; Lee, S.J.; Park, S.H.; Kim, N.; et al. Green tea extracts for the prevention of metachronous colorectal polyps among patients who underwent endoscopic removal of colorectal adenomas: A randomized clinical trial. *Clin. Nutr.* **2018**, *37*, 452–458. [CrossRef]
110. Joe, A.K.; Schnoll-Sussman, F.; Bresalier, R.S.; Abrams, J.A.; Hibshoosh, H.; Cheung, K.; Friedman, R.A.; Yang, C.S.; Milne, G.L.; Liu, D.D.; et al. Phase Ib Randomized, Double-Blinded, Placebo-Controlled, Dose Escalation Study of Polyphenon E in Patients with Barrett's Esophagus. *Cancer Prev. Res.* **2015**, *8*, 1131–1137. [CrossRef]
111. Cao, J.; Han, J.; Xiao, H.; Qiao, J.; Han, M. Effect of Tea Polyphenol Compounds on Anticancer Drugs in Terms of Anti-Tumor Activity, Toxicology, and Pharmacokinetics. *Nutrients* **2016**, *8*, 762. [CrossRef]
112. Wu, A.H.; Spicer, D.; Stanczyk, F.Z.; Tseng, C.C.; Yang, C.S.; Pike, M.C. Effect of 2-month controlled green tea intervention on lipoprotein cholesterol, glucose, and hormone levels in healthy postmenopausal women. *Cancer Prev. Res.* **2012**, *5*, 393–402. [CrossRef] [PubMed]
113. Samavat, H.; Newman, A.R.; Wang, R.; Yuan, J.M.; Wu, A.H.; Kurzer, M.S. Effects of green tea catechin extract on serum lipids in postmenopausal women: A randomized, placebo-controlled clinical trial. *Am. J. Clin. Nutr.* **2016**, *104*, 1671–1682. [CrossRef] [PubMed]
114. Dostal, A.M.; Samavat, H.; Bedell, S.; Torkelson, C.; Wang, R.; Swenson, K.; Le, C.; Wu, A.H.; Ursin, G.; Yuan, J.M.; et al. The safety of green tea extract supplementation in postmenopausal women at risk for breast cancer: Results of the Minnesota Green Tea Trial. *Food Chem. Toxicol.* **2015**, *83*, 26–35. [CrossRef] [PubMed]
115. Samavat, H.; Ursin, G.; Emory, T.H.; Lee, E.; Wang, R.; Torkelson, C.J.; Dostal, A.M.; Swenson, K.; Le, C.T.; Yang, C.S.; et al. A Randomized Controlled Trial of Green Tea Extract Supplementation and Mammographic Density in Postmenopausal Women at Increased Risk of Breast Cancer. *Cancer Prev. Res.* **2017**, *10*, 710–718. [CrossRef] [PubMed]
116. Shanafelt, T.D.; Call, T.G.; Zent, C.S.; Leis, J.F.; LaPlant, B.; Bowen, D.A.; Roos, M.; Laumann, K.; Ghosh, A.K.; Lesnick, C.; et al. Phase 2 trial of daily, oral Polyphenon E in patients with asymptomatic, Rai stage 0 to II chronic lymphocytic leukemia. *Cancer* **2013**, *119*, 363–370. [CrossRef] [PubMed]
117. Kumar, N.B.; Pow-Sang, J.; Egan, K.M.; Spiess, P.E.; Dickinson, S.; Salup, R.; Helal, M.; McLarty, J.; Williams, C.R.; Schreiber, F.; et al. Randomized, Placebo-Controlled Trial of Green Tea Catechins for Prostate Cancer Prevention. *Cancer Prev. Res.* **2015**, *8*, 879–887. [CrossRef]

118. McLarty, J.; Bigelow, R.L.; Smith, M.; Elmajian, D.; Ankem, M.; Cardelli, J.A. Tea polyphenols decrease serum levels of prostate-specific antigen, hepatocyte growth factor, and vascular endothelial growth factor in prostate cancer patients and inhibit production of hepatocyte growth factor and vascular endothelial growth factor in vitro. *Cancer Prev. Res.* **2009**, *2*, 673–682. [CrossRef]
119. Gee, J.R.; Saltzstein, D.R.; Kim, K.; Kolesar, J.; Huang, W.; Havighurst, T.C.; Wollmer, B.W.; Stublaski, J.; Downs, T.; Mukhtar, H.; et al. A Phase II Randomized, Double-blind, Presurgical Trial of Polyphenon E in Bladder Cancer Patients to Evaluate Pharmacodynamics and Bladder Tissue Biomarkers. *Cancer Prev. Res.* **2017**, *10*, 298–307. [CrossRef]
120. Zhao, H.; Zhu, W.; Xie, P.; Li, H.; Zhang, X.; Sun, X.; Yu, J.; Xing, L. A phase I study of concurrent chemotherapy and thoracic radiotherapy with oral epigallocatechin-3-gallate protection in patients with locally advanced stage III non-small-cell lung cancer. *Radiother. Oncol.* **2014**, *110*, 132–136. [CrossRef]
121. Zhao, H.; Xie, P.; Li, X.; Zhu, W.; Sun, X.; Sun, X.; Chen, X.; Xing, L.; Yu, J. A prospective phase II trial of EGCG in treatment of acute radiation-induced esophagitis for stage III lung cancer. *Radiother. Oncol.* **2015**, *114*, 351–356. [CrossRef]
122. Zhao, H.; Zhu, W.; Jia, L.; Sun, X.; Chen, G.; Zhao, X.; Li, X.; Meng, X.; Kong, L.; Xing, L.; et al. Phase I study of topical epigallocatechin-3-gallate (EGCG) in patients with breast cancer receiving adjuvant radiotherapy. *Brit. J. Radiol.* **2016**, *89*, 20150665. [CrossRef] [PubMed]

5

Divergent Effects of Daidzein and its Metabolites on Estrogen-Induced Survival of Breast Cancer Cells

Emiliano Montalesi, Manuela Cipolletti, Patrizio Cracco, Marco Fiocchetti and Maria Marino *

Department of Science, University Roma Tre, Viale Guglielmo Marconi 446, I-00146 Roma, Italy; emiliano.montalesi@uniroma3.it (E.M.); manuela.cipolletti@uniroma3.it (M.C.); patrizio.cracco95@live.it (P.C.); marco.fiocchetti@uniroma3.it (M.F.)

* Correspondence: maria.marino@uniroma3.it

Abstract: Although soy consumption is associated with breast cancer prevention, the low bioavailability and the extensive metabolism of soy-active components limit their clinical application. Here, the impact of daidzein (D) and its metabolites on estrogen-dependent anti-apoptotic pathway has been evaluated in breast cancer cells. In estrogen receptor α-positive breast cancer cells treated with D and its metabolites, single or in mixture, ERα activation and Neuroglobin (NGB) levels, an anti-apoptotic estrogen/ERα-inducible protein, were evaluated. Moreover, the apoptotic cascade activation, as well as the cell number after stimulation was assessed in the absence/presence of paclitaxel to determine the compound effects on cell susceptibility to a chemotherapeutic agent. Among the metabolites, only D-4′-sulfate maintains the anti-estrogenic effect of D, reducing the NGB levels and rendering breast cancer cells more prone to the paclitaxel treatment, whereas other metabolites showed estrogen mimetic effects, or even estrogen independent effects. Intriguingly, the co-stimulation of D and gut metabolites strongly reduced D effects. The results highlight the important and complex influence of metabolic transformation on isoflavones physiological effects and demonstrate the need to take biotransformation into account when assessing the potential health benefits of consumption of soy isoflavones in cancer.

Keywords: estrogen; estrogen receptor alpha; polyphenols; daidzein; daidzein metabolites; paclitaxel; apoptosis; breast cancer cells

---

1. Introduction

Plant-derived polyphenols are naturally occurring nonsteroidal compounds that play important roles in ecological functions such as pollinator attraction or protection from herbivores and UV irradiation [1]. Due to their molecular structure and size, some of these molecules, including lignans, flavonoids, and stilbenes, have a chemical structure that resembles that of human estrogens, in particular to 17-β-estradiol (E2) [2]. Among other, isoflavones, a class of flavonoids ranked among the most estrogenic compounds, bind to estrogen receptor subtypes (i.e., ERα and ERβ) [3,4] exerting estrogenic and/or antiestrogenic effects [1]. For isoflavones, the key to their bioactivity in human and animals seems to rely on their (anti)estrogenic activity. Indeed, due their antiestrogenic activities, isoflavone enriched diets are associated with a lower incidence of a variety of estrogen-related cancers, including breast, endometrial, and ovarian cancers [5,6].

The main dietary source of isoflavones in humans are soybean and soybean products, which contain mainly daidzein (7,4′-dihydroxyisoflavone, D) and genistein (7, 4′-dihydroxy-6-methoxyisoflavone), whose potential efficacy against breast cancer is well documented [7–12]. Although these data are promising for the use of these compounds as anticancer therapeutic agents, the therapeutic application of isoflavones is still limited, mainly due to their scarce bioavailability in human beings. In particular, D is almost completely metabolized by the gut microbiota and liver, resulting in water-soluble metabolites (e.g., equol, D-sulfates, O-desmethylangolensin) [13]. Thus, not only D has a low concentration and persistence in the bloodstream, even when consumed in high quantities, but also its metabolites strongly overcome the concentrations of the precursor probably affecting D biological activities [14–18]. Nowadays, the possibility that the metabolites may mimic the anti-carcinogenic effect of D in endocrine-related cancers or may act as synergistic or antagonistic molecules of their precursor is still unknown. Previously, the ability of D, metabolites, to modulate ERβ subtype activities activating a pro-apoptotic cascade in HeLa cancer cells transfected with ERβ expression vector, has been reported [19]. The possibility that a similar scenario could be found also in the modulation of ERα-dependent activities important for breast cancer cell progression is intriguing.

Breast cancer is one of the most common fatal diseases in women. A considerably higher ERα/ERβ ratio is reported in some breast cancer types, when compared to a healthy tissue, namely because of a reduction in the ERβ level [20,21]. The 70% of breast cancers are ERα-positive, where this subtype of receptor mediates E2-induced cancer cell survival and proliferation [22–25]. In particular, we recently demonstrated that E2 stimulation rapidly enhances the ERα activity (Ser118 phosphorylation and PI3K/AKT pathway activation) in breast cancer cells increasing the intracellular levels of an anti-apoptotic globin, neuroglobin (NGB) [22]. E2-induced NGB upregulation in cancer cells represents an inducible defense mechanism of E2-related human breast cancer rendering them insensitive to several injury including chemotherapy [22,26,27]. Indeed, NGB displays a pivotal role in the E2/ERα-induced anti-apoptotic pathway that abrogates the cell death induced by a chemotherapeutic agent (paclitaxel, Pacl) [22]. Intriguingly, the stilbene Resveratrol decreases NGB levels interfering with E2/ERα-induced NGB up-regulation potentiating Pacl pro-apoptotic effects [4]. In this study, we investigated the potential interference of daidzein on this pathway and evaluated if its metabolites produced mainly from gut microbiota (i.e., equol, Eq, and O-desmethylangolensin, O-DMA) and from both liver and gut enzymes (D-4′-sulfate, D4S, D-7-sulfate, D7S, and D-4′,7-disulfate, DDS) mimic D effect or may act as synergistic or antagonistic molecules. The ERα positive breast cancer cells, MCF-7 and T47D, have been used as the experimental models.

2. Results

2.1. *Effect of D and Its Metabolites on NGB Levels in Breast Cancer Cells*

NGB levels were evaluated in MCF-7 cells pre-treated for 24 h with different concentrations of D (Figure 1a) and its metabolites ranging between 0.1 and 10 μM (Figure 1). E2 (10 nM, 24 h) was used as positive control. Eq and O-DMA (Figure 1b) and D7S, D4S, and DDS (Figure 1c) were selected as prototypes of the D metabolites mainly produced by gut microbiota and the liver, respectively. The results clearly indicate that daidzein (1–10 μM) and D4S (0.1–1 μM) reduced the basal level of NGB levels in MCF-7 cells. On the other hand, Eq, O-DMA, D7S, and DDS, like E2, increased the level of NGB (Figure 1a,b). For the successive experiments, D and its mimetic sulphate metabolite (i.e., D4S) were selected. In addition, Eq, one gut metabolite, was selected as negative control. All compounds were used at 1 μM concentration in successive experiments.

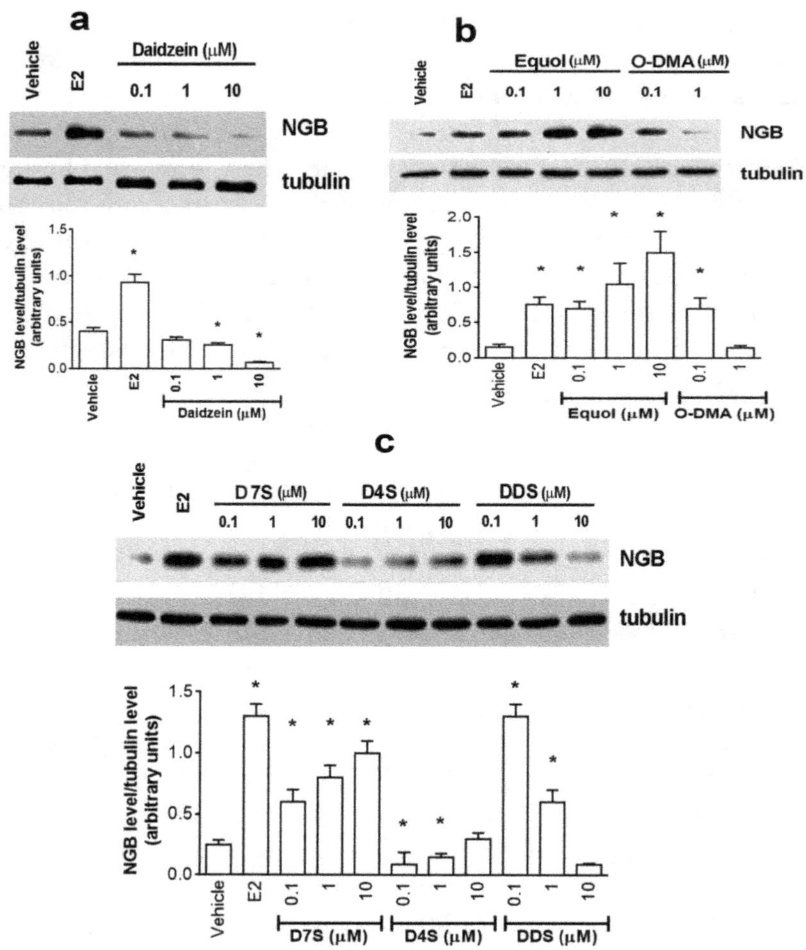

Figure 1. Effects of daidzein (**a**), equol and O-desmethylangolesin (**b**), daidzein-7-sulfate, daidzein-4′-sulfate and daidzein-7,4′-disulfate (**c**) on neuroglobin intracellular levels. (**a–c**) Western blot (top) and densitometric analyses (bottom) of NGB protein levels in MCF-7 cells treated for 24 h with the vehicle (DMSO), E2 (10 nM), D and its metabolites (0.1, 1.0, and 10 μM). The amount of proteins was normalized by comparison with tubulin levels. Data are the mean ± SD of four different experiments. $p < 0.001$ was determined with Student t test with respect to the vehicle (*) treated samples. E2: estradiol; NGB: neuroglobin; DMSO: dimethyl sulfoxide; D: daidzein; Eq: equol; O-DMA: O-desmethylangolesin; D7S: daidzein-7-sulfate; D4S: daidzein-4′-sulfate; DDS: daidzein-7,4′-disulfate.

The modulation of NGB levels by D, D4S, and Eq (1 μM, 24 h) was also confirmed in T47D cells (Figure 2). Indeed, also in these ERα-positive cells, D and D4S significantly reduced the basal level of NGB, whereas Eq, like E2, increased the globin level (Figure 2).

2.2. Mechanisms of D-, D4S-, and Eq Induced Modulation of NGB Levels

The involvement of ERα in the effects of D and its metabolites has been confirmed by pre-treating MCF-7 cells with 100 nM of the ERα inhibitor Endoxifen (Endo) before compound stimulation. As shown in Figure 3a, endoxifen pre-treatment completely impairs E2- and Eq-induced NGB up-regulation as well as D- and D4S-induced NGB down-regulation, strongly corroborating the necessity of an active ERα to modulate NGB levels. In particular, E2 rapidly down-regulates ERα levels maintaining high its phosphorylation status (Figure 3b) while neither D nor its metabolites modify the receptor levels but still increase ERα phosphorylation, although at lower level than E2 (Figure 3b). As expected, endoxifen pre-treatment completely prevents the ERα activation by all compounds considered (Figure 3b).

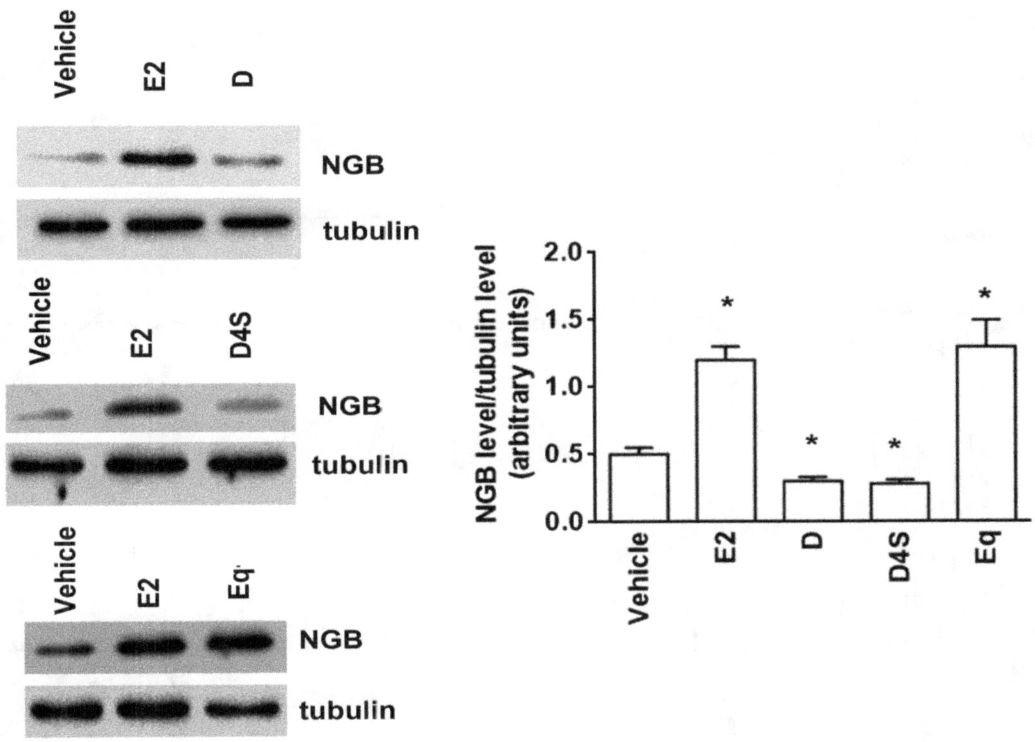

Figure 2. Effects of daidzein, daidzein-4′-sulfate and equol on neuroglobin intracellular levels in T47D cells. Western blot (left) and densitometric analyses (right) of NGB protein levels in T47D cells treated for 24 h with the vehicle (DMSO), E2 (10 nM), D (1 μM), D4S (1 μM), or Eq (1 μM). The amount of proteins was normalized by comparison with tubulin levels. Data are the mean ± SD of three different experiments. $p < 0.001$ was determined with Student t-test with respect to the vehicle (*) treated samples. DMSO: dimethyl sulfoxide; E2: estradiol; NGB: neuroglobin; D: daidzein; D4S: daidzein-4′-sulfate; Eq: equol.

ERα activation is the first step of a signal pathway triggered by E2 to enhance NGB levels. The activation of AKT is necessary to rapidly impair NGB degradation and assure NGB gene transcription via the CREBP transcription factor [28]. On the other hand, the ability of flavonoids (i.e., naringenin) to trigger the ERα-dependent activation of p38 has been demonstrated [29]. These evidences prompted us to evaluate if D and its metabolites trigger the activation of these kinases. Figure 4 shows that, as expected, E2 elicits the rapid and persistent activation of AKT enhancing its phosphorylation status in MCF-7 cells after both 1 h and 24 h of stimulation (Figure 4a,b). On the other hand, the hormone rapidly activates p38 phosphorylation (Figure 4c), but 24 h after stimulation, the phosphorylation status of p38 return similar to the control (Figure 4d). Completely different is the effect of D and its metabolites. Indeed, both D and D4S do not activate AKT phosphorylation, but these compounds, in particular D4S, trigger the rapid and persistent activation of p38 phosphorylation (Figure 4c,d). Endoxifen pretreatment prevents the D and D4S effects as well as that of E2, although 1 h after D4S stimulation the ER inhibitor does not completely impede p38 activation (Figure 4c), suggesting that an ERα-independent mechanism is at the root of the very high p38 phosphorylation induced by this sulphate metabolite. Similarly, Eq stimulation of MCF-7 cells rapidly activates AKT phosphorylation by an ERα-independent pathway, not prevented by endoxifen pre-treatment (Figure 4a). However, the Eq-induced AKT activation is transient, and indeed the level of kinase phosphorylation was similar to the control 24 h after Eq stimulation. Like D and D4S, Eq triggers the rapid and persistent ERα-dependent p38 activation (Figure 4c,d). As a whole, these data strongly sustain that daidzein does not share similar action mechanisms with all of its metabolites, at least 1 h after treatment.

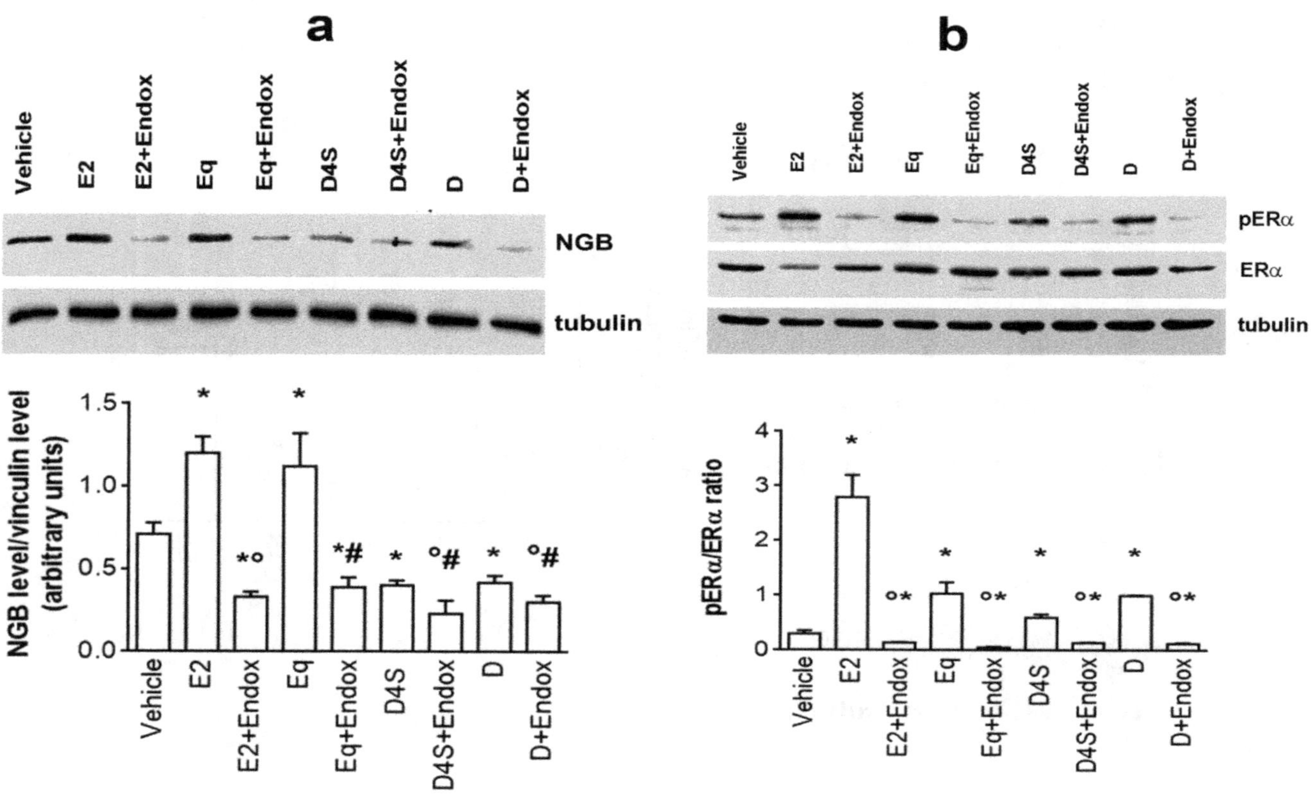

Figure 3. Daidzein, daidzein-4′-sulfate and equol effect on ERα activation status. (**a**) Western blot (top) and densitometric analyses (bottom) of NGB protein levels in MCF-7 cells treated for 24 h with either vehicle (DMSO) or E2 (10 nM) or D, D4S and Eq (1 μM) in presence or absence of the ERα inhibitor Endoxifen (1 μM; 30 min pretreatment). The amount of proteins was normalized by comparison with tubulin levels. Data are the mean ± SD of three different experiments. $p < 0.001$ was determined with Student's t test with respect to the vehicle (*) or E2-treated (°) samples. (**b**) ERα activation by daidzein, daidzein-4′-sulfate and equol. The panel represents the ERαSer118 phosphorylation status calculated as the ratio pERα/ERα). Determined by Western blot analysis in MCF-7 cells exposed for 1h to either vehicle (DMSO) or E2 (10 nM) or D, D4S and Eq (1 μM) in presence or absence of ERα inhibitor Endoxifen (1 μM; 30 min pretreatment). The nitrocellulose was stripped and then probed with anti-ERα antibody. The pERα/ERα ratio was calculated with respect to tubulin obtained by densitometric analyses of three different experiments (mean ± SD). $p < 0.001$ was determined by Student t test with respect to vehicle (*), E2-treated (°) or Endox-untreated samples (#). DMSO: dimethyl sulfoxide; E2: estradiol; Endox: endoxifen; ERα: estrogen receptor α; NGB: neuroglobin; D: daidzein; D4S: daidzein-4′-sulfate; Eq: equol.

2.3. Physiological Outcomes of D- and D4S-Induced E2/ERα/NGB Pathway Avoidance

We previously demonstrated that the ability of Resveratrol to impair NGB accumulation rendered cancer cells more prone to the anticancer effect of the chemotherapeutic agent paclitaxel (Pacl) [4]. This evidence prompted us to evaluate if D and D4S also exhibit this ability. As expected, Pacl treatment (100 nM) reduces NGB levels (Figure 5a–c) with the parallel increase of cleaved PARP-1 (i.e., 86 kDa band), a well-known biomarker of late apoptotic events (Figure 5d–f), and reduction of cell number (Figure 5g). Cell pre-treatment with E2 strongly prevents all Pacl effects in MCF-7 cells still enhancing NGB levels (Figure 5a–c), cell number (Figure 5g), and strongly reducing Pacl-induced PARP-1 cleavage (Figure 5d–f). Although neither D nor D4S pre-treatment affected Pacl effects, both these compounds restored Pacl effects in the presence of E2 (Figure 5). The ability of D and D4S to restore Pacl effects on cell number is also confirmed in T47D cell line (Figure 5h).

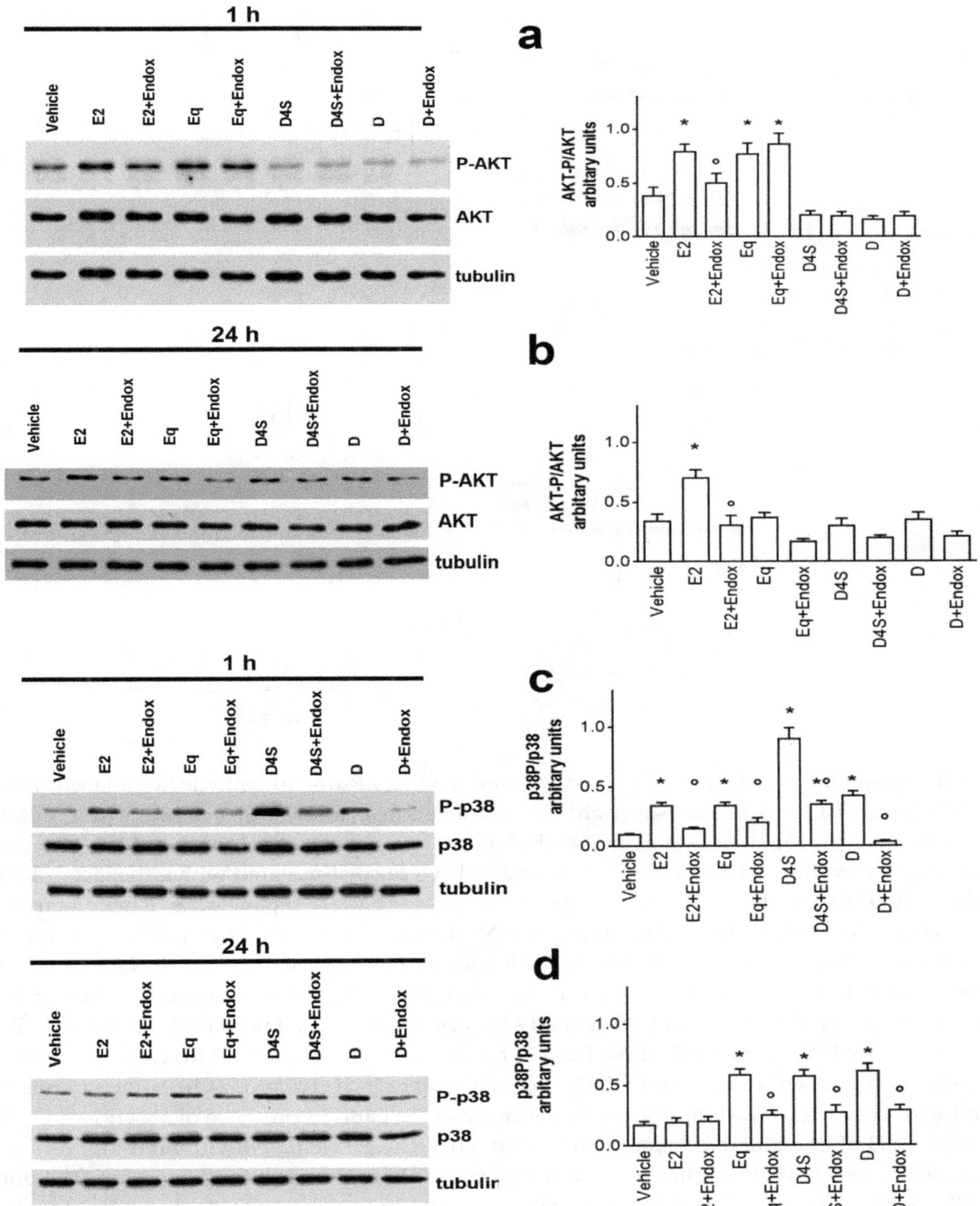

Figure 4. Daidzein, daidzein-4′-sulfate and equol action mechanism. The phosphorylation of the Ser473 residue of AKT (pAKT) (**a**,**b**) and Thr180/Tyr182 residues on P-38 (**c**,**d**) was determined by western blot analysis in MCF-7 cells exposed for 1 h (**a**,**c**) and 24 h (**b**,**d**) to either vehicle (DMSO) or E2 (10 nM) in presence or absence of D, D4S and Eq (1 μM). The nitrocellulose was stripped and then and then probed with anti-AKT or anti-P38 antibodies. In the panels, the pAKT/AKT (**a**,**b**) and pP38/P38 (**c**,**d**) ratios are represented. These ratios are calculated with respect to tubulin obtained by densitometric analyses of three different experiments (mean ± SD). $p < 0.001$ was determined by Student t-test with respect to vehicle (*) or Endox-untreated (°) samples. AKT: protein kinase B; E2: estradiol; Endox: endoxifen; ERα: estrogen receptor α; NGB: neuroglobin; p38: p38 mitogen-activated protein kinase; D: daidzein; D4S: daidzein-4′-sulfate; Eq: equol.

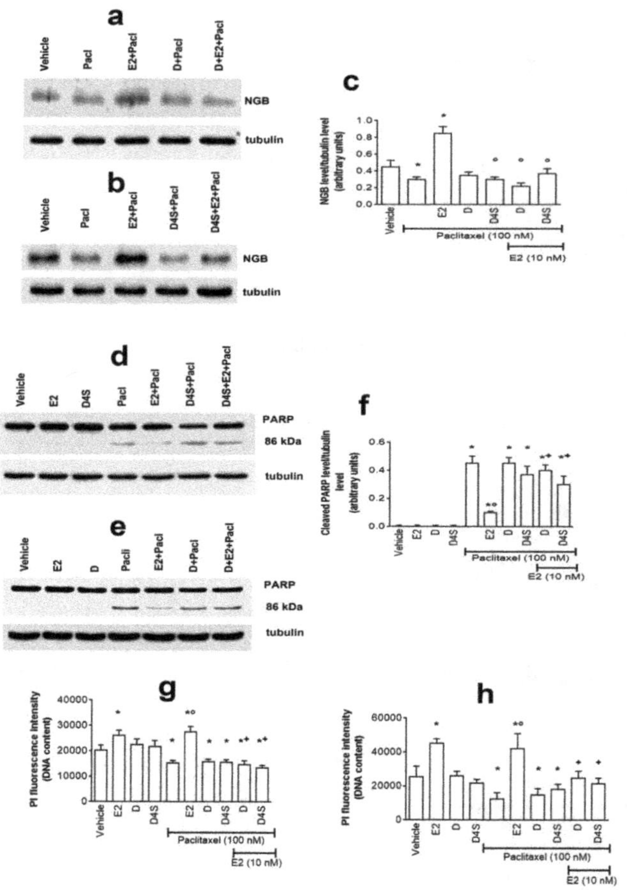

Figure 5. Physiological outcomes of D- and D4S-induced E2/ERα/NGB pathway avoidance. Western blot (left) and densitometric analyses (right) of NGB levels (**a**–**c**) and PARP-1 cleavage (**d**–**f**) in MCF-7 cells. Cells were treated with D (**a**,**e**) or D4S (**b**,**d**) (1 μM) in presence or absence of Pacl (100 nM) for 24 h, with either vehicle or E2; some Pacl treated cells were co-stimulated with either E2 or D or E2 together with D (**a**,**e**) or E2 or D4S or E2 together with D4S (**b**,**d**). (**c**,**f**) panels are densitometries that summarize the D- and D4S-induced modulation of NGB and PARP-1 cleavage respectively. The amount of protein was normalized by comparison with tubulin levels. Data are the mean ± SD of three different experiments. $p < 0.001$ was determined with Student t test with respect to the vehicle (*), Pacl-treated (°) samples or D- and D4S-treated samples, co-stimulated with Pacl but not with E2 (+). Effects of cellular DNA content obtained from PI assay on MCF-7 (**g**) or T47D (**h**) cells. The cells were treated for 24 h with either vehicle (DMSO) or E2 (10 nM) or Pacl (100 nM; 24 h); some samples were treated with D or D4S (1 μM) in presence or absence of Pacl and in presence of absence of E2. Data are mean ± SD of five different experiments. (*) $p < 0.001$ was calculated with Student t test versus vehicle or Pacl-treated (°) samples or D- and D4S-treated samples, co-stimulated with Pacl but not with E2 (+). E2: estradiol; NGB: neuroglobin; DMSO: dimethyl sulfoxide; D: daidzein; Eq: equol; D4S: daidzein-4′-sulfate; Pacl: paclitaxel.

2.4. Physiological Outcomes of D in Mixture with Its Metabolites

Due to its extensive biotransformation in the human body, D in circulation and in tissue is mainly present as a mixture with its metabolites. In order to evaluate if D maintains its anti-estrogenic actions described before, MCF-7 cells were treated with a mixture of compounds containing microbiota-produced metabolites (i.e., Eq and O-DMA, 1 μM each, gut metabolites) or metabolites produced by the gut and in liver enzymes (i.e., D7S, DDS, and D4S, 1 μM each, S metabolites) in presence or absence of D (1 μM). Figure 6a shows that the concentration of mixtures does not exert cytotoxic effects, indeed, the DNA content, and consequently the cell number, remain constant in MCF-7 cells stimulated with mixture or with the single compounds. D maintains the ability to reduce

NGB levels only in the co-stimulation with the mixture of sulphate metabolites (S metab), whereas this isoflavone effect is completely impaired by co-stimulation with the gut metabolites (Figure 6b). Notably, the mixture of S metabolites reduces NGB levels with respect to the control, while the mixture of gut metabolites increases NGB levels with respect to the control (Figure 6b). More intriguing is the effect of mixtures on Pacl-induced apoptosis (Figure 6c,d). Like the single compounds (Figure 5), neither sulphate nor gut metabolites induce the PARP cleavage at the concentration tested, however, sulphate metabolites preserve the Pacl-induced PARP-1 cleavage even in the presence of D or of E2 (Figure 6c), while gut metabolites reduce the Pacl effects even in the presence of D (Figure 6d). This latter effect is more evident in the presence of E2 (Figure 6d). As per other experiments, identical results have been obtained in T47D (data not showed), confirming that the mixture effects is not dependent on cellular context.

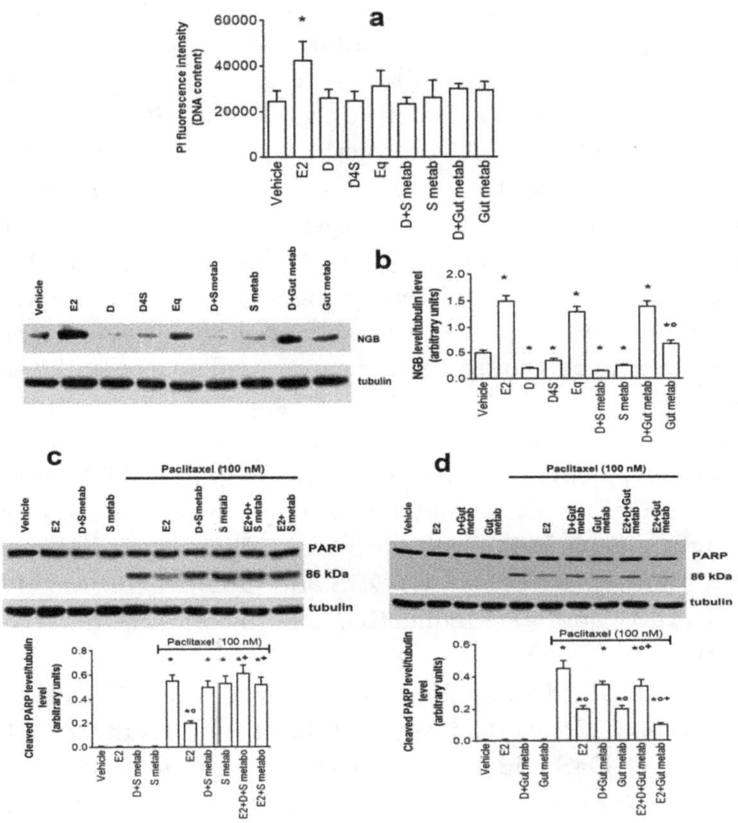

Figure 6. Physiological outcomes of D in mixture with its metabolites. (**a**) Analyses of cellular DNA content obtained from PI assay, Western blot (left) and densitometric analyses (right) of NGB levels (**b**) in MCF-7 cells. (**c**,**d**) Western blot (up) and densitometric analyses (bottom) of PARP-1 cleavage in MCF-7 cells. The MCF-7 cells were treated for 24 h with either vehicle (DMSO) or E2 (10 nM) or D, D4S or Eq (1 μM); some samples were treated with all the sulfate metabolites (D4S, D7S and DDS, 1 μM each) or all the gut metabolites (Eq and O-DMA, 1 μM each) in presence or absence of D (1 μM). Data are mean ± SD of three different experiments. (*) $p < 0.001$ was calculated with Student t test versus vehicle in (**a**). In **b**, data are the mean ± SD of five different experiments: $p < 0.001$ was determined with Student t test with respect to the vehicle (*) or to D-treated samples co-stimulated with metabolites (°). In (**c**,**d**), data are the mean ± SD of three different experiments. $p < 0.001$ was determined with Student *t* test with respect to the vehicle (*) or Pacl-treated (°) or E2 untreated samples co-stimulated with the metabolites (+). E2: estradiol; NGB: neuroglobin; DMSO: dimethyl sulfoxide; D: daidzein; Eq: equol; O-DMA: o-desmethylangolesin; D7S: daidzein-7-sulfate; D4S: daidzein-4′-sulfate; DDS: daidzein-7,4′-disulfate; Pacl: paclitaxel.

3. Discussion

Soy-derived isoflavones consumption has been largely recommended to the Western population for their possible vital role in maintaining human health through the regulation of metabolism and body weight, concurrent to the prevention of chronic and degenerative diseases including cancer and neurodegenerative disorders. Still, their short- and long-term effects have not been fully characterized, although some have cautioned that there may be harmful effects of overconsumption, especially in cases where compounds are isolated rather than consumed in a food matrix [30,31]. To further complicate this picture, isoflavones, once consumed as either aglycone or glycosides, enter a complex pathway of biotransformation that renders almost negligible the presence of the original molecule. The relative concentration of different metabolites in both plasma and tissues is determined by the specific contribution of intestinal microbiota and by de-conjugation/conjugation processes within the human body. Nowadays, available data on the estrogenic activity of D metabolites are restricted largely to Eq, whose production depends on the individual ability to host specific intestinal bacteria [32]. Once absorbed, daidzein is efficiently re-conjugated in the gut with either glucuronic acid or sulfate. Conjugation with sulfonic acid takes place also in the liver by hepatic sulfotransferase enzymes. Therefore, the plasma level of isoflavones in people on a soy-rich diet is very low (about 1–5 μM) [5,14], while they are present in the circulation predominantly in their glucuronide and sulfate forms [33].

Nowadays, the ability of D metabolites to maintain the effects of their precursor is largely unknown. The main aim of this study was to determine whether D metabolites produced by sulfotransferase and by microbiota enzymes maintain their anticancer effects, consisting in affecting ERα activities that are important for E2-induced resistance of breast cancer cells to chemotherapeutic injury. For this purpose, we utilized two human ERα positive breast cancer cells in which the pathway E2/ERα/NGB has been previously identified as pivotal for breast cancer cell susceptibility to the chemotherapeutic agent paclitaxel [22].

Our data indicate that, unlike E2 that induced NGB overexpression, 1–10 μM D reduced NGB levels under the basal level (i.e., vehicle -treated samples) in both MCF-7 and T47D breast cancer cells. This D effect was mimicked only by the D4S metabolite that reduced NGB levels at lower concentrations than D (i.e., 0.1–1 μM); while Eq and D7S showed an E2 like behavior, increasing NGB levels in a concentration dependent manner. Surprisingly, DDS and O-DMA increased NGB levels only at very low concentrations (i.e., 0.1 μM), and were ineffective at high concentrations (10 μM for DDS and 1 μM for O-DMA, respectively).

The differences between D and its metabolites in modulating NGB levels, as well as the different concentrations necessary to obtain the effect, suggest that D and its metabolites may trigger different signal transduction pathways. D4S and Eq were selected as representatives of the two contrasting effects to determine their mechanisms. Like E2, D, D4S, and Eq trigger ERαS118 phosphorylation, even if only E2 reduces the receptor levels, an important mechanism for E2-induced cancer cell proliferation [34]. Moreover, ERα is necessary for D and its metabolites to regulate NGB levels, confirming that D and its metabolites could bind to and activate ERα, as already reported [3]. However, downstream of ERα activation, D and its metabolites trigger divergent signal pathways. Indeed, differently from E2, D and D4S do not trigger AKT activation, which is pivotal for E2-induced NGB accumulation [28]. Instead, these compounds rapidly (1 h) and persistently (24 h) activate p38 kinase, whose activation is commonly shared among flavonoids (e.g., naringenin, quercetin) [29,35]. Upon receptor binding, naringenin modifies ERα conformation driving the receptor far from the plasma membrane (i.e., receptor de-palmitoylation) and decoupling its association with the active sub-unit of PI3K, but not with p38 kinase [24,29]. Consequently, AKT is not activated, whereas the persistent activation of p38 occurs, driving cancer cells to the activation of the apoptotic cascade that culminates with PARP cleavage [29]. A similar signal transduction pathway seems to be activated by D and D4S that at the concentrations used here (1 μM) do not affect the phosphorylation status of AKT, allowing the persistent p38 activation. On the other hand, Eq rapidly and transiently activates AKT phosphorylation that even if does not impair the persistent p38 activation, as E2 does, is sufficient to accumulate NGB into the cells. Note that the D4S-induced p38 and Eq-induced AKT phosphorylation is ERα-independent, at least partially for D4S, sustaining that these metabolites could bind to other cellular receptors, including the Arylic Receptor [36,37], which, in turn, can interfere with the estrogenic signal. As a whole, the chemical structure of D and its metabolites allows different ERα conformations that, in turn, drive cells to physiological outcomes that differ from that triggered by E2 [24,38,39].

Paclitaxel, a first line therapeutic agent for breast cancer, is a prototype of chemotherapeutic agents, which action mechanism is well known [4]. As reported above, E2/ERα-induced NGB accumulation in cancer cells represents an anti-apoptotic pathway, which abrogates the cell death induced by a chemotherapeutic agent (paclitaxel, Pacl) [4]. The ability of NGB accumulation to act as a shield against Pacl has been further confirmed here. In fact, E2 pretreatment impairs Pacl reduction of NGB as well as its ability to reduce cell number and activate PARP cleavage. Although at the selected concentrations (1 μM) they do not affect cell number or PARP cleavage, D and D4S completely prevent E2 effects, allowing the Pacl-induced activation of a pro-apoptotic cascade, even in the presence of the hormone, sustaining that the anti-estrogenic activity is pivotal for rendering cancer cells more vulnerable to the chemotherapeutic drug. The anti-proliferative action of isoflavones and other plant-derived polyphenols in cancer cells has been widely reported and disputed. Nowadays, it is quite accepted that only high concentrations of isoflavones (≤10 μM), very far from the concentration present in the plasma after a meal rich in polyphenols, could activate a mitochondrial-dependent apoptotic cascade, while low concentrations of these compounds result less active or, even, increase cancer cell proliferation [6–9]. Our data confirm that low concentrations of D and D4S are unable to trigger apoptosis or enhance Pacl effects, but acting as anti-estrogenic compounds, they can avoid the E2-induced anti-apoptotic effect on this chemotherapeutic drug.

The current study indicates, for the first time, that just D4S but no other metabolites retain the D anti-estrogenic activity. This effect is maintained when cancer cells were co-treated with D and mixtures of S metabolites, containing also D7S and DDS. On the contrary, the mixture of gut metabolites, containing Eq and O-DMA, completely impairs D effects, resulting in estrogen mimetic action. Identical results have been obtained in both MCF-7 and T47D (not completely reported), suggesting that the effect is not dependent on the cellular context. These results highlight the need to use physiologically relevant metabolites when investigating the putative beneficial properties of polyphenols against cancer.

4. Materials and Methods

4.1. Reagents

The Bradford protein assay and the chemiluminescence reagents for Western blot Clarity Western ECL Substrate were obtained from Bio-Rad Laboratories (Hercules, CA, USA). The anti-phospho-ERα (pERα Ser118) antibody and anti-phospho-AKT (pAKT Ser473) were purchased from Cell Signalling Technology Inc. (Beverly, MA, USA). The anti-α-tubulin and anti-NGB antibodies were purchased from Merck (Darmstadt, D). Specific antibodies against AKT, ERα (HC20), and poly [ADP-ribose] polymerase 1 (PARP-1) were obtained from Santa Cruz Biotechnology (Santa Cruz, CA, USA). The ERα inhibitor endoxifen was purchased from Tocris (Ballwin, MO, USA). All the other products were from Merck. Analytical and reagent grade products were used without further purification.

4.2. Cell Culture and Treatment

Human breast cancer cells MCF-7 and T47D (American Type Culture Collection, LGC Standards S.r.l., Milano, Italy) were grown in air containing 5% CO2 in either modified, phenol red free, Dulbecco's Modified Eagle's Medium (DMEM) medium. Ten percent (*v*/*v*) of charcoal-stripped fetal calf serum, L-glutamine (2 mM), gentamicin (0.1 mg/mL), and penicillin (100 U/mL) were added to the media before use. Cells were used at passage 4–8, as previously described [28]. Cell line authentication was periodically performed by the amplification of multiple short tandem repeat loci by BMR genomics

S.r.l (Padova, Italy). Cells were treated for 24 h with either vehicle (DMSO/phosphate-buffered saline, 1:10; *v/v*) or E2 (1 or 10 nM) or D and/or its metabolites (0.1, 1.0, and 10 μM) or Pacl (100 nM) or the metabolites mixtures. Two different metabolite mixtures were used for cell treatment, Sulphate metabolites (S metab) and Gut metabolites (Gut metab). The mixture of S metab was constituted by D4S (1 μM), D7S (1 μM) and DDS (1 μM), while that of Gut metab was constituted by Equol (1 μM) and O-DMA (1 μM). When indicated, endoxifen (1 μM) was added 30 min before compound administration, or E2 (10 nM) was added 4 h before Pacl addition (0.1, 1, and 100 nM) for 24 h. The E2 concentrations were selected on the bases of dose-response experiments already performed [40].

4.3. Western Blot Assay

Briefly, after the treatments, cells were lysed and proteins were solubilized in the YY buffer (50 mM HEPES at pH 7.5, 10% glycerol, 150 mM NaCl, 1% Triton X-100, 1 mM EDTA, and 1 mM EGTA) containing 0.70% (*w/v*) sodium dodecyl sulfate (SDS). Total proteins were quantified using the Bradford protein assay. Solubilized proteins (20 μg) were resolved by 7% or 15% SDS-polyacrylamide gel electrophoresis at 100 V for 1 h at 24.0 °C and then transferred to nitrocellulose with the Trans-Blot Turbo Transfer System (Bio-Rad) for 7 min. The nitrocellulose was treated with 5% (*w/v*) bovine serum albumin in 138.0 mM NaCl, 25.0 mM Tris, pH 8.0, at 24.0 °C for 1 h. Nitrocellulose was probed overnight at 4.0 °C with either anti-NGB (final dilution, 1:1000), or anti-pERα (final dilution, 1:1000), or anti-pAKT (final dilution, 1:1000), or anti p-38 (final dilution 1:1000), or anti-PARP-1 (final dilution, 1:1000) antibodies. The nitrocellulose was stripped by Restore Western Blot Stripping Buffer (Pierce Chemical, Rockford, IL) for 10 min at room temperature and then probed with either anti-ERα (final dilution, 1:1000) or anti-AKT (final dilution 1:1000) or anti-p38 (final dilution, 1:1000) or anti-α-tubulin (final dilution, 1:30,000) antibodies to normalize the protein loaded. The antibody reactivity was detected with ECL chemiluminescence Western blotting detection reagent using a ChemiDoc XRS+ Imaging System (Bio-Rad Laboratories, Hercules, CA, USA). Densitometric analyses were performed by the ImageJ software for Microsoft Windows (National Institute of Health, Bethesda, Rockville, MD, USA).

4.4. Cellular DNA Content, Propidium Iodide (PI) Assay

Cells were grown up to 80% confluence in 96-well plate and treated with the selected compounds. The cells were fixed and permeabilized with cold ethanol (EtOH) 70% for 15 min at −20 °C. EtOH solution were removed and the cells were incubated with PI buffer for 30 min in the dark. The solution was removed, and the cells were rinsed with PBS solution. The fluorescence was revealed (excitation wavelength: 537 nm; emission wavelength: 621 nm) with TECAN Spark 20 M multimode microplate reader (Life Science, Milano, Italy).

4.5. Statistical Analysis

The statistical analysis was performed by Student's t test to compare two sets of data by INSTAT software system for Windows. In all cases, $p < 0.05$ was considered significant.

5. Conclusions

Breast cancer, as well as lung, bronchial, and colorectal cancer, are estimated to be the three most commonly diagnosed types of malignancies. In particular, breast cancer alone accounts for 29% of all new cancers among women and the age of its onset is rapidly decreasing [41]. ERα activation status and signaling is considered one of the major drivers stimulating breast cancer proliferation, survival, and invasion [23–25]. The importance of ERα lies within its prognostic value, as it identifies patients that could benefit from the endocrine therapy [25]. Although the use of ERα antagonists has led to a considerable decline in breast cancer mortality, many patients become resistant to this therapy and developed metastatic tumors [24,41]. These observations have sparked the need for alternative approaches, increasing a sustained interest in soy isoflavones as a promising therapeutic option in breast cancer chemoprevention or as an adjuvant for chemotherapeutic agents. These claims lead patients with increased breast cancer risk to take into consideration supplementing their diet with soy or soy derivates, assuming that a high consumption might reduce the cancer risk [30,42]. Unfortunately, the increased economic interests in soy isoflavones has not yet been paralleled by the deciphering of the cellular and molecular mechanisms underlying their potential chemo-preventive role, which remains obscure.

The data reported here strongly sustain the need to examine in deep the effect and the action mechanisms of soy isoflavone. In particular, the activity of gut microbiota should be investigated in patients before isoflavone consumption, due to its key role in the metabolism and bioavailability of isoflavones [43], microflora influencing factors also require consideration. As examples, a high-carbohydrate milieu causes more extensive biotransformation, greatly enhancing Eq formation, and a *Clostridium* sp. strain that converts D principally to O-DMA has been identified from gut microbiota. These bio-transformations could render isoflavones less active [44] and reduce the efficacy of the chemotherapeutic treatment. Moreover, concerns could arise also among healthy individuals who regularly consume soy products. Indeed, Equol and O-DMA producer individuals may be subjected to a long exposure to potent estrogenic compounds. Those who are not, on the other hand, will be mostly exposed to anti-estrogenic compounds.

Author Contributions: Conceptualization, M.M. and E.M.; methodology, E.M., M.C., and P.C.; formal analysis, M.M. and E.M.; investigation, E.M., M.C., and P.C.; resources, M.M and M.F.; data curation, M.M. and E.M.; writing-original draft preparation, M.M.; writing-review and editing, M.M., M.C., M.F., E.M, and P.C.; supervision and funding acquisition, M.M. All authors have read and agreed to the published version of the manuscript.

References

1. Křížová, L.; Dadáková, K.; Kašparovská, J.; Kašparovský, T. Isoflavones. *Molecules* **2019**, *24*, 1076. [CrossRef]
2. Di Gioia, F.; Petropoulos, S.A. Phytoestrogens, phytosteroids and saponins in vegetables: Biosynthesis, functions, health effects and practical applications. *Adv. Food Nutr. Res.* **2019**, *90*, 351–421.
3. Lacroix, S.; Klicic Badoux, J.; Scott-Boyer, M.P.; Parolo, S.; Matone, A.; Priami, C.; Morine, M.J.; Kaput, J.; Moco, S. A computationally driven analysis of the polyphenol-protein interactome. *Sci. Rep.* **2018**, *8*, 2232. [CrossRef] [PubMed]
4. Cipolletti, M.; Montalesi, E.; Nuzzo, M.T.; Fiocchetti, M.; Ascenzi, P.; Marino, M. Potentiation of paclitaxel effect by resveratrol in human breast cancer cells by counteracting the 17β-estradiol/estrogen receptor α/neuroglobin pathway. *J. Cell. Physiol.* **2019**, *234*, 3147–3157. [CrossRef]
5. Sarkar, F.H.; Li, Y. Soy isoflavones and cancer prevention. *Cancer Investig.* **2003**, *21*, 744–757. [CrossRef] [PubMed]
6. Sahin, I.; Bilir, B.; Ali, S.; Sahin, K.; Kucuk, O. Soy Isoflavones in Integrative Oncology: Increased Efficacy and Decreased Toxicity of Cancer Therapy. *Integr. Cancer Ther.* **2019**, *18*. [CrossRef] [PubMed]
7. Guo, J.; Wang, Q.; Zhang, Y.; Sun, W.; Zhang, S.; Li, Y.; Wang, J.; Bao, Y. Functional daidzein enhances the anticancer effect of topotecan and reverses BCRP-mediated drug resistance in breast cancer. *Pharmacol. Res.* **2019**, *147*, 104387. [CrossRef]
8. Choi, E.J.; Kim, G.H. Antiproliferative activity of daidzein and genistein may be related to ERα/c-erbB-2 expression in human breast cancer cells. *Mol. Med. Rep.* **2013**, *7*, 781–784. [CrossRef]
9. Zhu, Y.; Yao, Y.; Shi, Z.; Everaert, N.; Ren, G. Synergistic Effect of Bioactive Anticarcinogens from Soybean on Anti-Proliferative Activity in MDA-MB-231 and MCF-7 Human Breast Cancer Cells In Vitro. *Molecules* **2018**, *23*, 1557. [CrossRef]
10. Bao, C.; Namgung, H.; Lee, J.; Park, H.C.; Ko, J.; Moon, H.; Ko, H.W.; Lee, H.J. Daidzein suppresses tumor necrosis factor-α induced migration and invasion by inhibiting hedgehog/Gli1 signaling in human breast cancer cells. *J. Agric. Food Chem.* **2014**, *62*, 3759–3767. [CrossRef]

11. Liu, X.; Suzuki, N.; Santosh Laxmi, Y.R.; Okamoto, Y.; Shibutani, S. Anti-breast cancer potential of daidzein in rodents. *Life Sci.* **2012**, *91*, 415–419. [CrossRef] [PubMed]
12. Jin, S.; Zhang, Q.Y.; Kang, X.M.; Wang, J.X.; Zhao, W.H. Daidzein induces MCF-7 breast cancer cell apoptosis via the mitochondrial pathway. *Ann. Oncol.* **2010**, *21*, 263–268. [CrossRef] [PubMed]
13. Heinonen, S.; Wähälä, K.; Adlercreutz, H. Identification of isoflavone metabolites Dihydrodaidzein, Dihydrogenistein, 6-OH-O-DMA, and cis-4-OH-equol in human urine by gas chromatography–mass spectroscopy using authentic reference compounds. *Anal. Biochem.* **1999**, *274*, 211–219. [CrossRef] [PubMed]
14. King, R.A.; Bursill, D.B. Plasma and urinary kinetics of the isoflavones daidzein and genistein after a single soy meal in humans. *Am. J. Clin. Nutr.* **1998**, *67*, 867–872. [CrossRef]
15. Gardana, C.; Canzi, E.; Simonetti, P. The role of diet in the metabolism of daidzein by human faecal microbiota sampled from Italian volunteers. *J. Nutr. Biochem.* **2009**, *20*, 940–947. [CrossRef]
16. Chang, Y.C.; Nair, M.G.; Nitiss, J.L. Metabolites of daidzein and genistein and their biological activities. *J. Nat. Prod.* **1995**, *58*, 1901–1905. [CrossRef]
17. Soukup, S.T.; Helppi, J.; Müller, D.R.; Zierau, O.; Watzl, B.; Vollmer, G.; Diel, P.; Bub, A.; Kulling, S.E. Phase II metabolism of the soy isoflavones genistein and daidzein in humans, rats and mice: A cross-species and sex comparison. *Arch. Toxicol.* **2016**, *90*, 1335–1347. [CrossRef]
18. Chang, Y.C.; Nair, M.G. Metabolism of daidzein and genistein by intestinal bacteria. *J. Nat. Prod.* **1995**, *58*, 1892–1896. [CrossRef]
19. Totta, P.; Acconcia, F.; Virgili, F.; Cassidy, A.; Weinberg, P.D.; Rimbach, G.; Marino, M. Daidzein-sulfate metabolites affect transcriptional and antiproliferative activities of estrogen receptor-beta in cultured human cancer cells. *J. Nutr.* **2005**, *135*, 2687–2693. [CrossRef]
20. Lazennec, G.; Bresson, D.; Lucas, A.; Chauveau, C.; Vignon, F. ERβ inhibits proliferation and invasion of breast cancer cells. *Endocrinology* **2001**, *142*, 4120–4130. [CrossRef]
21. Marino, M.; Ascenzi, P. Membrane association of estrogen receptor alpha and beta influences 17beta-estradiol-mediated cancer cell proliferation. *Steroids* **2008**, *73*, 853–858. [CrossRef]
22. Fiocchetti, M.; Cipolletti, M.; Leone, S.; Ascenzi, P.; Marino, M. Neuroglobin overexpression induced by the 17β-Estradiol-Estrogen receptor-α Pathway reduces the sensitivity of MCF-7 Breast cancer cell to paclitaxel. *IUBMB Life* **2016**, *68*, 645–651. [CrossRef] [PubMed]
23. Nilsson, S.; Gustafsson, J.-Å. Estrogen receptors: Therapies targeted to receptor subtypes. *Clin. Pharmacol. Ther.* **2011**, *89*, 44–55. [CrossRef] [PubMed]
24. Ascenzi, P.; Bocedi, A.; Marino, M. Structure-function relationship of estrogen receptor alpha and beta: Impact on human health. *Mol. Asp. Med.* **2006**, *27*, 299–402. [CrossRef] [PubMed]
25. Thomas, C.; Gustafsson, J.-Å. The different roles of ER subtypes in cancer biology and therapy. *Nat. Rev. Cancer* **2011**, *11*, 597–608. [CrossRef] [PubMed]
26. Fiocchetti, M.; Solar Fernandez, V.; Montalesi, E.; Marino, M. Neuroglobin: A novel player in the oxidative stress response of cancer cells. *Oxidative Med. Cell. Longev.* **2019**, *2019*, 6315034. [CrossRef] [PubMed]
27. Fiocchetti, M.; Cipolletti, M.; Leone, S.; Naldini, A.; Carraro, F.; Giordano, D.; Verde, C.; Ascenzi, P.; Marino, M. Neuroglobin in breast cancer cells: Effect of hypoxia and oxidative stress on protein level, localization, and anti-apoptotic function. *PLoS ONE* **2016**, *11*, e0154959. [CrossRef] [PubMed]
28. Fiocchetti, M.; Cipolletti, M.; Ascenzi, P.; Marino, M. Dissecting the 17β-estradiol pathways necessary for neuroglobin anti-apoptotic activity in breast cancer. *J. Cell. Physiol.* **2018**, *233*, 5087–5103. [CrossRef]
29. Galluzzo, P.; Ascenzi, P.; Bulzomi, P.; Marino, M. The nutritional flavanone naringenin triggers antiestrogenic effects by regulating estrogen receptor alpha-palmitoylation. *Endocrinology* **2008**, *149*, 2567–2575. [CrossRef]
30. Crowe, K.M.; Francis, C. Position of the academy of nutrition and dietetics: Functional foods. *J. Acad. Nutr. Diet.* **2013**, *113*, 1096–1103. [CrossRef]
31. Cory, H.; Passarelli, S.; Szeto, J.; Tamez, M.; Mattei, J. The role of polyphenols in human health and food systems: A mini-review. *Front. Nutr.* **2018**, *5*, 87. [CrossRef] [PubMed]
32. Selvaraj, V.; Zakroczymski, M.A.; Naaz, A.; Mukai, M.; Ju, Y.H.; Doerge, D.R.; Katzenellenbogen, J.A.; Helferich, W.G.; Cooke, P.S. Estrogenicity of the isoflavone metabolite equol on reproductive and non-reproductive organs in mice. *Biol. Reprod.* **2004**, *71*, 966–972. [CrossRef]
33. Karakaya, S. Bioavailability of phenolic compounds. *Crit. Rev. Food Sci. Nutr.* **2004**, *44*, 453–464. [CrossRef] [PubMed]

34. Acconcia, F.; Fiocchetti, M.; Marino, M. Xenoestrogen regulation of ERα/ERβ balance in hormone-associated cancers. *Mol. Cell. Endocrinol.* **2017**, *457*, 3–12. [CrossRef] [PubMed]
35. Bulzomi, P.; Galluzzo, P.; Bolli, A.; Leone, S.; Acconcia, F.; Marino, M. The pro-apoptotic effect of quercetin in cancer cell lines requires ERβ-dependent signals. *J. Cell. Physiol.* **2012**, *227*, 1891–1898. [CrossRef]
36. Park, H.; Jin, U.H.; Orr, A.A.; Echegaray, S.P.; Davidson, L.A.; Allred, C.D.; Chapkin, R.S.; Jayaraman, A.; Lee, K.; Tamamis, P.; et al. Isoflavones as Ah Receptor Agonists in Colon-Derived Cell Lines: Structure-Activity Relationships. *Chem. Res. Toxicol.* **2019**, *32*, 2353–2364. [CrossRef]
37. Lee, J.E.; Safe, S. 3′,4′-dimethoxyflavone as an aryl hydrocarbon receptor antagonist in human breast cancer cells. *Toxicol. Sci.* **2000**, *58*, 235–242. [CrossRef]
38. Marino, M.; Pellegrini, M.; La Rosa, P.; Acconcia, F. Susceptibility of estrogen receptor rapid responses to xenoestrogens: Physiological outcomes. *Steroids* **2012**, *77*, 910–917. [CrossRef]
39. La Rosa, P.; Pellegrini, M.; Totta, P.; Acconcia, F.; Marino, M. Xenoestrogens alter estrogen receptor (ER) α intracellular levels. *PLoS ONE* **2014**, *9*, e88961. [CrossRef]
40. Fiocchetti, M.; Nuzzo, M.T.; Totta, P.; Acconcia, F.; Ascenzi, P.; Marino, M. Neuroglobin, a pro-survival player in estrogen receptor α-positive cancer cells. *Cell Death Dis.* **2014**, *5*, e1449. [CrossRef]
41. Uifălean, A.; Schneider, S.; Ionescu, C.; Lalk, M.; Iuga, C.A. Soy Isoflavones and Breast Cancer Cell Lines: Molecular Mechanisms and Future Perspectives. *Molecules* **2015**, *21*, 13. [CrossRef] [PubMed]
42. Fang, C.Y.; Tseng, M.; Daly, M.B. Correlates of soy food consumption in women at increased risk for breast cancer. *J. Am. Diet. Assoc.* **2005**, *105*, 1552–1558. [CrossRef] [PubMed]
43. Rafii, F.; Davis, C.; Park, M.; Heinze, T.M.; Beger, R.D. Variations in metabolism of the soy isoflavonoid daidzein by human intestinal microfloras from different individuals. *Arch. Microbiol.* **2003**, *180*, 11–16. [CrossRef] [PubMed]
44. Hur, H.G.; Beger, R.D.; Heinze, T.M.; Lay, J.O., Jr.; Freeman, J.P.; Dore, J.; Rafii, F. Isolation of an anaerobic intestinal bacterium capable of cleaving the C-ring of the isoflavonoid daidzein. *Arch. Microbiol.* **2002**, *178*, 8–12. [CrossRef] [PubMed]

6

Nobiletin and Derivatives: Functional Compounds from Citrus Fruit Peel for Colon Cancer Chemoprevention

Joanna Xuan Hui Goh [1], Loh Teng-Hern Tan [2,3], Joo Kheng Goh [4], Kok Gan Chan [5,6,*], Priyia Pusparajah [7], Learn-Han Lee [2,8] and Bey-Hing Goh [1,8,*]

1 Biofunctional Molecule Exploratory (BMEX) Research Group, School of Pharmacy, Monash University Malaysia, Bandar Sunway 47500, Selangor Darul Ehsan, Malaysia; jxgoh2@student.monash.edu
2 Novel Bacteria and Drug Discovery (NBDD) Research Group, Microbiome and Bioresource Research Strength, Jeffrey Cheah School of Medicine and Health Sciences, Monash University Malaysia, Bandar Sunway 47500, Selangor Darul Ehsan, Malaysia; Loh.Tan@monash.edu (L.T.-H.T.); lee.learn.han@monash.edu (L.-H.L.)
3 Institute of Biomedical and Pharmaceutical Sciences, Guangdong University of Technology, Guangzhou 510006, China
4 School of Science, Monash University Malaysia, Jalan Lagoon Selatan, Bandar Sunway 47500, Selangor Darul Ehsan, Malaysia; goh.joo.kheng@monash.edu
5 Division of Genetics and Molecular Biology, Institute of Biological Sciences, Faculty of Science, University of Malaya, Kuala Lumpur 50603, Malaysia
6 International Genome Centre, Jiangsu University, Zhenjiang 212013, China
7 Medical Health and Translational Research Group, Jeffrey Cheah School of Medicine and Health Sciences, Monash University Malaysia, Bandar Sunway 47500, Selangor, Malaysia; priyia.pusparajah@monash.edu
8 Asian Centre for Evidence Synthesis in Population, Implementation and Clinical Outcomes (PICO), Health and Well-being Cluster, Global Asia in the 21st Century (GA21) Platform, Monash University Malaysia, Bandar Sunway, 47500, Malaysia
* Correspondence: kokgan@um.edu.my (K.G.C.); goh.bey.hing@monash.edu (B.-H.G.)

Abstract: The search for effective methods of cancer treatment and prevention has been a continuous effort since the disease was discovered. Recently, there has been increasing interest in exploring plants and fruits for molecules that may have potential as either adjuvants or as chemopreventive agents against cancer. One of the promising compounds under extensive research is nobiletin (NOB), a polymethoxyflavone (PMF) extracted exclusively from citrus peel. Not only does nobiletin itself exhibit anti-cancer properties, but its derivatives are also promising chemopreventive agents; examples of derivatives with anti-cancer activity include 3′-demethylnobiletin (3′-DMN), 4′-demethylnobiletin (4′-DMN), 3′,4′-didemethylnobiletin (3′,4′-DMN) and 5-demethylnobiletin (5-DMN). In vitro studies have demonstrated differential efficacies and mechanisms of NOB and its derivatives in inhibiting and killing of colon cancer cells. The chemopreventive potential of NOB has also been well demonstrated in several in vivo colon carcinogenesis animal models. NOB and its derivatives target multiple pathways in cancer progression and inhibit several of the hallmark features of colorectal cancer (CRC) pathophysiology, including arresting the cell cycle, inhibiting cell proliferation, inducing apoptosis, preventing tumour formation, reducing inflammatory effects and limiting angiogenesis. However, these substances have low oral bioavailability that limits their clinical utility, hence there have been numerous efforts exploring better drug delivery strategies for NOB and these are part of this review. We also reviewed data related to patents involving NOB to illustrate the extensiveness of each research area and its direction of commercialisation. Furthermore, this review also provides suggested directions for future research to advance NOB as the next promising candidate in CRC chemoprevention.

Keywords: nobiletin; colorectal cancer; chemoprevention; bioactivities

1. Introduction

Colorectal cancer (CRC) is the third most prevalent cancer reported in both men and women, ranking just after prostate or breast cancer and lung cancer [1]. Although in many cases there is no readily apparent cause of CRC, a number of factors have been found to be closely associated with this malignancy including gender, age, genetic predisposition, lifestyle, diet or as a complication from other diseases such as inflammatory bowel disease (IBD). Statistics showed that the death rate from CRC is 40% higher in males as compared to females, with the prevalence increasing with age, especially above 50 years old; however, there is a new and worrying trend of increasing incidence of colorectal cancer in the age group younger than 50, which, while slight, is still worrying [2,3].

The incidence of CRC has reduced as modern screening strategies have enabled much earlier detection of potentially malignant lesions, allowing for early intervention such as surgical excision of adenoma before it undergoes malignant transformation [4,5]. Although there has been a reduction, the high number of cases remains a major concern and the search for new and better treatments for CRC has been a key focus in pharmacological research. Standard therapy for cancer typically involves the triple regimen of surgery, chemotherapy, and radiation treatment. Efforts in exploring and developing new treatments are very much needed due to the limitations of the current treatment regimen—ranging from side effects, to complications and the development of drug resistance.

Researchers are attempting to explore multiple avenues for novel leads as anti-cancer agents with an increasing trend to focus on natural sources like plants and fruits [6–8]. However, while it is key to find new treatments to existing cancers, a crucial aspect that is also being explored is prevention of cancerous growths; in particular, this would be of benefit for those at risk due to the various factors outlined earlier. One of the effective strategies to control cancer is chemoprevention, which is defined as the use of a natural or synthetic agent to reverse, inhibit, or prevent the progression of cancer [9].

Plants and fruits are often part of a diet recommended to prevent various illnesses including cancer [10]. These beneficial properties may be from the chemicals they contain as well as their metabolites which enter our alimentary canal and eventually end up in our colon and rectum. If the compounds responsible can be isolated and purified for use as a treatment, this may be a milestone in new cancer therapies and prophylaxis. While an extensive review of polyphenols like apigenin and luteolin on anti-colorectal cancer effect can readily be found [11], this study highlights the potential chemopreventive effect on CRC of another flavonoid, namely nobiletin (NOB).

NOB, a polymethoxyflavone (PMF), is likely named after *Citrus nobilis*. This compound is one of the most ubiquitous flavones that can be isolated exclusively from the peel of citrus fruits [12]. Besides CRC, there is concurrently ongoing research looking into the effect of NOB on other types of cancers such as breast cancer [13,14], ovarian cancer [15], gastric cancer [16,17], lung cancer [18,19], liver cancer [20] and bone cancer [21]. There are also recent studies attesting to the benefits of NOB in anti-neurodegeneration [22,23], anti-diabetes [24], anti-obesity [25–27], antimicrobial [28], anti-allergy [29] and anti-inflammatory effects [30,31]. There are also a number of articles that support claims purporting to the role of NOB in reducing the risk of cardiovascular diseases [32,33] and osteoporosis [34,35].

Interestingly, this compound can be metabolised into a number of metabolites which also show significant anti-cancer effects. There are several recent reviews on the bioactivities of these citrus PMF [36] as well as the potential chemopreventive abilities of these PMFs toward cancers in general [37]. This review paper aims to gather the results of the in vivo and in vitro studies done in recent years and compile various molecular pathways by which the compound NOB and its derivatives act in CRC prevention which will in turn help to facilitate future research that targets these specific mechanisms.

2. Research Methodology

The main focus was to search for all relevant primary research papers published which looked into the use of NOB and its derivatives as a chemopreventive agent for CRC. A systematic search was performed to identify published literature on the chemopreventive potentials of NOB against CRC using Google Scholar. For studies published in foreign languages like Chinese, Japanese or Korean, an attempt was made to locate the translated version. The search strategy was performed using keywords 'nobiletin' and 'colorectal cancer' to locate relevant papers. This was also supplemented with keyword search of the terms 'cancer statistics', 'colorectal cancer', 'colon cancer', 'metabolites', 'synergism', 'biotransformation', 'mechanism', 'apoptosis', 'anti-inflammatory', 'inflammation', 'cell proliferation', 'cell cycle arrest', 'metastasis', 'tumour', 'angiogenesis', 'absorption', 'metabolism', 'toxicity', 'distribution', 'elimination', 'solubility' and 'delivery' combined using Boolean operators with 'nobiletin'. PubChem and EMBASE were used as alternatives to ensure inclusion of all relevant papers while SciFinder database was mainly used to locate patents related to NOB. The reference lists of relevant articles collected were also screened for additional studies to be included in the review.

3. Nobiletin and Its Derivatives

The compound nobiletin (NOB) can be extracted exclusively from citrus fruits, namely mandarin oranges (*Citrus reticulate*), sweet oranges or Valencia oranges (*Citrus sinesis*), Miaray mandarins (*Citrus miaray*) [38], flat lemons or Hayata (*Citrus depressa*) [39,40], tangerines (*Citrus tangerine*), bitter oranges (*Citrus aurantium*) [12], Unshu Mikans or Satsuma mandarins (*Citrus Unshiu arnicia indica*) [41,42], Cleopatra mandarins (*Citrus reshni*) [43], mandarin oranges (*Citrus tachibana*), Koji Oranges (*Citrus leiocarpa*), Natsu Mikans (*Citrus tardiva*), Jimikan (*Citrus succosa*), Kinokuni Mandarins (*Citrus Kinokuni*), Fukushu (*Citrus erythrosa*), Sunkat (*Citrus sunki*) and hybrids of the mandarin orange with pomelo (*Citrus deliciosa*) [44]. *Citrus tangerine* was reported to contain the highest content of NOB, approximately five times of that in *Citrus sinesis* [45].

PMF can be isolated from orange peel through different types of chemical extraction processes, for example, the supercritical fluid extraction, microwave assisted extraction [46] and Soxhlet method, which is capable of extracting large sample volumes [43]. Through the supercritical fluid extraction process, the supercritical fluid extractor is used to process the orange peel grinds that have been freeze-dried. Then, the extract is further treated with carbon dioxide and ethanol to concentrate the bioactive compound [47]. A special method to improve NOB yield through the supercritical fluid extraction method is currently patented in Korea [48]. It was found that the maximal yield of NOB occurs at a temperature of 80 °C and pressure of 30 MPa with an optimum sample particle size of 375 μm [40].

NOB is a PMF classified under the flavonoid family of polyphenols. The International Union of Pure and Applied Chemistry (IUPAC) nomenclature is 2-(3,4-dimethoxyphenyl)-5,6,7,8-tetramethoxychromen-4-one. It is also known as 5,6,7,8,3′,4′-hexamethoxyflavone or 2-(3,4-dimethoxyphenyl)-5,6,7,8-tetramethoxy-4H-1-benzopyran-4-one [12]. NOB has a molecular formula of $C_{21}H_{22}O_8$ and a molecular weight of 402.399 g/mol. The chemical structure of NOB is illustrated in Figure 1. This flavone has a distinct three aromatic ring structure (labelled A, B and C in Figure 1), with the ketone and ether group in ring C along with four methoxy groups at the 5, 6, 7 and 8 positions of ring A and 2 methoxy groups at the 3 and 4 positions of ring B. Under long-term storage, NOB can degrade into 5-demethylnobiletin (5-DMN), IUPAC name 5-hydroxy- 6,7,8,3′,4′-pentamethoxyflavone (structure illustrated in Figure 1), through the process of autohydrolysis [49]. It has also been proposed that 5-DMN could be formed through conversion of nobiletin by gastric acid after oral consumption [50].

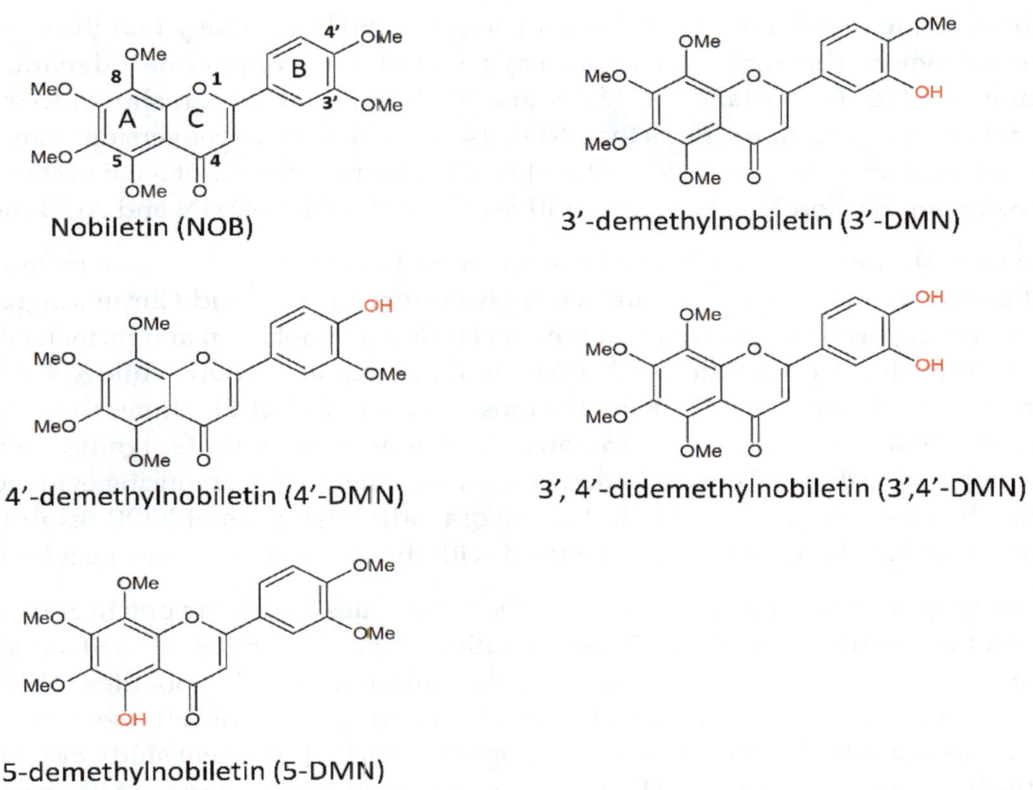

Figure 1. Chemical structures of nobiletin and its derivatives.

Both the NOB and 5-DMN undergo further transformation to form a number of metabolites in the body after ingestion [50,51]. More than 20 metabolites have been identified and the types vary significantly according to the species of citrus plants [12]. The three common phase I metabolites of NOB identified in urine after administration to rodents are 3′-DMN, 4′-DMN and 3′,4′-DMN [52,53]. Wu et al. successfully quantitated the amount of NOB, 3′-DMN, 4′-DMN and 3′,4′-DMN at 2.03, 3.28, 24.13 and 12.03 nmol/(gram of tissue of colonic mucosa) at the end of 20 weeks daily feeding of 500 ppm NOB to CD-1 mice [54].

After absorption, NOB generally undergoes Phase I and Phase II metabolism. In vivo tests show the Phase I demethylation of NOB is likely caused by the action of cytochrome P450 [55]. Koga et al. researched the enzymes involved in NOB metabolism and confirmed that CYP1A1, CYP1A2, CYP1B1 and CYP3A5 are involved in the conversion of NOB to 3′-DMN; further action from CYP1A1 and CYP1A2 is required to convert 3′-DMN to 3′,4′-DMN [56]. NOB was also found to undergo extensive Phase II metabolism in the small intestine involving glucuronides or sulphates. [57] Four phase II metabolites of NOB have been identified in rodent serum, bile and urine. These Phase II metabolites are formed from the glucuronidation/sulphation of the Phase I products, namely 4′-DMN and 3′,4′-DMN [58]. However, research on these Phase II metabolites are limited likely due to the fact that existing literature suggests a high likelihood that these substances have decreased activity. For example, Manthey et al. showed there was a reduced anti-inflammatory effect of the compound after glucuronidation [59].

In contrast to the dominant Phase II metabolites in the small intestines, the majority of the metabolites in the large intestine undergo deconjugation mainly through the action of the microflora in the gut. The microbiome produces enzymes such as C-deglycosidases, O-deglycosidases and hydrolases that break down the unabsorbed compounds from the small intestine. The microbiome also releases enzymes such as glucuronidases and sulphatases that hydrolyze the conjugate bonds, resulting in the reformation of free molecules that either undergo reuptake into the colonocytes or enter into the blood stream [60]. At present, only a limited species of the microbiome have been identified and further research is crucial to understand the in vivo biotransformation of the NOB compound resulting in the generation of multiple metabolites with different activities [61]. It is likely that the subtle variances in the gut microbiome in different individuals may result in different pharmacodynamic effects after administration of NOB. For instance, 4′-DMN and 3′,4′-DMN have been shown to exhibit higher anti-cancer and anti-inflammatory effects than NOB itself, but the rate of conversion from NOB to these metabolites may vary from one person to another [54,62]. The mechanisms of NOB in chemoprevention are elaborated under 'Section 5—Chemopreventive effects of NOB, 5-DMN and NOB-metabolites'.

Early in vitro studies using rat liver S9 extracts reveals 3′-DMN as the main metabolite of NOB after 24 h of treatment [42]. However, further High-Performance Liquid Chromatography (HPLC) analysis on in vivo experiments showed that the concentration of nobiletin and its metabolites differ in the colonic mucosa—the concentration of 3′-DMN is almost equal to NOB, while 3′,4′-DMN is about 5.9-fold more than NOB, and 4′-DMN being the most concentrated, at 11.9 times the concentration of NOB. Integrating these values, the concentration of NOB is actually 20 times significantly lower in the colon when compared to the total concentration of its metabolites [54]. Convincing evidence has shown that these metabolites generated in vivo following oral administration of NOB result in significant accumulation in colonic tissues which is associated with the chemopreventive effect for CRC.

Interestingly, growing evidence suggests that the metabolites have more potent anti-cancer activity than their parent compounds, and the high concentration of the metabolites of NOB found in the colon may indicate that anti-cancer effect of NOB is largely conferred by its metabolites. This is consistent with the findings of Wu et al. who discovered that by treating HCT116 cell lines with NOB and its metabolites results in a 3.3 to 7.6-fold increase in apoptotic cells [54]. A recent study by Chiou et al. also shows that the hydroxylated PMF, 5-DMN is more potent than NOB in terms of its chemopreventive effect on colon malignancy for both in vivo studies using xenograft mice and in vivo studies using three different colon cell lines. Chiou and colleagues reported that 5-DMN shows different levels of inhibition in different types of cell lines, with the highest efficacies in COLO205 cell lines, followed by HCT116 and HT-29 [49]. This is consistent with the findings of Qiu et al. stating that the half maximal inhibitory concentration (IC_{50}) required for 5-DMN to exert an inhibitory effect on the growth of HCT116 cells is 8.4 μM as compared to the notably higher value of 37 μM for NOB. Similarly, the IC_{50} required for 5-DMN against HT-29 cells is 22 μM as compared to the higher IC_{50} of 46.2 μM for NOB [63]. This may suggest that the hydroxyl group at the 5th position on the A ring is an important functional group involved in the molecular interactions [49].

4. Pathogenesis of Colorectal Cancer

The mechanisms leading to CRC development are part of a rather complex process. The pathogenesis of CRC is arbitrarily subdivided into three stages here: initiation, progression and metastasis. Each pathway is known to be regulated by chemical signals, called cytokines, which allow the progression from one stage to the next, whilst inflammation is the underlying result of each stage [11].

Cancer generally starts with a mutated cell which deviates from the normal cell growth cycle and progresses through the cell cycle rapidly with no differentiation of structure or function. It can be attributed to the down regulation of the regulatory genes or up-regulation of oncogenes. This gradually leads to the formation of a mass of undifferentiated cells called an adenoma. This lump of cells does not perform any specific function but competes with the surrounding normal cells for nutrients. In more than 60% of colorectal adenomas, the dysregulation of adenomatous polyposis coli gene resulting from the Wnt/β-catenin pathway is the major culprit in triggering this process [64].

The initial adenoma progresses on to an intermediate adenoma when the epidermal growth factor receptor (EGFR) is activated, which in turn triggers the phosphatidylinositol-3-kinase pathway and results in tumour formation [65]. Also, the inactivation of transforming growth factor-β (TGF-β) and the loss of function of p53 further aggravates tumour growth by preventing apoptosis [66,67].

Eventually, a tumour becomes malignant when angiogenesis occurs, and the cancer cells are released into the bloodstream and spread to other parts of the body through a process known as metastasis. Intercellular adhesion molecule-1 (ICAM-1) and matrix metalloproteinase (MMPs) are closely associated with the promotion of angiogenesis and metastasis. To illustrate, the MMP disrupts the integrity of the basal membrane allowing the cancer cells to enter the surrounding blood vessels and thus the blood stream through a process known as intravasation [68,69].

5. Chemopreventive Effects of Nobiletin, 5-DMN and NOB-Metabolites

In one of earliest in vitro studies, the antiproliferative effect of NOB was evaluated against HT-29 colon cancer cells [70]. The study determined that the IC_{50} and IC_{90} of NOB against HT-29 cell were 4.7 μM and 13.9 μM, respectively, via the 3H-thymidine uptake assay [70]. As a product of autohydrolysis of NOB, 5-DMN was also evaluated for its antiproliferative effect against colon cancer cells. In the H-thymidine uptake assay, the IC_{50} and IC_{90} of 5-DMN against HT-29 was reported to be 8.5 μM and 171 μM, respectively [70]. In the following years, NOB and 5-DMN were also reported to be cytotoxic towards different colon cancer cell lines, including HCT116, HT-29, SW489, COLO320, COLO205 and Caco-2 (Table 1). Despite the stronger anti-proliferative effect of NOB observed in the earlier study [70], recent studies increasingly showed that 5-DMN exhibits stronger cytotoxic effects against different colon cancer cells as compared to NOB [49,63]. These contradictory results are potentially due to the different aspects of cancer focused in each study. Based on these in vitro studies, NOB and 5-DMN were shown to exhibit their cytotoxic effects towards colon cancer cells, predominantly via cell cycle arrest and induction of apoptosis (Table 1).

Multiple in vivo studies demonstrated that NOB offers a protective effect against several carcinogens, such as the azoxymethane (AOM) and the 2-amino-1-methyl-6-phenylimidazo[4,5-b]pyridine (PhIP) (Table 2). AOM/DSS has been used to induce colitis in mice for the purpose of creating mouse models that replicate colitis induced CRC in humans [71]; however, PhIP, a heterocyclic amine, is a food-derived carcinogen that is abundantly released in the process of cooking fish and meat [72,73]. Administration of 0.01% wt of NOB to mice for five weeks in their diet resulted in the reduction of abnormal growths induced by colonic carcinogen AOM in the colons of the mice; there was a 50% reduction as compared to the controls [41].

Another similar study to determine the anti-adenocarcinoma effects of NOB also showed positive results but with lower efficacies, whereby 34 weeks administration of 0.01% or 0.05% wt. of NOB reduced the frequency of adenocarcinoma by 12% and 32%, respectively [74]. In addition to that, Wu et al. demonstrated that NOB treatment successfully reduced the rate of cell proliferation by 69%, tumour incidence by 40%, tumour multiplicity by 71%, and downregulated TNF-α, IL-1β and IL-6 by 65%, 69% and 45% respectively in AOM/DSS treated mice [54]. Consistent with the inhibitory effect against AOM induced colon carcinogenesis, NOB also showed significant reduction in the high density of colonic aberrant crypt foci (ACF) located in the transverse colon in PhlP-induced F344 rats [75]. This shows that NOB is effective in preventing CRC triggered by different types of carcinogens.

Further support for NOB as a prospective candidate for chemoprevention is that NOB is known to inhibit different pathways leading to cancer via a number of different mechanisms which includes inhibiting cell cycle progression [54,76], limiting inflammation [76], inducing apoptosis [54], preventing angiogenesis [77] and reducing tumour formation [49,54,78]. This subsection will describe the mechanism of action of NOB, its autohydrolysis product, 5-DMN and its three common metabolites, namely 3′-DMN, 4′-DMN and 3′,4′-DMN, in chemoprevention of CRC in detail.

Table 1. In vitro chemopreventive properties of NOB, 5-DMN and NOB-metabolites.

Compounds	Activities	Cell lines	Treatment/Assay (Treatment duration)	Assays/Results/Mechanisms	References
NOB 5-DMN	Anti-proliferative	HT-29	H-thymidine uptake assay	- IC_{50} of NOB = 4.7 µM - IC_{90} of NOB = 13.9 µM - IC_{50} of 5-DMN = 8.5 µM - IC_{90} of 5-DMN = 171 µM	[70]
NOB	Cytotoxicity	COLO320, SW480 and Caco-2	MTS viability assay (48 h)	- IC_{50} for COLO320 = 40.4 ± 9.1 µM - IC_{50} for SW480 = 245 ± 9.1 µM - IC_{50} for Caco-2 = 305.6 ± 41.9 µM	[79]
	Apoptosis-inducing		Apoptosis assays—DNA fragmentation - gel electrophoresis (48 h)	- DNA ladder pattern 200 µM—2-fold increase DNA fragmentation in COLO320	
	Anti-proliferative		BrdU labelling index	- 34.7 ± 4.7% BrdU-binding cells at 100 µM - 44.4 ± 6.4% BrdU-binding cells at 40 µM	
NOB	Anti-metastasis	HT-29	ELISA - proMMP-7 expression qPCR and Western blot	- At 100 µM, no detection of proMMP-7 in media, ~280 pg/mL proMMP-7 in media - >25 µM, reduced RNA and protein (both intracellular and supernatant) expression of proMMP-7	[77]
			AP-1 binding activity	- Inhibited binding activity of AP-1 (transcription factor for MMP-7 gene)	
NOB	Anti-proliferative	HT-29	Cell counting assay	- IC_{50} of NOB ≈ 50 µM - Inhibited cell proliferation in a time- and dose-dependent manner	[14]
	Cell cycle arrest		Cell cycle analysis - Propidium iodide staining	- Induced G1 phase cell cycle arrest (60 and 200 µM)	
	Apoptosis-inducing		Apoptosis assay	- No significant apoptosis detected at 60 and 100 µM	
			Resumption of proliferation	- Resumed proliferation within 24 h of removal of NOB and achieve the same stage of growth as compared to control after four days of removal of NOB	
NOB 5-DMN	Cytotoxicity	HCT116, HT-29	MTT viability assay (48 h)	- IC_{50} of NOB on HCT116 = 37 µM - IC_{50} of 5-DMN on HCT116 = 8.7 µM - IC_{50} of NOB on HT-29 = 46.2 µM - IC_{50} of 5-DMN on HT-29 = 22 µM	[63]
	Cell cycle arrest		Cell cycle analysis - Propidium iodide staining (24 h) Western blot	- At 8 µM, 5-DMN induced G2/M phase arrest in HCT116 - At 36 µM, 5-DMN induced G2/M phase arrest in HT-29 - At 16 µM, NOB reduced CDK-2 expression - At 4 µM and 8 µM, 5-DMN increased p21 and Rb, while decreased CDK-2 and p-Rb.	
	Apoptosis-inducing		Apoptosis assay Annexin-V/PI (48 h) Western blot	- At 8 µM, 5-DMN increased early apoptosis by 2.2-fold in HCT116 - At 36 µM, 5-DMN increased early apoptosis by ~2-fold in HT-29 - At 16 µM, NOB did not increase apoptotic cell population in HCT116/HT-29 - At 4 µM and 8 µM, 5-DMN increased expressions of cleaved caspase 8, cleaved caspase 3 and cleaved PARP.	

Table 1. *Cont.*

Compounds	Activities	Cell lines	Treatment/Assay (Treatment Duration)	Assays/Results/Mechanisms	References
5-DMN	Apoptosis-inducing	HCT116 (p53 $^{+/+}$) and HCT116 (p53 $^{-/-}$); HCT116 (Bax $^{+/-}$) and HCT116 (Bax $^{-/-}$);	Apoptosis assay Annexin-V/PI	- At 15 µM, 5-DMN increased late apoptotic/necrotic cell in HCT116 (p53 $^{-/-}$) > HCT115 (p53 $^{+/+}$), suggesting the apoptotic inducing action is independent of p53 - At 15 µM, 5-DMN increased early apoptotic cell in HCT116 (Bax $^{+/-}$), but not in HCT116 (Bax $^{-/-}$)	[80]
	Cell cycle arrest		Cell cycle analysis - Propidium iodide staining	- At 15 µM, 5-DMN arrested cells at G2/M and G0/G1 phases in HCT116 (p53 $^{+/+}$) cells, but only caused G2/M phase arrest in HCT116 (p53 $^{-/-}$) cells - G0/G1 is p53 dependent and G2/M is p53-independent	
NOB; 3′-DMN; 4′-DMN; 3′,4′-DMN	Cytotoxicity	HCT116, HT-29 HCT116 (p21 $^{-/-}$)	MTT viability assay	- At 2.03 µM and 3.28 µM, NOB and 3′-DMN, respectively showed no significant cytotoxicity against HCT116 and HT-29 - At 24.13 µM, 4′-DMN inhibited growth of HCT-116 by 45% and HT-29 by 33% - At 12.03 µM, 3′,4′-DMN inhibited growth of HCT116 by 30% and HT-29 by 9% - combination of all three NOB-metabolites inhibited growth of HCT116 by 64% and HT-29 by 62% (no significant difference to three NOB-metabolites + NOB)	[54]
	Cell cycle arrest		Cell cycle analysis - Propidium iodide staining (24 h)	- NOB (40 µM) arrested cells at G0/G1 phase in both HCT-116 and HT-29 - 3′-DMN (40 µM) arrested cells at both S phase and G2/M phase in HCT-116; while arrested cells at both G0/G1 and G2/M phase in HT-29 - 4′-DMN (40 µM) induced a stronger effect than NOB in arresting cells at G0/G1 phase in HCT-116 and HT-29 - 3′,4′-DMN (20 µM) arrested cells at both S phase and G2/M phase in HCT-116; while arrested cells at both G0/G1 and G2/M phase in HT-29	
	Apoptosis inducing		Western blot	- NOB and all three NOB-metabolites cause profound increase in expression of p21$^{Cip1/Waf1}$	
			Annexin-V/PI (48 h)	- NOB (40 µM) increased early apoptotic cell population by 3.3-fold, increased late apoptotic cell population by 4.2-fold in HCT116 - 3′-DMN (40 µM) increased early apoptotic cell population by 5.0-fold, increased late apoptotic cell population by 3.5-fold in HCT116 - 4′-DMN (40 µM) increased early apoptotic cell population by 4.9-fold, increased late apoptotic cell population by 7.1-fold in HCT116 - 3′,4′-DMN (20 µM) increased early apoptotic cell population by 7.6-fold, increase late apoptotic cell population by 4.5-fold in HCT116 -3′-DMN (40 µM) and 4′-DMN (40 µM) did not cause significant apoptosis in HT-29 - 3′,4′-DMN (20 µM) exhibits stronger apoptosis effect than NOB (40 µM) in HT-29	
			Western blot	- NOB (40 µM) only increased activation of caspase-9 and did not affect caspase-3 or PARP levels in HCT116 - NOB-metabolites increased activation of caspase-3, caspase-9 and other downstream proteins like PARP in HCT116	

Table 1. *Cont.*

Compounds	Activities	Cell lines	Treatment/Assay (Treatment duration)	Assays/Results/Mechanisms	References
NOB-Met (2.03 μM NOB: 3.28 μM 3′-DMN: 24.13 μM 4′-DMN: 12.03 μM 3′,4′-DMN	Anti-inflammatory	RAW264.7	Western Blot	- At 0.5× concentration of NOB-Met, supressed LPS-induced iNOS expression by 56.4% - At 1× and 2× concentration of NOB-Met, completely abrogated LPS-induced iNOS expression - At ×0.5, increased expression of NQO1 by 21% as compared to LPS-treated cells - At ×1, increased expression of HO-1 by 10%, increased expression of NQO1 by 34% as compared to LPS-treated cells - At ×2, increased expression of HO-1 by 37%, increased expression of NQO1 by 50% as compared to LPS-treated cells - Induced translocation of Nrf2	[76]
	Cell cycle arrest	HCT116	Cell cycle analysis - Propidium iodide staining Western blot	- At 1×, induced G0/G1 phase arrest; while at 2×, induced G0/G1 and G2/M phases arrest - Reduced expressions of CDK-2, CDK-4, CDK-6 and cyclin D, while increased expressions of p53 and p27	
NOB, 5-DMN	Cytotoxicity	HCT116, HT-29, COLO205	MTT viability assay	- At 40 μM, NOB significantly reduced viability of HCT116, HT-29 and COLO205 by ~20–30% - At >5 μM, 5-DMN significantly reduced viability of HCT116, HT-29 and COLO205	[49]
	Apoptosis inducing		Cell cycle analysis - SubG1 quantification Western	- At 20 μM, 5-DMN increased apoptosis ratio by ~26%, while no increased in subG1 population in NOB-treated COLO205 - At 10 and 20 μM, significantly increased expression of cleaved PARP in COLO205	
NOB	Anti-inflammatory	Human synovial fibroblast, mouse macrophage J774A.1	ELISA Western blot and qPCR qPCR Western blot	- At >4 μM, NOB inhibited PGE_2 induced by IL-1α in human synovial fibroblast - At >16 μM, NOB reduced mRNA of COX-2 induced by IL-1α in human synovial fibroblast - At 64 μM, NOB inhibited COX-2 protein expression induced by IL-1α in human synovial fibroblast - At 32 μM, NOB reduced mRNA of IL-1α, IL-1β, IL-6, TNF-α induced by LPS in J774A.1 - At >16 μM, NOB reduced proMMP-1 and proMMP-3 induced by IL-1α in human synovial fibroblast - At >16 μM, NOB enhanced TIMP-1 expression in response to IL-1α in human synovial fibroblast	[81]
NOB	Anti-inflammatory	Mouse adipocyte 3T3-L1	ELISA Western blot	- At 50 and 100 μM, NOB suppressed MCP-1 secretion induced by TNF-α IN 3T3-L1 adipocytes - At 50 and 100 μM, NOB reduced ERK phosphorylation in 3T3-L1 adipocytes treated with TNF-α	[82]

IC_{50}—half maximal inhibitory concentration; AP-1—activator protein-1; PI—propidium iodide; PARP—poly (ADP-ribosome) polymerase; CDK—cyclin-dependent kinase; Rb—retinoblastoma; LPS—lipopolysaccharide; iNOS—inducible NO synthase; NQO1—NAD(P)H quinone oxidoreductase 1; HO-1—heme oxygenase-1; PGE_2—prostaglandin E2; IL—interleukin; TNF—tumor necrosis factor; TIMP-1—tissue inhibitor metalloprotease-1; MCP-1—monocyte chemoattractant protein-1.

Table 2. In vivo studies of NOB for colon cancer chemoprevention.

Animal Models	Treatment/Dosage	Mechanisms	Detailed Results	References
Colitis-associated colon carcinogenesis model - AOM (12 mg/kg i.p.)/1% DSS in drinking water treated male CD-1 mice (5-week-old)	AIN93G diet containing 0.05% wt NOB (20 weeks)	Cell cycle arrest Anti-inflammatory effects	Protein expression in colonic mucosa by Western blot - Reduced levels of CDK-2, CDK-4, CDK-6, cyclin D and cyclin E - Increased levels of p21, p27 and p53 Immunohistochemical analysis - Reduced expression of iNOS reduced by 35% when compared to the positive control Protein expression in colonic mucosa by Western blot - Increased level of HO-1 - Increased level of NQO1 - Induced translocation of level of Nrf2 transcription factor (Nuclear fraction < Cytoplasmic fraction)	[76]
Colitis-associated colon carcinogenesis model - AOM/DSS treated AOM (12 mg/kg i.p.)/1% DSS in drinking water treated male CD-1 mice (5 week old)	AIN93G diet containing 0.05% wt NOB (20 weeks)	Inhibit AOM/DSS-induced colon carcinogenesis Anti-proliferative effect Apoptosis-inducing effect Anti-inflammatory effects	- Prevented shortening of colon length, reduced the increased colon weight/length ratio - Reduced tumor incidence by 40% and tumor multiplicity by 71% - Maintained histological characteristic of normal mucosa - Reduced PCNA-positive colonocytes by 69% in mucosal crypts - Increased cleaved caspase-3 positive cells by 2.3-fold in colonic tumor - Reduced levels of proinflammatory cytokines - ELISA showed reduction of TNF-α by 51%, IL-1ß by 92% and IL-6 by 69% compared - qRT-PCR analysis showed reduction of TNF-α by 65%, IL-1ß by 69% and IL-6 by 45%	[54]
Colon carcinogenesis model - AOM (15 mg/kg i.p.) treated male *db/db* mice	Diet containing 100 ppm NOB (0.1% wt) (10 weeks)	Inhibit AOM induced colon carcinogenesis	- Reduced frequency of preneoplastic lesions (colonic aberrant crypt foci (ACF) and β-catenin-accumulated crypts (BCAC)) - Reduced incidence of ACF by 68-91% and BCAC by 64–71% - Reduced PCNA-labeling index in ACF by 21% and BCAC by 19%	[83]
Colon carcinogenesis model - AOM (10 mg/kg i.p.)/1% DSS in drinking water treated male CD-1 mice	Diet containing 100 ppm NOB (0.1% wt) (for 17 weeks)	Inhibit AOM/DSS-induced colon carcinogenesis Inhibit leptin-induced colon carcinogenesis	- Suppressed incidence of neoplasms (adenoma and adenocarcinoma), lowered multiplicity of tumor - Suppressed serum levels of leptin by 75–84%	[84]
Colon carcinogenesis model - AOM (20 mg/kg s.c.) treated male F344 rats	Diet containing NOB (0.01% wt and 0.05% wt) (34 weeks)	Inhibit AOM induced colon carcinogenesis Anti-proliferative effect Anti-inflammatory effect	- Reduced incidence and multiplicity of colonic adenocarcinoma - Increased apoptosis index of adenocarcinoma - Reduced level of PGE_2 in colonic adenocarcinoma and surrounding mucosa	[74]

Table 2. *Cont.*

Animal Models	Treatment/Dosage	Mechanisms	Detailed Results	References
Colon carcinogenesis model - AOM (20 mg/kg s.c.) treated male F344 rats	Diet containing NOB (0.01% 0.01% wtwt and 0.05% wt) (5 weeks)	Inhibit AOM-induced colon carcinogenesis Anti-proliferative effect Anti-inflammatory effect	- Reduced the frequency of colonic aberrant crypt foci formation - Reduced number of ACF in proximal, middle and distal colon - Reduced MIB-5 labeling index of ACF but not of normal colonic crypts - Reduced level of PGE_2 in colonic mucosa	[41]
Colon carcinogenesis model - PhIP hydrochloride (100 mg/kg i.g.) treated F344 male rats (twice/week for 10 weeks)	Diet containing NOB (0.05% wt.) (50 weeks)	Inhibit PhIP-induced ACF in transverse colon	- Reduced the total colonic ACF indices in transverse colon	[75]
Colorectal cancer xenograft mouse model - COLO205 cells s.c.	NOB 100 mg/kg i.p. daily for 3 weeks 5-DMN 50 mg/kg and 100 mg/kg i.p. daily for 3 weeks	Anti-tumor effect Autophagy induction Anti-inflammatory effect Anti-angiogenesis	- NOB reduced tumor size and weight but not significant as compared to control - 5-DMN reduced tumor size and weight significantly as compared to control - 5-DMN increased LC3 expression - 5-DMN increased p53 expression - 5-DMN reduced COX-2 expression - 5-DMN reduced VEGF expression	[49]

AOM—azoxymethane; DSS—dextran sulfate sodium; i.p.—intraperitoneal injection; s.c.—subcutaneous injection; i.g.—intragastric administration; PCNA—proliferating cell nuclear antigen; ACF—aberrant crypt foci; BCAC—β-catenin-accumulated crypts; PhIP—1-Methyl-6-phenyl-1H-imidazo[4,5-b]pyridin-2-amine; LC3—microtubule-associated protein light chain 3; VEGF—vascular endothelial growth factor.

5.1. Cell Cycle Arrest

Uncontrolled cell growth that arises from genomic instability is known to contribute to tumorigenesis [85]. One way to counteract CRC is to halt its cell cycle progression. The cell cycle is akin to a biological growth clock that tightly regulates each stage of cell growth, where any mutated or abnormal cells will be arrested at either the G1 or G2 checkpoints; however, this mechanism is disrupted in cancerous conditions [86]. To progress through the stages, the regulatory protein cyclin acts like a key, as it needs to phosphorylate the cyclin-dependent kinase (CDK) complexes to allow progression to the next stage [87].

5.1.1. Action of NOB and Its Metabolites Inducing Cell Arrest

Notably, different metabolites of NOB work by different mechanisms against different cells. The flow cytometry test showed NOB and 4′-DMN arrest cells at G0/G1 phase in both HCT116 and HT-29 cell lines, despite the inhibitory effect of 4′-DMN being higher than that of NOB. Both 3′-DMN and 3′,4′-DMN arrest cells at both S phase and G2/M phase in HCT116 cell lines but arrest cells at both G0/G1 and G2/M phase in HT-29 cells. The inhibitory effect of 3′,4′-DMN is higher than that of 3′-DMN as only half the concentration is needed to induce a similar end result [54]. The fact that the metabolites 3′-DMN and 3′,4′-DMN exhibit more potent anti-cancer effects than NOB may suggest that demethylation at the 3′ and 4′-position significantly enhances its inhibitory effect [51].

In vitro tests using HCT116 cells reveal NOB and all three of the common metabolites increase the expression of CDK inhibitor, $p21^{Cip1/Waf1}$ [54]. $p21^{Cip1/Waf1}$, also known as p21 or P21/CDKN1A is a negative regulator for progression of the cell cycle that is responsible for the hypo-phosphorylation of retinoblastoma (Rb) proteins, leading to cell cycle arrest at the G1/S transition [86,88,89]. Although p21 is usually associated with the degradation of cyclin D1 [86], it is interesting to note that only 4′-DMN but not other metabolites nor the NOB itself causes significant reduction in cyclin D1 level. This may partly explain the strongest cell cycle arresting effect of 4′-DMN at the G0/G1 phase as compared to the other compounds aforementioned [54].

Proliferating cell nuclear antigen (PCNA) acts as a cofactor for DNA polymerase δ. It is an important marker commonly used to detect cell proliferation due to its increased expression through the G1 phase and S phase transition of cells [90,91]. Analysis from immunohistochemical tests recorded 69% reduction of cells with PCNA compared with the untreated controls [54]. Interestingly, evidence also reveals that p21 potentially suppresses action of PCNA. Interaction with the carboxy terminal of p21 inhibits PCNA from activating DNA polymerase δ, thus blocking DNA synthesis and preventing cell proliferation [92,93]. In this light, specific research of NOB on p21 and PCNA may be required to elucidate the pathways in further details.

Wu et al. studied the combinatory effect of NOB and its metabolites at different concentrations on HCT116 cells. At half the original concentration present in the colon, there is a decreasing trend of cells in S phase and G2/M phase but an increasing trend was noted in the G0/G1 phase. The cell cycle arrest effect seems to be dose dependent as flow cytometry recorded the population of cells arrested at the G0/G1 phase to be 57.8% higher than the untreated cells and significantly increased to 91.0% when the concentration of NOB and metabolites was doubled. To validate the findings, the levels of key signalling proteins were measured. Results showed that treatment with NOB and its metabolites lowered the levels of CDK-2, CDK-4, CDK-6 and cyclin D, raised the level of p52 and p27, but did not alter levels of p21 and cyclin E. In contrast, in vivo tests in AOM/DSS induced mice solely treated with NOB did document decreased expression of cyclin E and increased expression of CDK inhibitor p21. This difference is hypothesised to be due to the cell type specific response towards NOB, which is yet to be confirmed by further research [76]. The cell cycle is tightly regulated by key signalling proteins such as cyclins and cyclin dependent kinases (CDKs). To illustrate, complexes such as cyclin D-CDK-4/6 and cyclin E-CDK-2 facilitates the transition from G1 phase to S phase, while cell transition from G1 phase to S phase can be inhibited by tumour suppressor p53 and CDK inhibitors p21 and p27 [89,91].

It is also worth mentioning here that, at the effective concentration that arrests cell cycle, NOB produces a cytostatic effect, meaning it arrests growth without killing the cell [14]. As compared to other flavonoids like tangeretin (IC_{50} = 1.6 μM) and quercetin (IC_{50} = 0.84 μM), a slightly higher IC_{50} of 4.7 μM is required for the cell proliferation inhibition action by NOB in HT-29 cell lines and IC_{50} of 8.4 μM for 5-DMN [70]. However, the inhibitory effect of NOB may only be temporary. It is demonstrated that, with the removal of NOB, the treated cells resume cell proliferation within 24 h and regain similar growth status comparable to the control within 96 h [14]. This may also imply that, in order to sustain the inhibitory effect of NOB, the treatment with NOB has to be long-term to ensure continuous cell proliferation inhibition. This is possible as NOB is considered a natural compound and has no effect on healthy cells [83]. One might argue that the effect of NOB may be problematic for naturally fast-proliferating cells like healthy non-adenomatous intestinal lining cells. However, there is reassurance based on previous research that showed NOB is 10 times more selective towards transformed cancerous cells as compared to normal healthy cells [79].

5.1.2. Action of 5-DMN Inducing Cell Cycle Arrest

Treatment with 5-DMN also shows a similar increase of Rb in a dose dependent manner. Notably, 5-DMN does not affect the level of CDK-4, but there is a significant reduction of CDK-2 levels [63], hence indicating a reduced possibility of complex formation with cyclin A or cyclin E [94]. p21 is known to play a key role in arresting the cells at the cells at the G2/M phase through the inhibition of CDK-2/Cyclin E complex formation [95,96], and 5-DMN has been found to be able to arrest cell cycles at both the G0/G1 phase and G2/M phase in HCT116 (p53 $^{+/+}$), but is only able to accumulate cells at the G2/M phase in HCT116 (p53 $^{-/-}$). This suggests that G0/G1 arrest is dependent on p53 while G2/M is independent of p53 [80]. Using HT-29 cell lines, Qiu et al. reported that 5-DMN effectively causes cell cycle arrest at the G2/M phase [63]. This effect possibly arises from the downregulation of cdc25 protein expression, which is important to activate the cyc2/cyclin B1 through the process of dephosphorylating the inactive tyrosine residues Thr-14 and Thr-15 located in cdc2 ATP binding domain [97,98].

To sum up, different derivatives of NOB potentially arrest the cell at different stages of the cell cycle, mainly through downregulating the expression of proteins or kinases such as CDKs involved in the cell proliferation pathways and preventing the formation of cyclin complexes that allow cell cycle progression.

5.2. Programmed Cell Death

As growth of a cell is tightly regulated by the cell cycle, death of a damaged or aged cell also needs to be programmed to maintain homeostasis in our body. There are three models of programmed cell death (PCD), namely apoptosis, autophagy and necrosis [99]. A tumour mass of cancerous cells is formed when the cancerous cells develop the ability to evade cell death. Not responding to the death signal, the cells continue to grow and proliferate, leading to progression of cancer. Thus, NOB, being an agent that targets the key signalling pathways of programmed cell death, may help in chemoprevention of CRC. Apoptosis will be the main focus in this subsection, while autophagy will only be discussed briefly. Necrosis, the most abrupt death of all three, will not be discussed in this section as there are no data in this area. Although necrotic death is usually associated with inflammation, this does not exclude its possibility to be exploited as a means to eliminate cancerous cells [100].

Apoptosis can be induced by two core mechanisms, namely the extrinsic and the intrinsic pathway. The cell death signals in the extrinsic pathway come from external sources such as the Fas ligands or tumour necrosis factors [101]. The intrinsic pathway generally arises from the mitochondrial intracellular protein of the Bcl-2 family. Bcl-2 is an important regulator for apoptosis, which plays a role in mitochondrial disruption that activates the caspases [102]. High levels of Bcl-2 are expressed in various types of cancer and is associated with chemoresistance. Levels of Bcl-2 need to be lowered to promote apoptosis [103,104]. As a result of reduced Bcl-2 levels, a cascade of activity is activated in the cell leading to apoptosis with caspase-9 acting as the initiator caspase in the intrinsic pathway [105] and caspase-8 in the extrinsic pathway. It may also be crucial to mention here that the procaspase-8 forms a complex called Death Inducing Signalling Complex (DISC) before it is activated to caspase-8. The downstream effect would be the activation of the executioner caspase-3, and other caspases such as caspase-1, caspase-6 and caspase-7 [106,107] which then cleaves Poly (ADP-ribosome) polymerase (PARP) [108,109]. Soon after, the cell starts to bleb and shrink while its nucleus is condensed and fragmentised, proteolysis happens and the cell loses adhesion to the extracellular matrix and neighbouring cells [110,111]. Once the cell undergoes apoptosis, its contents are taken up by the body and recycled for new cell synthesis.

Action of NOB and Metabolites Inducing Programmed Cell Death

In vitro tests using different colon cell lines such as HCT116 and HT-29 reveals that the action of NOB and its various metabolites vary in different cell types. NOB was only shown to induce apoptosis of colon cancer cells when tested at high concentration. Zheng et al. [79] demonstrated that NOB increased DNA fragmentation in COLO302 only at 200 μM. Treatment with NOB, 3′-DMN, 4′-DMN and 3′,4′-DMN in HCT116 cell lines raise the early apoptotic cell population by 3.3-fold, 5.0-fold, 4.9-fold and 7.6-fold, respectively, while also resulting in 4.2-fold, 3.5-fold 7.1-fold and 4.5-fold increments in the late apoptotic cell population, respectively. In contrast, 3′-DMN and 4′-DMN did not cause any significant changes in apoptotic cell population in HT-29 cell lines, but the pro-apoptotic effect of 3′,4′-DMN was observed to be higher than that of NOB. An in vitro test using HCT116 shows that all three metabolites of NOB are able to induce the activation of caspase-3, caspase-9 and PARP, while NOB can only induce activation of caspase-9 but not that of caspase-3 or PARP. A negative result was also reported on the apoptosis inducing effect of NOB, whereby no apoptosis was detected when NOB was tested at concentrations of up to 100 μM in HT-29 [14]. In contrast, an in vivo test in AOM/DSS treated mice revealed a 2.3-fold increase of caspase-3 levels with NOB treatment [54]. Nevertheless, we can be certain that the metabolites of NOB render a higher proapoptotic effect as compared to their parent compound NOB.

Several previous works have demonstrated that NOB and its derivatives exhibit pro-apoptosis properties. However, this effect is known to be tissue specific. To illustrate, apoptosis is observed in colon cell lines but not the HL-60, promyelocytic leukaemia cell lines [79,112]. Interestingly, apoptosis could also be related to MMP-7. It has been discovered that cells that express MMP-7 are less sensitive to the Fas ligand-induced apoptosis as MMP-7 has a higher tendency to produce the non-apoptotic form of soluble Fas ligand by releasing the ligands in the cell membranes [77]. MMP will be further discussed in Section 5.4.

In vivo tests using xenograft mice show that 5-DMN triggers apoptosis at a concentration of 40 μM [49]. 5-DMN has been reported to increase levels of caspase-8, caspase-3 and PARP in a dose dependent manner, and results in 2.2-fold increase in the population of early apoptotic cells as compared to the control. In contrast, there is no apparent increase in the apoptotic effect even after doubling the concentration of NOB, suggesting NOB is required at a significantly higher concentration to induce a pro-apoptotic effect [14,63]. However, the effect of 5-DMN was notably distinct for different types of cancer cell lines. To illustrate, 5-DMN can induce early apoptosis in HCT116 colon cancer cell lines at a concentration as low as 8 μM while 5-DMN only slightly raises the apoptotic activities at a concentration as high as 36 μM in colon HT-29 cancer cell lines [63].

Annexin-V/PI analysis reveals that 5-DMN significantly increased the Annexin-V positive cells, especially in the late apoptotic or necrotic cell population among the HCT116 (p53 $^{-/-}$) cells, suggesting that the action of 5-DMN may be independent of p53 [80]. The fact that 5-DMN induces early apoptosis in HCT116 (Bax $^{+/+}$) cells but not in HCT116 (Bax $^{-/-}$) may suggest that Bax (Bcl-2 associated X protein) is important for apoptosis to occur. In other words, absence of Bax confers resistance to apoptosis [80,113,114]. A recent study by Chiou et al. proved that 5-DMN increases the expression of p53 proteins, which not only induces apoptosis, but also triggers cell death by autophagy that contributes to the prevention of tumour growth [49]. However, the detailed mechanism of how NOB prevents CRC development through the autophagy process is yet to be elucidated. From the current stage of knowledge, autophagy is known to exhibit both the pro-tumour and anti-tumour formation effects. In response to stress, autophagy acts as a protective mechanism for cell survival, which has already been elaborated in previous literature [115]. It is likely that overactivation of autophagy contributes to suppressing tumour formation by inhibiting the anti-autophagic-related genes (ATGs) in oncogenesis and activating the pro-ATG [116]. The effect of autophagy and apoptosis may be synergistic in chemoprevention of cancer [117,118].

To conclude, NOB was shown to be less effective in inducing apoptosis of colon cancer cells. Instead, the metabolites of NOB, 3′-DMN, 4′-DMN and 3′,4′-DMN were suggested to be responsible for the induction of apoptosis of colon and modulation of cancer cell growth in the colon carcinogenesis animal model [54] On top of that, the autohydrolysis product of NOB, 5-DMN could induce apoptosis in colon cancer cells at a lower concentration as compared to NOB.

5.3. Anti-Inflammation

Inflammation is a natural physiological response of our body, characterised by five main signs, namely loss of function, redness, pain, heat and swelling. Inflammation plays a significant role at times of infection and injury. It triggers the immune system to function and helps to protect our body through the release of chemical molecules called pro-inflammatory signals. However, too much inflammation is also not a good sign. There is increasing evidence narrating the interrelation between tumorigenesis and inflammation [119]. Whilst chronic inflammation is a hallmark of cancer, the inflammatory cytokines aggravate cancer progression by preventing differentiation of cells and promoting tumour formation [120]. The inflammatory cells release ROS after being activated, leading to the oxidative damage of DNA and p53 mutation [121–123]. The mechanism that triggers inflammation is a rather complex pathway and has been covered by previous literature [123,124]; only the anti-inflammatory effects mediated by NOB are discussed in this review.

Increasing evidence shows that progression of CRC can be accelerated by the upregulation of pro-inflammatory cytokines expressions—for example, TNF-α, IL-1α, IL-1β and IL-6 [81,119,125]. These proinflammatory cytokines enhance the secretion of inflammatory mediator PGE_2. Song et al. reported that treatment with NOB results in a noteworthy reduction of tumour size and frequency correlated with the significant lowering of IL-1, IL-6, iNOS and COX-2 levels [78]. ELISA test quantified the reduction of TNF-α, IL-1β and IL-6 at 51%, 92% and 69%, respectively, in the NOB treated group while real-time qRT-PCR quantified the reduction of the above pro-inflammatory cytokines at 65%, 69% and 45%, respectively, when compared to the control mice [54].

Anti-Inflammation Effect of NOB and Its Metabolites

Besides NOB, multiple studies have shown that its metabolites, especially, 4′-DMN and 3′,4′-DMN, also exhibit significant inhibitory effects towards nitric oxide production, iNOS and cyclooxygenase (COX) expressions in both in vivo and in vitro conditions [30,31,62,76,81,126]. However, the combined effect of NOB and its metabolites warrants further investigation [76]. Notably, NOB selectively inhibits COX-2 and did not affect COX-1 [81]. COX-2 is normally absent in healthy cells, but its release is triggered when the environment is inflammatory or hypoxic [127]. COX-2 is known to enhance CRC carcinogenesis, and inhibiting COX-2 also limits the production of PGE_2 [128], which may be associated with the inhibition of cell proliferation in colonic mucosa [41]. iNOS speeds up the conversion of L-arginine to NO through the process of oxidative deamination. NO is a potent inflammatory mediator that activates signalling molecules that trigger the process of inflammation and mutagenesis [129]. By inhibiting the iNOS and its downstream products, NOB helps in reducing the inflammation observed in chronic diseases like ulcerative colitis and CRC [130]. Introduction of NOB to colonic tissues harvested from mice treated with AOM/DSS results in a 35% reduction of cells expressing iNOS compared to the untreated tissue. This is consistent with the in vitro test. By administering NOB and its metabolites at a concentration equivalent to that found in the colons to the LPS-induced RAW 246.7

macrophages is shown to effectively and completely inhibits expression of iNOS, while, at half the concentration, the expression of iNOS was lowered by 56.4% compared to the untreated LPS-induced macrophages [76]. This shows that a similar process is likely to happen in the human body and NOB is indeed a promising anti-inflammatory agent.

Additionally, NOB also increases the release of the Nrf2-dependent enzymes which regulate Phase II enzyme production, such as heme oxygenase-1 (HO-1) and NQO1. HO-1 is an anti-oxidative enzyme that exhibits its anti-inflammatory effect by producing anti-oxidants like carbon monoxide and bilirubin. It is also important to note that HO-1 is not solely controlled by Nrf-2 [76]. NQO1 upregulation counteracts the increased expression of IL-1β and TNF-α induced by LPS [131]. This is consistent with the findings of Khor et al. reporting that a lower Nrf-2 expression greatly increases susceptibility of mice models to AOM-induced colitis [132]. The colonic mucosa of AOM/DSS-induced mice orally administrated with NOB was found to have increment of nuclear Nrf2 by 1.94-fold and reduction of cytoplasmic Nrf2 by 36% when compared to the AOM/DSS-treated mice. The upregulation and translocation of Nrf2 transcription factor is thought to be the cause for subsequent increment of HO-1 and NQO1 by 2.78-fold and 2.59-fold, respectively. This is consistent with the results from the combinatory effect of NOB and metabolites treatment on macrophages cell lines, which induces a 10% increase in the level of HO-1 and a 34% increase in the level of NQO1 when the concentration ratio of NOB and metabolites is equivalent to that in the colon [76]. In short, Nrf-2, which neutralises carcinogens and reactive oxygen species (ROS), is identified as a key signalling pathway to target in the effort to halt CRC progression [133,134].

5.4. Anti-Angiogenesis

Angiogenesis refers to the process by which new blood vessels are formed. This process is an important pathway that results in the progression of all types of cancer. This is because, when the tumour mass grows, it naturally needs more nutrients and nourishment to support its growth. To achieve this necessity, new blood vessels have to be formed surrounding the tumour mass to ensure a continuous supply of oxygen and glucose to support the growing cell mass [135,136].

Anti-Angiogenesis Effect of NOB

It is postulated that NOB prevents metastasis by inhibiting the activity of activator protein-1 (AP-1), a dimeric protein, thus preventing DNA binding [77]. Another hypothesis suggests that NOB acts via the Nuclear Factor-kappa B (NF-κB) pathway, altering the gene expression by modulating the promoter regions [126,137].

For angiogenesis to occur, the vascular endothelial growth factor (VEGF) plays a key role. VEGF not only acts as a signal to induce new blood vessel growth, but also inhibits the apoptosis induction. VEGF works by activating the mitogen activated protein kinase (MAPK). This kinase triggers the signal transduction and allows the endothelial cells to proliferate in order to form new blood vessels [138–140]. To elaborate on VEGF, it is necessary to mention leptin and insulin-like growth factor 1 (IGF-1) here. There is evidence suggesting that bidirectional cross talk exists between the leptin protein and IGF-1, a serum growth factor. Acting together, they not only catalyse the cell proliferation process, but also transactivate the epidermal growth factor receptor (EGFR), which enhances the migration and invasion power of the cancer malignancy [141].

Miyamoto et al. discovered that leptin, a protein that regulates energy balance and body mass has a positive correlation with CRC, where leptin is thought to be a mitogenic factor that leads to the development of colon cancer [84]. It induces cell proliferation by activating the nuclear factor κB, p38 MAPK and p42/44 MAPK [142]. Previous evidence demonstrates that introduction of 0.1 to 10 nM of leptin enhances the proliferation rate of HT-29 cells by 1.3 to 1.6 times [84] through c-Jun NH_2 terminal kinase and extracellular regulated kinase (ERK) 1/2 activation [143,144]. In other words, the chances of developing CRC can be reduced if leptin concentration is regulated. Treatment with NOB suppresses cell proliferation induced by leptin through inhibition of mitogen-activated protein/extracellular signal-regulated kinase (MEK) 1/2 [145]. Consistent with the in vitro findings, a reduction of 75% of leptin concentration by NOB, partly through the inactivation of the insulin signalling pathway, was reported at the end of the 17-week study in an in vivo model using Institute for Cancer Research (ICR) mice [83,84]. In this light, Miyamoto et al. conducted a study aiming to determine the prognosis of cancer in obese rats with flavonoid intervention. They reported that the flavonoids significantly reduced the incidence of β-catenin accumulated crypt (BCAC) by 64% to 71% and aberrant crypt foci (ACF) by 68% to 91% and proposed that this arises from the effect of NOB in downregulating the secretion of IGF-1 [83].

Metalloproteinase (MMP) plays a fundamental role in angiogenesis. MMP induces the protein that breaks down the extracellular matrix (ECM), thus making the blood vessel more permeable and allowing the cancerous cells to detach from the lump to flow, extravasate or invade the other parts of the body, causing the spread of tumour to other vital organs. This is a process called metastasis, leading to malignancy and cancer aggravation. The mortality rate greatly increases when cancerous cells metastasise to vital organs like the liver [146]. Similar to how a dexamethasone steroid acts, NOB is proven to be able to increase the expression of tissue inhibitor metalloprotease-1 (TIMP-1) in human synovial cells [81]. However, the benefit of upregulating TIMP-1 in CRC is debatable due to its bilateral role in cancer progression. Although TIMP-1 upregulation contributes to the anti-oncogenic effect, enhanced expression of it may lead to early phase tumour development via the pathways independent of MMPs. With this understanding, TIMP-1 glycosylation can function as a biomarker to aid in CRC staging [147].

There are more than 20 types of MMP involved in metastasis [148], with each one of them playing a distinct role [149]. However, whether MMP is produced by cancer cells or their surrounding stromal cells is still an ongoing debate [150]. Abnormally high levels of MMP-1, MMP-2, MMP-3, MMP-7, MMP-9 and MMP-13 have been implicated in CRC [150]. Treatment with NOB significantly inhibits release of pro-MMPs especially pro-MMP-7 (also known as metrilysin) mRNA in HT-29 cell lines. To illustrate, NOB at a concentration range of 25 μM to 100 μM, the proMMP-7 levels in the media diminishes significantly by 35% to 47% [77]. The maximal expression of MMP-7 arises from the β-catenin/TCF complex transcription factors formed in the presence of mutated APC genes [150–152]. Apart from MMP-7, the action of NOB on other MMPs in CRC is yet to be investigated. MMP-9, which is mainly secreted by inflammatory cells, is correlated with the transition phase from adenoma to adenocarcinoma, while the upregulation of MMP-3 usually suggests poor prognosis as it has a positive correlation with low microsatellite stability. On the other hand, high levels of MMP-12 reduces CRC mortality as it can potentially inhibit angiogenesis [150] by secreting angiostatin, a chemical that halts tumour progression and inhibits tumour neovascularisation [153–155]. As mentioned in the previous section, NOB suppresses MEK. This suppression of MEK then further diminishes the expression of pro-MMPs, which results in the reduction of MMP and subsequently confers anti-angiogenesis effect [144,145]. Briefly, NOB prevents angiogenesis and metastasis in CRC mainly via the inhibition of MMP, EGFR and VEGF through the regulation of leptin and IGF-1.

6. Pharmacokinetics, Bioavailability and Delivery Systems of NOB

The pharmacokinetic properties of NOB represent a key factor to be considered in an attempt to formulate it into a therapeutic product. Understanding the interactions between the compound and our body opens ways to creative strategies in solving the problem which require novel formulation in delivering NOB for chemoprevention purpose. For oral delivery, an important consideration is the bioavailability of the active compound. However, the bioavailability studies on NOB are limited [156]. Therefore, understanding the pharmacokinetic profile of NOB becomes even more crucial to assisting in the prediction of bioefficacy as the absorption, metabolism and elimination pattern indirectly affect its bioavailability.

There are many factors that affect the absorption of a compound; one important consideration is the molecular structure [157]. The proper absorption of any compound is depicted by its solubility and permeability across physiological barriers of which both properties are directly related to its molecular structure. Attributed to its unique chemical structure with multiple methoxy groups, NOB is lipophilic in nature and can easily pass through the cell membrane. Murakami et al. successfully demonstrated the relatively high permeation of NOB across differentiated Caco-2 cells which mimics the epithelial cells lining the small intestine. A significantly high 48.1% of NOB has been found to permeate through the basolateral compartment while another 39.3% remains on the apical compartment four hours after introduction of NOB in a Caco-2 monolayer trans-well permeability assay [158]. Parallel artificial membrane permeation assay (PAMPA) deciphered the permeability of NOB, 4′-DMN and 3′-DMN at 1.38×10^{-6} cm/s, 1.14×10^{-6} cm/s and 1.05×10^{-6} cm/s, respectively [159]. It was discovered that the methoxylated flavonoids show five to eight-fold higher permeability in the intestinal wall than its unmethoxylated counterparts [160]. The drawback is that PMF in general has limited solubility. Results from the high-throughput lyophilisation solubility assay (LYSA) reveal that NOB has a low solubility at 12 μg/mL, while its metabolites, 4′-DMN, 3′-DMN and 5-DMN exhibited two to three-fold higher solubilities of 22 μg/mL, 29 μg/mL and 32 μg/mL, respectively [156,161]. In general, the solubility increased with the number of hydroxyl group of the compound. This may also partly explain the higher activity of the derivatives of NOB as compared to its parent compound, which has a higher number of methoxy groups.

After absorption, NOB is found to be widely distributed throughout the body, as a significant amount of NOB could be detected in organs such as the stomach, small intestine, large intestine, brain, liver and kidney within four hours of single dose administration [162,163]. Interestingly, NOB was suggested to be absorbed through the muscularis layer of the gastrointestinal tract, especially the stomach tissue into the blood circulation given the distinctly higher concentration of NOB in the muscularis (390 ± 120 nmol/g) as compared to other organs [162]. Furthermore, it is also noteworthy that NOB was found to be distributed in the mucous membrane and muscularis from the large intestine (cecum, colon and rectum) of a rat at 4.3 ± 1.6 nmol/g after one hour of oral administration by gastric intubation [162]. More recent evidence demonstrated that the levels of NOB in the colonic mucosa of mice were 2.03 nmol/g of tissue after long-term oral administration of NOB (0.05 wt%) containing diet. Furthermore, Wu et al. [164] also suggested that the dose of NOB used (0.05 wt%) could be equivalent to approximately 100 mg/day for human oral consumption, which is achievable in humans.

After oral administration of NOB to rats, the mean plasma concentration of NOB was quantified in several pharmacokinetic studies. Wang et al. [163] reported that the plasma levels of total NOB and its metabolites could reach as high as 10 μg/mL (25 μM). Using a highly sensitive Liquid Chromatography-Mass Spectrometry/Mass Spectrometry-Electrospray ionisation (LC-MS/MS-ESI) method, the maximum concentration (C_{max}) of NOB in rat plasma was determined at 0.4 μg/mL (1 μM) after oral administration of 5 mg/kg NOB [165]. Meanwhile, a maximum concentration of 1.78 μg/mL (4.4 μM) was measured by a validated HPLC method in rat plasma after oral administration of 50 mg/kg NOB [166]. In addition, another study by Manthey et al. [167] reported that a peak of NOB serum level of 9.03 μg/mL (22.4 μM) was detected by HPLC-ESI-MS in rats after oral gavage of 50 mg/kg NOB. Nevertheless, these studies demonstrated a relatively early peak time (T_{max}) of 0.25 to one hour after oral administration of NOB in rats. This high rate of cellular uptake may be attributed to the highly hydrophobic nature of the compound rendered by the presence of six methoxy groups [162].

NOB undergoes extensive metabolism after being taken orally. As detailed in Section 3, NOB undergoes Phase I and Phase II metabolism after being absorbed in the small intestine where it may be conjugated to sulphate and glucuronide, and then again deconjugated by the microflora in the colon [60]. The three common phase I metabolites of NOB have been identified as 3′-DMN, 4′-DMN and 3′,4′-DMN [52,53]. Wang et al. found evidence of transformation of 3′-DMN and 4′-DMN into 3′,4′-DMN in the colon [163]. The liver is another important organ involved in metabolising NOB. Koga et al. identified three metabolites, demethylated at the 4, 6 or 7 positions respectively under the action of human liver microsomes when incubated aerobically with NADPH [56]. The metabolites exhibit distinct activity and distribution pattern in different areas of the body. It was found that 4′-DMN is the major metabolite present in the small intestine and liver while 3′,4′-DMN was predominantly present in the colon and spleen [163]. An in vitro test on NOB using rat liver S-9 extract shows that only 7% of NOB metabolites were detected towards the end of a 24 hour treatment, while 72.6% of NOB remains unchanged towards the end of the experiment [158]. This may be attributed to the slow rate of demethylation of NOB showed by Murakami et al. [162].

The elimination half-life of NOB from the blood plasma of a rat was reported as 1.8 h via a validated HPLC test [166] while Kumar et al. reported a terminal half-life of NOB at 4.75 ± 0.57 h following oral administration and a terminal half-life of 1.51 ± 0.61 h following parenteral administration using the LC-MS/MS-ESI method [165]. Despite the wide distribution throughout the body, concentration of NOB quickly diminishes with time and becomes undetectable in the serum, stomach, intestines, liver and kidney. Aside from the parent compound, mono-demethylated metabolites and conjugated NOB are detected in the urine, with the concentration of conjugated NOB revealing a time-dependent increment over a period of 24 h [162]. Since NOB is rapidly eliminated from the body, significant adverse effects reported after administration of NOB are rare.

Although the in vitro results were promising, most of the reported concentrations of NOB evaluated (>20 μM) were not achievable in physiological conditions as demonstrated by in vivo pharmacokinetic studies of NOB. Comparing the high experimental levels used against the relatively low peak plasma concentration—a mere 1.78 μg/mL (4.4 μM)—after one hour of oral administration of 50 mg/kg NOB [166] and the rapid elimination from the body [162] points out a limitation to utilizing NOB in its unaltered natural form as a clinical drug. In fact, the levels of NOB detected in the colonic mucosa ranged between 2 to 4 μM using the assumption that one gram of tissue is equivalent of 1 mL of volume [54,162]. However, there was a study demonstrating that NOB at lower concentration (≤5 μM) exhibited antiproliferative effects against colon cancer cells [70], perhaps indicating true promise for clinical use after all.

To further substantiate the notion of NOB for colon cancer chemoprevention, multiple in vivo studies have demonstrated that dietary treatment with NOB could inhibit colon carcinogenesis in rats [54,76]. As mentioned earlier, this may be related to the fact that, while bioavailability of NOB itself is low, much of its anti-CRC effect may be via its metabolites. Wu et al. [54] indicated that the NOB level in the colonic mucosa only accounted for <5% of the total levels of NOB and its metabolites after oral administration of NOB. The study further suggested that the NOB metabolites, which were formed as a result of phase I and II metabolism and biotransformation by gut microbiome, play an important role in colon carcinogenesis inhibition [54]. Although there is some suggestion that lower doses can have an effect on cancer, clearly, enhancement of NOB bioavailability is necessary and also represents a major challenge that needs to be addressed to achieve the desired therapeutic effect.

Given the importance of actually delivering adequate amounts of NOB to the target site to achieve chemopreventive activity, we also reviewed the delivery systems aiming to enhance the bioavailability of NOB in the gut. For chemoprevention of CRC, oral delivery represents the preferred route. There is a growing interest to formulate lipophilic natural compounds such as NOB into emulsion, as these systems not only improve the bioavailability of the active compound, but also reduce the rate of degradation during storage [168]. Yang et al. attempted to enhance the solubility of NOB by encapsulating NOB with citrus oil-based emulsion. The team discovered that dissolving NOB at a higher temperature and in an oil with log P close to NOB, such as bergamot oil, helps to increase solubility of the compound [169]. Yao et al. also experimented with the possibility of using self-microemulsifying drug delivery systems (SMEDDS) to improve the permeability of NOB in the rat intestines and reported that SMEDDS resulted in similar efficacies to micelles, but showed better absorption profile when compared to sub-microemulsions [170]. Self-assembled NOB proliposomes were also reported to improve the absorptive rate and confer longer mean residence time as compared to NOB suspension in rats [171].

Furthermore, Chen and colleagues demonstrated that, through the addition of hydroxypropyl methylcellulose (HPMC), the retention of NOB in nanoemulsion is increased by 25% [172]. Even though the fabrication of supersaturating nanoemulsion with the addition of HPMC aimed to improve the physical stability of NOB and prevent precipitation of NOB in the emulsion, the fabrication did not perform as expected at high NOB concentration where precipitation still occurred during storage and digestion process in the gut [172]. To address the issue of component precipitation in the emulsion system, a recent intervention of nanoemulsion-filled hydrogel matrix has been developed to stabilize NOB and prevent precipitation during delivery along the GI tract [173]. Interestingly, the hydrogels could provide a controlled release of NOB along the GI tract, thereby the hydrogel shrank at acidic condition pH 1.2 but swelled and burst at pH 7.4. Due to the lower bioaccessibility of NOB in hydrogel as compared to nanoemulsion during digestion, the nanoemulsion-filled hydrogel matrix could confer a sustainable absorption of NOB through a controlled release in the intestinal tract [173].

Aside from the liquid formulations, Onoue and colleagues proposed a solid formulation of NOB with the intention to further enhance the bioavailability in addition to solving the stability issues which showed a remarkable 13-fold increment in bioavailability compared to the nanosized NOB amorphous solid dispersion [174]. However, the results only quantitate the brain permeability, but the data for colon effect is still lacking. Further research is needed to establish the practicability and feasibility of each delivery method to address the bioavailability challenges before NOB can be used in aiding patients at high risk of CRC.

7. Toxicity

Although NOB is derived from a natural source, excessive intake of any substance might lead to some changes in the body. To illustrate, there are several case studies reporting that ingestion of products containing bitter orange causes adverse effects such as tachycardia and ventricular fibrillation [175]. To address this concern, a number of studies have been carried out to further evaluate this problem.

Body weight is commonly used as a surrogate marker for toxicity, whereby the weight is expected to reduce significantly if toxicity occurs. Wu et al. concluded there was no significant change in body weight, weight of liver, spleen appearance and behaviour throughout the length of their research, suggesting that the oral intake of NOB at the effective concentration 40 μM or 0.05% for a period of 3 to 20 weeks does not lead to adverse side effects [41,49,54]. This is consistent with the findings of Murakami et al. suggesting that NOB leads to no cytotoxic effects [42]. The action of NOB is more likely of a cytostatic nature rather than cytocidal as, at the concentration that inhibits cell proliferation, it does not trigger apoptosis. Furthermore, the treated cells continue to grow normally once the effect of NOB diminishes [14]. This shows that NOB could be a safer option for CRC treatment as it is less cytotoxic as compared to the available chemotherapy agents.

8. Commercial Uses

A search on Google Scholar using the keywords "nobiletin patents" gives about 1160 relevant results. This initial search was refined through the advanced search function for patents using the SciFinder database which helps to narrow down the number of patents directly and indirectly related to NOB to 300.

After a close analysis of the patents, we found that, among the 300 patents related to the concept of NOB, the largest portion of the total patents involves the usage of NOB in the medical, pharmaceutical and nutraceutical fields. The patents include both the application in traditional treatments and also western medications, where there are about 20 patents related to cardiovascular diseases [176–178], hypertension and hypercholesterolemia [179], roughly 10 patents targeting the central nervous system [180,181] or neurodegenerative disorders [182], diabetes [183,184] and obesity [185] each, and about five patents concerning body metabolism and hormonal functions, bone-related disorders [186], oral issues such as ulcer and halitosis [187,188], liver-related problems like hepatitis [189] and anti-infectives such as anti-bacterial, anti-viral [190] and vaccines, respectively. The patents also include a small number of

NOB usage in diseases like prostate disease, asthma [191,192], allergy [193], eye relief, prevention and improvements of conditions like hair fall [194], dysuria [195] and muscular atrophy [196].

A large proportion of the patents are related to anti-cancer treatments, which account for almost 13% of the total patents. The types of cancers covered are broad, ranging from the more prevalent ones like lung cancer [197] and breast cancer [198] to those lower down the prevalence indices like uterine, liver cancer, oral [199], and skin cancer [19]. Application wise, some major areas that involve the usage of NOB compounds include the synergistic effect of NOB with existing chemotherapeutic agents targeting the multidrug resistance cancer [200] which aim to increase therapeutic efficacy as well as aiming to address the side effects from conventional chemotherapeutic treatments, especially diarrhoea [201]. Some common cancer inhibition pathways leading to cancer that are targeted by the compound include anti-angiogenesis [202], anti-proliferation and anti-tumour or anti-neoplastic effects.

The usage of NOB in nutraceutical industries is also extensive; there are up to 20 patents of beverages that contain NOB, with some of the fortified drinks claiming to have pharmacological effects [203]. Next in the line, comprising one-fifth of the total patents, are the methods of extraction [204–206], purification [207,208], preparation [209,210], manufacturing [44,211,212] analysis [213], drug delivery and pharmacokinetics information such as ways to improve absorption, solubility and bioavailability.

Apart from that, the use of NOB in fields other than medicine is also very broad, which includes about 20 patents in cosmetics [214–216], another 20 patents in the food industry, which include its use as preservatives [217], flavourings or food additives [218], and four patents in the agricultural industry, of which mostly it is used as pesticide controls. Last but not least, there are also patents of NOB usage in stem cell technology and genetic analysis.

9. Future Directions

While NOB and its metabolites seem to have tremendous potential as chemopreventive agents, at this juncture of time, more intensive research is needed to resolve the challenges that arise from the limitations of this compound. As mentioned earlier, NOB showed dose dependent anti-cancer effects, but the challenge is to increase its bioavailability to enhance the chemopreventive effect. This is important as oral administration seems to be a more promising route of administration at the moment as intraperitoneal injection has been associated with severe side effects such as ischemic stroke [36]. In addition, given that the chemopreventive metabolites appear to be formed by via metabolism within the gut, the oral route seems to be a promising way of delivering drugs to the target site.

Although several effective delivery systems were developed to enhance the bioavailability of NOB, studies on targeted-delivery of NOB to the colon are still limited. Despite having delivery systems that enhance aqueous solubility and bioavailability, a colon-specific drug delivery system is highly desirable for efficient drug delivery of NOB to the colon or where the colorectal cancer reside. In 2012, a folate-modified self-microemulsifying drug delivery system (FSMEDDS) was developed with the aim to improve solubility of curcumin and specifically target colorectal cancer cells mediated by the binding of folate receptors in facilitating the endocytosis of the formulation [219]. Given the previous evidence of the successful preparation of NOB in SMEDDS [170], this intervention could be possible to be implemented to facilitate specific uptake of NOB into colorectal cancer cells via the FSMEDDS and further coated by Eudragit®S 100 (Evonik Industries AG, Essen, Germany), which prevent dissolution of the formulation under the condition of $pH < 7.5$ [219,220]. Recently, a dual stimuli-responsive Pickering emulsion (pH and magnetic- responsive) reported may hold immense potential for the biomedical field, particularly in the treatment of colorectal cancer [221,222]; to achieve an active targeting of specific sites, an external magnetic field could be utilized to direct the movement and accumulation of the drug carrier at the targeted sites to exert their therapeutic effects [223].

In addition to that, biotechnology can be applied to biosynthetically produce NOB in larger yields as citrus peel may only contain a limited amount of this bioactive product. In this regard, Itoh et al. successfully isolated five genes from *C. depressa* which encode the flavonoids by *O*-methyltransferases (FOMT), a precursor for a number of flavonoids. Quercetin has been synthesised via this method and it is highly likely that the same enzyme is also involved in the biosynthesis of NOB, suggesting that it may also be possible for NOB to be synthesised using this strategy [39]. However, the data on the effectiveness in this application is still lacking as there is limited research that uses this method to synthesise NOB. Apart from biotechnology, the introduction of reliable, efficient and economical validation methods such as ultraperformance liquid chromatography coupled with quadrupole time-of-flight mass spectrometry (UPLC-Q-TOP-MS) which allows high rate of separation of PMF compounds within 12 min also opens up more possibilities for NOB to be marketed [224].

In addition, another major challenge of chemotherapy that we are facing today is the development of drug resistance in cancer treatment. One possible cause that results in chemoresistance may be attributed to the cancer stem cell (CSC). CSCs are known to play a crucial role in tumour formation as they possess unique characteristics including unlimited cell renewal capacity and the ability to evade drug penetration [225,226]. Seeing the limitation of the single cell in vitro model [227], Silva et al. came up with a brilliant method of culturing cells into a three-dimensional block, which they named a 3D spheroid. At day seven, the 3D spheroids mimic the tumour lump, with the undifferentiated cells in the outer region surrounding the hypoxic inner core. Experiments showed that 2.9-fold higher concentration is needed to exhibit the same effect reported in the two-dimensional cell model [47].

Interestingly, the concomitant exposure of NOB and its metabolites gives rise to synergistic effects that are distinct from the response caused by NOB alone [228,229]. Therefore, the combinatory effect of NOB and its various metabolites should be explored in order to establish a solid foundation of understanding of the synergistic effect of NOB and its natural metabolites generated through the biotransformation process. Apart from that, compelling evidence showed that NOB produces a synergistic effect in tumour growth inhibition when co-administered with atorvastatin. When used together, only half the minimal effective concentration of each drug is required to achieve the targeted therapeutic outcome. Wu and co-authors reported a series of mechanisms by which this combination works, namely through altering important cellular signals that triggers inflammation, inhibiting cell cycle progression, inducing apoptosis and preventing angiogenesis and metastasis [164,230]. In this light, the drugs already in the market can be combined with NOB and tested for their synergistic effects in inhibiting CRC. In addition, the combinatory effect of NOB and its metabolites needs to be further elucidated to achieve a precisely targeted biological action in CRC chemoprevention. More clinical trials in human subjects with due ethical considerations are warranted as disparity will certainly exist if the data is solely extracted from in vitro or animal tests.

10. Conclusions

While there is a significant research focus on cancer, science is still at an early stage in understanding this noxious condition affecting people from every segment of society, but answers are critical as cancer's prevalence and variance are continuously on the rise. The current clinical practice in cancer treatment, which largely consists of the three broad fields, namely surgery, chemotherapy and radiotherapy, may be helpful to patients to some extent but more intensive and in-depth ongoing studies are needed in the quest for a panacea for cancer given the high mortality rates of this malady. Many more patients will be relieved from pain and suffering if scientific research can shine a light on the root causes of cancer and focus on its prevention so as to nip the problem in the bud before the need to treat it arises.

The advancement in science has allowed the discovery of numerous beneficial compounds offered by nature. It is reassuring to learn that NOB, a compound that is extracted from the ubiquitous citrus species confers a wide range of beneficial biological effects that includes cancer prevention. On top of that, the autohydrolysis product, 5-DMN and several metabolites of NOB such as 3′-DMN, 4′-DMN and 3′,4′-DMN, demonstrate more potent effects as compared to their parent compound NOB. It is apparent that NOB is indeed a prospective compound that exhibits a promising chemopreventive effect on CRC, especially for the types which are induced by carcinogens or associated with diseases such as colitis. In addition to that, this review also focuses on the underlying molecular mechanism of which NOB acts in CRC. The plus point is that NOB and its products target a number of different hallmarks of cancer. To illustrate, NOB is endowed with anti-proliferative, pro-apoptotic, anti-inflammatory and anti-angiogenesis effects, which renders it the potential to counteract the pathology of CRC in patients at various stages of cancer progression.

Besides NOB, many compounds under the polymethoxyflavones family are currently promising candidates in the field of cancer research, yet it is too early for science to conclude a best compound to formulate as the elixir. More studies, be it in vitro, in vivo or clinical studies, are needed to unravel the full potential of each possible compound. Furthermore, it would be worthwhile to explore the synergistic effect or possible interactions between NOB and well-known anti-cancer drugs by both experimental and clinical studies. The vast number of existing patents of NOB across various industries may suggest that this compound does have commercial value besides its noteworthy pharmacological benefits. Further research work needs to be intensified to overcome the current gap and limitation in formulation, for instance to increase the bioavailability and to enhance the efficacies of NOB in CRC chemoprevention. Although significant advances have been made, there is still a long way to go before NOB could truly become part of the arsenal of CRC chemoprevention.

Author Contributions: The literature searches and data collection was performed by J.X.H.G. & L.T.-H.T. The manuscript was written by J.X.H.G. and L.T.-H.T. The manuscript was critically reviewed and edited by J.X.H.G., L.T.-H.T., P.P., L.-H.L., J.K.G., K.G.C. and B.-H.G., B.-H.G. provided vital guidance and insight to the work. The project was conceptualized by B.-H.G.

Acknowledgments: This work was inspired by the Monash Pharmacy Degree Course, Unit PAC3512 entitled "Current aspects of pharmaceutical research".

References

1. Siegel, R.L.; Miller, K.D.; Jemal, A. Cancer statistics, 2017. *CA Cancer J. Clin.* **2017**, *67*, 7–30. [CrossRef] [PubMed]
2. Bernstein, C.N.; Blanchard, J.F.; Kliewer, E.; Wajda, A. Cancer risk in patients with inflammatory bowel disease: A population-based study. *Cancer* **2001**, *91*, 854–862. [CrossRef]
3. Rubin, D.C.; Shaker, A.; Levin, M.S. Chronic intestinal inflammation: Inflammatory bowel disease and colitis-associated colon cancer. *Front. Immunol.* **2012**, *3*, 107. [CrossRef] [PubMed]
4. Siegel, R.L.; Miller, K.D.; Fedewa, S.A.; Ahnen, D.J.; Meester, R.G.; Barzi, A.; Jemal, A. Colorectal cancer statistics, 2017. *CA Cancer J. Clin.* **2017**, *67*, 177–193. [CrossRef] [PubMed]
5. Simon, K. Colorectal cancer development and advances in screening. *Clin. Interv. Aging* **2016**, *11*, 967–976. [PubMed]
6. Tan, L.T.H.; Lee, L.H.; Yin, W.F.; Chan, C.K.; Abdul Kadir, H.; Chan, K.G.; Goh, B.H. Traditional Uses, Phytochemistry, and Bioactivities of Cananga odorata (Ylang-Ylang). *Evid. Based Complement. Altern. Med.* **2015**, *2015*, 30. [CrossRef]
7. Chan, W.-K.; Tan, L.T.-H.; Chan, K.-G.; Lee, L.-H.; Goh, B.-H. Nerolidol: A Sesquiterpene Alcohol with Multi-Faceted Pharmacological and Biological Activities. *Molecules* **2016**, *21*, 529. [CrossRef]
8. Tan, H.-L.; Chan, K.-G.; Pusparajah, P.; Saokaew, S.; Duangjai, A.; Lee, L.-H.; Goh, B.-H. Anti-Cancer Properties of the Naturally Occurring Aphrodisiacs: Icariin and Its Derivatives. *Front. Pharmacol.* **2016**, *7*. [CrossRef]
9. Steward, W.P.; Brown, K. Cancer chemoprevention: A rapidly evolving field. *Br. J. Cancer* **2013**, *109*, 1. [CrossRef]
10. Tang, C.; Hoo, P.C.-X.; Tan, L.T.-H.; Pusparajah, P.; Khan, T.M.; Lee, L.-H.; Goh, B.-H.; Chan, K.-G. Golden Needle Mushroom: A Culinary Medicine with Evidenced-Based Biological Activities and Health Promoting Properties. *Front. Pharmacol.* **2016**, *7*. [CrossRef]
11. Alam, M.N.; Almoyad, M.; Huq, F. Polyphenols in Colorectal Cancer: Current State of Knowledge including Clinical Trials and Molecular Mechanism of Action. *BioMed Res. Int.* **2018**, *2018*. [CrossRef] [PubMed]

12. Chen, S.; Cai, D.; Pearce, K.; Sun, P.Y.; Roberts, A.C.; Glanzman, D.L. Reinstatement of long-term memory following erasure of its behavioral and synaptic expression in Aplysia. *eLife* **2014**, *3*. [CrossRef] [PubMed]
13. Surichan, S.; Arroo, R.R.; Ruparelia, K.; Tsatsakis, A.M.; Androutsopoulos, V.P. Nobiletin bioactivation in MDA-MB-468 breast cancer cells by cytochrome P450 CYP1 enzymes. *Food Chem. Toxicol.* **2018**, *113*, 228–235. [CrossRef] [PubMed]
14. Morley, K.L.; Ferguson, P.J.; Koropatnick, J. Tangeretin and nobiletin induce G1 cell cycle arrest but not apoptosis in human breast and colon cancer cells. *Cancer Lett.* **2007**, *251*, 168–178. [CrossRef] [PubMed]
15. Jiang, Y.-P.; Guo, H.; Wang, X.-B. Nobiletin (NOB) suppresses autophagic degradation via over-expressing AKT pathway and enhances apoptosis in multidrug-resistant SKOV3/TAX ovarian cancer cells. *Biomed. Pharmacother.* **2018**, *103*, 29–37. [CrossRef] [PubMed]
16. Moon, J.Y.; Cho, M.; Ahn, K.S.; Cho, S.K. Nobiletin induces apoptosis and potentiates the effects of the anticancer drug 5-fluorouracil in p53-mutated SNU-16 human gastric cancer cells. *Nutr. Cancer* **2013**, *65*, 286–295. [CrossRef] [PubMed]
17. Moon, J.Y.; Cho, S.K. Nobiletin induces protective autophagy accompanied by ER-stress mediated apoptosis in human gastric cancer SNU-16 cells. *Molecules* **2016**, *21*, 914. [CrossRef] [PubMed]
18. Uesato, S.; Yamashita, H.; Maeda, R.; Hirata, Y.; Yamamoto, M.; Matsue, S.; Nagaoka, Y.; Shibano, M.; Taniguchi, M.; Baba, K. Synergistic antitumor effect of a combination of paclitaxel and carboplatin with nobiletin from Citrus depressa on non-small-cell lung cancer cell lines. *Planta Med.* **2014**, *80*, 452–457. [CrossRef]
19. Song, M.; Wu, X.; Charoensinphon, N.; Wang, M.; Zheng, J.; Gao, Z.; Xu, F.; Li, Z.; Li, F.; Zhou, J. Dietary 5-demethylnobiletin inhibits cigarette carcinogen NNK-induced lung tumorigenesis in mice. *Food Funct.* **2017**, *8*, 954–963. [CrossRef]
20. Ma, X.; Jin, S.; Zhang, Y.; Wan, L.; Zhao, Y.; Zhou, L. Inhibitory effects of nobiletin on hepatocellular carcinoma in vitro and in vivo. *Phytother. Res.* **2014**, *28*, 560–567. [CrossRef]
21. Cheng, H.-L.; Hsieh, M.-J.; Yang, J.-S.; Lin, C.-W.; Lue, K.-H.; Lu, K.-H.; Yang, S.-F. Nobiletin inhibits human osteosarcoma cells metastasis by blocking ERK and JNK-mediated MMPs expression. *Oncotarget* **2016**, *7*, 35208–35223. [CrossRef] [PubMed]
22. Braidy, N.; Behzad, S.; Habtemariam, S.; Ahmed, T.; Daglia, M.; Mohammad Nabavi, S.; Sobarzo-Sanchez, E.; Fazel Nabavi, S. Neuroprotective effects of citrus fruit-derived flavonoids, nobiletin and tangeretin in Alzheimer's and Parkinson's disease. *CNS Neurol. Disord. Drug Targets (Former. Curr. Drug Targets CNS Neurol. Disord.)* **2017**, *16*, 387–397. [CrossRef] [PubMed]
23. Qi, G.; Guo, R.; Tian, H.; Li, L.; Liu, H.; Mi, Y.; Liu, X. Nobiletin protects against insulin resistance and disorders of lipid metabolism by reprogramming of circadian clock in hepatocytes. *Biochim. Biophys. Acta Mol. Cell Biolo. Lipids* **2018**, *1863*, 549–562. [CrossRef] [PubMed]
24. Kumar, V.; Veeranjaneyulu, A. Complications of Diabetes and Role of a Citrus Flavonoid Nobiletin in Its Treatment. In *Herbs for Diabetes and Neurological Disease Management*; Apple Academic Press: Oakville, ON, Canada, 2018; pp. 197–224.
25. Morrow, N.M.; Telford, D.E.; Sutherland, B.G.; Edwards, J.Y.; Huff, M.W. Nobiletin Corrects Intestinal Lipid Metabolism in Ldlr-/-Mice Fed a High-Fat Diet. *Atheroscler. Suppl.* **2018**, *32*, 28. [CrossRef]
26. Yuk, T.; Kim, Y.; Yang, J.; Sung, J.; Jeong, H.S.; Lee, J. Nobiletin Inhibits Hepatic Lipogenesis via Activation of AMP-Activated Protein Kinase. *Evid. Based Complement. Altern. Med.* **2018**, *2018*. [CrossRef] [PubMed]
27. Tung, Y.-C.; Li, S.; Huang, Q.; Hung, W.-L.; Ho, C.-T.; Wei, G.-J.; Pan, M.-H. 5-Demethylnobiletin and 5-Acetoxy-6, 7, 8, 3′, 4′-pentamethoxyflavone Suppress Lipid Accumulation by Activating the LKB1-AMPK Pathway in 3T3-L1 Preadipocytes and High Fat Diet-Fed C57BL/6 Mice. *J. Agric. Food Chem.* **2016**, *64*, 3196–3205. [CrossRef] [PubMed]
28. Yao, X.; Zhu, X.; Pan, S.; Fang, Y.; Jiang, F.; Phillips, G.O.; Xu, X. Antimicrobial activity of nobiletin and tangeretin against Pseudomonas. *Food Chem.* **2012**, *132*, 1883–1890. [CrossRef]
29. Onishi, S.; Nishi, K.; Yasunaga, S.; Muranaka, A.; Maeyama, K.; Kadota, A.; Sugahara, T. Nobiletin, a polymethoxy flavonoid, exerts anti-allergic effect by suppressing activation of phosphoinositide 3-kinase. *J. Funct. Foods* **2014**, *6*, 606–614. [CrossRef]
30. Lai, C.-S.; Li, S.; Chai, C.-Y.; Lo, C.-Y.; Dushenkov, S.; Ho, C.-T.; Pan, M.-H.; Wang, Y.-J. Anti-inflammatory and antitumor promotional effects of a novel urinary metabolite, 3′, 4′-didemethylnobiletin, derived from nobiletin. *Carcinogenesis* **2008**, *29*, 2415–2424. [CrossRef]

31. Narayana, J.L.; Huang, H.-N.; Wu, C.-J.; Chen, J.-Y. Epinecidin-1 antimicrobial activity: In vitro membrane lysis and In vivo efficacy against Helicobacter pylori infection in a mouse model. *Biomaterials* **2015**, *61*, 41–51. [CrossRef]
32. Eguchi, A.; Murakami, A.; Li, S.; Ho, C.T.; Ohigashi, H. Suppressive effects of demethylated metabolites of nobiletin on phorbol ester-induced expression of scavenger receptor genes in THP-1 human monocytic cells. *Biofactors* **2007**, *31*, 107–116. [CrossRef] [PubMed]
33. Eguchi, A.; Murakami, A.; Ohigashi, H. Nobiletin, a citrus flavonoid, suppresses phorbol ester-induced expression of multiple scavenger receptor genes in THP-1 human monocytic cells. *FEBS Lett.* **2006**, *580*, 3321–3328. [CrossRef] [PubMed]
34. Lee, Y.-S.; Asai, M.; Choi, S.-S.; Yonezawa, T.; Teruya, T.; Nagai, K.; Woo, J.-T.; Cha, B.-Y. Nobiletin prevents body weight gain and bone loss in ovariectomized C57BL/6J mice. *Pharmaco. Pharm.* **2014**, *5*, 959–965. [CrossRef]
35. Tominari, T.; Hirata, M.; Matsumoto, C.; Inada, M.; Miyaura, C. Polymethoxy flavonoids, nobiletin and tangeretin, prevent lipopolysaccharide-induced inflammatory bone loss in an experimental model for periodontitis. *J. Pharmacol. Sci.* **2012**, *119*, 390–394. [CrossRef] [PubMed]
36. Gao, Z.; Gao, W.; Zeng, S.-L.; Li, P.; Liu, E.-H. Chemical structures, bioactivities and molecular mechanisms of citrus polymethoxyflavones. *J. Funct. Foods* **2018**, *40*, 498–509. [CrossRef]
37. Tung, Y.-C.; Chou, Y.-C.; Hung, W.-L.; Cheng, A.-C.; Yu, R.-C.; Ho, C.-T.; Pan, M.-H. Polymethoxyflavones: Chemistry and Molecular Mechanisms for Cancer Prevention and Treatment. *Curr. Pharmacol. Rep.* **2019**, *5*, 98–113. [CrossRef]
38. Uckoo, R.M.; Jayaprakasha, G.; Vikram, A.; Patil, B.S. Polymethoxyflavones isolated from the peel of Miaray Mandarin (Citrus miaray) have biofilm inhibitory activity in Vibrio harveyi. *J. Agric. Food Chem.* **2015**, *63*, 7180–7189. [CrossRef] [PubMed]
39. Itoh, N.; Iwata, C.; Toda, H. Molecular cloning and characterization of a flavonoid-O-methyltransferase with broad substrate specificity and regioselectivity from Citrus depressa. *BMC Plant Biol.* **2016**, *16*, 180. [CrossRef]
40. Lee, Y.-H.; Charles, A.L.; Kung, H.-F.; Ho, C.-T.; Huang, T.-C. Extraction of nobiletin and tangeretin from Citrus depressa Hayata by supercritical carbon dioxide with ethanol as modifier. *Ind. Crops Prod.* **2010**, *31*, 59–64. [CrossRef]
41. Kohno, H.; Yoshitani, S.-I.; Tsukio, Y.; Murakami, A.; Koshimizu, K.; Yano, M.; Tokuda, H.; Nishino, H.; Ohigashi, H.; Tanaka, T. Dietary administration of citrus nobiletin inhibits azoxymethane-induced colonic aberrant crypt foci in rats. *Life Sci.* **2001**, *69*, 901–913. [CrossRef]
42. Murakami, A.; Nakamura, Y.; Torikai, K.; Tanaka, T.; Koshiba, T.; Koshimizu, K.; Kuwahara, S.; Takahashi, Y.; Ogawa, K.; Yano, M. Inhibitory effect of citrus nobiletin on phorbol ester-induced skin inflammation, oxidative stress, and tumor promotion in mice. *Cancer Res.* **2000**, *60*, 5059–5066. [PubMed]
43. Uckoo, R.M.; Jayaprakasha, G.K.; Patil, B.S. Rapid separation method of polymethoxyflavones from citrus using flash chromatography. *Sep. Purif. Technol.* **2011**, *81*, 151–158. [CrossRef]
44. Teruya, T.; Teruya, Y.; Sueyoshi, K.; Yamano, A.; Jitai, Y. Manufacturing method of fermentation treated products containing high-content nobiletin and tangeretin. Patent JP 2015202065, 16 November 2015.
45. Kawaii, S.; Tomono, Y.; Katase, E.; Ogawa, K.; Yano, M. HL-60 differentiating activity and flavonoid content of the readily extractable fraction prepared from Citrus juices. *J. Agric. Food Chem.* **1999**, *47*, 128–135. [CrossRef]
46. Tsukayama, M.; Ichikawa, R.; Yamamoto, K.; Sasaki, T.; Kawamura, Y. Microwave-assisted rapid extraction of polymethoxyflavones from dried peels of Citrus yuko Hort. ex Tanaka. *J. Jpn. Soc. Food Sci. Technol.* **2009**, *56*, 359–362. [CrossRef]
47. Silva, I.; Estrada, M.F.; V. Pereira, C.; da Silva, A.B.; Bronze, M.R.; Alves, P.M.; Duarte, C.M.; Brito, C.; Serra, A.T. Polymethoxylated Flavones from Orange Peels Inhibit Cell Proliferation in a 3D Cell Model of Human Colorectal Cancer. *Nutr. Cancer* **2018**, *70*, 257–266. [CrossRef] [PubMed]
48. Seo, J.W.; Jang, D.R.; Kim, Y.U. Preparation Method of Citrus Peel Extract with Increased Polymethoxyflavone Content by Supercritical Fluid Extraction. Patent KR 1838266, 14 March 2018.
49. Chiou, Y.-S.; Zheng, Y.-N.; Tsai, M.-L.; Lai, C.-S.; Ho, C.-T.; Pan, M.-H. 5-Demethylnobiletin more potently inhibits colon cancer cell growth than nobiletin in vitro and in vivo. *J. Food Bioact.* **2018**, *2*, 91–97. [CrossRef]

50. Zheng, J.; Bi, J.; Johnson, D.; Sun, Y.; Song, M.; Qiu, P.; Dong, P.; Decker, E.; Xiao, H. Analysis of 10 metabolites of polymethoxyflavones with high sensitivity by electrochemical detection in high-performance liquid chromatography. *J. Agric. Food Chem.* **2015**, *63*, 509–516. [CrossRef]

51. Zheng, J.; Song, M.; Dong, P.; Qiu, P.; Guo, S.; Zhong, Z.; Li, S.; Ho, C.T.; Xiao, H. Identification of novel bioactive metabolites of 5-demethylnobiletin in mice. *Mol. Nutr. Food Res.* **2013**, *57*, 1999–2007. [CrossRef]

52. Li, S.; Wang, Z.; Sang, S.; Huang, M.T.; Ho, C.T. Identification of nobiletin metabolites in mouse urine. *Mol. Nutr. Food Res.* **2006**, *50*, 291–299. [CrossRef]

53. Yasuda, T.; Yoshimura, Y.; Yabuki, H.; Nakazawa, T.; Ohsawa, K.; Mimaki, Y.; Sashida, Y. Urinary metabolites of nobiletin orally administered to rats. *Chem. Pharm. Bull.* **2003**, *51*, 1426–1428. [CrossRef]

54. Wu, X.; Song, M.; Wang, M.; Zheng, J.; Gao, Z.; Xu, F.; Zhang, G.; Xiao, H. Chemopreventive effects of nobiletin and its colonic metabolites on colon carcinogenesis. *Mol. Nutr. Food Res.* **2015**, *59*, 2383–2394. [CrossRef] [PubMed]

55. Wang, Z.; Li, S.; Jonca, M.; Lambros, T.; Ferguson, S.; Goodnow, R.; Ho, C.T. Comparison of supercritical fluid chromatography and liquid chromatography for the separation of urinary metabolites of nobiletin with chiral and non-chiral stationary phases. *Biomed. Chromatogr.* **2006**, *20*, 1206–1215. [CrossRef] [PubMed]

56. Koga, N.; Ohta, C.; Kato, Y.; Haraguchi, K.; Endo, T.; Ogawa, K.; Ohta, H.; Yano, M. In vitro metabolism of nobiletin, a polymethoxy-flavonoid, by human liver microsomes and cytochrome P450. *Xenobiotica* **2011**, *41*, 927–933. [CrossRef] [PubMed]

57. Wang, M. Biotransformation of Polymethoxyflavones and Its Implication on Biological Activities. Ph.D. Thesis, University of Massachusetts, Amherst, MA, USA, 2017.

58. Xu, L.; He, Y.; Guo, X.; Lu, Y.; Wang, C.; Wang, Z. Identification of metabolites of nobiletin in rats using ultra-performance liquid chromatography coupled with triple-quadrupole mass spectrometry. *Yao Xue Xue Bao (Acta Pharm. Sin.)* **2011**, *46*, 1483–1487.

59. Manthey, J.A.; Bendele, P. Anti-inflammatory activity of an orange peel polymethoxylated flavone, 3′, 4′, 3, 5, 6, 7, 8-heptamethoxyflavone, in the rat carrageenan/paw edema and mouse lipopolysaccharide-challenge assays. *J. Agric. Food Chem.* **2008**, *56*, 9399–9403. [CrossRef] [PubMed]

60. Kemperman, R.A.; Bolca, S.; Roger, L.C.; Vaughan, E.E. Novel approaches for analysing gut microbes and dietary polyphenols: Challenges and opportunities. *Microbiology* **2010**, *156*, 3224–3231. [CrossRef] [PubMed]

61. Ma, C. Biotransformation of Polymethoxyflavones by Gut Microbiome and Molecular Characterization of Polymethoxyflavones by Surface Enhanced Raman Spectroscopy. Ph.D. Thesis, University of Massachusetts, Amherst, MA, USA, 2015.

62. Li, S.; Sang, S.; Pan, M.-H.; Lai, C.-S.; Lo, C.-Y.; Yang, C.S.; Ho, C.-T. Anti-inflammatory property of the urinary metabolites of nobiletin in mouse. *Bioorg. Med. Chem. Lett.* **2007**, *17*, 5177–5181. [CrossRef] [PubMed]

63. Qiu, P.; Dong, P.; Guan, H.; Li, S.; Ho, C.T.; Pan, M.H.; McClements, D.J.; Xiao, H. Inhibitory effects of 5-hydroxy polymethoxyflavones on colon cancer cells. *Mol. Nutr. Food Res.* **2010**, *54*, S244–S252. [CrossRef] [PubMed]

64. Fearon, E.R.; Vogelstein, B. A genetic model for colorectal tumorigenesis. *Cell* **1990**, *61*, 759–767. [CrossRef]

65. Ciardiello, F.; Tortora, G. EGFR antagonists in cancer treatment. *N. Engl. J. Med.* **2008**, *358*, 1160–1174. [CrossRef] [PubMed]

66. Shi, Y.; Massagué, J. Mechanisms of TGF-β signaling from cell membrane to the nucleus. *Cell* **2003**, *113*, 685–700. [CrossRef]

67. Neuzillet, C.; Tijeras-Raballand, A.; Cohen, R.; Cros, J.; Faivre, S.; Raymond, E.; de Gramont, A. Targeting the TGFβ pathway for cancer therapy. *Pharmacol. Ther.* **2015**, *147*, 22–31. [CrossRef] [PubMed]

68. Said, A.H.; Raufman, J.-P.; Xie, G. The role of matrix metalloproteinases in colorectal cancer. *Cancers* **2014**, *6*, 366–375. [CrossRef] [PubMed]

69. Maeda, K.; Kang, S.-M.; Sawada, T.; Nishiguchi, Y.; Yashiro, M.; Ogawa, Y.; Ohira, M.; Ishikawa, T.; Hirakawa-YS Chung, K. Expression of intercellular adhesion molecule-1 and prognosis in colorectal cancer. *Oncol. Rep.* **2002**, *9*, 511–514. [CrossRef] [PubMed]

70. Manthey, J.A.; Guthrie, N. Antiproliferative activities of citrus flavonoids against six human cancer cell lines. *J. Agric. Food Chem.* **2002**, *50*, 5837–5843. [CrossRef] [PubMed]

71. Parang, B.; Barrett, C.W.; Williams, C.S. AOM/DSS Model of Colitis-Associated Cancer. In *Gastrointestinal Physiology and Diseases*; Springer: Berlin/Heidelberg, Germany, 2016; pp. 297–307.
72. Ito, N.; Hasegawa, R.; Sano, M.; Tamano, S.; Esumi, H.; Takayama, S.; Sugimura, T. A new colon and mammary carcinogen in cooked food, 2-amino-1-methyl-6-phenylimidazo [4, 5-b] pyridine (PhIP). *Carcinogenesis* **1991**, *12*, 1503–1506. [CrossRef] [PubMed]
73. Nakagama, H.; Nakanishi, M.; Ochiai, M. Modeling human colon cancer in rodents using a food-borne carcinogen, PhIP. *Cancer Sci.* **2005**, *96*, 627–636. [CrossRef]
74. Suzuki, R.; Kohno, H.; Murakami, A.; Koshimizu, K.; Ohigashi, H.; Yano, M.; Tokuda, H.; Nishino, H.; Tanaka, T. Citrus nobiletin inhibits azoxymethane-induced large bowel carcinogenesis in rats. *Biofactors* **2004**, *21*, 111–114. [CrossRef]
75. Tang, M.X.; Ogawa, K.; Asamoto, M.; Chewonarin, T.; Suzuki, S.; Tanaka, T.; Shirai, T. Effects of nobiletin on PhIP-induced prostate and colon carcinogenesis in F344 rats. *Nutr. Cancer* **2011**, *63*, 227–233. [CrossRef]
76. Wu, X.; Song, M.; Gao, Z.; Sun, Y.; Wang, M.; Li, F.; Zheng, J.; Xiao, H. Nobiletin and its colonic metabolites suppress colitis-associated colon carcinogenesis by down-regulating iNOS, inducing antioxidative enzymes and arresting cell cycle progression. *J. Nutr. Biochem.* **2017**, *42*, 17–25. [CrossRef]
77. Kawabata, K.; Murakami, A.; Ohigashi, H. Nobiletin, a citrus flavonoid, down-regulates matrix metalloproteinase-7 (matrilysin) expression in HT-29 human colorectal cancer cells. *Biosci Biotechnol. Biochem.* **2005**, *69*, 307–314. [CrossRef] [PubMed]
78. Song, M.; Wu, X.; Zheng, J.; Xiao, H. 5-Demethylnobiletin inhibits colon carcinogenesis in azoxymethane/dextran sulfate sodium-treated mice (123.3). *FASEB J.* **2014**, *28*, 123.3.
79. Zheng, Q.; Hirose, Y.; Yoshimi, N.; Murakami, A.; Koshimizu, K.; Ohigashi, H.; Sakata, K.; Matsumoto, Y.; Sayama, Y.; Mori, H. Further investigation of the modifying effect of various chemopreventive agents on apoptosis and cell proliferation in human colon cancer cells. *J. Cancer Res. Clin. Oncol.* **2002**, *128*, 539–546. [CrossRef] [PubMed]
80. Qiu, P.; Guan, H.; Dong, P.; Li, S.; Ho, C.T.; Pan, M.H.; McClements, D.J.; Xiao, H. The p53-, Bax-and p21-dependent inhibition of colon cancer cell growth by 5-hydroxy polymethoxyflavones. *Mol. Nutr. Food Res.* **2011**, *55*, 613–622. [CrossRef] [PubMed]
81. Lin, N.; Sato, T.; Takayama, Y.; Mimaki, Y.; Sashida, Y.; Yano, M.; Ito, A. Novel anti-inflammatory actions of nobiletin, a citrus polymethoxy flavonoid, on human synovial fibroblasts and mouse macrophages. *Biochem. Pharmacol.* **2003**, *65*, 2065–2071. [CrossRef]
82. Yasunaga, S.; Domen, M.; Nishi, K.; Kadota, A.; Sugahara, T. Nobiletin suppresses monocyte chemoattractant protein-1 (MCP-1) expression by regulating MAPK signaling in 3T3-L1 cells. *J. Funct. Foods* **2016**, *27*, 406–415. [CrossRef]
83. Miyamoto, S.; Yasui, Y.; Ohigashi, H.; Tanaka, T.; Murakami, A. Dietary flavonoids suppress azoxymethane-induced colonic preneoplastic lesions in male C57BL/KsJ-db/db mice. *Chem. Biol. Interact.* **2010**, *183*, 276–283. [CrossRef]
84. Miyamoto, S.; Yasui, Y.; Tanaka, T.; Ohigashi, H.; Murakami, A. Suppressive effects of nobiletin on hyperleptinemia and colitis-related colon carcinogenesis in male ICR mice. *Carcinogenesis* **2008**, *29*, 1057–1063. [CrossRef]
85. Armaghany, T.; Wilson, J.D.; Chu, Q.; Mills, G. Genetic alterations in colorectal cancer. *Gastrointest. Cancer Res.* **2012**, *5*, 19.
86. Owa, T.; Yoshino, H.; Yoshimatsu, K.; Nagasu, T. Cell cycle regulation in the G1 phase: A promising target for the development of new chemotherapeutic anticancer agents. *Curr. Med. Chem.* **2001**, *8*, 1487–1503. [CrossRef]
87. Johnson, D.; Walker, C. Cyclins and cell cycle checkpoints. *Ann. Rev. Pharmacol. Toxicol.* **1999**, *39*, 295–312. [CrossRef] [PubMed]
88. Sherr, C.J. Cancer cell cycles. *Science* **1996**, *274*, 1672–1677. [CrossRef] [PubMed]
89. Malumbres, M.; Barbacid, M. Cell cycle, CDKs and cancer: A changing paradigm. *Nat. Rev. Cancer* **2009**, *9*, 153. [CrossRef] [PubMed]
90. Kurki, P.; Vanderlaan, M.; Dolbeare, F.; Gray, J.; Tan, E. Expression of proliferating cell nuclear antigen (PCNA)/cyclin during the cell cycle. *Exp. Cell Res.* **1986**, *166*, 209–219. [CrossRef]

91. McKay, J.A.; Douglas, J.J.; Ross, V.G.; Curran, S.; Loane, J.F.; Ahmed, F.Y.; Cassidy, J.; McLeod, H.L.; Murray, G.I. Analysis of key cell-cycle checkpoint proteins in colorectal tumours. *J. Pathol. J. Pathol. Soc. Great Br. Irel.* **2002**, *196*, 386–393. [CrossRef]
92. Kroker, A.J.; Bruning, J.B. p21 exploits residue Tyr151 as a tether for high-affinity PCNA binding. *Biochemistry* **2015**, *54*, 3483–3493. [CrossRef] [PubMed]
93. Soria, G.; Gottifredi, V. PCNA-coupled p21 degradation after DNA damage: The exception that confirms the rule? *DNA Repair* **2010**, *9*, 358–364. [CrossRef]
94. Morgan, D.O. Cyclin-dependent kinases: Engines, clocks, and microprocessors. *Annu. Rev. Cell Dev. Biol.* **1997**, *13*, 261–291. [CrossRef]
95. Karimian, A.; Ahmadi, Y.; Yousefi, B. Multiple functions of p21 in cell cycle, apoptosis and transcriptional regulation after DNA damage. *DNA Repair* **2016**, *42*, 63–71. [CrossRef]
96. Bertoli, C.; Skotheim, J.M.; De Bruin, R.A. Control of cell cycle transcription during G1 and S phases. *Nat. Rev. Mol. Cell Biol.* **2013**, *14*, 518–528. [CrossRef]
97. Taylor, W.R.; Stark, G.R. Regulation of the G2/M transition by p53. *Oncogene* **2001**, *20*, 1803–1815. [CrossRef] [PubMed]
98. Borgne, A.; Meijer, L. Sequential dephosphorylation of p34cdc2 on Thr-14 and Tyr-15 at the prophase/metaphase transition. *J. Biol. Chem.* **1996**, *271*, 27847–27854. [CrossRef] [PubMed]
99. Ouyang, L.; Shi, Z.; Zhao, S.; Wang, F.T.; Zhou, T.T.; Liu, B.; Bao, J.K. Programmed cell death pathways in cancer: A review of apoptosis, autophagy and programmed necrosis. *Cell Prolif.* **2012**, *45*, 487–498. [CrossRef] [PubMed]
100. Zong, W.-X.; Ditsworth, D.; Bauer, D.E.; Wang, Z.-Q.; Thompson, C.B. Alkylating DNA damage stimulates a regulated form of necrotic cell death. *Genes Dev.* **2004**, *18*, 1272–1282. [CrossRef] [PubMed]
101. Sayers, T.J. Targeting the extrinsic apoptosis signaling pathway for cancer therapy. *Cancer Immunol. Immunother* **2011**, *60*, 1173–1180. [CrossRef]
102. Wang, X. The expanding role of mitochondria in apoptosis. *Genes Dev.* **2001**, *15*, 2922–2933. [PubMed]
103. Llambi, F.; Green, D.R. Apoptosis and oncogenesis: Give and take in the BCL-2 family. *Curr. Opin. Genet. Dev.* **2011**, *21*, 12–20. [CrossRef]
104. Engel, T.; Henshall, D.C. Apoptosis, Bcl-2 family proteins and caspases: The ABCs of seizure-damage and epileptogenesis? *Int. J. Physiol. Pathophysiol. Pharmacol.* **2009**, *1*, 97–115.
105. Chan, C.K.; Supriady, H.; Goh, B.H.; Kadir, H.A. Elephantopus scaber induces apoptosis through ROS-dependent mitochondrial signaling pathway in HCT116 human colorectal carcinoma cells. *J. Ethnopharmacol.* **2015**, *168*, 291–304. [CrossRef]
106. Nuñez, G.; Benedict, M.A.; Hu, Y.; Inohara, N. Caspases: The proteases of the apoptotic pathway. *Oncogene* **1998**, *17*, 3237–3245. [CrossRef]
107. Fernandes-Alnemri, T.; Litwack, G.; Alnemri, E.S. CPP32, a novel human apoptotic protein with homology to Caenorhabditis elegans cell death protein Ced-3 and mammalian interleukin-1 beta-converting enzyme. *J. Biol. Chem.* **1994**, *269*, 30761–30764. [PubMed]
108. Kerr, J.F.; Wyllie, A.H.; Currie, A.R. Apoptosis: A basic biological phenomenon with wideranging implications in tissue kinetics. *Br. J. Cancer* **1972**, *26*, 239. [CrossRef] [PubMed]
109. Oliver, F.J.; de la Rubia, G.; Rolli, V.; Ruiz-Ruiz, M.C.; de Murcia, G.; Ménissier-de Murcia, J. Importance of poly (ADP-ribose) polymerase and its cleavage in apoptosis Lesson from an uncleavable mutant. *J. Biol. Chem.* **1998**, *273*, 33533–33539. [CrossRef] [PubMed]
110. Saraste, A.; Pulkki, K. Morphologic and biochemical hallmarks of apoptosis. *Cardiovasc. Res.* **2000**, *45*, 528–537. [CrossRef]
111. Martin, S.J.; Green, D.R. Protease activation during apoptosis: Death by a thousand cuts? *Cell* **1995**, *82*, 349–352. [CrossRef]
112. Lee, W.-R.; Shen, S.-C.; Lin, H.-Y.; Hou, W.-C.; Yang, L.-L.; Chen, Y.-C. Wogonin and fisetin induce apoptosis in human promyeloleukemic cells, accompanied by a decrease of reactive oxygen species, and activation of caspase 3 and Ca2+-dependent endonuclease. *Biochem. Pharmacol.* **2002**, *63*, 225–236. [CrossRef]
113. Fletcher, J.I.; Huang, D.C. Controlling the cell death mediators Bax and Bak: Puzzles and conundrums. *Cell Cycle* **2008**, *7*, 39–44. [CrossRef]

114. Wei, M.C.; Zong, W.-X.; Cheng, E.H.-Y.; Lindsten, T.; Panoutsakopoulou, V.; Ross, A.J.; Roth, K.A.; MacGregor, G.R.; Thompson, C.B.; Korsmeyer, S.J. Proapoptotic BAX and BAK: A requisite gateway to mitochondrial dysfunction and death. *Science* **2001**, *292*, 727–730. [CrossRef]
115. Wang, S.-Y.; Yu, Q.-J.; Zhang, R.-D.; Liu, B. Core signaling pathways of survival/death in autophagy-related cancer networks. *Int. J. Biochem. Cell Biol.* **2011**, *43*, 1263–1266. [CrossRef]
116. Kundu, M.; Thompson, C.B. Autophagy: Basic principles and relevance to disease. *Annu. Rev. Pathmechdis Mech. Dis.* **2008**, *3*, 427–455. [CrossRef]
117. Eum, K.-H.; Lee, M. Crosstalk between autophagy and apoptosis in the regulation of paclitaxel-induced cell death in v-Ha-ras-transformed fibroblasts. *Mol. Cell. Biochem.* **2011**, *348*, 61–68. [CrossRef] [PubMed]
118. Amelio, I.; Melino, G.; Knight, R.A. Cell death pathology: Cross-talk with autophagy and its clinical implications. *Biochem. Biophys. Res. Commun.* **2011**, *414*, 277–281. [CrossRef] [PubMed]
119. Terzić, J.; Grivennikov, S.; Karin, E.; Karin, M. Inflammation and colon cancer. *Gastroenterology* **2010**, *138*, 2101–2114.e5. [CrossRef] [PubMed]
120. Klampfer, L. Cytokines, inflammation and colon cancer. *Curr. Cancer Drug Targets* **2011**, *11*, 451–464. [CrossRef] [PubMed]
121. Meira, L.B.; Bugni, J.M.; Green, S.L.; Lee, C.-W.; Pang, B.; Borenshtein, D.; Rickman, B.H.; Rogers, A.B.; Moroski-Erkul, C.A.; McFaline, J.L. DNA damage induced by chronic inflammation contributes to colon carcinogenesis in mice. *J. Clin. Investig.* **2008**, *118*, 2516–2525. [CrossRef] [PubMed]
122. Westbrook, A.M.; Wei, B.; Braun, J.; Schiestl, R.H. Intestinal mucosal inflammation leads to systemic genotoxicity in mice. *Cancer Res.* **2009**, *69*, 4827–4834. [CrossRef]
123. Kraus, S.; Arber, N. Inflammation and colorectal cancer. *Curr. Opin. Pharmacol.* **2009**, *9*, 405–410. [CrossRef]
124. Itzkowitz, S.H.; Yio, X. Inflammation and cancer IV. Colorectal cancer in inflammatory bowel disease: The role of inflammation. *Am. J. Physiol. Gastrointest. Liver Physiol.* **2004**, *287*, G7–G17. [CrossRef]
125. Takahashi, M.; Wakabayashi, K. Gene mutations and altered gene expression in azoxymethane-induced colon carcinogenesis in rodents. *Cancer Sci.* **2004**, *95*, 475–480. [CrossRef]
126. Xiong, Y.; Chen, D.; Yu, C.; Lv, B.; Peng, J.; Wang, J.; Lin, Y. Citrus nobiletin ameliorates experimental colitis by reducing inflammation and restoring impaired intestinal barrier function. *Mol. Nutr. Food Res.* **2015**, *59*, 829–842. [CrossRef]
127. Kaidi, A.; Qualtrough, D.; Williams, A.C.; Paraskeva, C. Direct transcriptional up-regulation of cyclooxygenase-2 by hypoxia-inducible factor (HIF)-1 promotes colorectal tumor cell survival and enhances HIF-1 transcriptional activity during hypoxia. *Cancer Res.* **2006**, *66*, 6683–6691. [CrossRef] [PubMed]
128. Goodwin, J. Are prostaglandins proinflammatory, antiinflammatory, both or neither? *J. Rheumatol. Suppl.* **1991**, *28*, 26–29. [PubMed]
129. Surh, Y.-J.; Chun, K.-S.; Cha, H.-H.; Han, S.S.; Keum, Y.-S.; Park, K.-K.; Lee, S.S. Molecular mechanisms underlying chemopreventive activities of anti-inflammatory phytochemicals: Down-regulation of COX-2 and iNOS through suppression of NF-κB activation. *Mutat. Res./Fundam. Mol. Mech. Mutagen.* **2001**, *480*, 243–268. [CrossRef]
130. Rao, C.V. Nitric oxide signaling in colon cancer chemoprevention. *Mutat. Res./Fundam. Mol. Mech. Mutagen.* **2004**, *555*, 107–119. [CrossRef] [PubMed]
131. Rushworth, S.A.; MacEwan, D.J.; O'Connell, M.A. Lipopolysaccharide-induced expression of NAD (P) H: Quinone oxidoreductase 1 and heme oxygenase-1 protects against excessive inflammatory responses in human monocytes. *J. Immunol.* **2008**, *181*, 6730–6737. [CrossRef]
132. Khor, T.O.; Huang, M.-T.; Kwon, K.H.; Chan, J.Y.; Reddy, B.S.; Kong, A.-N. Nrf2-deficient mice have an increased susceptibility to dextran sulfate sodium–induced colitis. *Cancer Res.* **2006**, *66*, 11580–11584. [CrossRef]
133. Klaunig, J.E.; Kamendulis, L.M.; Hocevar, B.A. Oxidative stress and oxidative damage in carcinogenesis. *Toxicol. Pathol.* **2010**, *38*, 96–109. [CrossRef]
134. Kwak, M.-K.; Kensler, T.W. Targeting NRF2 signaling for cancer chemoprevention. *Toxicol. Appl. Pharmacol.* **2010**, *244*, 66–76. [CrossRef]
135. Nishida, N.; Yano, H.; Nishida, T.; Kamura, T.; Kojiro, M. Angiogenesis in cancer. *Vasc. Health Risk Manag.* **2006**, *2*, 213–219. [CrossRef]

136. Prager, G.; Poettler, M. Angiogenesis in cancer. *Hämostaseologie* **2012**, *32*, 105–114.
137. Park, M.H.; Hong, J.T. Roles of NF-κB in cancer and inflammatory diseases and their therapeutic approaches. *Cells* **2016**, *5*, 15. [CrossRef]
138. Ferrara, N.; Gerber, H.-P.; LeCouter, J. The biology of VEGF and its receptors. *Nat. Med.* **2003**, *9*, 669. [CrossRef] [PubMed]
139. Carmeliet, P. VEGF as a key mediator of angiogenesis in cancer. *Oncology* **2005**, *69*, 4–10. [CrossRef] [PubMed]
140. Berra, E.; Pagès, G.; Pouysségur, J. MAP kinases and hypoxia in the control of VEGF expression. *Cancer Metastasis Rev.* **2000**, *19*, 139–145. [CrossRef] [PubMed]
141. Saxena, N.K.; Taliaferro-Smith, L.; Knight, B.B.; Merlin, D.; Anania, F.A.; O'Regan, R.M.; Sharma, D. Bidirectional crosstalk between leptin and insulin-like growth factor-I signaling promotes invasion and migration of breast cancer cells via transactivation of epidermal growth factor receptor. *Cancer Res.* **2008**, *68*, 9712–9722. [CrossRef] [PubMed]
142. Fenton, J.I.; Hord, N.G.; Lavigne, J.A.; Perkins, S.N.; Hursting, S.D. Leptin, insulin-like growth factor-1, and insulin-like growth factor-2 are mitogens in ApcMin/+ but not Apc+/+ colonic epithelial cell lines. *Cancer Epidemiol. Prev. Biomark.* **2005**, *14*, 1646–1652. [CrossRef] [PubMed]
143. Rouet-Benzineb, P.; Aparicio, T.; Guilmeau, S.; Pouzet, C.; Descatoire, V.; Buyse, M.; Bado, A. Leptin counteracts sodium butyrate-induced apoptosis in human colon cancer HT-29 cells via NF-κB signaling. *J. Biol. Chem.* **2004**, *279*, 16495–16502. [CrossRef] [PubMed]
144. Miyata, Y.; Sato, T.; Yano, M.; Ito, A. Activation of protein kinase C βII/ε-c-Jun NH2-terminal kinase pathway and inhibition of mitogen-activated protein/extracellular signal-regulated kinase 1/2 phosphorylation in antitumor invasive activity induced by the polymethoxy flavonoid, nobiletin. *Mol. Cancer Ther.* **2004**, *3*, 839–847. [PubMed]
145. Miyata, Y.; Sato, T.; Imada, K.; Dobashi, A.; Yano, M.; Ito, A. A citrus polymethoxyflavonoid, nobiletin, is a novel MEK inhibitor that exhibits antitumor metastasis in human fibrosarcoma HT-1080 cells. *Biochem. Biophys. Res. Commun.* **2008**, *366*, 168–173. [CrossRef]
146. Fong, Y. Surgical therapy of hepatic colorectal metastasis. *CA Cancer J. Clin.* **1999**, *49*, 231–255. [CrossRef]
147. Kim, Y.-S.; Kim, S.-H.; Kang, J.-G.; Ko, J.-H. Expression level and glycan dynamics determine the net effects of TIMP-1 on cancer progression. *BMB Rep.* **2012**, *45*, 623–628. [CrossRef] [PubMed]
148. Chambers, A.F.; Matrisian, L.M. Changing views of the role of matrix metalloproteinases in metastasis. *J. Natl. Cancer Inst.* **1997**, *89*, 1260–1270. [CrossRef] [PubMed]
149. Waas, E.; Wobbes, T.; Lomme, R.; DeGroot, J.; Ruers, T.; Hendriks, T. Matrix metalloproteinase 2 and 9 activity in patients with colorectal cancer liver metastasis. *Br. J. Surg.* **2003**, *90*, 1556–1564. [CrossRef] [PubMed]
150. Zucker, S.; Vacirca, J. Role of matrix metalloproteinases (MMPs) in colorectal cancer. *Cancer Metastasis Rev.* **2004**, *23*, 101–117. [CrossRef] [PubMed]
151. Brabletz, T.; Jung, A.; Dag, S.; Hlubek, F.; Kirchner, T. β-Catenin regulates the expression of the matrix metalloproteinase-7 in human colorectal cancer. *Am. J. Pathol.* **1999**, *155*, 1033–1038. [CrossRef]
152. Crawford, H.C.; Fingleton, B.M.; Rudolph-Owen, L.A.; Goss, K.J.H.; Rubinfeld, B.; Polakis, P.; Matrisian, L.M. The metalloproteinase matrilysin is a target of β-catenin transactivation in intestinal tumors. *Oncogene* **1999**, *18*, 2883–2891. [CrossRef]
153. Egeblad, M.; Werb, Z. New functions for the matrix metalloproteinases in cancer progression. *Nat. Rev. Cancer* **2002**, *2*, 161–174. [CrossRef]
154. Bingle, á.; Brown, N.; Lewis, C. The role of tumour-associated macrophages in tumour progression: Implications for new anticancer therapies. *J. Pathol. J. Pathol. Soc. Great Br. Irel.* **2002**, *196*, 254–265. [CrossRef]
155. Kerkelä, E.; Ala-aho, R.; Klemi, P.; Grénman, S.; Shapiro, S.D.; Kähäri, V.M.; Saarialho-Kere, U. Metalloelastase (MMP-12) expression by tumour cells in squamous cell carcinoma of the vulva correlates with invasiveness, while that by macrophages predicts better outcome. *J. Pathol.* **2002**, *198*, 258–269. [CrossRef]
156. Li, S.; Pan, M.-H.; Lo, C.-Y.; Tan, D.; Wang, Y.; Shahidi, F.; Ho, C.-T. Chemistry and health effects of polymethoxyflavones and hydroxylated polymethoxyflavones. *J. Funct. Foods* **2009**, *1*, 2–12. [CrossRef]
157. Scholz; Williamson. Interactions affecting the bioavailability of dietary polyphenols in vivo. *Int. J. Vitam. Nutr. Res.* **2007**, *77*, 224–235. [CrossRef] [PubMed]
158. Murakami, A.; Kuwahara, S.; Takahashi, Y.; Ito, C.; Furukawa, H.; Ju-ichi, M.; Koshimizu, K.; OHIGASHI, H. In vitro absorption and metabolism of nobiletin, a chemopreventive polymethoxyflavonoid in citrus fruits. *Biosci. Biotechnol. Biochem.* **2001**, *65*, 194–197. [CrossRef] [PubMed]

159. Kansy, M.; Senner, F.; Gubernator, K. Physicochemical high throughput screening: Parallel artificial membrane permeation assay in the description of passive absorption processes. *J. Med. Chem.* **1998**, *41*, 1007–1010. [CrossRef] [PubMed]
160. Wen, X.; Walle, T. Methylated flavonoids have greatly improved intestinal absorption and metabolic stability. *Drug Metab. Dispos.* **2006**, *34*, 1786–1792. [CrossRef] [PubMed]
161. Van de Waterbeemd, H. Physico-Chemical Approaches to Drug Absorption. In *Drug Bioavailability: Estimation of Solubility, Permeability, Absorption and Bioavailability*; Wiley: Hoboken, NJ, USA, 2003; pp. 3–20.
162. Murakami, A.; Koshimizu, K.; Ohigashi, H.; Kuwahara, S.; Kuki, W.; Takahashi, Y.; Hosotani, K.; Kawahara, S.; Matsuoka, Y. Characteristic rat tissue accumulation of nobiletin, a chemopreventive polymethoxyflavonoid, in comparison with luteolin. *Biofactors* **2002**, *16*, 73–82. [CrossRef] [PubMed]
163. Wang, M.; Zheng, J.; Zhong, Z.; Song, M.; Wu, X. *Tissue Distribution of Nobiletin and Its Metabolites in Mice after Oral Administration of Nobiletin*; Federation of American Societies for Experimental Biology: Bethesda, MD, USA, 2013.
164. Wu, X.; Song, M.; Qiu, P.; Rakariyatham, K.; Li, F.; Gao, Z.; Cai, X.; Wang, M.; Xu, F.; Zheng, J. Synergistic chemopreventive effects of nobiletin and atorvastatin on colon carcinogenesis. *Carcinogenesis* **2017**, *38*, 455–464. [CrossRef] [PubMed]
165. Kumar, A.; Devaraj, V.; Giri, K.C.; Giri, S.; Rajagopal, S.; Mullangi, R. Development and validation of a highly sensitive LC-MS/MS-ESI method for the determination of nobiletin in rat plasma: Application to a pharmacokinetic study. *Biomed. Chromatogr.* **2012**, *26*, 1464–1471. [CrossRef] [PubMed]
166. Singh, S.P.; Tewari, D.; Patel, K.; Jain, G.K. Permeability determination and pharmacokinetic study of nobiletin in rat plasma and brain by validated high-performance liquid chromatography method. *Fitoterapia* **2011**, *82*, 1206–1214. [CrossRef] [PubMed]
167. Manthey, J.A.; Cesar, T.B.; Jackson, E.; Mertens-Talcott, S. Pharmacokinetic Study of Nobiletin and Tangeretin in Rat Serum by High-Performance Liquid Chromatography—Electrospray Ionization—Mass Spectrometry. *J. Agric. Food Chem.* **2011**, *59*, 145–151. [CrossRef]
168. McClements, D.J. Emulsion design to improve the delivery of functional lipophilic components. *Annu. Rev. Food Sci. Technol.* **2010**, *1*, 241–269. [CrossRef] [PubMed]
169. Yang, Y.; Zhao, C.; Chen, J.; Tian, G.; McClements, D.J.; Xiao, H.; Zheng, J. Encapsulation of polymethoxyflavones in citrus oil emulsion-based delivery systems. *J. Agric. Food Chem.* **2017**, *65*, 1732–1739. [CrossRef] [PubMed]
170. Yao, J.; Lu, Y.; Zhou, J.P. Preparation of nobiletin in self-microemulsifying systems and its intestinal permeability in rats. *J. Pharm. Pharm. Sci.* **2008**, *11*, 22–29. [CrossRef] [PubMed]
171. Lin, W.; Yao, J.; Zhou, J. Preparation of self-assemble nobiletin proliposomes and its pharmacokinetics in rats. *Yao Xue Xue Bao (Acta Pharm. Sin.)* **2009**, *44*, 192–196.
172. Chen, H.; An, Y.; Yan, X.; McClements, D.J.; Li, B.; Li, Y. Designing self-nanoemulsifying delivery systems to enhance bioaccessibility of hydrophobic bioactives (nobiletin): Influence of hydroxypropyl methylcellulose and thermal processing. *Food Hydrocoll.* **2015**, *51*, 395–404. [CrossRef]
173. Lei, L.; Zhang, Y.; He, L.; Wu, S.; Li, B.; Li, Y. Fabrication of nanoemulsion-filled alginate hydrogel to control the digestion behavior of hydrophobic nobiletin. *LWT Food Sci. Technol.* **2017**, *82*, 260–267. [CrossRef]
174. Onoue, S.; Uchida, A.; Takahashi, H.; Seto, Y.; Kawabata, Y.; Ogawa, K.; Yuminoki, K.; Hashimoto, N.; Yamada, S. Development of high-energy amorphous solid dispersion of nanosized nobiletin, a citrus polymethoxylated flavone, with improved oral bioavailability. *J. Pharm. Sci.* **2011**, *100*, 3793–3801. [CrossRef] [PubMed]
175. Jordan, S.; Murty, M.; Pilon, K. Products containing bitter orange or synephrine: Suspected cardiovascular adverse reactions. *Can. Med. Assoc. J.* **2004**, *171*, 993–994.
176. Yang, G.; Li, S.; Long, T.; Yang, Y.; Li, Y. Application of Polymethoxylflavone in Preparation of Prevention Drug for Cardiovascular Inflammation. Patent CN 107281179, 24 October 2017.
177. Wu, X.; Zheng, D.; Qin, Y.; Liu, Z.; Zhu, X. Application of Nobiletin in Medicine for Preventing or Treating Heart Failure. Patent CN 106924241, 7 July 2017.
178. Morimoto, T.; Hasegawa, K.; Murakami, A.; Fukuda, H.; Takahashi, K. Cardiac Disease Treatment Agents Containing Nobiletin. Patent JP 2011037798, 24 February 2011.
179. Caramelli, G. Product with Blood Lipid-Lowering Activity. Patent IT 2008RM0232, 2 August 2008.

180. Ohizumi, Y.; Kajima, K.; Maruyama, K.; Ishibashi, M. Pharmaceutical Composition and Food Containing Citrus Butanol Extract for Preventing and/or Treating Central Nervous System Disease. Patent WO 2017208869, 7 December 2017.
181. Ohizumi, Y.; Kajima, K.; Maruyama, K. Pharmaceutical and food composition containing Anredera cordifolia and nobiletin. Patent JP 6238089, 29 November 2017.
182. Jeon, M.R.; L, S.A.; Yoon, G.J.; Park, J.H. Composition for Preventing or Treating Neurodegenerative Disease Comprising Nobiletin as Active Ingredient. Patent KR 2017090073, 25 September 2017.
183. Wu, X.; Mei, Z.; Zheng, D.; Liu, Z.; Zhu, X.; Zhou, Y.; Zeng, L.; Liang, Z. Application of Nobiletin in Preparation or Screening of Diabetic Cardiomyopathy Drug. Patent CN 108403684, 17 August 2018.
184. Guthrie, N. Compositions Comprising at Least one Polymethoxyflavone, Flavonoid, Liminoid, and/or Tocotrienol Useful in Combination Therapies for Treating Diabetes. Patent WO 2014203059, 24 December 2014.
185. Kim, T.J.; Kim, H.G.; Kwon, Y.I.; Lee, J.U. Obesity inhibiting Composition Comprising Powder of Citrus Grandis Cultivated by Eco Friendly Method as Active Ingredient. Patent KR 2016111554, 27 September 2016.
186. Miyaura, C.; Inada, M. Preventive or Therapeutic Compositions Containing Heptamethoxyflavone for Bone Diseases. Patent JP 2012232916, 22 October 2012.
187. Liao, X. Manufacture Method of Chinese Medicine Composition for Treatment of Halitosis. Patent CN 105434729, 30 March 2016.
188. Wang, L.; Tian, A.; Li, S.; Chen, J.; Li, B. Mouth Smell-Improving Agent and Its Preparation Method. Patent CN 103893334, 2 July 2014.
189. Huang, R.L.; Hsu, S.W. Polymethoxylated Flavone for Manufacturing Drugs Against Hepatitis-B with Drug Resistance. Patent TW I535439, 1 June 2016.
190. Kim, D.H.; Han, M.J.; Cho, E.H.; Kim, Y.R. Natural Products for Treating Cancer and HIV-Related diseases. Patent KR 2012011169, 7 February 2012.
191. Zhang, T.; Liao, M.; Gong, S.; Xie, X.; Sun, W.; Wang, L.; Zheng, Y. Application of Total Flavonoid Extract from Citrus Aurantium in Manufacturing Medicines for Treating Asthma. Patent CN 102935131, 20 February 2013.
192. Li, K. Application of Nobiletin in Medicine for Treating Allergic Asthma. Patent CN 102552242, 11 July 2012.
193. Sugawara, T.; Kadota, A.; Kikuchi, T. Antiallergic Oral Composition Containing β-Lactoglobulin and Nobiletin. Patent JP 2015036369, 23 February 2015.
194. Seo, J.W.; Choi, B.G.; Cheng, J.H.; Cho, M.J. Citrus Pericarp Extracts for Preventing Hair Loss and Promoting Hair Growth. Patent KR 1651833, 19 September 2016.
195. Ito, Y.; Hikiyama, E.; Yamada, S.; Woo, J.-T.; Teruya, Y.; Sugaya, K.; Nishijima, S.; Wakuda, H.; Shinozuka, K. Medicinal Composition for Preventing or Improving Dysuria, Antagonist Against Dysuria-Related Receptor, and Method for Preventing or Improving Dysuria Using Medicinal Composition or Antagonist. Patent WO 2016075960, 19 May 2016.
196. Sakata, Y.; Nakamura, H.; Oshio, K. Muscular Atrophy Preventing Agent Containing Citrus Depressa Extract. Patent WO 2013099982, 4 July 2013.
197. Li, S.; Yang, G.; Long, T. Application of (demethyl) polymethoxyflavone and taxol medicine in producing the medicine for treating non-small cell lung cancer. Patent CN 106562954, 19 April 2017.
198. Nakano, S.; Ono, M.; Hayashi, C. Agent and Method for Inhibiting Breast Cancer Cell Proliferation Comprising Nobiletin. Patent JP 2016017042, 4 February 2016.
199. Chen, G.; Wang, H. Application of Nobiletin in the Preparation of Health Products or Medicines for Preventing and/or Treating Oral Cancer. Patent CN 105030559, 11 November 2015.
200. Ma, W.-Z.; Feng, S.-L.; Yao, X.-J.; Yuan, Z.-W.; Liu, L.; Xie, Y. Use of Nobiletin in Cancer Treatment. Patent AU 2015101287, 22 October 2015.
201. Zhang, Z. Chinese Medicinal Composition Containing Extracts from Citrus and Scutellaria for Treating Cancer Chemotherapy Related Diarrhea. Patent CN 103655835, 26 March 2014.
202. Li, M.; Jin, H.; Yang, Z.; Xu, G.; Lin, Y.; Lin, Q.; Zhang, Z. Medical Application of Flavonoids of Citrus Reticulata Pericarp as Angiogenesis Inhibitor. Patent CN 101947215, 19 January 2011.
203. Zhou, H.; Xie, B.; Zang, X.; Cheng, L.; Liang, G. A Multiple Index Component content Determination, Fingerprint Construction and Preparation Method for Liver-Tonifying Eyesight-Improving Oral Liquid [Machine Translation]. Patent CN 105510452, 20 April 2016.
204. Guo, J.; Liang, L.; Song, J.; Li, H.; Yang, J.; Chen, B.; Wang, S. Method for Extracting Nobiletin and Hesperetin from Citrus. Patent CN 106632196, 10 May 2017.

205. Cao, J.; Hu, S.; Liu, X.; Cao, W.; Pang, X.; Dai, H.; Da, J. A method of Extracting Flavonoids active Ingredients in Citrus Reticulata Pericarp. Patent CN 104297026, 21 January 2015.
206. Yamaguchi, K.; Mogami, K.; Yamaguchi, Y.; Hitomi, N.; Murata, K.; Tani, Y. Manufacture of Nobiletin by Solvent Extraction and Nobiletin-Containing Extract. Patent JP 2012056938, 22 March 2012.
207. Sun, C.; Wang, Y.; Chen, K.; Li, X.; Cao, J. Process Forextn. And Purifn. of Polymethoxylated Flavonoids Compound from Fruit of Citrus Reticulate. Patent CN 107011308, 4 August 2017.
208. Li, X.; Zhang, J.; Sun, C.; Chen, K. Method for Isolating and Purifying Seven Flavonoids from Citrus Tangerina oil Cell Layer. Patent CN 103610800, 5 March 2014.
209. Liang, H.; Wu, D.; Li, B.; Li, Y.; Li, J. Stable Nobiletin liquid Preparation and Preparation Method Thereof. Patent CN 107998073, 8 May 2018.
210. Yang, W.; Song, Y.; Chen, H.; Luo, X.; Yuan, J. A Technique Based on Multi-Solvents for Preparing Nobiletin. Patent CN 105669626, 15 June 2016.
211. Iwashita, M.; Umehara, M.; Onishi, S.; Yamamoto, M.; Yamagami, K.; Ishigami, T. Method for Manufacturing Nobiletin-Containing Solid Dispersion. Patent WO 2018025871, 8 February 2018.
212. Woo, J.T.; Komaki, M. Polymethoxyflavonoid Dissolved Composition and its Manufacturing Method. Patent JP 2015221761, 10 December 2015.
213. Chen, Y.; Yu, Y.; Yang, D.; Wei, W.; He, Z.; Lin, X.; Xie, H. Measurement Method for Seventeen Kinds of Phenol Substances in Grape and Citrus Fruit Using High Performance Liquid Chromatography (HPLC). Patent CN 102706980, 3 October 2012.
214. Kusano, S.; Tamasu, S. Composition Containing 4′-Demethylnobiletin for skin Whitening Cosmetics, Medicines, Foods and Drinks. Patent JP 2017226612, 28 December 2017.
215. Choi, B.G.; Lee, D.R. Skin Moisturizers Containing Citrus Peel Extracts. Patent KR 2017000068, 6 January 2017.
216. Karabey, F. Nobiletin Molecules in Cosmetic Preparationsuse. Patent TR 2014000324, 2015.
217. Zhang, X.; Chen, S.; Wang, X.; Xie, F.; Liu, X.; Wang, J.; Yan, A.; Gao, N.; Li, F. A Snap Bean Preservative [Machine Translation]. Patent CN 106172719, 7 December 2016.
218. Krohn, M.; Seibert, S.; Kleber, A.; Wonschik, J. Sweetener and/or Sweetness Enhancer, Sweetener Composition, Methods of Making the Same and Consumables Containing the Same. Patent WO 2012107203, 16 August 2012.
219. Zhang, L.; Zhu, W.; Yang, C.; Guo, H.; Yu, A.; Ji, J.; Gao, Y.; Sun, M.; Zhai, G. A novel folate-modified self-microemulsifying drug delivery system of curcumin for colon targeting. *Int. J. Nanomed.* **2012**, *7*, 151–162. [CrossRef]
220. Bansode, S.T.; Kshirsagar, S.J.; Madgulkar, A.R.; Bhalekar, M.R.; Bandivadekar, M.M. Design and development of SMEDDS for colon-specific drug delivery. *Drug Dev. Ind. Pharm.* **2016**, *42*, 611–623. [CrossRef]
221. Low, L.E.; Tan, L.T.-H.; Goh, B.-H.; Tey, B.T.; Ong, B.H.; Tang, S.Y. Magnetic cellulose nanocrystal stabilized Pickering emulsions for enhanced bioactive release and human colon cancer therapy. *Int. J. Biol. Macromol.* **2019**, *127*, 76–84. [CrossRef] [PubMed]
222. Low, L.E.; Tey, B.T.; Ong, B.H.; Chan, E.S.; Tang, S.Y. Palm olein-in-water Pickering emulsion stabilized by Fe_3O_4-cellulose nanocrystal nanocomposites and their responses to pH. *Carbohydr. Polym.* **2017**, *155*, 391–399. [CrossRef] [PubMed]
223. Vangijzegem, T.; Stanicki, D.; Laurent, S. Magnetic iron oxide nanoparticles for drug delivery: Applications and characteristics. *Exp. Opin. Drug Deliv.* **2019**, *16*, 69–78. [CrossRef] [PubMed]
224. Xing, T.T.; Zhao, X.J.; Zhang, Y.D.; Li, Y.F. Fast separation and sensitive quantitation of polymethoxylated flavonoids in the peels of citrus using UPLC-Q-TOF-MS. *J. Agric. Food Chem.* **2017**, *65*, 2615–2627. [CrossRef] [PubMed]
225. Yang, T.; Rycaj, K.; Liu, Z.-M.; Tang, D.G. *Cancer Stem Cells: Constantly Evolving and Functionally Heterogeneous Therapeutic Targets*; AACR: Philadelphia, PA, USA, 2014.
226. Chen, K.; Huang, Y.-H.; Chen, J.-L. Understanding and targeting cancer stem cells: Therapeutic implications and challenges. *Acta Pharmacol. Sin.* **2013**, *34*, 732–740. [CrossRef] [PubMed]
227. Tan, L.T.H.; Low, L.E.; Tang, S.Y.; Yap, W.H.; Chuah, L.H.; Chan, C.K.; Lee, L.H.; Goh, B.H. A reliable and affordable 3D tumor spheroid model for natural product drug discovery: A case study of curcumin. *Prog. Drug Discov. Biomed. Sci.* **2019**, *2*, 1–5.
228. DiMarco-Crook, C.; Xiao, H. Diet-based strategies for cancer chemoprevention: The role of combination regimens using dietary bioactive components. *Annu. Rev. Food Sci. Technol.* **2015**, *6*, 505–526. [CrossRef]

229. Funaro, A.; Wu, X.; Song, M.; Zheng, J.; Guo, S.; Rakariyatham, K.; Rodriguez-Estrada, M.T.; Xiao, H. Enhanced Anti-Inflammatory Activities by the Combination of Luteolin and Tangeretin. *J. Food Sci.* **2016**, *81*, H1320–H1327. [CrossRef]

230. Wu, X.; Song, M.; Qiu, P.; Li, F.; Wang, M.; Zheng, J.; Wang, Q.; Xu, F.; Xiao, H. A metabolite of nobiletin, 4′-demethylnobiletin and atorvastatin synergistically inhibits human colon cancer cell growth by inducing G0/G1 cell cycle arrest and apoptosis. *Food Funct.* **2018**, *9*, 87–95. [CrossRef]

7

Fatty Acid Synthase Inhibitor G28 Shows Anticancer Activity in EGFR Tyrosine Kinase Inhibitor Resistant Lung Adenocarcinoma Models

Emma Polonio-Alcalá [1,2,†], Sònia Palomeras [1,†], Daniel Torres-Oteros [3], Joana Relat [3,4,5], Marta Planas [6], Lidia Feliu [6], Joaquim Ciurana [2], Santiago Ruiz-Martínez [1,*] and Teresa Puig [1,*]

1 New Therapeutic Targets Laboratory (TargetsLab)-Oncology Unit, Department of Medical Sciences, Faculty of Medicine, University of Girona, 17003 Girona, Spain; emma.polonio@udg.edu (E.P.-A.); sonia.palomeras@udg.edu (S.P.)
2 Product, Process and Production Engineering Research Group (GREP), Department of Mechanical Engineering and Industrial Construction, University of Girona, 17003 Girona, Spain; quim.ciurana@udg.edu
3 Department of Nutrition, Food Sciences and Gastronomy, School of Pharmacy and Food Sciences, Food Torribera Campus, University of Barcelona, E-08921 Santa Coloma de Gramanet, Spain; danytoot@hotmail.com (D.T.-O.); jrelat@ub.edu (J.R.)
4 Institute of Nutrition and Food Safety of the University of Barcelona (INSA-UB), E-08921 Santa Coloma de Gramenet, Spain
5 CIBER Physiopathology of Obesity and Nutrition (CIBER-OBN), Instituto de Salud Carlos III, E-28029 Madrid, Spain
6 LIPPSO, Department of Chemistry, University of Girona, 17003 Girona, Spain; marta.planas@udg.edu (M.P.); lidia.feliu@udg.edu (L.F.)
* Correspondence: santiago.ruiz@udg.edu (S.R.-M.); teresa.puig@udg.edu (T.P.);

† These authors contributed equally to this work.

Abstract: Epidermal growth factor receptor (EGFR) tyrosine kinases inhibitors (TKIs) are effective therapies for non-small cell lung cancer (NSCLC) patients whose tumors harbor an EGFR activating mutation. However, this treatment is not curative due to primary and secondary resistance such as T790M mutation in exon 20. Recently, activation of transducer and activator of transcription 3 (STAT3) in NSCLC appeared as an alternative resistance mechanism allowing cancer cells to elude the EGFR signaling. Overexpression of fatty acid synthase (FASN), a multifunctional enzyme essential for endogenous lipogenesis, has been related to resistance and the regulation of the EGFR/Jak2/STAT signaling pathways. Using EGFR mutated (EGFRm) NSCLC sensitive and EGFR TKIs' resistant models (Gefitinib Resistant, GR) we studied the role of the natural polyphenolic anti-FASN compound (−)-epigallocatechin-3-gallate (EGCG), and its derivative G28 to overcome EGFR TKIs' resistance. We show that G28's cytotoxicity is independent of TKIs' resistance mechanisms displaying synergistic effects in combination with gefitinib and osimertinib in the resistant T790M negative (T790M−) model and showing a reduction of activated EGFR and STAT3 in T790M positive (T790M+) models. Our results provide the bases for further investigation of G28 in combination with TKIs to overcome the EGFR TKI resistance in NSCLC.

Keywords: NSCLC; EGFR TKI; FASN inhibitors; resistance; STAT3; EGCG

---

1. Introduction

Lung cancer is the most incident and the leading cause of cancer death worldwide. Non-small cell lung cancer (NSCLC) subtype is the most common and it represents 80–85% of lung cancers diagnosed.

Early-stage NSCLC patients have long-term survival after surgery. However, approximately 75% of patients are diagnosed in advanced stages [1,2].

Gefitinib is a first generation epidermal growth factor receptor (EGFR) tyrosine kinase inhibitor (TKI). It was approved in 2003 by the Food and Drug Administration (FDA) for the treatment of patients whose tumors harbor an EGFR sensitizing/activating mutation (EGFRm) i.e., exon 19 deletion (ΔE746-A750) or the point mutation in exon 21 that leads to the amino acid substitution L858R [3–5]. Despite this therapy represents a breakthrough in the treatment of EGFRm NSCLC patients, in a median time of 9–16 months nearly all patients do not achieve a complete response. One of the most common resistance mechanisms described is the EGFR point mutation in exon 20 that leads to the replacement of threonine 790 by methionine (T790M), which normally derives to lethal disease progression [6]. Osimertinib is an irreversible third generation TKI effective in EGFRm T790M positive (T790M+) patients. However, the point mutation C797S in exon 20 has appeared as the main resistance mechanism to the latest FDA-approved TKI [6]. Other mechanisms for EGFR TKI resistance include Met amplification, phosphatidylinositol-4,5-bisphosphate 3-kinase catalytic subunit alpha (PI3KCA) mutations, appearance of stem-like properties as evidenced by increase in epithelial–mesenchymal transition (EMT) and histological transformation, epidermal growth factor receptor type 2 (ErbB2) gene amplification, increase of insulin-like growth factor 1 receptor (IGF-1R) signaling pathway through the loss of inhibitory insulin-like growth factor-binding protein (IGF-BP) and loss or reduction of phosphatase and tensin homolog (PTEN), activation of AXL tyrosine kinase receptor or B-Raf proto-oncogene, and serine/threonine kinase (BRAF) mutations [6–12].

Recently, the activation of a signal transducer and activator of transcription 3 (STAT3) has been described as an alternative resistance mechanism allowing cancer cells to escape the EGFR signaling or the TKI suppression [13]. STAT3 is involved in the transcription of many genes related to cell differentiation, proliferation, resistance to apoptosis, angiogenesis, metastasis, and immune response [14–16]. Besides being phosphorylated by EGFR [17], STAT3 can also be activated in response to different cytokines and growth factors such as interleukin 6 (IL-6), interferon-alpha (IFN-α) or epidermal growth factor (EGF), among others [18]. Approximately 60% of patients show STAT3 activation, which correlates with poorly differentiated tumors, the presence of metastasis, and the late clinical stage [19,20]. STAT3 phosphorylation has been related to disease progression in a small cohort of patients after EGFR TKI treatment [21]. Additionally, neither gefitinib nor osimertinib are able to inhibit STAT3 activation [22,23].

Energy metabolism deregulation has been described as a hallmark of cancer, allowing cell growth and proliferation [24]. Fatty acid synthase (FASN) is an essential enzyme for the de novo synthesis of long-chain fatty acids from acetyl-CoA, malonyl-CoA, and NADPH [25]. Unlike most normal cells, highly-proliferative cancer cells overexpress this lipogenic enzyme, being an interesting target in cancer therapy [26,27]. FASN is strongly associated to poor prognosis and resistance to treatment in different human tumors such as breast [28], bladder [29], pancreatic [30], or lung cancer [31]. Moreover, FASN overexpression has also been proposed as a multidrug resistance mechanism, protecting cells from drug-induced apoptosis through the overproduction of palmitic acid [32]. The natural compound (−)-epigallocatechin-3-gallate (EGCG) is a polyphenolic flavonoid from green tea that has been broadly studied for its cardiovascular, neuroprotective, anticancer, and antimicrobial properties [33,34]. EGCG has been reported to compete with NADPH to bind the β-ketoacyl reductase domain of FASN [35]. The ability of several FASN inhibitors to regulate the canonical EGFR/Jak2/STAT pathway has also been stated in the literature [36,37]. We and others have shown that FASN inhibition is mainly related to EGFR/HER2 signaling pathways, leading to cytotoxic effects in vitro and in vivo in a wide range of carcinomas, including breast and lung [38–42]. To date, many EGCG derivatives have been developed to improve efficacy and increase stability in physiological conditions. Among them, the naphthalene derivative G28 has shown interesting antiproliferative features against sensitive and resistant breast cancer cells [38,43,44].

The purpose of this work was to study the role of FASN inhibitors (EGCG and G28) to overcome TKI resistance in NSCLC. FASN inhibitors were tested alone and in combination with EGFR TKIs (gefitinib and osimertinib) in EGFRm NSCLC models resistant to EGFR TKIs (Gefitinib Resistant, GR). In addition, we also evaluated gene and protein expression changes of FASN, EGFR, and STAT3 resulting from treatments with FASN inhibitors and EGFR TKIs alone or in combination. We show that FASN inhibitor G28 cytotoxicity is independent of EGFR TKI resistance mechanisms. Interestingly, G28 compound exhibited a cytotoxic effect in combination with gefitinib showing changes in EGFR/STAT3 pathway in T790M positive (T790M+) GR models and strong synergism in combination with gefitinib or osimertinib in T790M negative (T790M−) GR model.

2. Results

2.1. EGFRm GR NSCLC Models Are Sensitive to FASN Inhibition

In order to study the role of FASN in the acquisition of EGFR TKI resistance in NSCLC, we used the sensitive PC9 cell line carrying the EGFR exon 19 deletion (ELREA) and three GR models, two T790M+ models (PC9-GR1 and PC9-GR4), and one T790M− model (PC9-GR3) [45].

2.1.1. EGFRm NSCLC Models Overexpress FASN

Firstly, we determined whether EGFRm NSCLC models express FASN enzyme. Hence, FASN protein (Figure 1a) and mRNA expression levels (Figure 1b) were analyzed by immunoblotting and quantitative real time PCR (qRT-PCR), respectively.

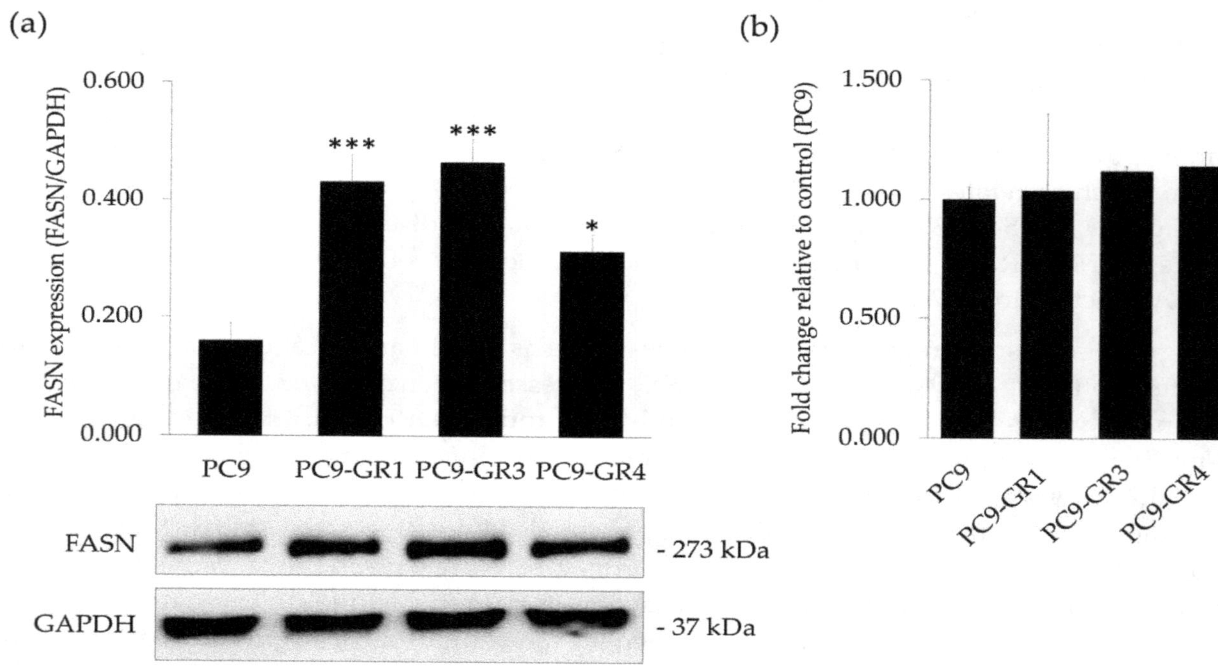

Figure 1. FASN protein and mRNA expression levels in sensitive (PC9) and Gefitinib Resistant (GR) models (PC9-GR1, PC9-GR3, and PC9-GR4). (**a**) Western blot analysis (quantification in upper panel and bands in lower panel) of FASN protein expression. GAPDH was used as a loading control. Results shown are representative from at least three independent experiments. (**b**) FASN endogenous mRNA levels were obtained by qRT-PCR and normalized against the GAPDH gene. FASN expression in the sensitive cells was normalized to 1 an expressed as a fold change, to which all other conditions were compared. Results shown are mean ± SE from three independent experiments. * $p < 0.050$, *** $p < 0.001$ indicate levels of statistically significance.

All models showed FASN protein and mRNA expression. Despite no differences in mRNA, GR models presented significantly higher protein expression levels (PC9-GR1 $p = 8.710 \times 10^{-4}$; PC9-GR3 $p = 3.160 \times 10^{-4}$, and PC9-GR4 $p = 0.049$) in comparison to PC9.

2.1.2. PC9-GR3 Model Is Resistant to Gefitinib and Osimertinib

We confirmed the resistance to EGFR TKIs in PC9 and GR models. For that, we measured the cytotoxic effect of gefitinib and osimertinib on all models by determining the half-maximal inhibitory concentration (IC_{50}) using the MTT assay (Figure 2).

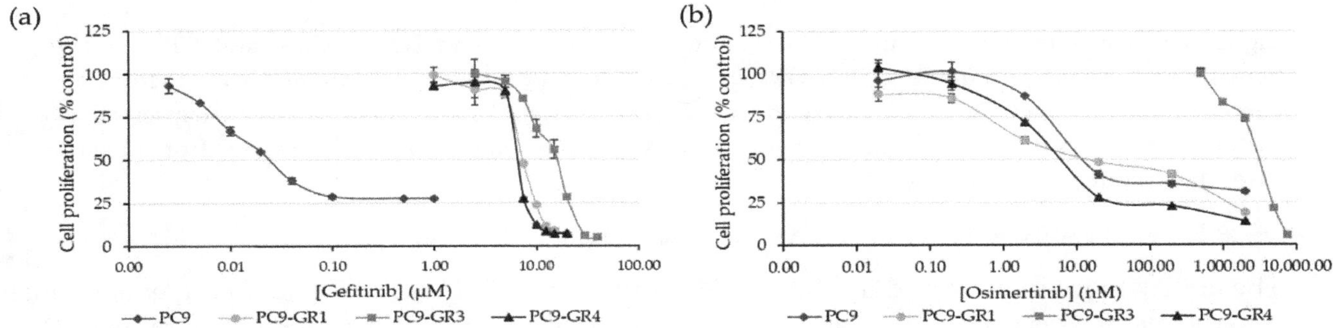

Figure 2. Cell proliferation inhibition of EGFR TKIs (gefitinib and osimertinib) in parental and Gefitinib Resistant (GR) models. Sensitive (PC9) and GR models (PC9-GR1, PC9-GR3, and PC9-GR4) were treated with increasing concentrations of (**a**) gefitinib (from 2.5×10^{-3} to 1 μM for PC9 and 1–40 μM for GR models) and (**b**) osimertinib (0.02–2000 nM for PC9, PC9-GR1, and PC9-GR4 and 500–7500 nM for PC9-GR3) for 72 h. Results shown are expressed as percentage of surviving cells after drug treatment (mean ± SE) and are representative from at least three independent experiments.

As expected, GR models were significantly more resistant to gefitinib with IC_{50} values in the micromolar range compared to the nanomolar IC_{50} found in the PC9 cell line (PC9-GR1 $p = 2.793 \times 10^{-7}$; PC9-GR3 $p = 1.631 \times 10^{-10}$, and PC9-GR4 $p = 1.000 \times 10^{-6}$). Although no significant differences were found in the IC_{50} value for gefitinib between the two T790M+ GR models, the IC_{50} value of the PC9-GR3 model for gefitinib was significantly greater than PC9-GR1 ($p = 7.953 \times 10^{-7}$) and PC9-GR4 ($p = 1.659 \times 10^{-7}$). PC9-GR3 model was also resistant to osimertinib compared to other models (PC9 $p = 2.799 \times 10^{-9}$; PC9-GR1 $p = 3.749 \times 10^{-8}$, and PC9-GR4 $p = 5.200 \times 10^{-9}$).

2.1.3. FASN Inhibitors Present Cytotoxic Effects in NSCLC Models

Cancer cells have been described to increase the de novo lipogenesis through the activation of FASN and its inhibition has proven to cause cell death. Therefore, this enzyme has become a promising candidate for the development of new anticancer therapies. Here we tested the cytotoxic activity of the two FASN inhibitors, EGCG and its derivative G28. MTT cell viability assays showed that the natural polyphenolic compound EGCG was cytotoxic for PC9 ($IC_{50} = 77.9 \pm 1.9$ μM), PC9-GR1 ($IC_{50} = 74.3 \pm 4.3$ μM), PC9-GR3 ($IC_{50} = 91.0 \pm 5.5$ μM), and PC9-GR4 ($IC_{50} = 75.6 \pm 2.4$ μM) NSCLC models with no significant differences ($p = 0.358$; Figure 3a).

The synthetic EGCG derivative G28 showed higher cytotoxicity in all tested models with IC_{50} of 12.8 ± 1.3 μM for PC9, 12.0 ± 0.8 μM for PC9-GR1, 17.8 ± 1.3 μM for PC9-GR3, and 11.2 ± 1.2 μM for PC9-GR4 (Figure 3b). Besides, only PC9-GR3 showed a significantly higher IC_{50} value compared to PC9 ($p = 0.030$), PC9-GR1 ($p = 0.005$), and PC9-GR4 ($p = 0.002$).

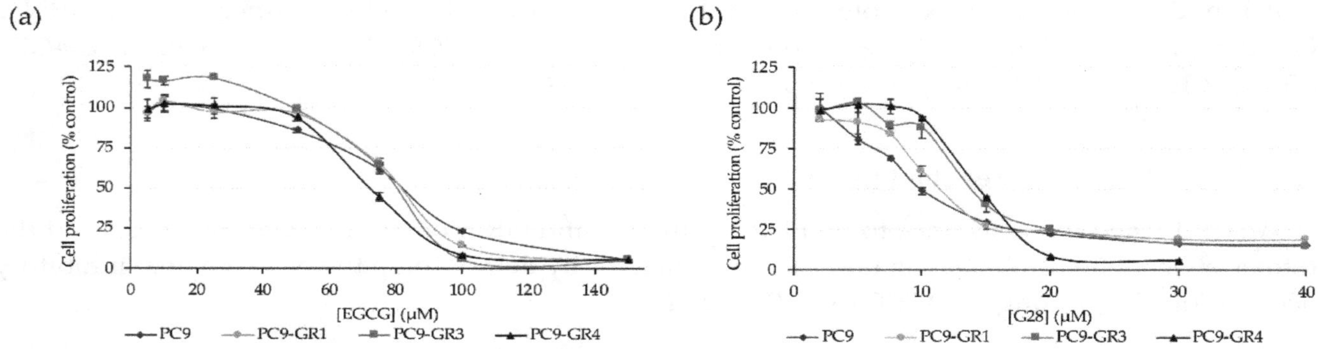

Figure 3. Cell proliferation inhibition of FASN inhibitors in parental and Gefitinib Resistant (GR) models. Sensitive (PC9) and GR models (PC9-GR1, PC9-GR3, and PC9-GR4) were treated with increasing concentrations of (**a**) EGCG (5–150 μM) and (**b**) G28 (2–40 μM) for 72 h. Results shown are expressed as the percentage of surviving cells after drug treatment (mean ± SE) and are representative from at least three independent experiments.

2.1.4. G28 Inhibits FASN in EGFRm NSCLC Models

The ability to internalize and inhibit FASN activity of EGCG and G28 after being exogenously added to the media was tested in sensitive and GR models (Figure 4). EGCG and G28 inhibited FASN in PC9 cells, resulting in a similar FASN activity reduction of roughly 80% ($p = 0.265$). Moreover, G28 significantly reduced FASN activity in all GR models in comparison with EGCG (PC9-GR1 $p = 3.000 \times 10^{-5}$; PC9-GR3 $p = 0.001$; PC9-GR4 $p = 0.008$) while the EGCG compound was not able to diminish FASN activity.

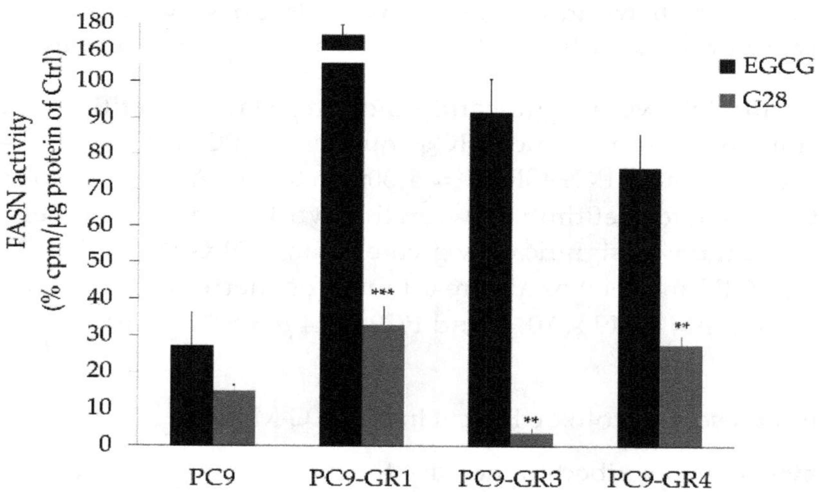

Figure 4. G28 compound inhibits FASN activity in Gefitinib Resistant (GR) models. Cells were treated for 72 h with EGCG or G28 at a concentration equal to their IC_{50} and with DMSO as control. FASN activity was assayed by counting radiolabeled fatty acids synthesized de novo. Bars represent the remaining activity as a percentage in treated versus untreated cells (control, Ctrl). Data are mean ± SE from at least three independent experiments. ** $p < 0.010$, *** $p < 0.001$ indicate levels of statistically significance.

2.1.5. Apoptosis Induction of FASN Inhibitors and EGFR TKIs Treatments

We also investigated whether the cell death caused by treatment with EGFR TKIs or FASN inhibitors was the result of apoptosis induction in both sensitive and GR models. Poly(ADP-ribose) polymerase (PARP) terminal proapoptotic protein activated after cleavage was used as an apoptosis marker. The effects of all compounds on PARP was determined by Western blot analysis in all models (Figure 5). The uncropped Western blots can be found in Figure S2a.

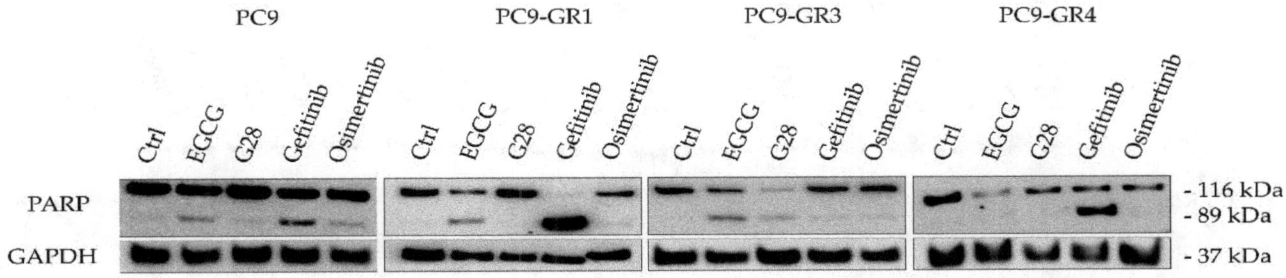

Figure 5. Effects of FASN inhibitors and EGFR TKIs on apoptosis determined by PARP cleavage. Sensitive (PC9) and Gefitinib Resistant (GR) models (PC9-GR1, PC9-GR3, and PC9-GR4) were treated for 72 h with a concentration equivalent to IC_{50} of each drug. Untreated cells were used as an internal control (Ctrl) and GAPDH as a loading control. Results shown are representative from at least three independent experiments.

The cleaved form of PARP (89 kDa) appeared in either sensitive or resistant T790M− models after treatment with the IC_{50} concentration of both EGFR TKIs (gefitinib and osimertinib) and FASN inhibitors (EGCG and G28), indicating the induction of apoptosis. Gefitinib treatment led to PARP cleavage in T790M+ GR models. Additionally, EGCG and osimertinib led to the formation of cleaved PARP in PC9-GR1 model.

2.2. *G28 Increases EGFR Activation in EGFRm NSCLC Models*

FASN has been previously related to AKT/ERK/EGFR signaling pathways [46] and the inhibition of the transcription factor STAT3 [36] in lung adenocarcinomas. Thus, differences in FASN, EGFR, and STAT3 protein and mRNA expression levels after FASN inhibitors or EGFR TKIs treatment were analyzed through immunoblotting (Figure 6a) and qRT-PCR (Figure 6b) in PC9 and GR models. The uncropped Western blots can be found in Figure S2b.

A reduction of FASN mRNA expression levels was observed in sensitive and GR models treated with FASN inhibitors, being statistically significant in the PC9-GR4 treated with G28 ($p = 0.004$) and PC9 cells treated with G28 ($p = 7.370 \times 10^{-4}$) and gefitinib ($p = 3.210 \times 10^{-4}$). T790M+ GR models presented a basal hyperactivation of EGFR that was inhibited after treatment with EGFR TKIs. Regarding FASN inhibitors, EGCG and G28 increased its activation in PC9 cells contrary to the PC9-GR1 model, while no changes were observed in PC9-GR3 and PC9-GR4 models.

EGCG reduced EGFR protein levels in sensitive and T790M+ GR models that did not correlate with mRNA expression levels. Contrary, G28 significantly increased EGFR mRNA expression in all models, without protein level modification. No changes in EGFR mRNA levels were observed after gefitinib treatment, however higher protein levels were detected in T790M− GR models. Osimertinib treatment did not lead to EGFR protein nor mRNA expression alteration. EGFR TKIs treatment increased STAT3 activation in all GR models. Gefitinib increased p-STAT3 levels in sensitive cells, while the highest STAT3 activation in GR models was found with osimertinib treatment. No STAT3 protein or mRNA expression differences were found in any of the models and treatments assayed.

Lung carcinomas are highly proliferative and resistance acquisition after EGFR TKI-based therapy is a major problem. Overproduction of palmitic acid by FASN emerges as a resistance mechanism, protecting cells from drug-induced apoptosis [47]. The combination of these drugs with a different mechanism of action may decrease resistance development and improve treatment response.

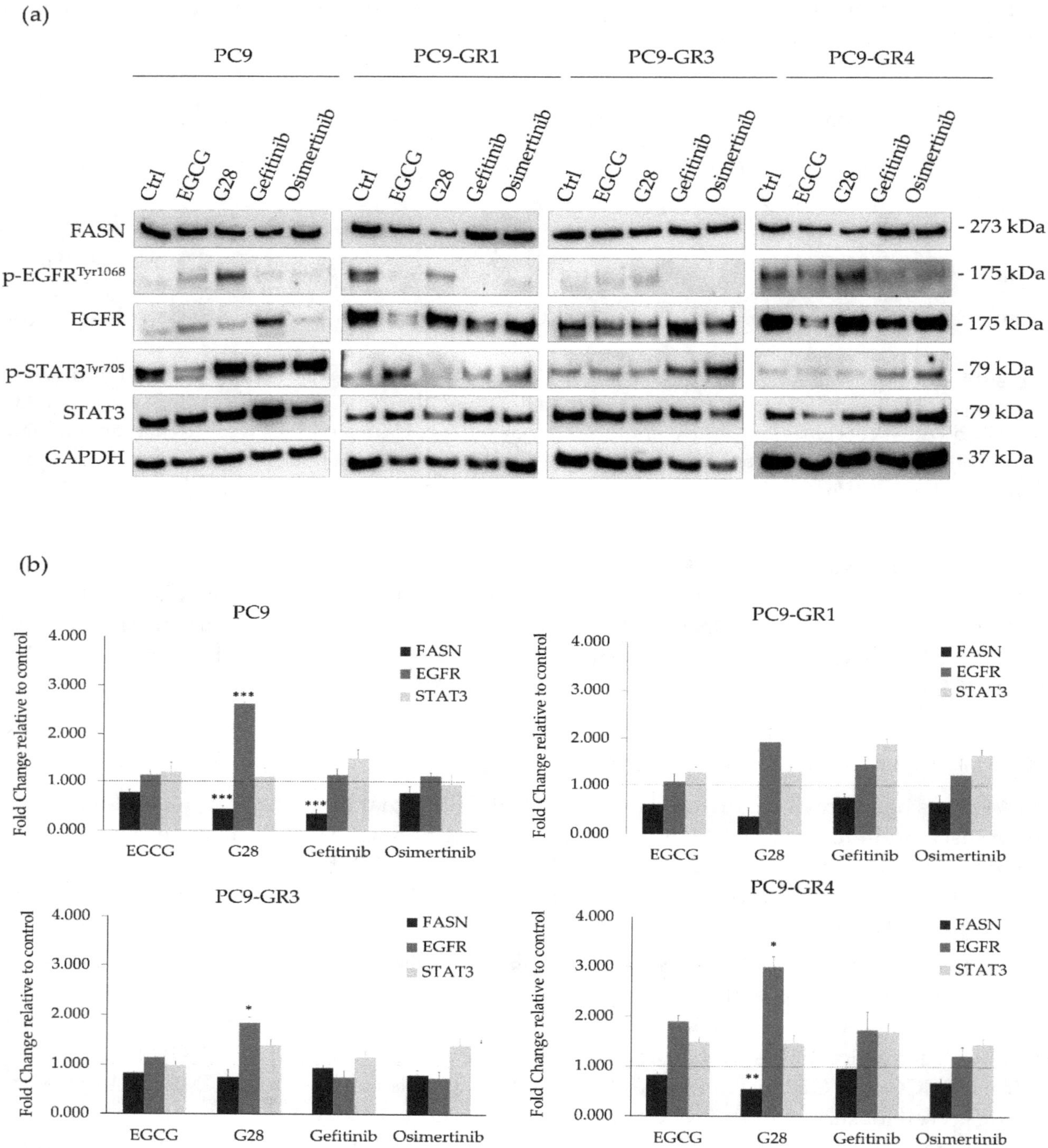

Figure 6. FASN, EGFR, and STAT3 protein and mRNA expression levels after FASN inhibitors (EGCG and G28) and EGFR TKIs (gefitinib and osimertinib) treatment in sensitive (PC9) and Gefitinib Resistant (GR) models (PC9-GR1, PC9-GR3, and PC9-GR4). (**a**) Western blot analysis of FASN, EGFR, and STAT3 protein expression after 72 h of FASN inhibitors (IC_{50}) and EGFR TKIs (IC_{50}) treatment in EGFR TKI sensitive and GR models. Untreated cells were used as an internal control (Ctrl) and GAPDH as a loading control. Results shown are representative from at least three independent experiments. (**b**) FASN, EGFR, and STAT3 mRNA levels after treatment with FASN inhibitors and EGFR TKIs in sensitive and GR models. mRNA levels were obtained by qRT-PCR and normalized against the GAPDH gene. All conditions were compared to control (untreated cells), which was normalized to 1 (indicated by the dotted line) and expressed as a fold change. Experiments were performed at least three times. * $p < 0.050$, ** $p < 0.010$, *** $p < 0.001$, indicate levels of statistically significance.2.3. G28 Combined with EGFR TKIs Outcomes in Synergistic Effects.

Once the effects of FASN inhibitors and EGFR TKIs alone were analyzed in all models, the combinatorial treatment between FASN inhibitors and EGFR TKIs was also studied in order to evaluate the possible synergistic interactions (Figure 7 and Figure S1). Despite the fact that EGCG did not reduce FASN activity in GR models, no IC_{50} differences were found in comparison with sensitive cells. Therefore, GR models were treated with EGCG or G28 in combination with the EGFR TKI to which they were resistant. Three EGFR TKIs concentrations were chosen based on MTT assays (vide supra). The combination of EGCG with either gefitinib or osimertinib resulted in mostly additive effect as shown by the combination index (CI; Figure 7a).

The combination of G28 with gefitinib generally led to additivism in T790M+ GR models, with some synergism found in G28 concentrations ranging from 10 to 20 μM. Remarkably, T790M− GR model treated with G28 combined with gefitinib or osimertinib showed greater synergistic effects (Figure 7b).

2.3. *G28 Reduces STAT3 Activation in T790M+ GR Models Alone or in Combination with Gefitinib*

In order to discern whether G28 is able to reduce the STAT3 activation produced by EGFR TKIs, a combinatorial analysis was performed (Figure 8). As before, FASN, EGFR, and STAT3 protein and mRNA levels were analyzed using Western blot (Figure 8a) and qRT-PCR (Figure 8b) in GR models treated with synergistic drug concentrations (all of them under the IC_{50} value). The uncropped Western blots can be found in Figure S2c. Therefore, GR models were treated with G28 at 15 μM in combination with 1 μM gefitinib, which is the highest clinically achievable plasma concentration [5]. Osimertinib-resistant PC9-GR3 model was co-treated with 15 μM G28 and 0.5 μM osimertinib. All concentrations were also used in single-treatment to elucidate the effects produced by the combination.

T790M+ GR models treated with G28 alone and in combination with gefitinib showed both FASN protein and mRNA expression decrease. In the PC9-GR3 model, the FASN protein was slightly diminished in mono- and co-treatments. This decrease is in accordance to FASN mRNA expression, which was significantly reduced in combination with osimertinib. Although G28 alone showed more activated EGFR compared to control in all GR models, the combination of G28 with both EGFR TKIs decreased p-EGFR levels. Regarding the total EGFR, co-treatment resulted in higher protein levels compared to monotreatment in all GR models.

However, only T790M+ GR models treated with G28 in combination with gefitinib presented significantly higher EGFR mRNA expression (PC9-GR1 $p = 0.036$ and PC9-GR4 $p = 0.040$). Moreover, G28 both alone and in combination with gefitinib reduced STAT3 activation in T790M+ GR models. No changes in STAT3 activation were seen in PC9-GR3 in any treatment. None of the models analyzed showed alterations in the STAT3 protein or mRNA expression levels.

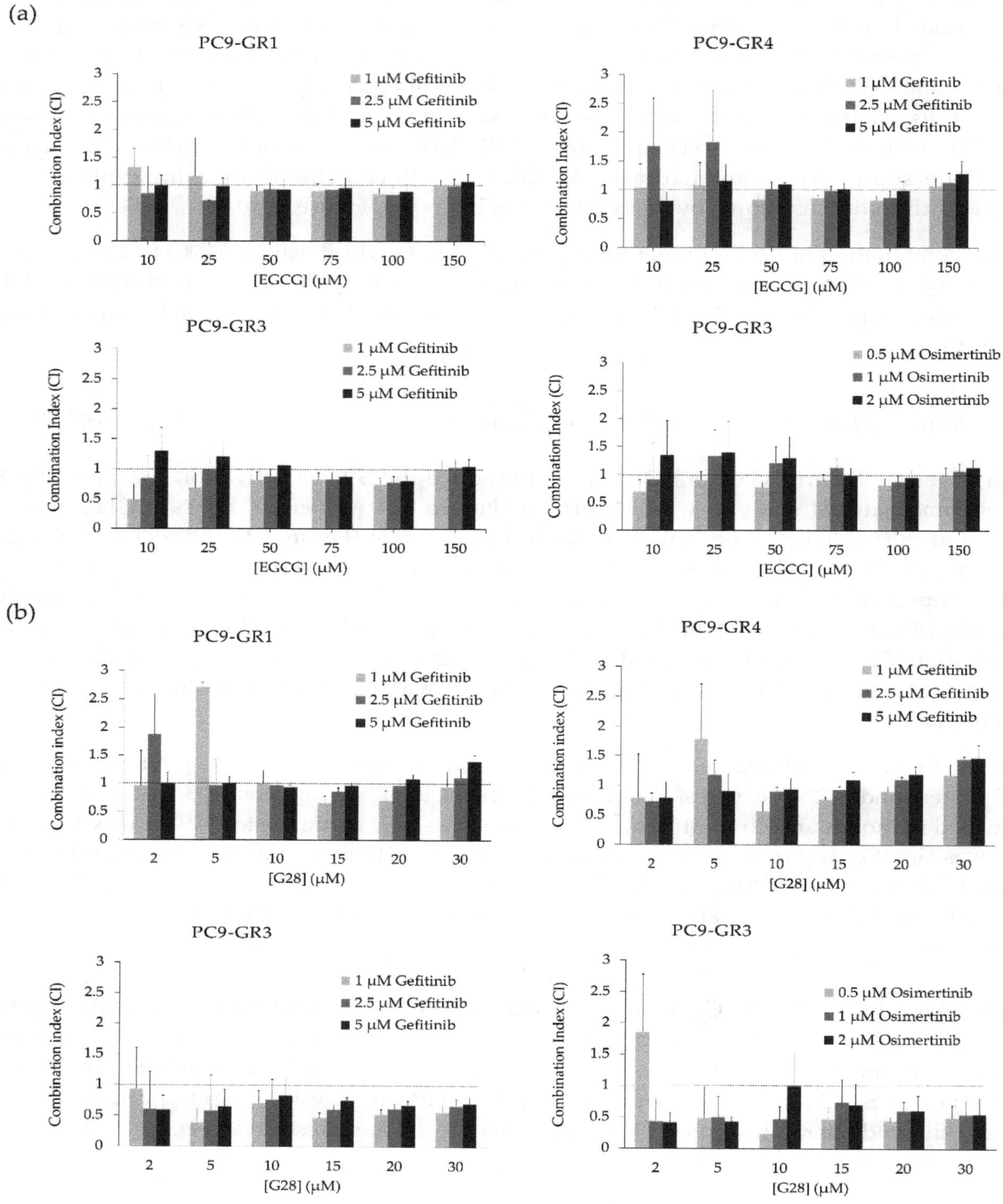

Figure 7. Combination index (CI) of FASN inhibitors (EGCG and G28) and EGFR TKIs (gefitinib and osimertinib) treatment in Gefitinib Resistant (GR) models (PC9-GR1, PC9-GR3, and PC9-GR4). (**a**) CI of EGCG and gefitinib in PC9-GR1, PC9-GR3, and PC9-GR4 models or osimertinib in PC9-GR3. (**b**) CI of G28 and gefitinib in PC9-GR1, PC9-GR3, and PC9-GR4 models or osimertinib in PC9-GR3. PC9-GR1, PC9-GR3, and PC9-GR4 models were treated with EGCG (10–150 μM) or G28 (2-30 μM) in combination with gefitinib (1, 2.5, and 5 μM) for 72 h. PC9-GR3 cells were also treated with EGCG (10–150 μM) or G28 (2–30 μM) in combination with osimertinib (0.5, 1, and 2 μM) for 72 h. Results were determined using the MTT assay and are expressed as the CI based on the Chou and Talalay method [48]. The dotted line indicates additivism (CI approximately equal to 1). CI > 1 designates antagonistic effects and CI < 1 synergistic effects. Experiments were performed at least three times. Results shown are mean ± SE.

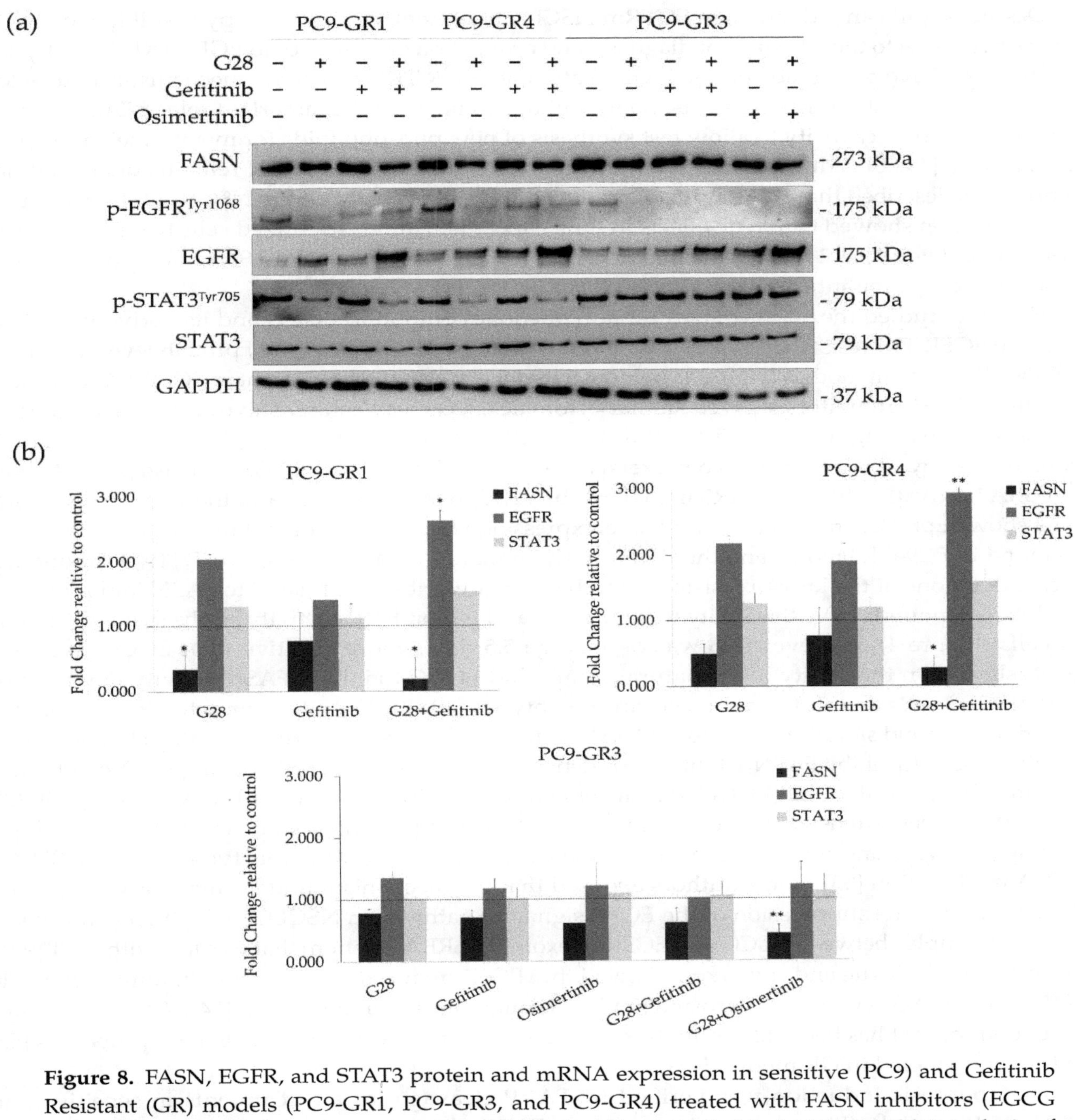

Figure 8. FASN, EGFR, and STAT3 protein and mRNA expression in sensitive (PC9) and Gefitinib Resistant (GR) models (PC9-GR1, PC9-GR3, and PC9-GR4) treated with FASN inhibitors (EGCG and G28) in combination with EGFR TKIs (gefitinib and osimertinib). (**a**) Western blot analysis of FASN, EGFR, and STAT3 in PC9-GR1, PC9-GR3, and PC9-GR4 models treated with G28 alone and in combination with gefitinib, and PC9-GR3 treated with G28 and osimertinib for 72 h. Results shown are representative from three independent experiments. Untreated cells are used as internal control (Ctrl) and GAPDH as a loading control. (**b**) FASN, EGFR, and STAT3 mRNA levels analysis in PC9-GR1, PC9-GR3, and PC9-GR4 models treated with G28 in combination with gefitinib, PC9-GR3 model treated with the combination G28 and osimertinib for 72 h. mRNA levels were obtained by qRT-PCR and normalized against the GAPDH gene. All conditions were compared to the control (untreated cells), which was normalized to 1 (indicated by the dotted line) and expressed as a fold change. Experiments were performed at least three times. * $p < 0.050$, ** $p < 0.010$, *** $p < 0.001$ indicate levels of statistical significance.

3. Discussion

Despite significant advances in EGFRm NSCLC treatment, current therapy is still ineffective to many patients due to the late stage of diagnosis and acquisition of resistance to EGFR TKIs [2,6]. Hence, several efforts have been made on the identification of EGFR TKIs resistance mechanisms to develop an effective treatment for these patients. Some authors pointed out the important role of FASN in drug resistance due to its capacity to allow fast synthesis of new phospholipids for membrane remodeling and plasticity [49,50]. Although the relationship between EGFR and FASN remains unclear, it has recently been described that EGFR upregulates FASN in TKI-resistant EGFRm NSCLC [41]. In addition, FASN inhibition showed cytotoxic effects in lung cancer [40] and resensitized cells to chemotherapy, anti-EGFR and anti-HER2 therapies in breast cancer [38,51]. Therefore, the FASN enzyme may become a promising target for anticancer therapy in EGFRm NSCLC.

Here we studied the effects of natural polyphenolic compound EGCG and its derivative G28 to overcome EGFR TKI resistance in sensitive and GR models. The higher FASN protein levels observed in EGFR TKI resistant models (Figure 1) demonstrated its potential involvement in EGFR TKI resistance acquisition. FASN inhibitors showed similar cytotoxic effects between sensitive and resistant models with IC_{50} values ranging from 75 to 90 μM for EGCG and from 12 to 18 μM for G28 (Figure 3). As determined by K. Jacobsen and coworkers, PC9-GR1 is a T790M+ GR model that also presents MET and EphA2 activation, the PC9-GR3 model exhibits AXL overexpression, and the T790M+ PC9-GR4 model shows EphA2 activation and AXL overexpression [45]. In correlation with this, the higher G28 IC_{50} found in PC9-GR3 model and the significantly similar IC_{50} values in the two T790M+ GR models indicate that none of the known resistance mechanisms described are related to FASN inhibition.

Both compounds have the ability to internalize and inhibit FASN activity as observed in parental PC9 cells (Figure 4), however G28 was of average 5.5 times more effective than EGCG. We have previously shown the ability of the natural compound EGCG to inhibit FASN activity in wild type EGFR NSCLC cells and different breast cancer subtypes [40,43]. Despite their cytotoxicity, only the synthetic compound significantly reduced FASN activity in GR models (Figure 4). Other studies proved the ability of G28 to inhibit FASN activity in triple-negative breast cancer (TNBC) cells [43]. Nevertheless, our study demonstrated that EGCG anticancer activity was independent of FASN inhibition in GR models. It has been extensively described that EGCG has multiple targets and it is involved in multiple signaling pathways and transcription factors, membrane-associated receptors tyrosine kinase (RTKs), or DNA methylation [33]. Some authors exposed that the mechanism underlying EGCG antitumor potency is due to the suppression of the EGFR signaling pathway in NSCLC [52]. Others observed a very stable complex between EGCG and EGFRm (exon 19 ELREA deletion) that was lost with the T790M substitution [53]. Kozue and coworkers showed that EGCG reduced stemness and immunogenicity in EGFR wild type NSCLC cells in vitro and in vivo through the inhibition of AXL [54]. AXL is a tyrosine kinase receptor that has been related to drug resistance and the induction of malignant properties [55] and is overexpressed in GR models [45].

The apoptosis induction was verified by PARP cleavage for all treatments in sensitive and T790M− GR models (Figure 5). However, no PARP cleavage was observed through Western blot analysis in T790M+ GR models after G28 treatment. These results suggest that G28 might cause an apoptosis-independent proliferation reduction in T790M+ GR models as found by others in NSCLC wild-type EGFR models treated with the natural plant polyphenol resveratrol (3,5,40-trihydroxystilben) [56]. The anticancer activity of polyphenols has been shown to be mediated by numerous mechanisms including cell cycle arrest. EGCG, among other natural compounds, showed down-regulation of cyclin-dependent kinases (CDK) and modulation in CDK inhibitors in different human carcinomas [33,57]. The lack of PARP cleavage in some of the treatments and models could be due to the activation of other programmed cell death mechanisms such as autophagy [58].

Alteration in EGFR expression was observed after treatment with FASN inhibitors. EGCG produced a decrease in EGFR protein levels in T790M+ GR models, which is in agreement with

Ali et al., who observed an EGFR decrease in sensitive and resistant PC9 cells treated with Orlistat, a FDA-approved FASN inhibitor for obesity management [41]. The synthetic G28 compound increased EGFR mRNA levels in all models, indicating that EGFR overexpression could be an alternative pathway to FASN inhibition. The EGFR activation after FASN gene overexpression in epithelial breast cells has been previously shown [42]. Furthermore, our results suggest that the EGFR pathway could be implicated in FASN regulation at a transcriptional or translational level as exposed before [40]. Despite all models increased EGFR mRNA expression after G28 treatment, only PC9 cells seemed to compensate the effect of G28 by increasing EGFR activation. Therefore, cell proliferation reduction found in all models after FASN inhibition (Figure 3) could be due to the lack of post-translational palmitoylation substrate [41].

It seems increasingly clear that persistent STAT3 activation is related to EGFR-based therapies resistance [13]. STAT3 is under the control of different cytokines and growth factors playing an important role in metastasis, proliferation, survival, invasion, migration, and angiogenesis [14–16]. Natural polyphenols, normally multitarget inhibitors, are now emerging as promising STAT3 inhibitors or its upstream signaling molecules Src, gp130, or NFκB [18]. Among them, EGCG has been reported to reduce STAT3 phosphorylation in head and neck carcinomas [59] and pancreatic cancer [60]. Based on the above, we hypothesized that EGCG and its derivative G28 would diminish the STAT3 activation produced by EGFR TKIs in NSCLC cells. Both compounds reduced p-STAT3 levels in a dose-dependent manner when used alone in comparison to control samples. In agreement with previous studies, STAT3 was activated by EGFR TKIs (Figure 6) [22].

Combinatorial treatments of EGCG and G28 with EGFR TKIs were performed in order to study their effects on GR models (Figure S1). The combination of gefitinib and osimertinib with EGCG showed additivism whereas synergistic effects were identified in combination with G28 (Figure 7). Other authors have previously reported synergistic outcomes after co-treatment with a STAT3 inhibitor (TPCA-1) and EGFR TKI in EGFRm NSCLC models [61]. Previous results from our group demonstrated that G28 compound had a synergistic interaction with pertuzumab and temsirolimus in HER2+ breast cancer cells [38] and EGCG with cetuximab in TNBC [51]. Interestingly, G28 in combination with gefitinib decreased the activation of STAT3 to the same extent as when used alone in T790M+ GR models. Thus, other mechanisms must be involved in the synergistic effects found. On the other hand, no differences in p-STAT3 were observed in PC9-GR3. This could be, in part, due to the multiple pathways that can be altered in the acquisition of gefitinib and osimertinib double-resistance in PC9-GR3 model such as mutations in EGFR/STAT3 or other related up- or downstream signaling molecules, leading to the constitutive activation of STAT3. The analysis of the main genes regulated by the STAT3 transcription factor could provide relevant information to identify some pathways alterations after FASN inhibitors treatment. The synergistic effects found in GR models co-treated with FASN inhibitor G28 and EGFR TKIs supports the idea that EGFR palmitoylation mediated by FASN leads to TKI resistance acquisition in EGFRm NSCLC [41].

However, the specific G28 mechanism of action and possible targets are still unknown and further studies are needed. Wu et al. suggested that FASN inhibition may cause an imbalance in the membrane lipids levels, which may produce a membrane localization decrease of IGF-1R, and the inactivation of the downstream STAT3 signaling pathway [36]. Furthermore, the IGF-1R is a transmembrane tyrosine kinase linked to MAPK and PI3K/AKT pathways, shared with EGFR, which could explain the effects found only in T790M+ GR models [62].

Taken together, our observations suggest that FASN has a key role in acquired TKI-resistant EGFRm NSCLC. The inhibition of this enzyme resensitizes cells to EGFR TKIs treatments. These results encourage for further studies to analyze the combinatorial treatment of FASN inhibitors and EGFR TKIs to overcome the EGFR TKI resistance in NSCLC.

4. Materials and Methods

4.1. Cell Lines and Culture Conditions

Human adenocarcinoma PC9 cells and its gefitinib resistant derivatives PC9-GR1, PC9-GR3, and PC9-GR4 models [45] were kindly provided by Dr. R. Rosell and Dr. M. A. Molina (Barcelona, Spain). All cells were routinely grown in RPMI-1640 medium (Lonza, Basel, Switzerland), supplemented with 10% fetal bovine serum (FBS; HyClone Laboratories, GE Healthcare, Chicago, IL, USA), 50 U/mL penicillin, and 50 µg/mL streptomycin (Lonza). In all cases, the cells were used immediately after resuscitation and were maintained at 37 °C in a humidified atmosphere with 5% CO_2, propagated following established protocols, remaining free of mycoplasma throughout the experiments.

4.2. Cell Proliferation Assays

To investigate the effect of EGFR TKIs or FASN inhibitors cells were seeded into 96-well plates at the appropriate density in their growth medium. Gefitinib and osimertinib were kindly provided by AstraZeneca. EGCG was purchased from Sigma (USA) and G28 was synthesized as described elsewhere [43]. For monotreatment assays, after 24 h cells were treated with different concentrations of each drug for 72 h. Cell viability was determined by the 3-(4,5-dimethyl-2-thiazolyl)-2,5-diphenyl-tetrazolium bromide (MTT) assay (Sigma) as described elsewhere [44]. For drug combination experiments, cells were treated with three fixed concentrations of gefitinib (1, 2.5, and 5 µM) or osimertinib (0.5, 1, and 2 µM) in combination of a series of increasing concentrations of EGCG or G28 for 72 h. Following treatment, cell proliferation was measured using the standard colorimetric MTT assay. Using the multi-well plate reader Benchmark Plus (Bio-Rad Laboratories, Inc., CA, USA), absorbance was determined at 570 nm. Combinatorial effects were evaluated using the combination index (CI) based on the Chou and Talalay method [48] using the CompuSyn™ software (Biosoft, MO, USA). CompuSyn™ calculates the CI values; if the value equals 1 the effect is considered additive, if above 1 antagonistic and below 1 synergistic. Data presented are from three separate wells per assay, and the assay was performed at least three times.

4.3. Western Blot Analysis of Cell Lysates

Gefitinib-sensitive and -resistant models were treated with EGFR TKI, FASN inhibitor, or the combination of both drugs for 72 h. Afterwards, attached and floating cells were harvested and lysed in ice-cold lysis buffer (Cell Signaling Technology Inc., MA, USA) containing 100 µg/mL phenylmethylsulfonylfluoride (PMSF; Sigma) by vortexing every 5 min for 30 min. Protein concentration was determined by the Lowry method (DC Protein Assay, Bio-Rad Laboratories, Inc.). Equal amounts of protein were heated in lithium dodecyl sulfate (LDS) sample buffer with a sample reducing agent (Invitrogen, CA, USA) for 10 min at 70 °C, separated by SDS-PAGE and transferred to nitrocellulose membranes (ThermoFisher Scientific Inc., MA, USA). Membranes were incubated for 1 h at room temperature in blocking buffer (5% skim milk powder in Tris-buffered saline (TBS)) 0.05% Tween (TBS-T) and overnight at 4 °C with the following primary antibodies diluted in blocking buffer: FASN (Cell Signaling Technology Inc.; #3180), p-STAT3^{Tyr705} (Cell Signaling Technology Inc.; #9131), p-EGFR^{Tyr1068} (Cell Signaling Technology Inc.; #2234), PARP (Cell Signaling Technology Inc.; #9542), EGFR (Cell Signaling Technology Inc.; #2232), STAT3 (Cell Signaling Technology Inc.; #4904), and GAPDH (Proteintech, Manchester, UK; #60004-1-IG). Specific horseradish peroxidase (HRP)-conjugated secondary antibodies were incubated for 1 h at room temperature. The immune complexes were detected using chemiluminescent HRP substrate Clarity™ Western ECL Substrate (Bio-Rad Laboratories, Inc.) or West Femto Maximum Sensitivity Substrate (ThermoFisher Scientific Inc.) in a Bio-Rad ChemiDoc™ MP Imaging System (Bio-Rad Laboratories, Inc.). Western blot analyses were repeated at least three times and representative results are shown.

4.4. *Quantitative Real-Time PCR (qRT-PCR) Analysis*

Cells were treated with EGFR TKIs or FASN inhibitors as a single agent or in combination for 72 h. Then, cells were PBS washed and resuspended in 1 mL of Qiazol (Qiagen, Hilden, Germany). GeneJET RNA Purification Kit (ThermoFisher Scientific Inc.) was used to isolate total RNA following the manufacturer's instructions. RNA samples were quantified using a Nano-Drop 2000 Spectophotometer (ThermoFisher Scientific). Total RNA was reverse-transcribed into complementary DNA (cDNA) using a High Capacity cDNA Archive Kit (Applied Biosystems, CA, USA). Different gene expression levels were determined using QuantStudio3 Real-time PCR System (ThermoFisher Scientific Inc.) with qPCRBIO SyGreen Mix Lo-Rox real-time PCR (PCR Biosystems Inc., PA, USA), following manufacture instructions. Primers used are shown in Table 1. qRT-PCR analyses were performed at least four times and each gene was run in triplicate. Gene expression levels were quantified using the standard formula $2^{\hat{}dCT}$ and normalized to the housekeeping GAPDH ($2^{\hat{}dCT}$).

Table 1. Primer design.

FASN	Forward	CAGGCACACACGATGGAC
	Reverse	CGGAGTGAATCTGGGTTGAT
STAT3	Forward	CACCTTCAGGATGTCCGGAA
	Reverse	ATCCTGGAGATTCTCTACCACTTTCA
EGFR7	Forward	CATGTCGATGGACTTCCAGA
	Reverse	GGGACAGCTTGGATCACACT
GAPDH	Forward	TCTTCCAGGAGCGAGATC
	Reverse	CAGAGATGATGACCCTTTTG

4.5. *Inhibition of Fatty Acid Synthase Activity*

Cells were seeded in 24-well plates at a density of 3×10^4 cells/well in RPMI supplemented with 10% fetal bovine serum (FBS). 24 h later, the maintenance medium was replaced by the treatment medium (RPMI-1640 supplemented with 1% lipoprotein-deficient FBS (Sigma-Aldrich)) along with the assayed compounds or vehicle (dimethyl sulfoxide, DMSO, Sigma-Aldrich). Cells were treated with a concentration corresponding to the previously determined IC_{50} for 72 h. For the last 6 h (1,2-14C) acetic acid sodium salt (53.9 mCi/mmol, Perkin Elmer Biosciences, Waltham, MA, USA) was added to the medium (0.5 μCi/mL). The lipid extraction was performed as previously described [43]. Cells were washed twice with phosphate-buffered saline (PBS, HyClone Laboratories, Logan, UT, USA) and once with MeOH/PBS (2:3). Cell pellets were resuspended in 0.2 M NaCl and lysed with freeze (liquid N_2)—thaw (37 °C) cycles. Then, lipids were extracted with $CHCl_3$/MeOH (2:1) and 0.1 M KOH. The organic phase was washed with $CHCl_3$/MeOH/H_2O (3:48:47) and the solvents were evaporated under vacuum conditions. Finally, pellets were resuspended in EtOH and counted by scintillation. The total protein content was quantified by the Bradford assay (Sigma-Aldrich).

4.6. *Statistical Analysis*

Parametric data were analyzed by the Student's t test when comparing two groups or the one-way analysis of variance (ANOVA) followed by Bonferroni or Tamhane's T2 post hoc test for multiple comparisons. The non-parametric data were analyzed with the Mann–Whitney U tests for non-normally independent variables; otherwise, the Kruskal–Wallis test was used for more than two groups. All data are expressed as mean ± SE. Levels of significance were set at $p < 0.050$ and are represented by asterisks, as follows: $p < 0.050$ (denoted as *), $p < 0.010$ (denoted as **), and $p < 0.001$ (denoted as ***). The statistical analysis was performed using the IBM SPSS software (Version 21.0; SPSS Inc., IL, USA).

5. Conclusions

The need to find more effective and less toxic therapeutic treatments for EGFRm NSCLC patients is one of the major challenges in lung cancer research. Natural compounds are emerging as potential anticancer candidates for their safety and multitarget intrinsic features. Improvement of the properties of natural compounds through the design of synthetic derivatives is aimed at maintaining these features while increasing, efficacy, bioavailability, and stability in physiological conditions.

Here we show additive and synergistic effects of the polyphenolic plant-derived EGCG compound and its derivative G28, respectively, in combination with EGFR TKIs in GR models. Despite the exact mechanism by which these compounds are cytotoxic is still unknown, our results shed light on their ability to modulate FASN/EGFR/STAT3 pathways. The capacity to affect multiple pathways might prove useful in overcoming other drug resistances. Further analyses are required to completely understand the mechanism of action.

Taken together, this paper supports the inhibition of the metabolic enzyme FASN by G28 compound in combination with EGFR TKIs as a new potential strategy for resistant EGFRm NSCLC.

Author Contributions: Conceptualization, T.P. and S.R.-M.; methodology, E.P.-A., S.P., S.R.-M., J.R., D.T.-O., M.P., L.F.; validation, E.P.-A., S.P., S.R.-M.; resources, T.P., and J.C.; writing—original draft preparation, E.P.-A., S.P., S.R.-M.; writing—review and editing, E.P.-A., S.P., S.R.-M., T.P. and J.C.; supervision, T.P. and S.R.-M.; funding acquisition, T.P. and J.C. All authors have read and agreed to the published version of the manuscript.

Acknowledgments: Authors thank R. Rosell and M. A. Molina from laboratory of Oncology Pangaea (Barcelona, Spain) for kindly provided PC9 models and AstraZeneca (London, UK) for supplying gefitinib and osimertinib.

References

1. Testa, U.; Castelli, G.; Pelosi, E. Lung Cancers: Molecular Characterization, Clonal Heterogeneity and Evolution, and Cancer Stem Cells. *Cancers* **2018**, *10*. [CrossRef] [PubMed]
2. Sun, W.; Song, L.; Ai, T.; Zhang, Y.; Gao, Y.; Cui, J. Prognostic value of MET, cyclin D1 and MET gene copy number in non-small cell lung cancer. *J. Biomed. Res.* **2013**, *27*, 220. [CrossRef] [PubMed]
3. Choo, J.R.E.; Tan, C.S.; Soo, R.A. Treatment of EGFR T790M−Positive Non-Small Cell Lung Cancer. *Target. Oncol.* **2018**, *13*, 141–156. [CrossRef] [PubMed]
4. Lynch, T.J.; Bell, D.W.; Sordella, R.; Gurubhagavatula, S.; Okimoto, R.A.; Brannigan, B.W.; Harris, P.L.; Haserlat, S.M.; Supko, J.G.; Haluska, F.G.; et al. Activating Mutations in the Epidermal Growth Factor Receptor Underlying Responsiveness of Non–Small-Cell Lung Cancer to Gefitinib. *N. Engl. J. Med.* **2004**, *350*, 2129–2139. [CrossRef] [PubMed]
5. Cohen, M.H.; Williams, G.A.; Sridhara, R.; Chen, G.; McGuinn, W.D.; Morse, D.; Abraham, S.; Rahman, A.; Liang, C.; Lostritto, R.; et al. United States Food and Drug Administration Drug Approval summary: Gefitinib (ZD1839; Iressa) tablets. *Clin. Cancer Res.* **2004**, *10*, 1212–1218. [CrossRef]
6. Barnes, T.A.; O'Kane, G.M.; Vincent, M.D.; Leighl, N.B. Third-Generation Tyrosine Kinase Inhibitors Targeting Epidermal Growth Factor Receptor Mutations in Non-Small Cell Lung Cancer. *Front. Oncol.* **2017**, *7*, 113. [CrossRef]
7. Bean, J.; Brennan, C.; Shih, J.-Y.; Riely, G.; Viale, A.; Wang, L.; Chitale, D.; Motoi, N.; Szoke, J.; Broderick, S.; et al. MET amplification occurs with or without T790M mutations in EGFR mutant lung tumors with acquired resistance to gefitinib or erlotinib. *Proc. Natl. Acad. Sci. USA* **2007**, *104*, 20932–20937. [CrossRef]
8. Marks, J.L.; Gong, Y.; Chitale, D.; Golas, B.; McLellan, M.D.; Kasai, Y.; Ding, L.; Mardis, E.R.; Wilson, R.K.; Solit, D.; et al. Novel MEK1 mutation identified by mutational analysis of epidermal growth factor receptor signaling pathway genes in lung adenocarcinoma. *Cancer Res.* **2008**, *68*, 5524–5528. [CrossRef]
9. Shien, K.; Toyooka, S.; Yamamoto, H.; Soh, J.; Jida, M.; Thu, K.L.; Hashida, S.; Maki, Y.; Ichihara, E.; Asano, H.; et al. Acquired Resistance to EGFR Inhibitors Is Associated with a Manifestation of Stem cell–like Properties in Cancer Cells. *Cancer Res.* **2013**, *73*, 3051. [CrossRef]

10. Byers, L.A.; Diao, L.; Wang, J.; Saintigny, P.; Girard, L.; Peyton, M.; Shen, L.; Fan, Y.; Giri, U.; Tumula, P.K.; et al. An Epithelial-Mesenchymal Transition Gene Signature Predicts Resistance to EGFR and PI3K Inhibitors and Identifies Axl as a Therapeutic Target for Overcoming EGFR Inhibitor Resistance. *Clin. Cancer Res.* **2013**, *19*, 279–290. [CrossRef]
11. Takezawa, K.; Pirazzoli, V.; Arcila, M.E.; Nebhan, C.A.; Song, X.; de Stanchina, E.; Ohashi, K.; Janjigian, Y.Y.; Spitzler, P.J.; Melnick, M.A.; et al. HER2 amplification: A potential mechanism of acquired resistance to EGFR inhibition in EGFR-mutant lung cancers that lack the second-site EGFR T790M mutation. *Cancer Discov.* **2012**, *2*, 922–933. [CrossRef] [PubMed]
12. Ohashi, K.; Sequist, L.V.; Arcila, M.E.; Moran, T.; Chmielecki, J.; Lin, Y.-L.; Pan, Y.; Wang, L.; de Stanchina, E.; Shien, K.; et al. Lung cancers with acquired resistance to EGFR inhibitors occasionally harbor BRAF gene mutations but lack mutations in KRAS, NRAS, or MEK1. *Proc. Natl. Acad. Sci. USA* **2012**, *109*, E2127–E2133. [CrossRef] [PubMed]
13. Zulkifli, A.A.; Tan, F.H.; Putoczki, T.L.; Stylli, S.S.; Luwor, R.B. STAT3 signaling mediates tumour resistance to EGFR targeted therapeutics. *Mol. Cell. Endocrinol.* **2017**, *451*, 15–23. [CrossRef] [PubMed]
14. Germain, D.; Frank, D.A. Targeting the Cytoplasmic and Nuclear Functions of Signal Transducers and Activators of Transcription 3 for Cancer Therapy. *Clin. Cancer Res.* **2007**, *13*, 5665–5669. [CrossRef]
15. Frank, D.A. STAT3 as a central mediator of neoplastic cellular transformation. *Cancer Lett.* **2007**, *251*, 199–210. [CrossRef]
16. Aggarwal, B.B.; Kunnumakkara, A.B.; Harikumar, K.B.; Gupta, S.R.; Tharakan, S.T.; Koca, C.; Dey, S.; Sung, B. Signal transducer and activator of transcription-3, inflammation, and cancer: How intimate is the relationship? *Ann. N. Y. Acad. Sci.* **2009**, *1171*, 59–76. [CrossRef]
17. Rosell, R.; Karachaliou, N. Large-scale screening for somatic mutations in lung cancer. *Lancet* **2016**, *387*, 1354–1356. [CrossRef]
18. Levy, D.E.; Darnell, J.E. Stats: Transcriptional control and biological impact. *Nat. Rev. Mol. Cell Biol.* **2002**, *3*, 651–662. [CrossRef]
19. Yu, Y.; Zhao, Q.; Wang, Z.; Liu, X.Y. Activated STAT3 correlates with prognosis of non-small cell lung cancer and indicates new anticancer strategies. *Cancer Chemother. Pharmacol.* **2015**, *75*, 917–922. [CrossRef]
20. Xu, Y.H.; Lu, S. A meta-analysis of STAT3 and phospho-STAT3 expression and survival of patients with non-small-cell lung cancer. *Eur. J. Surg. Oncol.* **2014**, *40*, 311–317. [CrossRef]
21. Lee, H.J.; Zhuang, G.; Cao, Y.; Du, P.; Kim, H.J.; Settleman, J. Drug resistance via feedback activation of stat3 in oncogene-addicted cancer cells. *Cancer Cell* **2014**, *26*, 207–221. [CrossRef]
22. Ninomiya, T.; Takigawa, N.; Ichihara, E.; Ochi, N.; Murakami, T.; Honda, Y.; Kubo, T.; Minami, D.; Kudo, K.; Tanimoto, M.; et al. Afatinib Prolongs Survival Compared with Gefitinib in an Epidermal Growth Factor Receptor-Driven Lung Cancer Model. *Mol. Cancer Ther.* **2013**, *12*, 589–597. [CrossRef] [PubMed]
23. Chaib, I.; Karachaliou, N.; Pilotto, S.; Servat, J.C.; Cai, X.; Li, X.; Drozdowskyj, A.; Servat, C.C.; Yang, J.; Hu, C.; et al. Co-activation of STAT3 and YES-Associated Protein 1 (YAP1) Pathway in EGFR-Mutant NSCLC. *J. Natl. Cancer Inst.* **2017**, *109*, 1–12. [CrossRef] [PubMed]
24. Hanahan, D.; Weinberg, R.A.A. Hallmarks of cancer: The next generation. *Cell* **2011**, *144*, 646–674. [CrossRef] [PubMed]
25. Jayakumar, A.; Tai, M.H.; Huang, W.Y.; al-Feel, W.; Hsu, M.; Abu-Elheiga, L.; Chirala, S.S.; Wakil, S.J. Human fatty acid synthase: Properties and molecular cloning. *Proc. Natl. Acad. Sci. USA* **1995**, *92*, 8695–8699. [CrossRef] [PubMed]
26. Kuhajda, F.P. Fatty acid synthase and cancer: New application of an old pathway. *Cancer Res.* **2006**, *66*, 5977–5980. [CrossRef] [PubMed]
27. Liu, H.; Liu, J.-Y.; Wu, X.; Zhang, J.-T. Biochemistry, molecular biology, and pharmacology of fatty acid synthase, an emerging therapeutic target and diagnosis/prognosis marker. *Int. J. Biochem. Mol. Biol.* **2010**, *1*, 69–89.
28. Puig, T.; Vázquez-Martín, A.; Relat, J.; Pétriz, J.; Menéndez, J.A.; Porta, R.; Casals, G.; Marrero, P.F.; Haro, D.; Brunet, J.; et al. Fatty acid metabolism in breast cancer cells: Differential inhibitory effects of epigallocatechin gallate (EGCG) and C75. *Breast Cancer Res. Treat.* **2008**, *109*, 471–479. [CrossRef]
29. Jiang, B.; Li, E.-H.; Lu, Y.-Y.; Jiang, Q.; Cui, D.; Jing, Y.-F.; Xia, S.-J. Inhibition of Fatty-acid Synthase Suppresses P-AKT and Induces Apoptosis in Bladder Cancer. *Urology* **2012**, *80*, 484.e9–484.e15. [CrossRef]

30. Yang, Y.; Liu, H.; Li, Z.; Zhao, Z.; Yip-Schneider, M.; Fan, Q.; Schmidt, C.M.; Chiorean, E.G.; Xie, J.; Cheng, L.; et al. Role of fatty acid synthase in gemcitabine and radiation resistance of pancreatic cancers. *Int. J. Biochem. Mol. Biol.* **2011**, *2*, 89–98.
31. Zhan, N.; Li, B.; Xu, X.; Xu, J.; Hu, S. Inhibition of FASN expression enhances radiosensitivity in human non-small cell lung cancer. *Oncol. Lett.* **2018**, *15*, 4578–4584. [CrossRef] [PubMed]
32. Flavin, R.; Peluso, S.; Nguyen, P.L.; Loda, M. Fatty acid synthase as a potential therapeutic target in cancer. *Futur. Oncol.* **2010**, *6*, 551–562. [CrossRef] [PubMed]
33. Colomer, R.; Sarrats, A.; Lupu, R.; Puig, T. Natural Polyphenols and their Synthetic Analogs as Emerging Anticancer Agents. *Curr. Drug Targets* **2016**, *18*, 147–159. [CrossRef] [PubMed]
34. Chakrawarti, L.; Agrawal, R.; Dang, S.; Gupta, S.; Gabrani, R. Therapeutic effects of EGCG: A patent review. *Expert Opin. Ther. Pat.* **2016**, *26*, 907–916. [CrossRef]
35. Wang, X.; Tian, W. Green Tea Epigallocatechin Gallate: A Natural Inhibitor of Fatty-Acid Synthase. *Biochem. Biophys. Res. Commun.* **2001**, *288*, 1200–1206. [CrossRef]
36. Wu, J.; Du, J.; Fu, X.; Liu, B.; Cao, H.; Li, T.; Su, T.; Xu, J.; Tse, A.K.-W.; Yu, Z.-L. Icaritin, a novel FASN inhibitor, exerts anti-melanoma activities through IGF-1R / STAT3 signaling. *Oncotarget* **2016**, *7*, 51251–51269. [CrossRef]
37. Ou, Y.-C.; Li, J.-R.; Kuan, Y.-H.; Raung, S.-L.; Wang, C.-C.; Hung, Y.-Y.; Pan, P.-H.; Lu, H.-C.; Chen, C.-J. Luteolin sensitizes human 786-O renal cell carcinoma cells to TRAIL-induced apoptosis. *Life Sci.* **2014**, *100*, 110–117. [CrossRef]
38. Blancafort, A.; Giró-Perafita, A.; Oliveras, G.; Palomeras, S.; Turrado, C.; Campuzano, Ò.; Carrión-Salip, D.; Massaguer, A.; Brugada, R.; Palafox, M.; et al. Dual fatty acid synthase and HER2 signaling blockade shows marked antitumor activity against breast cancer models resistant to anti-HER2 drugs. *PLoS ONE* **2015**, *10*, e0131241. [CrossRef]
39. Giró-Perafita, A.; Rabionet, M.; Puig, T.; Ciurana, J. Optimization of Poli(ϵ-caprolactone) Scaffolds Suitable for 3D Cancer Cell Culture. *Procedia CIRP* **2016**, *49*, 61–66. [CrossRef]
40. Relat, J.; Blancafort, A.; Oliveras, G.; Cufí, S.; Haro, D.; Marrero, P.F.; Puig, T. Different fatty acid metabolism effects of (-)-epigallocatechin-3-gallate and C75 in adenocarcinoma lung cancer. *BMC Cancer* **2012**, *12*, 280. [CrossRef]
41. Ali, A.; Levantini, E.; Teo, J.T.; Goggi, J.; Clohessy, J.G.; Wu, C.S.; Chen, L.; Yang, H.; Krishnan, I.; Kocher, O.; et al. Fatty acid synthase mediates EGFR palmitoylation in EGFR mutated non-small cell lung cancer. *EMBO Mol. Med.* **2018**, *10*. [CrossRef] [PubMed]
42. Vazquez-Martin, A.; Colomer, R.; Brunet, J.; Lupu, R.; Menendez, J.A. Overexpression of fatty acid synthase gene activates HER1/HER2 tyrosine kinase receptors in human breast epithelial cells. *Cell Prolif.* **2008**, *41*, 59–85. [CrossRef] [PubMed]
43. Crous-Masó, J.; Palomeras, S.; Relat, J.; Camó, C.; Martínez-Garza, Ú.; Planas, M.; Feliu, L.; Puig, T. (−)-Epigallocatechin 3-gallate synthetic analogues inhibit fatty acid synthase and show anticancer activity in triple negative breast cancer. *Molecules* **2018**, *23*. [CrossRef]
44. Giró-Perafita, A.; Rabionet, M.; Planas, M.; Feliu, L.; Ciurana, J.; Ruiz-Martínez, S.; Puig, T. EGCG-Derivative G28 Shows High Efficacy Inhibiting the Mammosphere-Forming Capacity of Sensitive and Resistant TNBC Models. *Molecules* **2019**, *24*, 1027. [CrossRef]
45. Jacobsen, K.; Bertran-Alamillo, J.; Molina, M.A.; Teixidó, C.; Karachaliou, N.; Pedersen, M.H.; Castellví, J.; Garzón, M.; Codony-Servat, C.; Codony-Servat, J.; et al. Convergent Akt activation drives acquired EGFR inhibitor resistance in lung cancer. *Nat. Commun.* **2017**, *8*. [CrossRef] [PubMed]
46. Chang, L.; Fang, S.; Chen, Y.; Yang, Z.; Yuan, Y.; Zhang, J.; Ye, L.; Gu, W. Inhibition of FASN suppresses the malignant biological behavior of non-small cell lung cancer cells via deregulating glucose metabolism and AKT/ERK pathway. *Lipids Health Dis.* **2019**, *18*, 118. [CrossRef]
47. Liu, H.; Liu, Y.; Zhang, J.-T. A new mechanism of drug resistance in breast cancer cells: Fatty acid synthase overexpression-mediated palmitate overproduction. *Mol. Cancer Ther.* **2008**, *7*, 263–270. [CrossRef]
48. Chou, T.C.; Talalay, P. Quantitative analysis of dose-effect relationships: The combined effects of multiple drugs or enzyme inhibitors. *Adv. Enzym. Regul.* **1984**, *22*, 27–55. [CrossRef]
49. Wu, X.; Qin, L.; Fako, V.; Zhang, J.-T. Molecular mechanisms of fatty acid synthase (FASN)-mediated resistance to anti-cancer treatments. *Adv. Biol. Regul.* **2014**, *54*, 214–221. [CrossRef]

50. Liu, H.; Wu, X.; Dong, Z.; Luo, Z.; Zhao, Z.; Xu, Y.; Zhang, J.-T. Fatty acid synthase causes drug resistance by inhibiting TNF-α and ceramide production. *J. Lipid Res.* **2013**, *54*, 776–785. [CrossRef]
51. Giró-Perafita, A.; Palomeras, S.; Lum, D.H.; Blancafort, A.; Viñas, G.; Oliveras, G.; Pérez-Bueno, F.; Sarrats, A.; Welm, A.L.; Puig, T. Preclinical Evaluation of Fatty Acid Synthase and EGFR Inhibition in Triple Negative Breast Cancer. *Clin. Cancer Res.* **2016**, *22*, 4687–4697. [CrossRef] [PubMed]
52. Ma, Y.C.; Li, C.; Gao, F.; Xu, Y.; Jiang, Z.B.; Liu, J.X.; Jin, L.Y. Epigallocatechin gallate inhibits the growth of human lung cancer by directly targeting the EGFR signaling pathway. *Oncol. Rep.* **2014**, *31*, 1343–1349. [CrossRef] [PubMed]
53. Minnelli, C.; Laudadio, E.; Mobbili, G.; Galeazzi, R. Conformational Insight on WT- and Mutated-EGFR Receptor Activation and Inhibition by Epigallocatechin-3-Gallate: Over a Rational Basis for the Design of Selective Non-Small-Cell Lung Anticancer Agents. *Int. J. Mol. Sci.* **2020**, *21*, 1721. [CrossRef] [PubMed]
54. Namiki, K.; Wongsirisin, P.; Yokoyama, S.; Sato, M.; Rawangkan, A.; Sakai, R.; Iida, K.; Suganuma, M. (−)-Epigallocatechin gallate inhibits stemness and tumourigenicity stimulated by AXL receptor tyrosine kinase in human lung cancer cells. *Sci. Rep.* **2020**, *10*, 1–11. [CrossRef] [PubMed]
55. Zhu, C.; Wei, Y.; Wei, X. AXL receptor tyrosine kinase as a promising anti-cancer approach: Functions, molecular mechanisms and clinical applications. *Mol. Cancer* **2019**, *18*. [CrossRef] [PubMed]
56. Yousef, M.; Vlachogiannis, I.; Tsiani, E. Effects of Resveratrol against Lung Cancer: In Vitro and In Vivo Studies. *Nutrients* **2017**, *9*, 1231. [CrossRef]
57. Bailon-Moscoso, N.; Cevallos-Solorzano, G.; Romero-Benavides, J.C.; Orellana, M.I.R. Natural Compounds as Modulators of Cell Cycle Arrest: Application for Anticancer Chemotherapies. *Curr. Genom.* **2017**, *18*, 106–131. [CrossRef]
58. Hasima, N.; Ozpolat, B. Regulation of autophagy by polyphenolic compounds as a potential therapeutic strategy for cancer. *Cell Death Dis.* **2014**, *5*, e1509. [CrossRef]
59. Lin, H.-Y.; Hou, S.-C.; Chen, S.-C.; Kao, M.-C.; Yu, C.-C.; Funayama, S.; Ho, C.-T.; Way, T.-D. (−)-Epigallocatechin Gallate Induces Fas/CD95-Mediated Apoptosis through Inhibiting Constitutive and IL-6-Induced JAK/STAT3 Signaling in Head and Neck Squamous Cell Carcinoma Cells. *J. Agric. Food Chem.* **2012**, *60*, 2480–2489. [CrossRef]
60. Tang, S.-N.; Fu, J.; Shankar, S.; Srivastava, R.K. EGCG Enhances the Therapeutic Potential of Gemcitabine and CP690550 by Inhibiting STAT3 Signaling Pathway in Human Pancreatic Cancer. *PLoS ONE* **2012**, *7*, e31067. [CrossRef]
61. Codony-servat, C.; Codony-servat, J.; Karachaliou, N.; Angel, M.; Chaib, I.; Ramirez, J.L.; Gil, M.D.L.L.; Solca, F. Activation of signal transducer and activator of transcription 3 (STAT3) signaling in EGFR mutant non-small-cell lung cancer (NSCLC). *Oncotarget* **2017**, *8*, 47305–47316. [CrossRef] [PubMed]
62. Steelman, L.S.; Chappell, W.H.; Abrams, S.L.; Kempf, C.R.; Long, J.; Laidler, P.; Mijatovic, S.; Maksimovic-Ivanic, D.; Stivala, F.; Mazzarino, M.C.; et al. Roles of the Raf/MEK/ERK and PI3K/PTEN/Akt/mTOR pathways in controlling growth and sensitivity to therapy-implications for cancer and aging. *Aging (Albany. N.Y.)* **2011**, *3*, 192–222. [CrossRef] [PubMed]

8

Targeting Glucose Transporters for Breast Cancer Therapy: The Effect of Natural and Synthetic Compounds

Ana M. Barbosa [1] and Fátima Martel [2,3,*]

[1] Instituto de Ciências Biomédicas Abel Salazar, University of Porto, 4169-007 Porto, Portugal; anamargabarbosa@gmail.com

[2] Unit of Biochemistry, Department of Biomedicine, Faculty of Medicine, University of Porto, 4200-319 Porto, Portugal

[3] Instituto de Investigação e Inovação em Saúde, University of Porto, 4200-135 Porto, Portugal

* Correspondence: fmartel@med.up.pt

Abstract: Reprogramming of cellular energy metabolism is widely accepted to be a cancer hallmark. The deviant energetic metabolism of cancer cells-known as the Warburg effect-consists in much higher rates of glucose uptake and glycolytic oxidation coupled with the production of lactic acid, even in the presence of oxygen. Consequently, cancer cells have higher glucose needs and thus display a higher sensitivity to glucose deprivation-induced death than normal cells. So, inhibitors of glucose uptake are potential therapeutic targets in cancer. Breast cancer is the most commonly diagnosed cancer and a leading cause of cancer death in women worldwide. Overexpression of facilitative glucose transporters (GLUT), mainly GLUT1, in breast cancer cells is firmly established, and the consequences of GLUT inhibition and/or knockout are under investigation. Herein we review the compounds, both of natural and synthetic origin, found to interfere with uptake of glucose by breast cancer cells, and the consequences of interference with that mechanism on breast cancer cell biology. We will also present data where the interaction with GLUT is exploited in order to increase the efficiency or selectivity of anticancer agents, in breast cancer cells.

Keywords: breast cancer; glucose transport; drugs; natural compounds

---

1. Introduction

According to the last Global Cancer Statistics (GLOBOCAN 2018), breast cancer represented 12% of all cancers, being the second most frequent cancer worldwide, after lung cancer, and caused about 7% of the total cancer deaths in 2018 [1]. In women, breast cancer is the leading type of cancer and the leading cause of cancer death worldwide [1].

Screening programs and adjuvant chemotherapy have had a significant impact on the prognosis of breast cancer patients, having significantly improved their overall survival, disease-free survival, and death rates related to breast-cancer since the early 1990s [2,3]. Nevertheless, efforts must continue in order to reduce not only the incidence but also the mortality and treatment-associated morbidities associated with this disease. In this context, discovery of new molecular targets and the refinement of lead compounds constitute a priority in breast cancer research.

2. Metabolic Reprogramming in Cancer Cells

Metabolic reprogramming and altered energetics is firmly established as a hallmark of cancer and constitutes an active area of basic, translational, and clinical cancer research in recent years [4].

One of the cancer metabolic hallmarks is a deviant energetic metabolism-known as the Warburg effect-characterized by a very high rate of glycolysis and production of lactate, even in the presence of oxygen [5]. Cancer cells have a high dependence on the glycolytic pathway to supply their need of high amounts of adenosine triphosphate (ATP) and also of metabolic intermediates that contribute to several biosynthetic pathways, crucial for cancer progression [4] and to compensate for excess metabolic production of reactive oxygen species (ROS) [6]. So, they shift their main ATP-producing process from oxidative phosphorylation to glucose fermentation, even in aerobic conditions [4]. This altered metabolism may be not only a consequence of genetic mutations, but also a contributing factor or cause of tumorigenesis [7].

More recently, a 'two-compartment' model, also named 'the reverse Warburg effect' or "metabolic coupling", has been proposed to reconsider metabolism in tumors, because it was realized that another type of metabolism occurs in certain types of cancers, having high mitochondrial respiration and low glycolysis rate [8]. According to this model, tumor cells and adjacent stromal fibroblasts form a two-compartment model of cancer metabolism, in which fibroblasts perform aerobic glycolysis (because of the acidic microenvironment induced by cancer cells), and the generated metabolites (such as pyruvate, ketone bodies, fatty acids, and lactate), are transferred to tumor cells, to fuel the Krebs cycle and maintain ATP generation [9]. This metabolic coupling is found in some forms of breast cancer [10], and may contribute drug resistance and therapeutic failure in some types of cancers [11], as observed with tamoxifen-resistance in breast cancer MCF7 cells [12].

3. Upregulation of Glucose Transport in Breast Cancer Cells

Since the energetic metabolic shift in cancer cells produces less ATP per glucose molecule, the demand for glucose in these cells is higher than in normal cells. Therefore, cancer cells rely on higher rates of glucose uptake in order to support their increased energy, biosynthesis and redox needs. This increased rates of cellular uptake of glucose is met by overexpression of glucose transporters, which is observed in most cancer cells [13].

Two families of glucose transporters mediate glucose uptake in mammalian cells: the Na^+-dependent glucose co-transporters (SGLTs) and the facilitative glucose transporters (GLUTs).

The SGLT family (gene symbol *SLC5A*) are secondary active transporters that transfer glucose against its concentration gradient coupled with Na^+ transport down its concentration gradient, which is maintained by the Na^+/K^+ pump. For every glucose molecule that is transported, two Na^+ are also transported. SGLT transporters have 14 transmembrane domains and a high affinity for glucose. At physiological extracellular Na^+ concentration and membrane potential, an apparent Km of 0.5 mM of SGLT1 for glucose was described, but glucose is transported with a lower affinity when the plasma membrane is depolarized and/or the extracellular Na^+ concentration is low [14,15]. SGLT1 and SGLT2 overexpression is present in some types of cancer, such as pancreas, prostate, lung, liver, and ovarian cancer, but these transporters have not been described in breast cancer [16].

The GLUT family (gene symbol *SLC2A*) are facilitative transporters that mediate the transport of glucose down its concentration gradient. This family of transporters is composed of 14 members: GLUT1-GLUT12, GLUT14, and the H^+/myo-inositol transporter. All GLUTs are predicted to have 12 transmembrane domains connected by hydrophilic loops. Each of the GLUT transport protein possesses different affinities for glucose and other hexoses such as fructose. GLUT1, GLUT3, and GLUT4 have a high affinity for glucose (e.g., the Km of GLUT1 for glucose is 1–3 mM), allowing transport of glucose at a high rate under normal physiological conditions [17].

Increased cellular uptake of glucose in tumor cells is associated with increased and deregulated expression of GLUT transporters [13]. Among GLUT family members, overexpression of GLUT1 has been consistently observed in many different cancers, including breast, lung, renal, colorectal, and pancreatic cancers [13,18,19]. Consistent with its overexpression, GLUT1 is crucial for uptake of glucose by breast cancer cells [20–22] and is also the main glucose transporter in breast cancer cell lines (e.g., MCF-7 and MDA-MB-231) [21,23]. GLUT1 is a transporter ubiquitously expressed in most mammalian tissues (abundantly in brain and erythrocytes), being responsible for basal glucose cellular uptake in the majority of tissues [16,17]; it is also the predominant isoform present in human and bovine mammary glands [24,25]. Glucose uptake mediated by GLUT1 appears to be especially critical in the early stages of breast cancer development, affecting cell transformation and tumor formation [26,27]. Indeed, GLUT1 overexpression, which occurs early during the transformation process, induces a change in breast epithelial cell metabolism that precedes morphological changes in breast cancer, and thus may be a fundamental part of the neoplastic process [18]. Interestingly, the loss of even a single GLUT1 allele is sufficient to impose a strong break in breast tumor development in a mouse model [26]. A strong correlation between *GLUT1* gene expression and breast cancers of higher grade and proliferative index and lower degree of differentiation [28] and higher malignant potential, invasiveness, and consequently poorer prognosis [29] exists. GLUT1 is thus considered an oncogene [18–20,30].

One of the factors responsible for the upregulation of GLUT1 in breast tumor cells is hypoxia. The promoters of GLUT1 contain hypoxia-response elements, which bind the hypoxia-inducible factor (HIF-1) to facilitate transcription. Since an increase in the levels of HIF-1α protein is a phenomenon seen in most cancers, it provides a molecular mechanism for cancer-associated overexpression of GLUT1 [18,31]. Additionally, hypoxia appears to increase GLUT1 transport activity in the MCF-7 breast cancer cell line, independently of changes in transporter expression [32]. Besides HIF-1, the ovarian hormone estrogen is also known to induce GLUT1 expression in breast cancer [18,33]. Moreover, the histone deacetylase SIRT6, the cellular oncogene product c-MYC (V-Myc Avian Myelocytomatosis Viral Oncogene Homolog), the pro-survival protein kinase Akt (Protein Kinase B) and mutant p53, all of which induce the expression of GLUT1 [31,34], can also be involved in GLUT1 overexpression in breast cancer.

In addition to GLUT1, which is consistently found to be expressed in breast tumors and cell lines, other GLUT family members can also contribute to glucose uptake by breast cancer cells. More specifically, GLUT2 [19,23] and GLUT3 [18] are also expressed in several breast cancer cell lines. Additionally, GLUT4 expression [30,35–37] and insulin-stimulated glucose uptake were also described in some cancer cell lines [38–40]. Moreover, the involvement of GLUT4 in basal glucose uptake was described in two breast cancer cell lines [41]. Finally, a second insulin-stimulated transporter, GLUT12, was also described in MCF-7 cells [18,42]. Similar to GLUT1, the expression of GLUT3 and GLUT12 correlate with poor prognosis [18,19]. Importantly, increased expression of GLUT1 and GLUT3 was also associated with resistance of cancer cells to radio or chemotherapy [43–45], but the underlying mechanisms linking GLUT and chemo- or radio-resistance remain largely unknown.

Increased glucose uptake by cancer cells has been exploited clinically in diagnosis and follows up of cancer via the use of ^{18}fluoro-2-deoxy-D-glucose (FDG), a radiolabeled glucose analogue, in Positron Emission Tomography (PET) [46]. This radiotracer enters cells via GLUTs, being then phosphorylated by hexokinases into FDG-6-phosphate that cannot be further metabolized and thus accumulates in the cytoplasm. Importantly, the sensitivity of this technique varies depending on the type of cancer, and this heterogeneity has been particularly associated with GLUT1 or GLUT3 tumor expression [23,47].

4. Glucose Transporters as Therapeutic Targets in Breast Cancer

Since cancer cells depend on increased utilization of glucose as compared to normal healthy cells, glucose deprivation is considered an effective anticancer therapy and as a potential strategy for cancer prevention, and many compounds targeting cancer cell energy metabolism are currently on trial or approved as therapeutic agents against cancer [48,49]. These include specific inhibitors of monocarboxylate transporter 1, hexokinase II, glyceraldehyde-3-phosphate dehydrogenase (GAPDH), pyruvate dehydrogenase, pyruvate dehydrogenase kinase 1, cancer-specific mutant isocitrate dehydrogenase, lactate dehydrogenase A, phosphoglycerate mutase 1, phosphofructokinase, or pyruvate kinase M2 [48,50]. In support of glucose deprivation as a molecular target in cancer, high-fat and low-carbohydrate diet appear to provide therapeutic benefits for increased survival by reducing angiogenesis, peri-tumoral edema, cancer migration, and invasion [51]. According to some authors, inhibition of glucose metabolism will not only deplete cancer cells of ATP, but also will lead to enhanced oxidative stress-related cytotoxicity [6].

Additionally, because tumor cells have an increased dependence in relation to extracellular glucose, GLUTs constitute also an anticancer target [18,52–54]. A direct approach to this therapeutic target is to block GLUT-mediated glucose uptake, which would abolish entry of glucose into the cancer cell. Alternatively, new approaches consist in the design and development of "GLUT-transportable anticancer agents", or the use of GLUT antibodies to selectively deliver an anticancer agent to cancer cells.

In this review, we will list compounds, both of natural and synthetic origin, found to interfere with glucose uptake by breast cancer cells, and present the consequences of GLUT inhibition and/or knockout on breast cancer cell biology. We will also present data where the interaction of defined molecules with GLUT is exploited in order to increase its efficiency or selectivity, in breast cancer cells.

5. Effect of Synthetic and Natural Compounds on Glucose Uptake by Breast Cancer Cells

5.1. Effect of Synthetic Compounds

5.1.1. GLUT Inhibitors

WZB117 and STF-31

The effect of two recently described GLUT1 inhibitors, WZB117 and STF-31, on breast cancer cells was studied by some authors. WZB117 is a representative of a group of novel small compounds that were recently reported to inhibit basal glucose transport and cell growth in vitro and in vivo [55,56]. STF-31 is a small molecule that was firstly reported to selectively target von Hippel-Lindau (VHL)-deficient renal cell carcinoma (RCC) cells [55].

These two GLUT1 inhibitors were able to inhibit cell proliferation and induce apoptosis in several breast cancer cell lines (MCF-7, MDA-MB-231, HBL100, and BT549), and these effects were accompanied by interference with cellular glucose handling, increasing the levels of extracellular glucose, and decreasing the levels of extracellular lactate, suggesting an inhibitory effect upon glucose uptake and/or glycolysis. Of interest, STF31 (30 μM) potentiated the antiproliferative effect of metformin (3 mM) in MDA-MB-231 cells [57]. Although the effect on glucose uptake was not studied, GLUT1 inhibition (with WZB117) blocked transformation of MCF10A-ERBB2 cells (a breast epithelial cell line used as a model to study the early events leading to transformation) induced by activated ERBB2 through reduced cell proliferation [26] (Table 1).

In addition of testing these GLUT1 inhibitors alone as a targeted therapy, GLUT1 inhibition in combination with other cancer therapeutics has also been evaluated (Table 1). In one study, WZB117 was found to reduce GLUT1 mRNA and protein levels and glucose uptake and lactate production in two breast cancer cell lines (MCF-7 and MDA-MB-231). The interaction of this agent with radiation was investigated. Glucose metabolism and GLUT1 expression were found to be significantly stimulated by radiotherapy. Interestingly, radioresistant breast cancer cells exhibited upregulated GLUT1 expression and glucose metabolism but combination of WZB117 and radiation re-sensitized the radioresistant cancer cells to radiation [58]. A synergic antitumoral effect was also found between WZB117 and the anticancer drugs cisplatin and paclitaxel, in MCF-7 cells [59]. Finally, the possibility that a combined treatment with a GLUT1 inhibitor could overcome resistance to another breast cancer therapeutic agent (adriamycin) was also investigated. Resistance to adriamycin is a common obstacle occurring during therapy of breast cancer patients. WZB117 was found to resensitize MCF-7/ADR cells (adriamycin-resistant) to adriamycin [60]. Therefore, GLUT1 inhibition could overcome resistance to adriamycin and radiation.

WZB27 and WZB115

Two other GLUT1 inhibitors, WZB27 and WZB115, were synthesized and tested against several cell types, including a breast cancer cell line (MCF-7). These compounds reduced basal glucose uptake and cell proliferation, induced apoptosis, and led to cell cycle arrest in G1/S phase, without affecting much the normal cell line MCF12A. Importantly, their inhibitory effect on cancer cell growth was ameliorated when additional glucose was present, suggesting that the inhibition was due, at least in part, to inhibition of basal glucose uptake. Moreover, when used in combination, the test compounds demonstrated synergistic effects with the anticancer drugs cisplatin and paclitaxel (Table 1) [56].

Bay876

BAY-876 is a highly selective GLUT1 inhibitor under preclinical study for oncolytic treatment [61]. In a recent report, the interaction between GLUT1 and bromodomains (BRDs) was investigated. BRDs are conserved protein interaction modules, which recognize acetyl-lysine modifications, and BRD-containing proteins are components of the transcription factor and chromatin-modifying complexes and determinants of epigenetic memory [62]. BAY876 decreased glucose uptake by a triple-negative breast cancer cell line, and a vulnerability of these breast cancer cells to inhibition of BRPF2/3 BRDs, under conditions of glucose deprivation or GLUT1 inhibition, was reported (Table 1) [63].

2-deoxy-D-glucose

2-deoxy-D-glucose (2-DG) is a synthetic non-metabolizable glucose analogue. 2-DG inhibits the glycolytic pathway, because the product of its phosphorylation by hexokinase cannot be further metabolized and, additionally, is a non-competitive inhibitor of hexokinase, thus causing ATP depletion. Additionally, 2-DG competes with glucose for GLUT [64]. In a triple-negative breast cancer cell line (MDA-MB-231), but not in an estrogen receptor (ER)-positive cell line (MCF-7), 2-DG was able to reduce glucose uptake (Table 1) [65].

GLUT1 shRNA

Another strategy that is being tested to target GLUT1 is by RNA interference (RNAi) using short hairpin RNA (shRNA). Silencing of GLUT1 expression with an shRNA led to a significant decrease in glucose uptake in vitro in both a triple-negative (MDA-MB-468) and a HER2-positive cell line (SK-BR3), together with a decrease of the growth of xenograft tumors (MDA-MB-468 cells) [66]. Similarly, shRNA targeting GLUT1 decreased glucose transport and consumption, reduced lactate secretion, and inhibited growth of the mouse mammary tumor cell line 78617GL, both in vitro and in vivo (Table 1) [27].

A similar negative effect of GLUT1 shRNA on glucose uptake was found in two other triple-negative breast cancer cell lines (MDA-MB-231 and Hs578T), together with a decrease in cell proliferation, migration, and invasion, which was concluded to result from GLUT1-mediated modulation of Epidermal Growth Factor Receptor (EGFR)/Mitogen-Activated Protein Kinase (MAPK), and integrin β1/Src/FAK signaling pathways [67]. However, the same group verified that, contrary to the expected, ablation of GLUT1 attenuated apoptosis and increased drug resistance in triple-negative breast cancer cells (MDA-MB-231 cells), via upregulation of p-Akt/p-GSK-3β (Ser9)/β-catenin/surviving (Table 1) [52]. Not only is the prognostic of triple-negative breast cancer (TNBC) usually poor due to aggressive tumor phenotypes, but also because conventional chemotherapy cannot be used. Therefore, and because TNBC have higher levels of GLUT1, this transporter is seen as a potential therapeutic target, sensitizing cells to chemotherapy. The results of this later study, however, indicate that the potential of GLUT1 as a therapeutic target in TNBC should be carefully re-evaluated [68].

Anti-GLUT1-antibody

An anti-GLUT1 monoclonal antibody was able to decrease glucose uptake in breast cancer cells (MDA-MB-231), and to reduce cell proliferation and stimulate apoptosis (MCF-1 and T47D). Importantly, when associated with chemotherapeutic agents (5 μM cisplatin, 5 μM paclitaxel, or 10 μM gefitinib), it potentiated the anti-proliferative and pro-apoptotic effects of these agents in MCF-7 cells (Table 1). The authors concluded that the use of antibodies to GLUT1 may be a viable but an as yet unexplored therapeutic strategy in tumors that overexpress GLUT1 [69].

GLUT4 shRNA

By stably silencing GLUT4 expression by lentiviral expression of a GLUT4 shRNA, GLUT4 was concluded to have a prominent role in basal glucose uptake in MCF7 and MDA-MB-231 breast cancer cells (Table 1). Moreover, GLUT4 specific downregulation in these two different breast cancer cell lines, with different degrees of malignancy and differentiation, promoted metabolic reprogramming and affected cell proliferation and viability. According to these authors, their study provides proof-of-principle for the feasibility of using pharmacological approaches to inhibit GLUT4 in order to induce metabolic reprogramming in vivo in breast cancer models [41].

5.1.2. Antidiabetics

Biguanides, including metformin and phenformin, are inhibitors of mitochondrial respiratory chain complex I, and have been shown to reduce cancer incidence and cancer-related death [68].

Metformin

Metformin is the most prescribed oral antidiabetic drug used for the treatment of diabetes mellitus. Metformin was associated with reduced risk of developing cancer in diabetic patients in 2005 [70]. Since then, a large amount of studies confirmed this observation, and the role of metformin in breast cancer has been evaluated [71,72]. In this context, the effect of metformin on glucose uptake and metabolism by breast cancer cells has been evaluated in a few studies (Table 1).

In a first study, metformin was found to decrease glucose utilization both in vitro (MDA-MB-231) and in vivo (using MDA-MB-231 cells orthotopically implanted in a mammary fat pad). However, this effect was concluded to be related to a direct inhibitory effect on the glycolytic enzyme hexokinase and drug effects on transmembrane glucose transport were excluded, because glucose uptake and glucose transporters expression levels were not affected by metformin [73].

In the study by Amaral et al. [65], short-term exposure to metformin inhibited glucose uptake, probably by direct inhibition of GLUT1, and, in contrast, long-term exposure to metformin led to a significant increase in glucose uptake, which was not associated with changes in GLUT1 mRNA levels. It was suggested that the increase in glucose uptake induced by long-term metformin, is a compensatory mechanism in response to cellular ATP depletion resulting from its inhibitory effect on oxidative phosphorylation and that this metformin-induced dependence on glycolytic pathway, associated with an anticarcinogenic effect of the drug, provides a biochemical basis for the design of new therapeutic strategies. The increase in glucose uptake after a long-term exposure to metformin, to compensate for the reduced mitochondrial ATP generation, was corroborated in another study, using two triple-negative breast cancer cell lines (MDA-MB-231 and MDA-MB-436) [74]. Lastly, the interaction between metformin and PPARδ (peroxisome-proliferator-activated receptor δ), known to have a role in inflammation, metabolism, and cancer, was recently evaluated [75]. Metformin was able to block the increase in GLUT1 and SGLT1 mRNA and protein levels, glucose uptake, glucose consumption, and lactate production caused by the PPARδ agonist GW501516 in MCF-7 cells. The effect of metformin in reducing the expression of GLUT1 and SGLT1 was not present with metformin alone; rather, it results from metformin-mediated inhibition of PPARδ activity. Therefore, metformin can block the effect of GW501516, but has no effect of its own in reduction of glucose transporters levels, which is in concordance with the previous studies.

Phenformin

A recent study showed that glucose uptake and utilization affects cancer cell sensitivity to phenformin treatment. More specifically, a correlation between low expression of glucose transporters, including GLUT1, and both a defective glucose uptake/utilization and an increased sensitivity to phenformin treatment was found in several cancer cell lines. Moreover, restoration of GLUT1 expression attenuated the phenformin-sensitivity in the corresponding cancer cells [76]. Additionally, Liu and Gan [77], by using the MDA-MB-231 cell line, demonstrated that phenformin upregulates GLUT1 levels, causing increased glucose uptake and production of lactate. Importantly, they verified that this effect of phenformin is dependent on NBR2 (neighbor of *BRCA1* gene 2), a glucose starvation-induced long non-coding RNA that interacts with AMP-Activated Protein Kinase (AMPK) and regulates AMPK activity. They thus concluded that the NBR2-GLUT1 axis may serve as an adaptive response in breast cancer cells to survive in response to phenformin treatment (Table 1) [77].

Troglitazone

Another antidiabetic drug also associated with an anticarcinogenic effect [78], troglitazone, belongs to the class of thiazolidinediones, which activate peroxisome proliferator-activated receptor-γ (PPARγ), although it has been withdrawn from the market due to its hepatotoxicity. Unlike the antidiabetic effects of this drug, many other actions of troglitazone are thought to occur in a PPARγ-independent manner. Since troglitazone is known to cause mitochondrial dysfunction, its effect on glucose metabolism was investigated [79]. Troglitazone enhanced uptake of glucose in several breast cancer cell lines, but changes in GLUT levels do not seem to play a role in this effect, that rather appears to involve MAPK, AMPK, and EGFR. Interestingly, troglitazone reduced T-47D cell content, and this effect was potentiated by restriction of glucose availability. So, it was concluded that troglitazone stimulates uptake of glucose by cancer cells and shifts its metabolism toward glycolysis, likely as an adaptive response to impaired mitochondrial oxidative respiration (Table 1) [80].

5.1.3. Chemotherapeutic Agents

Cisplatin

Cisplatin (cis-diamminedichloroplatinum II) is a very common used chemotherapeutic agent. It is a platinum-derived agent that interferes with DNA replication, and has also been associated with mitochondrial damage. Wang et al [36] used the MDA-MB-231 cell line in order to study cisplatin's metabolic effects. The compound decreased glucose uptake and lactate production and the expression levels of GLUT1 and GLUT4 (Table 1). Cisplatin downregulation of integrin β5 (ITGB5)/FAK signaling pathway was concluded to be responsible for its effect on the expression of GLUT1 and GLUT4 [36].

Sorafenib

The bisarylurea sorafenib is a multi-kinase inhibitor with anti-proliferative and anti-angiogenic activity, currently under evaluation in a variety of solid tumors. Evidence has shown that sorafenib can inhibit oxidative phosphorylation in some types of cancer cell lines [80,81], and the question if it also affects glucose metabolism was then addressed [82]. In this work, the effect of sorafenib on glucose uptake, utilization, lactate production, and GLUT1 expression was investigated in several breast cancer cell lines. Sorafenib produced distinct early and long-term effects on glucose uptake, metabolism, and GLUT1 expression in MCF-7 (ERα-positive), MDA-MB-231 (triple negative), and SKBR3 (ERα-negative/HER2-positive) cell lines. Fasentin (a GLUT1 inhibitor) inhibited the initial GLUT1 overexpression caused by sorafenib and, importantly, its cytotoxic effect (Table 1). It was concluded that the early-term effects were dependent on AMPK and thought to compensate for the loss of mitochondrial ATP, but that persistent activation of AMPK by sorafenib finally led to the impairment of glucose metabolism in all the cell lines, resulting in cell death [82].

Trastuzumab

Trastuzumab, effective in about 15% of women with breast cancer, targets Human Epidermal Growth Factor Receptor 2 (HER2) and downregulates signaling through Akt/phosphoinositide 3-kinase (PI3K) and MAPK pathways. These pathways modulate glucose metabolism and so it was evaluated if trastuzumab decreased glucose uptake in breast cancer cells. For this, xenografts derived from HER2-overexpressing MDA-MB-453 human breast tumor cells were grown in severe combined immunodeficient mice. Xenografts were significantly smaller and [^{18}F] FDG uptake was also reduced in trastuzumab-treated mice. This observation was accompanied by lower GLUT1 protein levels (Table 1) [83].

Doxorubicin (DOX) and 5-fluorouracil (5FU)

The effect of these two chemotherapeutic agents on the expression and activity of GLUT1 and hexokinase and on glucose uptake by the MCF-7 breast cancer cell line was evaluated [84]. Both agents induced a decrease in glucose uptake together with an increase in GLUT1 mRNA levels. The effect on GLUT1 protein levels were not as marked, which suggest posttranslational alterations in GLUT1. It was concluded that after DOX or 5FU therapy, the relationship between glucose and viable cell number can become disjointed, with transient declines in glucose uptake in excess of the decline in cell number despite increased GLUT1 mRNA levels [84]. In another work, DOX and selenium, either free or in PLGA (poly (d, l-lactide-co-glycolide)) nanoparticles were described to reduce the cellular uptake of glucose by MCF-7 and MDA-MB-231 cells, based on measurements of medium glucose levels [85]. So, no direct measurement of glucose uptake was made (Table 1).

Palbociclib

Dysregulation of the cell cycle is a hallmark of cancer that leads to aberrant cellular proliferation and inhibition of cell cycle regulators such as Cyclin-Dependent Kinase 4 (CDK4) and 6 (CDK6) has become a new therapeutic target for the treatment of breast cancer. Palbociclib, an orally-available inhibitor of CDK4 and CDK6, represents the most widely studied compound among cell cycle inhibitors [86]. Interestingly, palbociclib also seems to be able to inhibit GLUT1 mediated glucose uptake and metabolism in TNBC cells [87,88]. Moreover, combination of palbociclib with a chemotherapeutic agent currently used for the treatment of TNBC patients (paclitaxel) inhibited cell proliferation and increased cell death more efficiently than single treatments, associated with a more marked effect on glucose uptake and consumption and on GLUT1 protein levels [87]. Additionally, combination of palbociclib with a PI3K/mTOR inhibitor (BYL719) enhanced the antitumoral effect of these agents and the negative effect of each of these drugs on glucose uptake and consumption and on GLUT1 protein levels (Table 1) [88].

5.1.4. Other Drugs

Propranolol

Another type of drug that has been getting attention for its recently found anticarcinogenic effect are beta-blockers, more specifically propranolol (PROP). Clinical evidence has strongly indicated that PROP can inhibit cancer growth, metastasis development, and tumor recurrence in breast cancer patients [89]. Treatment with PROP decreased hexokinase-2 expression in vitro and 18F-FDG uptake in vivo, but GLUT1 levels were not affected. This indicates that GLUT1 is not involved in the anticarcinogenic effect of PROP (Table 1) [90].

Saracatinib

Prevention of estrogen receptor negative (ER-) and tamoxifen-resistant (TamR) breast cancer remains an important demand due to gaps in pathobiological understanding of this type of cancer. Transforming (sarcoma-inducing) Gene of Rous Sarcoma Virus (Src) activation appears to be a key signaling event driving ER- and TamR breast cancer progression and thus, targeting Src may prevent ER- breast cancer [91]. Accordingly, Src-targeting agents such as the tyrosine kinase inhibitor saracatinib, have been extensively tested in the clinic for treatment of metastatic breast cancer [92]. In the report by Jain et al. [93], activation of Src kinase was investigated as an early signaling alteration in premalignant breast lesions of women who did not respond to tamoxifen, a widely used ER antagonist for hormonal therapy of breast cancer. They verified that Src plays an essential role in regulating glucose uptake, because knocking down Src significantly reduced glucose uptake. Moreover, they showed that saracatinib inhibited glucose uptake in premalignant breast cell lines (MCF-10A and MCF12A) with or without HER-2 overexpression (Table 1).

P53 Modulators

The tumor protein p53, a well-recognized tumor suppressor, is a key regulator of energy metabolism, playing an important role in preventing the cell from reprogramming its energetic metabolic pathway [94]. The p53-reactivating compound RITA (Reactivating p53 and Inducing Tumor Apoptosis) activates p53 in cells expressing oncogenes, whereas its effect in non-transformed cells is almost negligible [95]. This agent decreased GLUT1 mRNA expression in MCF-7 cells. Further, another p53 activator, nutlin3a [96], also caused repression of GLUT1 mRNA expression. Interestingly, the p53 inhibitor pifithrin-α p53 [95] induced the expression of GLUT1 mRNA and abolished the effect of RITA upon GLUT1 mRNA levels (Table 1) [94]. This study shows that reinstatement of p53 function targets the dependence of cancer cells on glycolysis, which can contribute to the selective killing of cancer cells by pharmacologically activated p53.

Akt Inhibitors

The protein kinase Akt is involved in various cellular processes, including cell proliferation, growth and metabolism, and hyperactivation of Akt is commonly observed in human tumors [97]. Three non-ATP-competitive allosteric Akt inhibitors (Akt1i, Akt2i, and Akt1/2i) reduced glucose transport into T-47D breast cancer cells, by interfering with a process distinct from the Akt signaling pathway (involved in movement of GLUT4 to the plasma membrane, e.g., in adipocytes). Among other evidences, the PI3K inhibitor wortmannin was devoid of effect on glucose uptake. It was concluded that these drugs, at least in part, inhibit tumorigenesis through inhibition of glucose transport in tumor cells (Table 1) [98].

PGC1β and HKDC1 shRNA

The peroxisome proliferator-activated receptor-γ (PPARγ) co-activator-1b (PGC1b) promotes tumorigenesis by modulation of mitochondrial function and glycolysis metabolism [99]. On the other hand, hexokinase domain component 1 (HKDC1), recently discovered as a putative hexokinase [100], may be a novel potential therapeutic target for cancer [101]. A recent study demonstrated that knockdown of either PGC1β or HKDC1 resulted in a decrease in glucose uptake in MCF-7 cells (Table 1) [102].

miRNA-34a Inhibitor

miRNA-34a is a tumor suppressor that is expressed in a variety of different types of cancer, including breast cancer. A recent report showed that miRNA-34a inhibition promoted cancer cell proliferation, accelerated glucose uptake and upregulated GLUT1 expression in two triple-negative breast cancer cell lines used, but interestingly, was devoid of effect in the normal human breast epithelial cell line (Table 1) [103].

miRNA-186-3p

Recently, it was verified that systemic delivery of cholesterol-modified agomiR-186-3p to mice bearing tamoxifen-resistant breast tumors effectively attenuates both tumor growth and ^{18}F-FDG uptake (Table 1) [104].

Table 1. Effect of synthetic compounds on glucose uptake by breast cancer cells.

Compound	Concentration (Time)	Cell Line/Model	Effect	Mechanism of Action	Ref
GLUT inhibitors					
WZB117	3–30 μM (24 h)	MCF-7, HBL100	↑ extracellular glucose levels ↔ (HBL100) or ↓ (MCF-7) extracellular lactate levels	-	[57]
WZB117	0.6 μM (16 h)	MCF-7, MDA-MB-231	↓ glucose uptake, lactate production and extracellular levels	↓ GLUT1 mRNA and protein levels	[58]
STF31	0.01–1 μM (24 h)	MCF-7, HBL100	↓ glucose and ↔ lactate in the extracellular medium (HBL100) ↑ glucose and ↓ lactate in the extracellular medium (MCF-7)	-	[57]
WZB27 and WZB115	30 μM and 10 μM, respectively (15 min)	MCF-7	↓ glucose uptake	-	[56]
2-deoxy-D-glucose	2 mM (24 h)	MCF-7 MDA-MB-231	↔ glucose uptake ↓ glucose uptake	- -	[65]
GLUT4 shRNA	transfection	MCF-7	↓ glucose uptake	-	[41]
GLUT1 shRNA	transfection	SK-BR3, MDA-MB-468	↓ glucose uptake and lactate production	-	[66]
GLUT1 shRNA	transfection	78617GL	↓ glucose uptake, consumption and lactate production	-	[27]
GLUT1 shRNA	transfection	MDA-MB-231, Hs578T	↓ glucose uptake	-	[67]
BAY 876	3 μM (5 days)	MDA-MB-436	↓ glucose uptake	-	[63]
Anti-GLUT1 antibody	0.1 mg/mlL (18 h)	MDA-MB-231	↓ glucose uptake	-	[69]
Anti-diabetics					
Metformin	1–10 mM (24–48 h)	MDA-MB-231 Orthotopically implanted MDA-MB-231 cells in mice	↔ glucose uptake	↔ GLUT1, GLUT2, GLUT3, and GLUT4 mRNA levels	[73]
Metformin	0.05–5 mM (26 min) 0.5–1 mM (24 h)	MCF-7, MDA-MB-231	↓ glucose uptake ↑ glucose uptake and lactate production	- ↔ GLUT1 mRNA levels	[65]
Metformin	10 mM (12 h)	MCF-7	↔ GLUT1 and SGLT1 protein levels	↓ PPARδ agonist-induced ↑ glucose uptake, consumption, lactate production and GLUT1 and SGLT1 mRNA and protein levels	[75]
Metformin	2 mM (8 weeks)	MDA-MB-231, MDA-MB-436	↑ glucose uptake	-	[74]
Phenformin	2 mM (12 h)	MDA-MB-231	↑glucose uptake, lactate production	↑ GLUT1 mRNA and protein levels NBR2-dependent	[77]
Troglitazone	20 μM (1 h)	MCF-7, MDA-MB-231, MDA-MB-468, T47D	↑ glucose uptake and lactate production	↔ GLUT1 protein levels PPARγ-independent, MAPK-, AMPK-, and EGFR-dependent	[79]

Table 1. *Cont.*

Compound	Concentration (Time)	Cell Line/Model	Effect	Mechanism of Action	Ref
Chemotherapeutic agents					
Cisplatin	20 µM (48 h)	MDA-MB-231	↓ glucose uptake, lactate production and GLUT1 and GLUT4 mRNA levels	↓ integrin β5/FAK signaling pathway ↓ GLUT1 and GLUT4 mRNA levels	[36]
Sorafenib	7.5 µM (6–24–48 h)	MCF-7 MDA-MB-231 SKBR3	6 h: ↑ glucose uptake, utilization, lactate production (MCF-7 and SKBR3), no effect (MDA-MB-231) 24 h: ↓ glucose uptake and utilization (MCF-7 and SKBR3), ↑ glucose uptake and utilization (MDA-MB-231)	6 h: ↑ GLUT1 protein levels (MCF-7 and SKBR3), no effect (MDA-MB-231) 24 h: ↓ GLUT1 protein levels (MCF-7 and SKBR3), ↑ GLUT1 protein levels (MDA-MB-231) 48: ↓ GLUT1 protein levels (all cell lines) AMPK-dependent inhibition of mTORC1 pathway	[82]
Trastuzumab	initial dose of 4 mg/kg and 2 mg/kg on the 8th and 15th day	xenografts derived from HER2-overexpressing MDA-MB-453 human breast tumour grown in SCID mice	↓ glucose uptake	↓ GLUT1 protein levels	[83]
Doxorrubicin	1 µM (24 h); analysis for 3 d	MCF-7	↓ glucose uptake	↑ GLUT1 mRNA and protein levels	[84]
5-Fluorouracil	200 µM (24 h); analysis for 3 d	MCF-7	↓ glucose uptake	↑ GLUT1 mRNA and protein levels	[84]
Selenium and doxorubicin, free and nanoparticles	Se, nano-Se: 10 µM (24 h) DOX, nano-DOX: 50 µM (24 h)	MCF-7, MDA-MB-231	↑ extracelular glucose levels	-	[85]
Palbociclib + BYL719	0.5 µM palbociclib and 5 µM BYL719 alone or in combination; normoxic or hypoxic conditions (24 h)	MDA-MB-231	Alone: ↓ glucose uptake and consumption When combined: enhancement of effect, in both normoxic and hypoxic conditions	Alone: ↓ GLUT1 protein levels When combined: enhancement of effect, in both normoxic and hypoxic conditions The greater efficacy of the combination ascribed to inhibition of both PI3K/mTOR signaling and c-myc expression	[88]
Palbociclib + paclitaxel	0.5 µM palbociclib and 10 nM paclitaxel alone (48 h) or palbociclib (24 h) + paclitaxel (24 h); normoxic or hypoxic conditions	MDA-MB-231	Alone: ↓ glucose uptake and consumption When combined: enhancement of effect, in both normoxic and hypoxic conditions	Alone: ↓ GLUT1 protein levels When combined: enhancement of effect, in both normoxic and hypoxic conditions The greater efficacy of the combination ascribed to enhancement of inhibition of Rb/E2F/c-myc signaling	[87]
Others					
Tamoxifen	2 µM (72 h)	MCF-7	-	↓ of the ↑ in GLUT1 protein levels induced by E2	[33]
Saracatinib	0.5–1 µM	MCF-10A, MCF12A, with or without HER-2 overexpression	↓ glucose uptake	↓ of ERK1/2-MNK1-eIF4E-mediated cap-dependent translation of c-Myc and transcription of the glucose transporter GLUT1	[93]

Table 1. *Cont.*

Compound	Concentration (Time)	Cell Line/Model	Effect	Mechanism of Action	Ref
RITA, nutlin 3a (P53 activating compounds)	1 μM (8 h)	MCF-7	-	↓ GLUT1 mRNA levels Not related to induction of apoptosis	[94]
Pifithrin-α (PFTα; P53 inhibitor)	Not mentioned	MCF-7	-	↑ GLUT1 mRNA levels, abolishes the effect of RITA on GLUT1 mRNA levels Not related to apoptosis induction	[94]
Wortmannin (PI3K inhibitor)	100 nM (30 min)	T-47D	↔ glucose uptake	-	[98]
Akt1i, Akt2i, Akt1/2i (Akt inhibitors)	10 μM (30 min)	T-47D	↓ glucose uptake	Akt signaling pathway-independent	[98]
PGC1b or HKDC1 shRNA	transfection	MCF-7	↓ glucose uptake	-	[102]
miRNA-34a inhibitor	transfection	BT-20, MDA-MB-231	↓ glucose uptake and GLUT1 protein levels	Inhibition of miRNA34a	[103]
agomiR-186-3p	Systemic delivery of cholesterol-modified agomiR-186-3p	Mice bearing tamoxifen-resistant breast tumors	↓ tumor growth and ^{18}F-FDG uptake	EREG (agonist of EGFR)-mediated	[104]

Legend: ↑, increase; ↓, decrease; ↔ no effect; - not studied.

5.2. *Effect of Endogenous Compounds*

5.2.1. Hormones

Melatonin

Melatonin is produced and secreted by the pineal gland, and modulates several biological pathways in cancer [105]. Interestingly, GLUT1 appears to be involved in the uptake of melatonin into cancer cells and melatonin appears to bind the glucose binding site of the transporter [106]. Despite the lack of reports elucidating the effects of melatonin targeting the Warburg effect in breast cancer cells, an important study using a xenograft breast cancer model found that glucose uptake and lactate production were inversely correlated with melatonin levels during the 12:12 light:dark cycle [107]. In this context, a recent report evaluated the effect of low pH (6.7) on human breast cancer cell lines (MCF-7 and MDA-MB-231), and the effectiveness of melatonin in the acid tumor microenvironment. Melatonin was able to decrease GLUT1 protein expression levels in both cell lines, both at normal (7.2) and acidic pH (6.7). It was concluded that melatonin treatment increases apoptosis and decreases proliferation and GLUT1 protein expression under acute acidosis conditions in breast cancer cell lines [108] (Table 2).

17β-oestradiol

17β-oestradiol or E2 is a steroid hormone, being the main female sexual hormone. Besides its physiological effects, such as maintenance of reproductive cycle and secondary female characteristics, it plays a major role in the carcinogenesis of breast cancer. A few studies evaluated the effect of E2 on glucose uptake be breast cancer cells (Table 2). In a study using MCF-7 cells, E2 was concluded to have no effect on glucose cellular uptake. In this study, E2 increased culture growth, proliferation rates, cellular viability, and lactate production, but did not affect the uptake of glucose nor GLUT1 mRNA levels. So, it was concluded that the pro-proliferative and cytoprotective effects of E2 are not dependent of stimulation of glucose cellular uptake [109]. In contrast, previous studies found E2 to increase the rate of glucose utilization (although glucose uptake levels were not really measured) [110], to increase glucose uptake and expression/translocation of GLUT4 into the plasma membrane (although E2 showed no effect on the expression/translocation of GLUT1) [30,35], and to increase the expression of GLUT1 [33], or to have no effect on GLUT1 expression levels, although higher rates of glucose uptake were found [111]. So, the effect of E2 on glucose uptake and transporter expression needs to be further clarified. Of note, in the work of Rivenzon-Segal et al. [33], tamoxifen had an opposite effect on GLUT1 and treatment of the cells with both E2 and tamoxifen resulted in a partial (±50%) abolishment of the effect of E2 on GLUT1, demonstrating thus the antiestrogenic activity of tamoxifen with regard to GLUT1 expression.

Progesterone

In the work by Medina et al. [30] the effect of progesterone, which also increases the risk of breast cancer, on GLUT expression levels and glucose uptake by ZR-75-1 cells was analyzed (Table 2). This hormone was found to increase glucose uptake and the expression levels of GLUT1, GLUT3 and GLUT4 [30].

Glucocorticoids

Stress has a vast variety of effects in the human body, one of them being the stimulation of the production of adrenocorticotropic hormone by the anterior pituitary gland. This increases secretion of glucocorticoids, steroid hormones that modulate inflammation and the immune system, cell differentiation, and metabolism [112]. Glucocorticoids are often prescribed in chemotherapy treatments in order to avoid hypersensitivity reactions. Therefore, it is important to investigate if it affects treatment. Additionally, glucocorticoids such as dexamethasone may be involved in resistance processes (chemotherapy desensitization) in various types of solid neoplasms, including breast cancer [113]. Dexamethasone (10.7–10.8 μM; 3 days) showed antiproliferative properties on MCF-7 cells [114]. The antiproliferative effect of dexamethasone in MCF-7 cells was confirmed in a later study; this effect was associated with a slight increase in glucose uptake, a strong increase in GLUT4 expression levels and with the formation of adipocyte-like vesicles. In contrast, dexamethasone did not affect MDA-MB-231 cells proliferation, although it slightly increased glucose uptake and strongly increased GLUT4 expression levels. The authors concluded that dexamethasone treatment induces inhibition of cell growth of dexamethasone-sensitive cancer cells by stimulation of differentiation into adipocyte-like cells [112] (Table 2).

KL1

Klotho is a transmembrane protein that can be shed and act as a circulating hormone in three forms: soluble klotho, KL1, and KL2 [115]. Klotho was proposed to be implicated in aging through inhibition of the Insulin-like Growth Factor 1 (IGF-1) pathway, but it also functions as a tumor suppressor in several types of cancer, including breast cancer [116]. This hormone was recently found to decrease glucose uptake and glycolytic flux in MCF-7 cells, but the mechanism of action was not reported [117] (Table 2).

Insulin

Insulin a peptide hormone secreted by the β cells of the pancreatic islets of Langerhans, with an important role in the maintenance of glucose blood levels. Additionally, insulin exhibits potent anabolic properties and has been implicated in many malignancies, including breast cancer [118]. Insulin is also known to be a modifier of cancer cell metabolism. Indeed, it regulates carbohydrate and lipid metabolism, stimulates DNA synthesis, modulates transcription [118], and stimulates the cellular uptake of various nutrients, including glucose, by facilitated diffusion [119]. Agrawal et al. studied the effect of insulin on the sensitivity of a breast cancer cell line (MCF-7) to 5-fluorouracil (5FU) and cyclophosphamide (CPA) [120]. The chemotherapeutic agents 5FU and CPA are widely used in the clinic and incorporated in the treatment of several cancer, including breast cancer, being associated with increased levels of chemoresistance. Insulin was found to increase the cytotoxic effects of 5FU and CPA in vitro up to two-fold. This effect of insulin was linked to enhancement of apoptosis, activation of apoptotic and autophagic pathways, and to overexpression of GLUT1 and GLUT3 as well as to inhibition of cell proliferation and motility (Table 2). Therefore, it was concluded that insulin sensitization before chemotherapy treatment could overcome chemoresistance [120]. The effect of insulin upon GLUT1 and GLUT3 protein expression levels were hypothesized to be mediated by the PI3K-Akt pathway, but the hypothesis was not tested.

5.2.2. Other Endogenous Compounds

Lactic Acid

Besides being a metabolic fuel, lactate is an important signaling molecule in cancer. This compound induces angiogenesis [121], induces HIF1α, which is associated with cancer cell growth and poor prognosis [122], and stimulates folate uptake by breast cancer cells [38]. Lactic acid interferes also with glucose uptake by breast cancer cells, but either a stimulatory [38] or an inhibitory effect [123] were described (Table 2). In the interesting paper of Turkcan et al, single cells from the core of 4T1 and MDA-MB-231 mice large tumors (>8 mm diameter) grafts were found to take up less glucose than those from the periphery. The authors were able to show that this difference was attributed to an inhibitory effect of lactic acid on glucose uptake [123].

Interleukin-4

Cytokines and chemokines in the tumor microenvironment promote breast cancer progression and metastasis. The interleukin-4 (IL4)/IL4Rα immune signaling axis is a direct promoter of survival and proliferation in breast cancer cells [124]. Venmar et al. [124] investigated whether IL4R-mediated metabolic reprogramming could support tumor growth. They verified that promotion of tumor cell survival and proliferation by IL4 involved an increase in glucose uptake and lactate production by murine 4T1 breast cancer cells, associated with an increase in GLUT1 expression, both in vivo and in vitro (Table 2). Moreover, that concluded that, in addition to IL4, there may also be a role for the second IL4Rα-binding cytokine, IL13, in promoting GLUT1 expression through IL4Rα. Importantly, this effect of IL4 on glucose uptake and transporter expression in murine breast cancer cells was not observed in the human MDA-MB-231 cells [124].

Epidermal Growth Factor

Breast cancer that expresses epidermal growth factor receptors (EGFR) is associated with poor patient prognosis, both in TNBC and in non-TNBC subtypes [125]. In breast cancer patients, EGFR expression is strongly correlated with tumor uptake of the glucose analogue, ^{18}F-FDG [126]. An in vitro study with three breast cancer cell lines showed that Epidermal Growth Factor (EGF) stimulated glucose uptake in EGFR-positive T-47D and MDA-MB-468 cells, but not in the weakly EGFR-positive MCF-7 cells. In T-47D cells, the effect was accompanied by upregulated GLUT1 expression and increased lactate production. EGFR stimulation also increased T47D cell proliferation [127] (Table 2).

Table 2. Effect of endogenous compounds on glucose uptake by breast cancer cells.

Compound	Concentration (Time)	Cell Line/Model	Effect	Mechanism of Action	Ref
Hormones					
Melatonin	1 mM (24 h)	MCF-7, MDA-MB-231	-	↓ GLUT1 protein levels (normal and acidic conditions)	[108]
17β-estradiol	3×10^{-8} M (7 days)	T47D-clone 11	↑ glucose utilization	-	[110]
17β-estradiol	10 nM (24 h)	ZR-75-1	↑ glucose (0.1 mM) uptake ↔ glucose (15 mM) uptake	↔ GLUT1, GLUT2, GLUT3 and GLUT4 mRNA levels ↔ GLUT1, GLUT2, GLUT3 protein levels, ↑ GLUT4 protein levels	[30]
17β-estradiol	3×10^{-8}M (72 h)	MCF-7, T47D, ZR-75-1	-	↑ GLUT1 protein levels	[33]
17β-estradiol	10 nM (24 h)	T-47D MDA-MB-231 and MDA-MB-468	↑ glucose uptake and lactate production ↔ glucose uptake	↔ GLUT1 protein levels ER- and PI3K–Akt-dependent Non-genomic, membrane-initiated action	[111]
17β-estradiol	10 nM (25–45 min)	MCF-7	↑ glucose uptake	↑ GLUT4 in plasma membrane (but not total protein levels) ↔ GLUT1 (total and plasma membrane protein levels) ERα- and PI3K-dependent Non-genomic, membrane-initiated action	[35]
17β-estradiol	100 nM (48 h)	MCF-7	↔ glucose uptake	↔ GLUT1 mRNA levels	[109]
Progesterone	10 nM (24 h)	ZR-75-1	↑ glucose (0.1 mM) uptake ↔ glucose (15 mM) uptake	↑ GLUT1 and GLUT3 mRNA levels, ↔ GLUT2 and GLUT4 mRNA levels ↑ GLUT1, GLUT3, and GLUT4 protein levels, ↔ GLUT2 protein levels	[30]
Dexamethasone	1 µg/mL (2 weeks)	MCF-7, MDA-MB-231	Small ↑ in glucose uptake	↑ GLUT4 mRNA levels	[112]
KL-1	Not mentioned	MCF-7	↓ glucose uptake and lactate production	-	[117]
Insulin	40 µg/mL (8 h)	MCF-7	-	↑ GLUT1 and GLUT3 protein levels	[120]
Others					
Lactic acid	10–25 mM (48 h)	Single cells isolated from 4T1 and MDA-MB-231 tumors grafts in mice 4T1 and MDA-MB-231	Single cells from the core of tumors grafts took up less glucose than those from the periphery Lactic acid levels were higher in the core of the tumor ↓ glucose uptake	-	[123]
Lactic acid	10 mM (26 min)	T-47D	↑ glucose uptake	-	[38]
Epidermal growth factor	100 ng/mL (24 h)	T-47D, MDA-MB-468, MCF-7	↑ glucose uptake (T-47D, MDA-MB-468), ↔ glucose uptake (MCF-7) ↑ lactate production (T47D)	↑ GLUT1 protein levels (T47D) PI3 kinase (PI3K) activation	[127]

Legend: ↑, increase; ↓, decrease; ↔ no effect; - not studied.

5.3. *Effect of Exogenous Natural Compounds*

5.3.1. Polyphenols

A large class of GLUT inhibitors is represented by polyphenols, a heterogeneous and large family of natural compounds widely distributed in plants and in the human diet (e.g., in fruits, vegetables and beverages such as tea and wine) [128]. Many of these compounds show an appreciable activity on several distinct membrane transporters, including GLUTs [129,130]. Polyphenols possess anticancer effects in relation to several cancer types, including breast cancer. Several distinct mechanisms are involved in their anticarcinogenic effect in breast cancer: interference with redox balance, pro-apoptotic effect, cell cycle arrest, activation of autophagy, inhibition of angiogenesis, anti-inflammatory effect, anti-estrogenic effect, changes in ER expression, aromatase modulation, interference with HER2 signaling, and effect on microbiota [131,132]. Additionally, some polyphenols interfere with glucose cellular uptake by breast cancer cells [133,134], as next described.

Gossypol

This polyphenolic bisnaphthalene aldehyde obtained from the cotton plant markedly increased both glucose consumption and lactate production in MCF-7 cells, but the increase in glucose consumption may not related to an increase in glucose uptake, and rather be the consequence of increased glycolytic rates or increased rates of glycose oxidation not related to glycolysis (e.g., pentose phosphate pathway) [135] (Table 3).

Naringenin

This grapefruit flavanone inhibited both basal and insulin-stimulated glucose uptake in two breast cancer cell lines (MCF-7 and T-47D). The reduction in insulin-stimulated glucose uptake was not associated with changes in GLUT4 protein levels but rather with inhibition of insulin-stimulated PIP3/Akt and p44/p42 MAPK activity [39]. The antiproliferative effect of naringenin was mimicked by low glucose conditions and so it was concluded that it was dependent on impairment of glucose uptake [39] (Table 3).

Genistein

The flavonoid genistein, found in soybean, reduced glucose uptake in both estrogen receptor-positive MCF-7 and -negative (MDA-MB-231) breast cancer cell lines [136]. The inhibitory effect of genistein upon glucose uptake by MCF-7 cells was later confirmed in two studies. In the first, the effect of genistein, daidzein, and a soy seed extract on two distinct breast cancer cell lines were investigated. In MCF-7 cells, these compounds presented an inhibitory effect on cell proliferation that correlated with a decrease in glucose cellular uptake [137]. In the second, exposure to several polyphenols, including genistein (myricetin, genistein, resveratrol, and kaempferol), was shown to reduce glucose uptake by MCF-7 cells, and genistein inhibited glucose uptake with a 50% Inhibitory Concentration (IC_{50}) of 39 μM [138] (Table 3).

Kaempferol

In the work of Azevedo et al. [138], kaempferol was found to be the most potent inhibitor of glucose uptake, with an IC_{50} of 4 μM. Kaempferol (30 μM) decreased glucose uptake and the GLUT1 transcription level. Moreover, low extracellular glucose mimicked, and high extracellular glucose conditions prevented, the antiproliferative and cytotoxic properties of kaempferol. So, it was suggested that inhibition of GLUT1-mediated glucose cellular uptake mediates the anticancer effect of kaempferol in MCF-7 cells [138] (Table 3).

Resveratrol

An inhibitory effect of resveratrol (IC_{50} = 67 μM), found in fruits such as grapes and berries, upon glucose uptake by breast cancer cells was also described in the work by Azevedo et al. [138]. Moreover, an inhibitory effect of this stilbene was previously described in another breast cancer cell line. Resveratrol (150 μM), suppressed uptake of glucose and glycolysis in T-47D breast cancer cells, associated with a reduction in GLUT1 expression and dependent on a reduction in intracellular ROS levels, which decreases HIF-1α accumulation [139] (Table 3).

Hesperitin

This flavanone, found in citrus fruits, reduced both basal and insulin-stimulated glucose uptake in MDA-MB-231 cells. Of note, the negative effect of hesperitin on basal glucose uptake was associated with GLUT1 downregulation, whereas the negative effect on insulin-induced glucose uptake was associated with impaired GLUT4 translocation to the cell membrane [37] (Table 3).

Quercetin and epigallocatechin-3-gallate (EGCG)

The flavonoids quercetin and EGCG (26 min) concentration-dependently inhibited glucose uptake by MCF-7 (IC_{50} = 11–23 μM) and MDA-MB-231 (IC_{50} = 44–16 μM) cells, respectively, associated with a decrease in lactate production. The effects of quercetin and EGCG were independent of estrogen signaling and did not involve Protein Kinase A (PKA), C (PKC), G (PKG) and calcium-calmodulin. A 4 h exposure to quercetin or EGCG induced also a decrease in glucose uptake, which was associated with an increase in GLUT1 transcription rates. Moreover, an antiproliferative and cytotoxic effect of both compounds was described in MCF-7 cells, which was more potent when extracellular glucose was present. So, inhibition of basal glucose uptake and consequently lactate production were concluded to be determinants of the cytotoxic and antiproliferative effects of quercetin and EGCG in breast cancer cells [40]. The inhibitory effect of quercetin on glucose uptake by breast cancer cells was confirmed in later studies, as shown next. Xintaropoulou et al. [57] verified that inhibition of growth of the HBL100 breast cancer cell line by quercetin (50–150 μM) is associated with an increase in the amount of extracellular glucose and a reduction in lactate production, suggesting inhibition of glucose uptake [57]. Quercetin was also found to decrease the mobility of MCF-7 and MDA-MB-231 cells, associated with a decrease glucose uptake, lactate production and GLUT1 protein levels [140], and to decrease glucose uptake and GLUT1 protein levels in MDA-MB-231 cells [141] (Table 3).

In relation to EGCG, a recent study using rodent 4T1 breast carcinoma cancer cells showed that EGCG inhibits breast cancer growth, both in vitro and in vivo, associated with a reduction in glucose and lactic acid levels and GLUT1 mRNA levels in these cells [142] (Table 3).

Phloretin and Phloridzin

The dihydrochalcone phloretin is found primarily in apples and pears and can also be produced when its glycoside phlorizin is consumed and subsequently nearly entirely converted into phloretin by hydrolytic enzymes in the small intestine. Several studies present evidence for an inhibitory effect of phloretin (and also its glycone phloridzin) in relation to glucose uptake by breast cancer cells. Phloretin and phloridzin were found to decrease glucose uptake by a rat breast adenocarcinoma cell line, both in vivo and in vitro [143]. Phloretin was also suggested to decrease glucose uptake (as assessed by the increase in the amount of extracellular glucose and the decrease in the amount of lactate produced) associated with an antiproliferative effect in HBL100, but not MCF-7 cell line [57]. Finally, inhibition of GLUT2 by phloretin was concluded to potentially suppress MDA-MB-231 cell growth and metastasis, although phloretin was found to increase GLUT2 protein levels. The authors concluded that phloretin treatment inhibited uptake of glucose, and, as a consequence, increased GLUT2 protein expression was required for cancer cell survival [63]. In relation to phloridzin, it reduced glucose uptake in several breast cancer cell lines, either alone [38,40] or associated with cytochalasin B [138] (Table 3).

Glabridin

This flavonoid decreased glucose uptake and lactate production, possibly mediated by a decrease in GLUT1 protein levels, in MDA-MB-231 cells [141] (Table 3).

(+)-Catechin

The anticancer efficacy of polyphenols can be enhanced by combining them with compounds such as amino acids and vitamins [144]. In this context, a catechin:Lys complex (Cat:Lys 1:2) was recently tested in MCF-7 and MDA-MB-231 breast cancer cell lines and in the non-tumorigenic breast (MCF12A) cell line. Cat:Lys (24 h) decreased glucose uptake and lactate production in MCF-7 cells but increased glucose uptake and lactate production in MDA-MB-231 and MCF12A cells. Cat:lys (24 h) was also found to increase GLUT1 mRNA expression levels in MDA-MB-231 cells. In contrast, a shorter-term exposure (26 min) of these cell lines to Cat:Lys caused an increase in glucose uptake in MDA-MB-231 and MCF12A cells but no effect on MCF-7 cells [145]. In contrast, (+)-catechin was found to increase glucose uptake by MCF-7 cells [138]. Moreover, in the work of Silva et al. [145], by using a GLUT inhibitor, it was concluded that: (a) there is a contribution of a GLUT-mediated mechanism in glucose uptake in the three breast cell lines, (b) Cat:Lys stimulates GLUT-mediated glucose uptake in MDA-MB-231 and MCF12A cell lines, and (c) Cat:Lys inhibits non-GLUT-mediated glucose uptake in MCF-7 cells, a conclusion that was supported by the results of GLUT1 mRNA expression. So, Cat:Lys shows no consistent effects on glucose uptake by the breast cell lines (Table 3). Thus, apparently, its antitumoral effect is not related to an effect on glucose uptake, because Cat:Lys showed a similar antiproliferative, cytotoxic, antimigratory, and proapoptotic effect on both cancer cell lines and a much less evident effect in the non-tumorigenic cell line [145].

Polyphenolic Esters

Zhang et al. [146] reported inhibition of basal glucose transport in MCF-7 cells and other cell lines (including H1299 lung cancer cell line) by synthesized polyphenolic esters. Although not tested in breast cancer cells, these basal glucose transport inhibitors also inhibited H1299 cell growth, and these two activities appear to be correlated (Table 3).

Curcumin

Very recently, the effect of curcumin (diferuloylmethane), a well-known phytopolyphenolic compound isolated from rhizome of the plant *Curcuma longa* was evaluated and this compound was found to reduce glucose uptake and lactate production in a variety of cancer cell lines, including in MCF-7 cells [147]. Curcumin was concluded to inhibit aerobic glycolysis by downregulating pyruvate kinase M2 expression, which drives the Warburg effect and thus is essential for survival of cancer cells. Nevertheless, a direct effect of curcumin on glucose transporters was not investigated [147] (Table 3).

Cardamonin

This chalcone, isolated from *Alpiniae katsumadai*, reduced glucose uptake as well as lactate production and efflux in the breast cancer MDA-MB-231 cell line [148] (Table 3).

Plant Extracts

Some studies have investigated the effect of plant extracts rather than the effect of individual compounds (Table 3). In one study, *Baeckea frutescens* leaves extracts were found to decrease glucose uptake in two breast cancer cell lines (MCF-7 and MDA-MB-231), associated with a cytotoxic and proapoptotic effect. Importantly, the extracts were devoid of cytotoxic effect in the non-tumoral breast cell line MCF10A and were also devoid of effect on glucose uptake [149]. In another study, an extract of *Petiveria alliacea* leaves and stems reduced glucose uptake and lactate production in the 4T1 breast cell line. However, glucose levels in supernatant, rather than direct measurement of glucose uptake, were measured [150]. Finally, an extract of Kudingcha leaves, one of the *Ligustrum robustum* species, was described to concentration-dependently reduce GLUT1 and GLUT3 protein expression levels and lactate production in two triple-negative breast cancer cell lines [151].

5.3.2. Other Exogenous Natural Compounds

Cytochalasin B

The macrocyclic mycotoxin cytochalasin B is a known GLUT inhibitor used extensively in the literature of GLUT investigation. Cytochalasin is a GLUT1, GLUT2, and GLUT4 inhibitor [152,153]. This compound has been described to interfere also with glucose uptake in several breast cancer cell lines: T-47D [38,98] and MCF-7 and MDA-MB-231 [40] (Table 3).

Genipin

Genipin, an aglycone derived from an iridoid glycoside called geniposide extracted from gardenia fruits, caused a decrease in glucose uptake by the breast cancer cells T-47D and MDA-MB-435, although no effect on MCF-7 and MDA-MB-231 cells was found (Table 3). The effect of genipin was most pronounced in the T-47D cell line; in this cell line, an IC_{50} = 61 μM was calculated and a decrease in lactate production was also found. In this report, genipin was concluded to decrease cancer cell glucose uptake by reducing both glycolytic flux and mitochondrial oxidative phosphorylation, an effect that was related to inhibition of Uncoupling Protein 2 (UCP2)-mediated dissipation of energy and restriction of ROS production through proton leakage [154]. However, an effect of genipin on glucose transporters cannot be excluded.

Cantharidin

This sesquiterpenoid bioactive compound is secreted by beetles of the family of Meloidae [155]. Although it has been available for almost a century, its use has not been approved due to its high toxicity to the gastrointestinal tract. However, new anticarcinogenic properties have been found. In a recent study, cantharidin was found to inhibit aerobic glycolysis, associated with a decrease in GLUT1 protein expression levels. It was concluded that cantharidin inhibits nuclear translocation of pyruvate kinase isoform M2 (PKM2), which promotes the transcription of GLUT1. So, cantharidin interferes with the glycolytic metabolic loop between GLUT1 and PKM2 [155] (Table 3).

Betulinic Acid (BA)

BA is a natural pentacyclic terpene reported to be capable of inhibiting various malignancies. BA was recently reported to decrease the viability of breast cancer cell lines MCF-7 and MDA-MB-231, being ineffective against the non-malignant mammary epithelial cell line MCF-10A, indicating that BA might be a highly selective killing agent toward malignant cells. BA was shown to decrease glucose uptake and lactate production in the two cancer cell lines, but it was concluded that suppression of the glycolytic activity mainly occurred at the intracellular level, and no further investigation of its effect upon glucose uptake was done [156] (Table 3).

Benzyl Isothiocyanate (BITC)

Data from numerous preclinical studies advocate BITC, an aromatic isothiocyanate, which occurs naturally in edible cruciferous vegetables, promising for breast cancer chemoprevention [157]. This compound was described to increase glucose uptake by breast cancer cells, both in vivo and in vitro. This effect is probably a compensatory mechanism in response to inhibition of complex III of the mitochondrial respiratory chain and of oxidative phosphorylation caused by this compound [158]. Moreover the effect of BITC upon glucose uptake was found to be dependent on Akt activation (Table 3). So, these results indicate that BITC increased glucose uptake/metabolism in breast cancer cells and suggest that breast cancer chemoprevention by BITC may be augmented by pharmacological inhibition of Akt [159].

Docosahexaenoic Acid (DHA)

n-3 polyunsaturated fatty acids (PUFAs) have been proposed to have anticancer properties, and the effects on cancer cell metabolism constitutes one possible mechanism contributing to their anticancer effect [160]. The effect of DHA on breast cancer and non-cancer cell lines was evaluated (Table 3). It was concluded that DHA contributes to impaired cancer cell growth and survival by altering cancer cell metabolism, including by causing a decrease in glucose uptake, while not affecting non-transformed cells [161].

Vitamin D3 (VD3)

VD3, the bioactive form of Vitamin D, is known to be an important modulator of bone metabolism and diabetes, amongst many other effects. Low levels of VD3 are linked with an increased risk of cancer, whilst high levels of vitamin D3 usually promise better prognosis [162]. Although its positive effects have been shown, not much is known as to the mechanisms involved. Santos et al [163] tested the effect of VD3 on MCF-7 and MDA-MB-231 cells. VD3 significantly reduced GLUT1 mRNA and protein levels and glucose uptake in both cell types. Moreover, lactate production in the highly metastatic MDA-MB-231 cells was significantly reduced (Table 3). This study proved that VD3 decreased breast cancer cell viability along with reduced expression of GLUT1 and key glycolytic enzymes (hexokinase II and lactate dehydrogenase A), causing a decrease in glucose uptake.

γ-Tocotrienol

This member of the vitamin E family of compounds displays potent anticancer effects at doses having little or no effect on normal cell viability [164]. To test the role of glycolysis in the effect caused by γ-tocotrienol, Parajuli et al. [165] used the MCF-7 breast cancer cell line. γ-tocotrienol was found to decrease MCF-7 cell growth, coincident with a concentration-dependent decrease in glucose consumption and lactate production. This effect was correlated with a decrease in the expression of glycolytic enzymes (HK-II, PFK, PKM2, and LDHA) and MCT1, but the compound did not affect GLUT1 expression levels. So, GLUT1 reduction was not considered the mediator of the glycolysis inhibition caused by γ-tocotrienol [165] (Table 3).

d-Allose

This compound, a C-3 epimer of d-glucose with 80% of the sweetness of sucrose, exists in small quantities in nature. This compound is known to possess anticarcinogenic properties via upregulation of thioredoxin interacting protein (TXNIP) [166]. A study involving breast adenocarcinoma, hepatocellular carcinoma, and neuroblastoma cell lines concluded that d-allose downregulates GLUT1 expression and consequently glucose uptake, thus suppressing cancer cell growth, as a result of overexpression of TXNIP [166] (Table 3).

Table 3. Effect of exogenous compounds on glucose uptake by breast cancer cells.

Compound	Concentration (Time)	Cell Line/Model	Effect	Mechanism of Action	Ref
Polyphenols					
Gossypol	10 μM (25 h)	MCF-7	↑ glucose consumption and lactate production ↔ ratio lactate produced/glucose consumed	Quasi-competitive inhibition	[135]
Naringenin	10 μM (15 min)	MCF-7, T-47D	↓ basal and insulin-stimulated glucose uptake	Inhibition of PI3K, Akt, and MAPK pathways	[39]
Genistein	10–100 μM (10 min)	MCF-7, MDA-MB-231	↓ glucose uptake	-	[136]
Genistein, daidzein and a soy seed extract	22 μM, 52 μM and 166 μg/mL, respectively (72 h)	MCF-7, MDA-MB-231	↓ glucose uptake	-	[137]
Myricetin, resveratrol genistein, kaempferol	10–100 μM (26 min)	MCF-7	↓ glucose uptake	Mixed-type inhibition for kaempferol	[138]
Catechin	100 μM (26 min)	MCF-7	↑ glucose uptake	-	[138]
Resveratrol	150 μM (24 h)	T-47D	↓ glucose uptake	↓ GLUT 1 protein levels ↓ intracellular ROS causing ↓ of HIF-1α accumulation	[139]
Hesperetin	50–100 μM (24 h)	MDA-MB-231	↓ basal glucose uptake ↓ insulin-stimulated glucose uptake	↓ GLUT 1 mRNA and protein levels ↓ GLUT4 cell membrane translocation	[37]
Quercetin and EGCG	1–500 μM (26 min) 1–100 μM (4 h)	MCF-7, MDA-MB-231	↓ glucose uptake	Competitive, independent of PKA, PKC, PKG, and calcium-calmodulin intracellular pathways	[40]
Quercetin, Phloretin	50–150 μM (24 h)	HBL100	↓ glucose uptake	-	[57]
Quercetin	30 μM (6.5 h)	MCF-7, MDA-MB-231	↓ glucose uptake, ↓ lactate production	↓ GLUT1 protein levels	[140]
Quercetin	Not mentioned	MDA-MB-231	↓ glucose uptake, ↔ lactate production	↓ GLUT1 protein levels	[141]
Glabridin	Not mentioned	MDA-MB-231	↓ glucose uptake, ↓ lactate production	↓ GLUT1 protein levels	[141]
Phloretin and phloridzin	Not mentioned	Rat mammary adenocarcinoma	↓ glucose uptake in vitro and in vivo	-	[143]
Phloretin	10–150 μM (16 h)	MDA-MB-231	-	↑ GLUT2 protein levels	[167]
Phloridzin	1 mM (26 min)	T-47D	↓ glucose uptake	-	[38]
Phloridzin	0.5–1 mM (26 min)	MCF-7, MDA-MB-231	↓ glucose uptake	-	[40]

Table 3. *Cont.*

Compound	Concentration (Time)	Cell Line/Model	Effect	Mechanism of Action	Ref
Phloridzin + Cytochalasin B	0.5 mM and 50 µM, respectively (26 min)	MCF-7	↓ glucose uptake	-	[138]
EGCG	20–240 µM (24 h) 20–80 µM (24 h) 20 mg/kg (mice)	4T1	↓ glucose and lactic acid levels ↓ glucose and lactic acid levels in tumour	↓ GLUT1 mRNA levels	[142]
Cat:Lys (1:2) complex	0.01–5 mM (26 min)	MCF-7, MDA-MB-231 and MCF12A	↑ glucose uptake (MDA-MB-231 and MCF12A) ↔ glucose uptake (MCF-7)	-	[145]
Cat:Lys (1:2) complex	0.01–1 mM (24 h)	MCF-7, MDA-MB-231 and MCF12A	↑ glucose uptake and lactate production (MDA-MB-231 and MCF12A) ↓ glucose uptake and lactate production (MCF-7)	↑ GLUT1 mRNA levels (MDA-MB-231) ↔ GLUT1 mRNA levels (MCF-7 and MCF12A)	[145]
Compound 1a and 2a (polyphenolic esters)	30 µM (15 min)	MCF-7	↓ glucose uptake	-	[146]
Curcumin	20 µM (24 h)	MCF-7	↓ glucose uptake and lactate production	-	[147]
Cardamonin	20–80 µM (6 h)	MDA-MB-231	↓ glucose uptake and lactate production	-	[148]
Baeckea frutescens extracts	IC50 = 10–127 µg/mL (MCF-7 cells; 72 h)	MCF-7, MDA-MB-231	↓ glucose uptake	-	[149]
Petiveria alliacea extract	3 µg/mL (48 h)	4T1	↓ glucose uptake	-	[150]
Kudingcha extract	100–200 µg/mL (48 h)	MDA-MB-231, HCC1806	- Decrease in lactate levels	↓ GLUT1 and GLUT3 protein levels	[151]
Others					
Cytochalasin B	25 µM (30 min)	T-47D	↓ glucose uptake	-	[98]
Cytochalasin B	50–100 µM (26 min)	T-47D	↓ glucose uptake	-	[38]
Cytochalasin B	10–50 µM (26 min)	MCF-7, MDA-MB-231	↓ glucose uptake	-	[40]
Cantharidin	0.5–2 µM (24 h)	MCF-7, MDA-MB-231	↓ glucose consumption and lactate production	↓ GLUT1 protein levels	[155]
Betulinic acid	5–40 µM (3 h)	MCF-7, MDA-MB-231	↓ glucose uptake and lactate production	-	[156]
Genipin	50–100 µM (24 h)	T-47D, MDA-MB-435 MCF-7, MDA-MB-231	↓ glucose uptake ↔ glucose uptake	-	[154]
Benzyl isothiocyanate	3 mmol/kg diet 2.5 µM (24 h)	MMTV-neu mice mammary tumours MDA-MB-231, SUM159	↑ glucose uptake ↑ glucose uptake	↑ GLUT1 total and membrane-located protein levels Dependent on Akt activation	[159]

Table 3. *Cont.*

Compound	Concentration (Time)	Cell Line/Model	Effect	Mechanism of Action	Ref
Docosahexaenoic acid	100 μM (48 h)	MDA-MB-231, BT-474, MCF-10A	↓ glucose uptake and metabolism (MDA-MB-231, BT-474) ↔ glucose uptake and metabolism (MCF10A)	-	[161]
Vitamin D_3	0.5–1 μM (24 h)	MCF-7, MDA-MB-231	↓ glucose uptake (both cell lines) ↓ lactate production (MDA-MB-231 cells)	↓ GLUT1 mRNA and protein levels (both cell lines) AMPK-dependent inhibition of mTOR (?)	[163]
γ-Tocotrienol	6–8 μM (96 h)	MCF-7	↓ glucose consumption and lactate production	↔ GLUT1 mRNA levels	[165]
d-allose	50 mM (7 days)	MDA-MB-231	-	↑ GLUT1 mRNA and protein levels Mediated by overexpression of TXNIP	[166]

Legend: ↑, increase; ↓, decrease; ↔ no effect; - not studied.

6. Effect of Stimulation of the Interaction of Anticancer Agents with GLUT

Conjugation of anticancer agents with glucose or other sugars is a widely exploited technique to design therapeutic agents, in order to improve their uptake into highly glycolytic cancer cells overexpressing GLUTs, thus increasing efficacy while reducing side effects. One possibility is to develop sugar-conjugated agents that can be transported into cancer cells through GLUT without inhibiting GLUTs themselves [168]. Another possibility is to promote interaction of anticancer agents with GLUT by their conjugation with an anti-GLUT antibody. Some of these agents have been tested in breast cancer cell lines, as shown next.

6.1. Adriamycin

Adriamycin (doxorubicin) is effective against many types of solid tumors in clinical applications. However, its use is limited because of systemic toxicity and multidrug resistance. Adriamycin conjugated with a glucose analogue (2-amino-2-deoxy-d-glucose) and succinic acid (2DG-SUC-ADM) was designed to target tumor cells through GLUT1, thus enhancing the selectivity of doxorubicin against cancer cells while reducing its toxicity to healthy cells [169]. In a work using several cancer cell lines, including MCF-7 and MDA-MB-231 cell lines, the complex showed better inhibition to tumor cells and lower toxicity to normal cells, and, most importantly, displayed a potential to reverse multidrug resistance. In vivo experiments also showed that this new complex could significantly decrease organ toxicity and enhance the antitumor efficacy compared with free ADM, indicating 2DG-SUC-ADM as a promising drug for targeted cancer therapy [169]. The GLUT1-mediated transport into the cells explained the specificity of 2DG-SUC-ADM, because uptake of free doxorubicin mainly occurred through diffusion, whereas the uptake of 2DG-SUC-ADM was mostly GLUT1-mediated [169].

Sztandera et al. [170] developed a glucose-modified PAMAM dendrimer for the delivery of doxorubicin (dox) to breast cancer cells, designed to specifically enter tumor cell with enhanced glucose uptake. They verified that PAMAM-dox-glucose conjugate exhibited pH-dependent drug release and an increased cytotoxic activity compared to free drug in MCF-7 cells, in the absence of glucose. They also verified that GLUT1 inhibition eliminated the toxic effect of the conjugate. So, they concluded that the cytotoxic effect of PAMAM-dox-glucose depends on presence of a functional GLUT1, suggesting specific, transporter-dependent internalization as a main route of cellular uptake of glucose-conjugated PAMAM dendrimers [170].

6.2. Paclitaxel

This drug is widely used for the treatment of breast, ovarian, and lung carcinomas, but its low water solubility severely reduces its clinical application. In this context, a new prodrug was designed to enhance its solubility and its selective delivery to cancer by a preferential uptake via GLUTs. More specifically, the glycoconjugation of paclitaxel led to a derivative in which the drug was linked to 1-methyl glucose via a short succinic acid linker. The resulting compound, whose transport was mediated at least in part by GLUT1, showed a comparable cytotoxicity against several cancer cells without toxicity on normal cells. Of note, paclitaxel linked to succinic acid resulted in a lower toxicity against MCF-7 cells than the parent compound, suggesting that the presence of glucose improved its cytotoxicity [171].

6.3. Oxiplatin

The platinum antitumor drug oxaliplatin is a commonly used chemotherapeutic agent; however, its multiple side effects severely limit its benefits. The conjugation with sugar portions was introduced as a strategy to improve the tumor-targeting ability of the drug and also to enhance its water solubility, allowing renal excretion and lower systemic toxicity. A glycosylated (trans-R,R-cyclohexane-1,2-diamine)-malonatoplatinum(II) derivative showed increased cytotoxicity compared to oxaliplatin in all the tested human carcinoma cell lines. Its potency was prevented when human colon cancer (HT29) and breast cancer (MCF-7) cells, which overexpress GLUTs, were treated with the GLUT inhibitor phlorizin, thus confirming that the uptake and the antiproliferative activity of this compound are GLUT-mediated [172].

In summary, a great potential of GLUT-mediated transport of therapeutics into cancer cells opens new roads for targeted delivery of anticancer drugs.

7. Conclusions and Future Perspectives

Despite the high-survival rate in breast cancer patients and the availability of well-designed and effective therapeutic strategies, especially for hormone receptor or HER2-positive breast cancer, more drug research is still needed, particularly regarding triple-negative breast cancer, because of its unresponsiveness to hormone or anti-HER2 therapy. In this context, metabolic targeting of tumors, and more specifically targeting GLUT1-mediated glucose transport, constitutes an interesting approach. In addition to GLUT1, there are a several other potential cancer therapies that target the cellular energetic metabolism pathway in tumors. Indeed, many compounds targeting energy metabolism are currently in trial or approved as therapeutic agents for cancer [48,49]. Preclinical data from these inhibitors are encouraging; therefore, they represent additional options for targeting the enhanced aerobic glycolysis in cancer.

In this review, we show that a wide range of compounds, ranging from endogenous to dietary compounds and synthetic compounds, are able to interfere with glucose uptake by breast cancer cells. Moreover, for some of the presented compounds, their antitumoral effect is concluded to result from the effect on glucose uptake. Since cancer cells are highly dependent on glucose, even if these compounds possess other anticancer-inducing mechanisms, their effect on glucose uptake certainly contributes to their antitumoral effect.

The mechanisms underlying the modulatory effect of the compounds upon glucose uptake are very diverse, ranging from a direct effect upon the transporter, inhibition of transporter gene expression or protein synthesis, impairment of membrane insertion of the transporter, and redox balance modulation. Additionally, the effect of compounds on glucose uptake may be secondary to a decrease in the activity of glycolytic enzymes or signaling pathways. However, it should be pointed out that, for most of the presented compounds, the mechanisms underlying their modulatory effect upon glucose uptake by breast cancer cells have not been investigated. So, more research is needed in this area. A better knowledge of the mechanisms able to interfere with glucose transporter function in cancer cells may open new windows for therapeutic targets in breast cancer.

Most studies on GLUTs in cancer are focused on their role and regulation in the tumor cells. However, solid tumors are composed of several cell types, forming a dynamic and complex network. In this context, a role for GLUT1 in glycolytic reprograming enabling survival, growth, and expansion of effector T lymphocytes has been demonstrated [173]. T lymphocytes in tumors constitute a primary cellular target for immunotherapies including adoptive T cell therapy and immune checkpoint blockade. Moreover, GLUT1 induction was observed in human fibroblasts placed in contact with prostate cancer cells [174]. Cancer-associated fibroblasts (CAFs) are known to promote tumor growth, invasion, chemoresistance, and angiogenesis. So, the requirements for glucose entry and usage by cancer-supporting or cancer-antagonizing cells add on to the complexity of metabolic rewiring in cancer.

Metabolic targeting of tumors using GLUT inhibitors has attracted more and more attention in the past years, which can be demonstrated by the growing number and more recent publications on this subject. Most therapeutic strategies that are being developed to target GLUTs in cancer are in the preclinical phase of drug development. These preclinical data suggest that inactivation of GLUT1, leading to glucose starvation that ultimately leads to cell death, is a viable drug target for cancer therapy [52,175].

Regrettably, therapies designed to target this pathway have not been fully translated to the clinic yet, and clinical trials in cancer patients using GLUT inhibitors to ensure their safety and/or efficacy are still largely lacking. One of the major obstacles to the success of GLUT1-based therapies is the potential systemic toxicity, because GLUT1 is ubiquitously expressed in mammalian tissues. Although it is expected that targeting GLUT1-mediated glucose uptake will have a much more marked effect on cancer cells than in non-cancer cells, because cancer cells are much more sensitive to glucose deprivation than normal cells, a certain degree of side effects may be expected, especially those occurring in organs characterized by high glucose-consumption rates such as the brain, immune system and stem cells. One example is the observation that several glucose transport inhibitors, tested in phase I clinical trials for hepatocellular and prostate cancer, were associated with significant side effects [176]. So, selective blockade of GLUTs in tumor cells still remains a key challenge and research on this subject should be fostered in the near future.

In this context, important points should be considered in future research:

(1). Development of cancer-specific and potent GLUT inhibitors that minimize side effects;

(2). Development of selective targeted delivery of GLUT inhibitors (using recent imaging technology) directly into the tumor or intra-arterially near the tumor, or micro-encapsulation of the inhibitor [52];

(3). More studies on GLUT regulation and function in vivo should be conducted;

(4). Studies on multi-targeted inhibition, allowing lower doses of GLUT inhibitors to be used. For instance, the preliminary results from clinical trials of 2-DG as a monotherapy are inconclusive and ambiguous, with toxic and side effects being reported [49,177]. Currently, 2-DG was reintroduced for use in combination approach, as reported in more recent preclinical and clinical studies, using 2-DG at lower doses to produce synergistic anticancer effects with other chemotherapeutic agents or irradiation. Thus, combination treatments using 2-DG may have encouraging outcomes providing a new opportunity for cancer combination therapy [52,175];

(5). An accurate verification and analysis of the transporter expression profiles, because cancers are extremely heterogeneous diseases and they have unique metabolic features. Moreover, abnormal glycolysis due to defects of mitochondrial oxidative phosphorylation is not absolutely common in spontaneous tumors [8,178];

(6). Many natural compounds interfere with glucose uptake at higher than dietary/physiological concentrations (e.g., polyphenols). For some dietary compounds, these concentrations are not attainable even after the consumption of food supplements due to reduced bioavailability and/or metabolism of these compounds. For these compounds (a) improvement of their bioavailability and delivery, as it would result in the improvement of their biological effects in vivo, (b) the use of natural or synthetic analogs that have better bioavailability or more potency, or (c) combination with other glucose transport inhibitors or with conventional therapy, resulting in a synergistic effect or in improvements of its bioavailability [144,179] are possible strategies.

(7). Resistance resulting from the treatment with GLUT inhibitors, involving development of different routes for energy supply using other energy substrates, is another issue that should not be underestimated. Indeed, cancer cells display metabolic plasticity and can overcome the inhibition of a specific metabolic pathway via the expression or up-regulation of alternative pathways. Moreover, adjacent cells such as fibroblasts can offer metabolic intermediates for the needs of cancer cells. To overcome this problem, combination of other targeted therapy drugs with GLUT inhibitors may be an effective way [180]. Alternatively, combination of two or more antimetabolic agents inhibiting different metabolic pathways simultaneously would decrease resistance and prevent relapse [52].

(8). Research focused on the design of GLUT-transportable chemotherapeutics, which may provide therapeutic selectivity [180];

(9). Characterization of glucose transporters in tumors treated with immunotherapies, to determine if their expression in tumor cells or cells of the tumor environment changes upon treatment, and if their activity is linked to the outcome of therapy [181];

(10). Research focused on overcoming side effects that are expected, especially those occurring in organs such as the brain. In this context, it is known that, in starvation, ketone bodies can replace glucose as fuel for the brain. Therefore, a combined administration of GLUT-interfering agents with either a ketogenic diet or dietary supplements such as triheptanoin (which is currently being tested for the treatment of GLUT1 deficiency [182]), should improve the safety profile of these compounds [53].

In conclusion, in this review we show that several chemically distinct compounds interfere with glucose uptake by breast cancer cells, and these GLUT inhibitors should be used as starting point in future research, which should focus in developing new compounds/combinations/delivery methods to solve specific problems already identified.

References

1. Bray, F.F.J.; Soerjomataram, I.; Siegel, R.L.; Torre, L.A.; Jemal, A. GLOBOCAN estimates of incidence and mortality worldwide for 36 cancers in 185 countries. *CA Cancer J. Clin.* **2018**, *68*, 394–424. [CrossRef] [PubMed]
2. Rossi, L.; Stevens, D.; Pierga, J.Y.; Lerebours, F.; Reyal, F.; Robain, M.; Asselain, B.; Rouzier, R. Impact of adjuvant chemotherapy on breast cancer survival: A real-world population. *PLoS ONE* **2015**, *10*, e0132853. [CrossRef] [PubMed]
3. Coleman, M.P.; Quaresma, M.; Berrino, F.; Lutz, J.M.; de Angelis, R.; Capocaccia, R.; Baili, P.; Rachet, B.; Gatta, G.; Hakulinen, T.; et al. Cancer survival in five continents: A worldwide population-based study (CONCORD). *Lancet Oncol.* **2008**, *9*, 730–756. [CrossRef]
4. Hanahan, D.; Weinberg, R.A. Hallmarks of cancer: The next generation. *Cell* **2011**, *144*, 646–674. [CrossRef]
5. Warburg, O. On the origin of cancer cells. *Science* **1956**, *123*, 309–314. [CrossRef]
6. Aykin-Burns, N.; Ahmad, I.M.; Zhu, Y.; Oberley, L.W.; Spitz, D.R. Increased levels of superoxide and H_2O_2 mediate the differential susceptibility of cancer cells versus normal cells to glucose deprivation. *Biochem. J.* **2009**, *418*, 29–37. [CrossRef]
7. Yun, J.; Rago, C.; Cheong, I.; Pagliarini, R.; Angenendt, P.; Rajagopalan, H.; Schmidt, K.; Willson, J.K.; Markowitz, S.; Zhou, S.; et al. Glucose deprivation contributes to the development of KRAS pathway mutations in tumor cells. *Science* **2009**, *325*, 1555–1559. [CrossRef]
8. Pavlides, S.; Whitaker-Menezes, D.; Castello-Cros, R.; Flomenberg, N.; Witkiewicz, A.K.; Frank, P.G.; Casimiro, M.C.; Wang, C.; Fortina, P.; Addya, S.; et al. The reverse Warburg effect: Aerobic glycolysis in cancer associated fibroblasts and the tumor stroma. *Cell Cycle* **2009**, *8*, 3984–4001. [CrossRef]
9. Sotgia, F.; Martinez-Outschoorn, U.E.; Pavlides, S.; Howell, A.; Pestell, R.G.; Lisanti, M.P. Understanding the Warburg effect and the prognostic value of stromal caveolin-1 as a marker of a lethal tumor microenvironment. *Breast Cancer Res.* **2011**, *13*, e213. [CrossRef]
10. Sun, K.; Tang, S.; Hou, Y.; Xi, L.; Chen, Y.; Yin, J.; Peng, M.; Zhao, M.; Cui, X.; Liu, M. Oxidized ATM-mediated glycolysis enhancement in breast cancer-associated fibroblasts contributes to tumor invasion through lactate as metabolic coupling. *EBioMedicine* **2019**, *41*, 370–383. [CrossRef]
11. Gonzalez, C.D.; Alvarez, S.; Ropolo, A.; Rosenzvit, C.; Bagnes, M.F.; Vaccaro, M.I. Autophagy, Warburg, and Warburg reverse effects in human cancer. *Biomed Res. Int.* **2014**, *2014*, e926729. [CrossRef] [PubMed]
12. Martinez-Outschoorn, U.E.; Lin, Z.; Ko, Y.H.; Goldberg, A.F.; Flomenberg, N.; Wang, C.; Pavlides, S.; Pestell, R.G.; Howell, A.; Sotgia, F.; et al. Understanding the metabolic basis of drug resistance: Therapeutic induction of the Warburg effect kills cancer cells. *Cell Cycle* **2011**, *10*, 2521–2528. [CrossRef] [PubMed]
13. Szablewski, L. Expression of glucose transporters in cancers. *Biochim. Biophys. Acta* **2013**, *1835*, 164–169. [CrossRef] [PubMed]
14. Wright, E.M.; Loo, D.D.; Hirayama, B.A. Biology of human sodium glucose transporters. *Physiol. Rev.* **2011**, *91*, 733–794. [CrossRef]

15. Wright, E.M.; Turk, E. The sodium/glucose cotransport family SLC5. *Pflugers Arch.* **2004**, *447*, 510–518. [CrossRef]
16. Koepsell, H. The Na(+)-D-glucose cotransporters SGLT1 and SGLT2 are targets for the treatment of diabetes and cancer. *Pharmacol. Ther.* **2017**, *170*, 148–165. [CrossRef]
17. Mueckler, M.; Thorens, B. The SLC2 (GLUT) family of membrane transporters. *Mol. Aspects Med.* **2013**, *34*, 121–138. [CrossRef]
18. Macheda, M.L.; Rogers, S.; Best, J.D. Molecular and cellular regulation of glucose transporter (GLUT) proteins in cancer. *J. Cell Physiol.* **2005**, *202*, 654–662. [CrossRef]
19. Medina, R.A.; Owen, G.I. Glucose transporters: Expression, regulation and cancer. *Biol. Res.* **2002**, *35*, 9–26. [CrossRef]
20. Furuta, E.; Okuda, H.; Kobayashi, A.; Watabe, K. Metabolic genes in cancer: Their roles in tumor progression and clinical implications. *Biochim. Biophys. Acta* **2010**, *1805*, 141–152. [CrossRef]
21. Grover-McKay, M.; Walsh, S.A.; Seftor, E.A.; Thomas, P.A.; Hendrix, M.J. Role for glucose transporter 1 protein in human breast cancer. *Pathol. Oncol. Res.* **1998**, *4*, 115–120. [CrossRef] [PubMed]
22. Lopez-Lazaro, M. The Warburg effect: Why and how do cancer cells activate glycolysis in the presence of oxygen? *Anticancer Agents Med. Chem.* **2008**, *8*, 305–312. [CrossRef] [PubMed]
23. Wuest, M.; Hamann, I.; Bouvet, V.; Glubrecht, D.; Marshall, A.; Trayner, B.; Soueidan, O.M.; Krys, D.; Wagner, M.; Cheeseman, C.; et al. Molecular Imaging of GLUT1 and GLUT5 in breast cancer: A multitracer positron emission tomography imaging study in mice. *Mol. Pharmacol.* **2018**, *93*, 79–89. [CrossRef]
24. Zhao, F.Q. Biology of glucose transport in the mammary gland. *J. Mammary Gland Biol. Neoplasia* **2014**, *19*, 3–17. [CrossRef] [PubMed]
25. Zhao, F.Q.; Keating, A.F. Expression and regulation of glucose transporters in the bovine mammary gland. *J. Dairy Sci.* **2007**, *90* (Suppl. 1), 76–86. [CrossRef]
26. Wellberg, E.A.; Johnson, S.; Finlay-Schultz, J.; Lewis, A.S.; Terrell, K.L.; Sartorius, C.A.; Abel, E.D.; Muller, W.J.; Anderson, S.M. The glucose transporter GLUT1 is required for ErbB2-induced mammary tumorigenesis. *Breast Cancer Res.* **2016**, *18*, e131. [CrossRef]
27. Young, C.D.; Lewis, A.S.; Rudolph, M.C.; Ruehle, M.D.; Jackman, M.R.; Yun, U.J.; Ilkun, O.; Pereira, R.; Abel, E.D.; Anderson, S.M. Modulation of glucose transporter 1 (GLUT1) expression levels alters mouse mammary tumor cell growth in vitro and in vivo. *PLoS ONE* **2011**, *6*, e23205. [CrossRef]
28. Pinheiro, C.; Sousa, B.; Albergaria, A.; Paredes, J.; Dufloth, R.; Vieira, D.; Schmitt, F.; Baltazar, F. GLUT1 and CAIX expression profiles in breast cancer correlate with adverse prognostic factors and MCT1 overexpression. *Histol. Histopathol.* **2011**, *26*, 1279–1286.
29. Krzeslak, A.; Wojcik-Krowiranda, K.; Forma, E.; Jozwiak, P.; Romanowicz, H.; Bienkiewicz, A.; Brys, M. Expression of GLUT1 and GLUT3 glucose transporters in endometrial and breast cancers. *Pathol. Oncol. Res.* **2012**, *18*, 721–728. [CrossRef]
30. Medina, R.A.; Meneses, A.M.; Vera, J.C.; Guzman, C.; Nualart, F.; Astuya, A.; Garcia, M.A.; Kato, S.; Carvajal, A.; Pinto, M.; et al. Estrogen and progesterone up-regulate glucose transporter expression in ZR-75-1 human breast cancer cells. *Endocrinology* **2003**, *144*, 4527–4535. [CrossRef]
31. Ganapathy, V.; Thangaraju, M.; Prasad, P.D. Nutrient transporters in cancer: Relevance to Warburg hypothesis and beyond. *Pharmacol. Ther.* **2009**, *121*, 29–40. [CrossRef] [PubMed]
32. Burgman, P.; Odonoghue, J.A.; Humm, J.L.; Ling, C.C. Hypoxia-Induced increase in FDG uptake in MCF7 cells. *J. Nucl. Med.* **2001**, *42*, 170–175. [PubMed]
33. Rivenzon-Segal, D.; Boldin-Adamsky, S.; Seger, D.; Seger, R.; Degani, H. Glycolysis and glucose transporter 1 as markers of response to hormonal therapy in breast cancer. *Int. J. Cancer* **2003**, *107*, 177–182. [CrossRef] [PubMed]
34. Kato, Y.; Maeda, T.; Suzuki, A.; Baba, Y. Cancer metabolism: New insights into classic characteristics. *Jpn. Dent. Sci. Rev.* **2018**, *54*, 8–21. [CrossRef] [PubMed]
35. Garrido, P.; Moran, J.; Alonso, A.; Gonzalez, S.; Gonzalez, C. 17beta-estradiol activates glucose uptake via GLUT4 translocation and PI3K/Akt signaling pathway in MCF-7 cells. *Endocrinology* **2013**, *154*, 1979–1989. [CrossRef] [PubMed]
36. Wang, S.; Xie, J.; Li, J.; Liu, F.; Wu, X.; Wang, Z. Cisplatin suppresses the growth and proliferation of breast and cervical cancer cell lines by inhibiting integrin beta5-mediated glycolysis. *Am. J. Cancer Res.* **2016**, *6*, 1108–1117. [PubMed]

37. Yang, Y.; Wolfram, J.; Boom, K.; Fang, X.; Shen, H.; Ferrari, M. Hesperetin impairs glucose uptake and inhibits proliferation of breast cancer cells. *Cell Biochem. Funct.* **2013**, *31*, 374–379. [CrossRef]
38. Guedes, M.; Araujo, J.R.; Correia-Branco, A.; Gregorio, I.; Martel, F.; Keating, E. Modulation of the uptake of critical nutrients by breast cancer cells by lactate: Impact on cell survival, proliferation and migration. *Exp. Cell Res.* **2016**, *341*, 111–122. [CrossRef]
39. Harmon, A.W.; Patel, Y.M. Naringenin inhibits glucose uptake in MCF-7 breast cancer cells: A mechanism for impaired cellular proliferation. *Breast Cancer Res. Treat.* **2004**, *85*, 103–110. [CrossRef]
40. Moreira, L.; Araujo, I.; Costa, T.; Correia-Branco, A.; Faria, A.; Martel, F.; Keating, E. Quercetin and epigallocatechin gallate inhibit glucose uptake and metabolism by breast cancer cells by an estrogen receptor-independent mechanism. *Exp. Cell Res.* **2013**, *319*, 1784–1795. [CrossRef]
41. Garrido, P.; Osorio, F.G.; Moran, J.; Cabello, E.; Alonso, A.; Freije, J.M.; Gonzalez, C. Loss of GLUT4 induces metabolic reprogramming and impairs viability of breast cancer cells. *J. Cell Physiol.* **2015**, *230*, 191–198. [CrossRef] [PubMed]
42. Rogers, S.; Macheda, M.L.; Docherty, S.E.; Carty, M.D.; Henderson, M.A.; Soeller, W.C.; Gibbs, E.M.; James, D.E.; Best, J.D. Identification of a novel glucose transporter-like protein-GLUT-12. *Am. J. Physiol. Endocrinol. Metab.* **2002**, *282*, 733–738. [CrossRef] [PubMed]
43. Evans, A.; Bates, V.; Troy, H.; Hewitt, S.; Holbeck, S.; Chung, Y.L.; Phillips, R.; Stubbs, M.; Griffiths, J.; Airley, R. Glut-1 as a therapeutic target: Increased chemoresistance and HIF-1-independent link with cell turnover is revealed through COMPARE analysis and metabolomic studies. *Cancer Chemother. Pharmacol.* **2008**, *61*, 377–393. [CrossRef] [PubMed]
44. Housman, G.; Byler, S.; Heerboth, S.; Lapinska, K.; Longacre, M.; Snyder, N.; Sarkar, S. Drug resistance in cancer: An overview. *Cancers* **2014**, *6*, 1769–1792. [CrossRef] [PubMed]
45. Kuang, R.; Jahangiri, A.; Mascharak, S.; Nguyen, A.; Chandra, A.; Flanigan, P.M.; Yagnik, G.; Wagner, J.R.; de Lay, M.; Carrera, D.; et al. GLUT3 upregulation promotes metabolic reprogramming associated with antiangiogenic therapy resistance. *JCI Insight* **2017**, *2*, e88815. [CrossRef] [PubMed]
46. Bomanji, J.B.; Costa, D.C.; Ell, P.J. Clinical role of positron emission tomography in oncology. *Lancet Oncol.* **2001**, *2*, 157–164. [CrossRef]
47. Zhu, A.; Lee, D.; Shim, H. Metabolic positron emission tomography imaging in cancer detection and therapy response. *Semin. Oncol.* **2011**, *38*, 55–69. [CrossRef]
48. Luengo, A.; Gui, D.Y.; Heiden, M.G.V. Targeting metabolism for cancer therapy. *Cell Chem. Biol.* **2017**, *24*, 1161–1180. [CrossRef]
49. Qian, Y.; Wang, X.; Chen, X. Inhibitors of glucose transport and glycolysis as novel anticancer therapeutics. *World J. Transl. Med.* **2014**, *3*, 37–57. [CrossRef]
50. Michelakis, E.D.; Webster, L.; Mackey, J.R. Dichloroacetate (DCA) as a potential metabolic-targeting therapy for cancer. *Br. J. Cancer* **2008**, *99*, 989–994. [CrossRef]
51. Woolf, E.C.; Syed, N.; Scheck, A.C. Tumor metabolism, the ketogenic diet and beta-hydroxybutyrate: Novel approaches to adjuvant brain tumor therapy. *Front. Mol. Neurosci.* **2016**, *9*, e122. [CrossRef] [PubMed]
52. Abdel-Wahab, A.F.; Mahmoud, W.; Al-Harizy, R.M. Targeting glucose metabolism to suppress cancer progression: Prospective of anti-glycolytic cancer therapy. *Pharmacol. Res.* **2019**, *150*, e104511. [CrossRef] [PubMed]
53. Granchi, C.; Fortunato, S.; Minutolo, F. Anticancer agents interacting with membrane glucose transporters. *Medchemcomm* **2016**, *7*, 1716–1729. [CrossRef] [PubMed]
54. Rodriguez-Enriquez, S.; Marin-Hernandez, A.; Gallardo-Perez, J.C.; Carreno-Fuentes, L.; Moreno-Sanchez, R. Targeting of cancer energy metabolism. *Mol. Nutr. Food Res.* **2009**, *53*, 29–48. [CrossRef] [PubMed]
55. Chan, D.A.; Sutphin, P.D.; Nguyen, P.; Turcotte, S.; Lai, E.W.; Banh, A.; Reynolds, G.E.; Chi, J.T.; Wu, J.; Solow-Cordero, D.E.; et al. Targeting GLUT1 and the Warburg effect in renal cell carcinoma by chemical synthetic lethality. *Sci. Transl. Med.* **2011**, *3*, 94ra70. [CrossRef]
56. Liu, Y.; Zhang, W.; Cao, Y.; Liu, Y.; Bergmeier, S.; Chen, X. Small compound inhibitors of basal glucose transport inhibit cell proliferation and induce apoptosis in cancer cells via glucose-deprivation-like mechanisms. *Cancer Lett.* **2010**, *298*, 176–185. [CrossRef]
57. Xintaropoulou, C.; Ward, C.; Wise, A.; Marston, H.; Turnbull, A.; Langdon, S.P. A comparative analysis of inhibitors of the glycolysis pathway in breast and ovarian cancer cell line models. *Oncotarget* **2015**, *6*, 25677–25695. [CrossRef]

58. Zhao, F.; Ming, J.; Zhou, Y.; Fan, L. Inhibition of Glut1 by WZB117 sensitizes radioresistant breast cancer cells to irradiation. *Cancer Chemother. Pharmacol.* **2016**, *77*, 963–972. [CrossRef]
59. Liu, Y.; Cao, Y.; Zhang, W.; Bergmeier, S.; Qian, Y.; Akbar, H.; Colvin, R.; Ding, J.; Tong, L.; Wu, S.; et al. A small-molecule inhibitor of glucose transporter 1 downregulates glycolysis, induces cell-cycle arrest, and inhibits cancer cell growth in vitro and in vivo. *Mol. Cancer Ther.* **2012**, *11*, 1672–1682. [CrossRef]
60. Chen, Q.; Meng, Y.Q.; Xu, X.F.; Gu, J. Blockade of GLUT1 by WZB117 resensitizes breast cancer cells to adriamycin. *Anticancer Drugs* **2017**, *28*, 880–887. [CrossRef]
61. Siebeneicher, H.; Cleve, A.; Rehwinkel, H.; Neuhaus, R.; Heisler, I.; Muller, T.; Bauser, M.; Buchmann, B. Identification and Optimization of the First Highly Selective GLUT1 Inhibitor BAY-876. *ChemMedChem* **2016**, *11*, 2261–2271. [CrossRef] [PubMed]
62. Zeng, L.; Zhou, M.M. Bromodomain: An acetyl-lysine binding domain. *FEBS Lett.* **2002**, *513*, 124–128. [CrossRef]
63. Wu, Q.; Heidenreich, D.; Zhou, S.; Ackloo, S.; Kramer, A.; Nakka, K.; Lima-Fernandes, E.; Deblois, G.; Duan, S.; Vellanki, R.N.; et al. A chemical toolbox for the study of bromodomains and epigenetic signaling. *Nat. Commun.* **2019**, *10*, e1915. [CrossRef] [PubMed]
64. Kuntz, S.; Mazerbourg, S.; Boisbrun, M.; Cerella, C.; Diederich, M.; Grillier-Vuissoz, I.; Flament, S. Energy restriction mimetic agents to target cancer cells: Comparison between 2-deoxyglucose and thiazolidinediones. *Biochem. Pharmacol.* **2014**, *92*, 102–111. [CrossRef]
65. Amaral, I.; Silva, C.; Correia-Branco, A.; Martel, F. Effect of metformin on estrogen and progesterone receptor-positive (MCF-7) and triple-negative (MDA-MB-231) breast cancer cells. *Biomed. Pharmacother.* **2018**, *102*, 94–101. [CrossRef]
66. Zhang, C.; Liu, J.; Liang, Y.; Wu, R.; Zhao, Y.; Hong, X.; Lin, M.; Yu, H.; Liu, L.; Levine, A.J.; et al. Tumour-associated mutant p53 drives the Warburg effect. *Nat. Commun.* **2013**, *4*, e2935. [CrossRef]
67. Oh, S.; Kim, H.; Nam, K.; Shin, I. Glut1 promotes cell proliferation, migration and invasion by regulating epidermal growth factor receptor and integrin signaling in triple-negative breast cancer cells. *BMB Rep.* **2017**, *50*, 132–137. [CrossRef]
68. Oh, S.; Kim, H.; Nam, K.; Shin, I. Silencing of Glut1 induces chemoresistance via modulation of Akt/GSK-3beta/beta-catenin/survivin signaling pathway in breast cancer cells. *Arch. Biochem. Biophys.* **2017**, *636*, 110–122. [CrossRef]
69. Rastogi, S.; Banerjee, S.; Chellappan, S.; Simon, G.R. Glut-1 antibodies induce growth arrest and apoptosis in human cancer cell lines. *Cancer Lett.* **2007**, *257*, 244–251. [CrossRef]
70. Evans, J.M.; Donnelly, L.A.; Emslie-Smith, A.M.; Alessi, D.R.; Morris, A.D. Metformin and reduced risk of cancer in diabetic patients. *BMJ* **2005**, *330*, 1304–1305. [CrossRef]
71. Grossmann, M.E.; Yang, D.Q.; Guo, Z.; Potter, D.A.; Cleary, M.P. Metformin treatment for the prevention and/or treatment of breast/mammary tumorigenesis. *Curr. Pharmacol. Rep.* **2015**, *1*, 312–323. [CrossRef] [PubMed]
72. Wysocki, P.J.; Wierusz-Wysocka, B. Obesity, hyperinsulinemia and breast cancer: Novel targets and a novel role for metformin. *Expert Rev. Mol. Diagn.* **2010**, *10*, 509–519. [CrossRef] [PubMed]
73. Marini, C.; Salani, B.; Massollo, M.; Amaro, A.; Esposito, A.I.; Orengo, A.M.; Capitanio, S.; Emionite, L.; Riondato, M.; Bottoni, G.; et al. Direct inhibition of hexokinase activity by metformin at least partially impairs glucose metabolism and tumor growth in experimental breast cancer. *Cell Cycle* **2013**, *12*, 3490–3499. [CrossRef] [PubMed]
74. Banerjee, A.; Birts, C.N.; Darley, M.; Parker, R.; Mirnezami, A.H.; West, J.; Cutress, R.I.; Beers, S.A.; Rose-Zerilli, M.J.J.; Blaydes, J.P. Stem cell-like breast cancer cells with acquired resistance to metformin are sensitive to inhibitors of NADH-dependent CtBP dimerization. *Carcinogenesis* **2019**, *40*, 871–882. [CrossRef] [PubMed]
75. Ding, J.; Gou, Q.; Jin, J.; Shi, J.; Liu, Q.; Hou, Y. Metformin inhibits PPARdelta agonist-mediated tumor growth by reducing Glut1 and SLC1A5 expressions of cancer cells. *Eur. J. Pharmacol.* **2019**, *857*, e172425. [CrossRef] [PubMed]
76. Birsoy, K.; Possemato, R.; Lorbeer, F.K.; Bayraktar, E.C.; Thiru, P.; Yucel, B.; Wang, T.; Chen, W.W.; Clish, C.B.; Sabatini, D.M. Metabolic determinants of cancer cell sensitivity to glucose limitation and biguanides. *Nature* **2014**, *508*, 108–112. [CrossRef] [PubMed]

77. Liu, X.; Gan, B. lncRNA NBR2 modulates cancer cell sensitivity to phenformin through GLUT1. *Cell Cycle* **2016**, *15*, 3471–3481. [CrossRef]
78. Elstner, E.; Muller, C.; Koshizuka, K.; Williamson, E.A.; Park, D.; Asou, H.; Shintaku, P.; Said, J.W.; Heber, D.; Koeffler, H.P. Ligands for peroxisome proliferator-activated receptorgamma and retinoic acid receptor inhibit growth and induce apoptosis of human breast cancer cells in vitro and in BNX mice. *Proc. Natl. Acad. Sci. USA* **1998**, *95*, 8806–8811. [CrossRef]
79. Moon, S.H.; Lee, S.J.; Jung, K.H.; Quach, C.H.; Park, J.W.; Lee, J.H.; Cho, Y.S.; Lee, K.H. Troglitazone stimulates cancer cell uptake of ^{18}F-FDG by suppressing mitochondrial respiration and augments sensitivity to glucose restriction. *J. Nucl. Med.* **2016**, *57*, 129–135. [CrossRef]
80. Fiume, L.; Manerba, M.; Vettraino, M.; di Stefano, G. Effect of sorafenib on the energy metabolism of hepatocellular carcinoma cells. *Eur. J. Pharmacol.* **2011**, *670*, 39–43. [CrossRef]
81. Bull, V.H.; Rajalingam, K.; Thiede, B. Sorafenib-induced mitochondrial complex I inactivation and cell death in human neuroblastoma cells. *J. Proteome Res.* **2012**, *11*, 1609–1620. [CrossRef] [PubMed]
82. Fumarola, C.; Caffarra, C.; la Monica, S.; Galetti, M.; Alfieri, R.R.; Cavazzoni, A.; Galvani, E.; Generali, D.; Petronini, P.G.; Bonelli, M.A. Effects of sorafenib on energy metabolism in breast cancer cells: Role of AMPK-mTORC1 signaling. *Breast Cancer Res. Treat.* **2013**, *141*, 67–78. [CrossRef] [PubMed]
83. Smith, T.A.; Appleyard, M.V.; Sharp, S.; Fleming, I.N.; Murray, K.; Thompson, A.M. Response to trastuzumab by HER2 expressing breast tumour xenografts is accompanied by decreased Hexokinase II, glut1 and [18F]-FDG incorporation and changes in ^{31}P-NMR-detectable phosphomonoesters. *Cancer Chemother. Pharmacol.* **2013**, *71*, 473–480. [CrossRef] [PubMed]
84. Engles, J.M.; Quarless, S.A.; Mambo, E.; Ishimori, T.; Cho, S.Y.; Wahl, R.L. Stunning and its effect on ^{3}H-FDG uptake and key gene expression in breast cancer cells undergoing chemotherapy. *J. Nucl. Med.* **2006**, *47*, 603–608.
85. Abd-Rabou, A.A.; Ahmed, H.H.; Shalby, A.B. Selenium overcomes doxorubicin resistance in their nano-platforms against breast and colon cancers. *Biol. Trace Elem. Res.* **2019**. [CrossRef]
86. DeMichele, A.; Clark, A.S.; Tan, K.S.; Heitjan, D.F.; Gramlich, K.; Gallagher, M.; Lal, P.; Feldman, M.; Zhang, P.; Colameco, C.; et al. CDK 4/6 inhibitor palbociclib (PD0332991) in Rb+ advanced breast cancer: Phase II activity, safety, and predictive biomarker assessment. *Clin. Cancer Res.* **2015**, *21*, 995–1001. [CrossRef]
87. Cretella, D.; Fumarola, C.; Bonelli, M.; Alfieri, R.; la Monica, S.; Digiacomo, G.; Cavazzoni, A.; Galetti, M.; Generali, D.; Petronini, P.G. Pre-treatment with the CDK4/6 inhibitor palbociclib improves the efficacy of paclitaxel in TNBC cells. *Sci. Rep.* **2019**, *9*, e13014. [CrossRef]
88. Cretella, D.; Ravelli, A.; Fumarola, C.; la Monica, S.; Digiacomo, G.; Cavazzoni, A.; Alfieri, R.; Biondi, A.; Generali, D.; Bonelli, M.; et al. The anti-tumor efficacy of CDK4/6 inhibition is enhanced by the combination with PI3K/AKT/mTOR inhibitors through impairment of glucose metabolism in TNBC cells. *J. Exp. Clin. Cancer. Res.* **2018**, *37*, e72. [CrossRef]
89. Powe, D.G.; Voss, M.J.; Zanker, K.S.; Habashy, H.O.; Green, A.R.; Ellis, I.O.; Entschladen, F. Beta-blocker drug therapy reduces secondary cancer formation in breast cancer and improves cancer specific survival. *Oncotarget* **2010**, *1*, 628–638. [CrossRef]
90. Kang, F.; Ma, W.; Ma, X.; Shao, Y.; Yang, W.; Chen, X.; Li, L.; Wang, J. Propranolol inhibits glucose metabolism and 18F-FDG uptake of breast cancer through posttranscriptional downregulation of hexokinase-2. *J. Nucl. Med.* **2014**, *55*, 439–445. [CrossRef]
91. Zheng, X.; Resnick, R.J.; Shalloway, D. Apoptosis of estrogen-receptor negative breast cancer and colon cancer cell lines by PTP alpha and src RNAi. *Int. J. Cancer* **2008**, *122*, 1999–2007. [CrossRef] [PubMed]
92. Puls, L.N.; Eadens, M.; Messersmith, W. Current status of SRC inhibitors in solid tumor malignancies. *Oncologist* **2011**, *16*, 566–578. [CrossRef] [PubMed]
93. Jain, S.; Wang, X.; Chang, C.C.; Ibarra-Drendall, C.; Wang, H.; Zhang, Q.; Brady, S.W.; Li, P.; Zhao, H.; Dobbs, J.; et al. Src inhibition blocks c-Myc translation and glucose metabolism to prevent the development of breast cancer. *Cancer Res.* **2015**, *75*, 4863–4875. [CrossRef] [PubMed]
94. Zawacka-Pankau, J.; Grinkevich, V.V.; Hunten, S.; Nikulenkov, F.; Gluch, A.; Li, H.; Enge, M.; Kel, A.; Selivanova, G. Inhibition of glycolytic enzymes mediated by pharmacologically activated p53: Targeting Warburg effect to fight cancer. *J. Biol. Chem.* **2011**, *286*, 41600–41615. [CrossRef] [PubMed]

95. Grinkevich, V.V.; Nikulenkov, F.; Shi, Y.; Enge, M.; Bao, W.; Maljukova, A.; Gluch, A.; Kel, A.; Sangfelt, O.; Selivanova, G. Ablation of key oncogenic pathways by RITA-reactivated p53 is required for efficient apoptosis. *Cancer Cell* **2009**, *15*, 441–453. [CrossRef]
96. Vassilev, L.T.; Vu, B.T.; Graves, B.; Carvajal, D.; Podlaski, F.; Filipovic, Z.; Kong, N.; Kammlott, U.; Lukacs, C.; Klein, C.; et al. In vivo activation of the p53 pathway by small-molecule antagonists of MDM2. *Science* **2004**, *303*, 844–848. [CrossRef]
97. Vivanco, I.; Sawyers, C.L. The phosphatidylinositol 3-Kinase AKT pathway in human cancer. *Nat. Rev. Cancer* **2002**, *2*, 489–501. [CrossRef]
98. Tan, S.X.; Ng, Y.; James, D.E. Akt inhibitors reduce glucose uptake independently of their effects on Akt. *Biochem. J.* **2010**, *432*, 191–197. [CrossRef]
99. Deblois, G.; St-Pierre, J.; Giguere, V. The PGC-1/ERR signaling axis in cancer. *Oncogene* **2013**, *32*, 3483–3490. [CrossRef]
100. Ludvik, A.E.; Pusec, C.M.; Priyadarshini, M.; Angueira, A.R.; Guo, C.; Lo, A.; Hershenhouse, K.S.; Yang, G.Y.; Ding, X.; Reddy, T.E.; et al. HKDC1 is a novel hexokinase involved in whole-body glucose use. *Endocrinology* **2016**, *157*, 3452–3461. [CrossRef]
101. Li, G.H.; Huang, J.F. Inferring therapeutic targets from heterogeneous data: HKDC1 is a novel potential therapeutic target for cancer. *Bioinformatics* **2014**, *30*, 748–752. [CrossRef] [PubMed]
102. Chen, X.; Lv, Y.; Sun, Y.; Zhang, H.; Xie, W.; Zhong, L.; Chen, Q.; Li, M.; Li, L.; Feng, J.; et al. PGC1beta regulates breast tumor growth and metastasis by SREBP1-mediated HKDC1 expression. *Front. Oncol.* **2019**, *9*, e290. [CrossRef] [PubMed]
103. Li, Z.; Gong, X.; Zhang, W.; Zhang, J.; Ding, L.; Li, H.; Tu, D.; Tang, J. Inhibition of miRNA-34a promotes triple negative cancer cell proliferation by promoting glucose uptake. *Exp. Ther. Med.* **2019**, *18*, 3936–3942. [CrossRef] [PubMed]
104. He, M.; Jin, Q.; Chen, C.; Liu, Y.; Ye, X.; Jiang, Y.; Ji, F.; Qian, H.; Gan, D.; Yue, S.; et al. The miR-186-3p/EREG axis orchestrates tamoxifen resistance and aerobic glycolysis in breast cancer cells. *Oncogene* **2019**, *38*, 5551–5565. [CrossRef]
105. de Almeida Chuffa, L.G.; Seiva, F.R.F.; Cucielo, M.S.; Silveira, H.S.; Reiter, R.J.; Lupi, L.A. Mitochondrial functions and melatonin: A tour of the reproductive cancers. *Cell Mol. Life Sci.* **2019**, *76*, 837–863. [CrossRef]
106. Hevia, D.; Gonzalez-Menendez, P.; Quiros-Gonzalez, I.; Miar, A.; Rodriguez-Garcia, A.; Tan, D.X.; Reiter, R.J.; Mayo, J.C.; Sainz, R.M. Melatonin uptake through glucose transporters: A new target for melatonin inhibition of cancer. *J. Pineal Res.* **2015**, *58*, 234–250. [CrossRef]
107. Blask, D.E.; Dauchy, R.T.; Dauchy, E.M.; Mao, L.; Hill, S.M.; Greene, M.W.; Belancio, V.P.; Sauer, L.A.; Davidson, L. Light exposure at night disrupts host/cancer circadian regulatory dynamics: Impact on the Warburg effect, lipid signaling and tumor growth prevention. *PLoS ONE* **2014**, *9*, e102776. [CrossRef]
108. Sonehara, N.M.; Lacerda, J.Z.; Jardim-Perassi, B.V.; de Paula, R., Jr.; Moschetta-Pinheiro, M.G.; Souza, Y.S.T.; de Andrade, J.C.J.; De Campos Zuccari, D.A.P. Melatonin regulates tumor aggressiveness under acidosis condition in breast cancer cell lines. *Oncol. Lett.* **2019**, *17*, 1635–1645. [CrossRef]
109. Nunes, C.; Silva, C.; Correia-Branco, A.; Martel, F. Lack of effect of the procarcinogenic 17beta-estradiol on nutrient uptake by the MCF-7 breast cancer cell line. *Biomed. Pharmacother.* **2017**, *90*, 287–294. [CrossRef]
110. Neeman, M.; Degani, H. Metabolic studies of estrogen- and tamoxifen-treated human breast cancer cells by nuclear magnetic resonance spectroscopy. *Cancer Res.* **1989**, *49*, 589–594.
111. Ko, B.H.; Paik, J.Y.; Jung, K.H.; Lee, K.H. 17beta-estradiol augments ^{18}F-FDG uptake and glycolysis of T47D breast cancer cells via membrane-initiated rapid PI3K-Akt activation. *J. Nucl. Med.* **2010**, *51*, 1740–1747. [CrossRef]
112. Kim, H.I.; Moon, S.H.; Lee, W.C.; Lee, H.J.; Shivakumar, S.B.; Lee, S.H.; Park, B.W.; Rho, G.J.; Jeon, B.G. Inhibition of cell growth by cellular differentiation into adipocyte-like cells in dexamethasone sensitive cancer cell lines. *Anim. Cells Syst.* **2018**, *22*, 178–188. [CrossRef] [PubMed]
113. Zhang, C.; Beckermann, B.; Kallifatidis, G.; Liu, Z.; Rittgen, W.; Edler, L.; Buchler, P.; Debatin, K.M.; Buchler, M.W.; Friess, H.; et al. Corticosteroids induce chemotherapy resistance in the majority of tumour cells from bone, brain, breast, cervix, melanoma and neuroblastoma. *Int. J. Oncol.* **2006**, *29*, 1295–1301. [CrossRef] [PubMed]
114. Buxant, F.; Kindt, N.; Laurent, G.; Noel, J.C.; Saussez, S. Antiproliferative effect of dexamethasone in the MCF-7 breast cancer cell line. *Mol. Med. Rep.* **2015**, *12*, 4051–4054. [CrossRef]

115. Dalton, G.D.; Xie, J.; An, S.W.; Huang, C.L. New insights into the mechanism of action of soluble Klotho. *Front. Endocrinol.* **2017**, *8*, e323. [CrossRef]
116. Wolf, I.; Levanon-Cohen, S.; Bose, S.; Ligumsky, H.; Sredni, B.; Kanety, H.; Kuro-o, M.; Karlan, B.; Kaufman, B.; Koeffler, H.P.; et al. Klotho: A tumor suppressor and a modulator of the IGF-1 and FGF pathways in human breast cancer. *Oncogene* **2008**, *27*, 7094–7105. [CrossRef]
117. Davidov, B.; Shmulevich, R.; Shabtay, A.; Rubinek, T.; Wolf, I. The hormone KL1: A regulator of breast cancer cell metabolism. *Isr. Med. Assoc. J.* **2019**, *21*, e504.
118. Pollak, M. Insulin and insulin-like growth factor signalling in neoplasia. *Nat. Rev. Cancer* **2008**, *8*, 915–928. [CrossRef]
119. Acevedo, C.G.; Marquez, J.L.; Rojas, S.; Bravo, I. Insulin and nitric oxide stimulates glucose transport in human placenta. *Life Sci.* **2005**, *76*, 2643–2653. [CrossRef]
120. Agrawal, S.; Luc, M.; Ziolkowski, P.; Agrawal, A.K.; Pielka, E.; Walaszek, K.; Zduniak, K.; Wozniak, M. Insulin-induced enhancement of MCF-7 breast cancer cell response to 5-fluorouracil and cyclophosphamide. *Tumour Biol.* **2017**, *39*. [CrossRef]
121. Beckert, S.; Farrahi, F.; Aslam, R.S.; Scheuenstuhl, H.; Konigsrainer, A.; Hussain, M.Z.; Hunt, T.K. Lactate stimulates endothelial cell migration. *Wound Repair Regen.* **2006**, *14*, 321–324. [CrossRef] [PubMed]
122. Lu, H.; Forbes, R.A.; Verma, A. Hypoxia-inducible factor 1 activation by aerobic glycolysis implicates the Warburg effect in carcinogenesis. *J. Biol. Chem.* **2002**, *277*, 23111–23115. [CrossRef] [PubMed]
123. Turkcan, S.; Kiru, L.; Naczynski, D.J.; Sasportas, L.S.; Pratx, G. Lactic acid accumulation in the tumor microenvironment suppresses (18)F-FDG uptake. *Cancer Res.* **2019**, *79*, 410–419. [CrossRef] [PubMed]
124. Venmar, K.T.; Kimmel, D.W.; Cliffel, D.E.; Fingleton, B. IL4 receptor alpha mediates enhanced glucose and glutamine metabolism to support breast cancer growth. *Biochim. Biophys. Acta* **2015**, *1853*, 1219–1228. [CrossRef]
125. Masuda, H.; Zhang, D.; Bartholomeusz, C.; Doihara, H.; Hortobagyi, G.N.; Ueno, N.T. Role of epidermal growth factor receptor in breast cancer. *Breast Cancer Res. Treat.* **2012**, *136*, 331–345. [CrossRef]
126. Lee, J.; Lee, E.J.; Moon, S.H.; Kim, S.; Hyun, S.H.; Cho, Y.S.; Choi, J.Y.; Kim, B.T.; Lee, K.H. Strong association of epidermal growth factor receptor status with breast cancer FDG uptake. *Eur. J. Nucl. Med. Mol. Imaging* **2017**, *44*, 1438–1447. [CrossRef]
127. Jung, K.H.; Lee, E.J.; Park, J.W.; Lee, J.H.; Moon, S.H.; Cho, Y.S.; Lee, K.H. EGF receptor stimulation shifts breast cancer cell glucose metabolism toward glycolytic flux through PI3 kinase signaling. *PLoS ONE* **2019**, *14*, e0221294. [CrossRef]
128. Williamson, G. The role of polyphenols in modern nutrition. *Nutr. Bull.* **2017**, *42*, 226–235. [CrossRef]
129. Hussain, S.A.; Sulaiman, A.A.; Alhaddad, H.; Alhadidi, Q. Natural polyphenols: Influence on membrane transporters. *J. Intercult. Ethnopharmacol.* **2016**, *5*, 97–104. [CrossRef]
130. Williamson, G. Possible effects of dietary polyphenols on sugar absorption and digestion. *Mol. Nutr. Food Res.* **2013**, *57*, 48–57. [CrossRef]
131. Losada-Echeberria, M.; Herranz-Lopez, M.; Micol, V.; Barrajon-Catalan, E. Polyphenols as promising drugs against main breast cancer signatures. *Antioxidants* **2017**, *6*, 88. [CrossRef] [PubMed]
132. Mocanu, M.M.; Nagy, P.; Szollosi, J. Chemoprevention of breast cancer by dietary polyphenols. *Molecules* **2015**, *20*, 22578–22620. [CrossRef] [PubMed]
133. Keating, E.; Martel, F. Antimetabolic effects of polyphenols in breast cancer cells: Focus on glucose uptake and metabolism. *Front. Nutr.* **2018**, *5*, e25. [CrossRef]
134. Martel, F.; Guedes, M.; Keating, E. Effect of polyphenols on glucose and lactate transport by breast cancer cells. *Breast Cancer Res. Treat.* **2016**, *157*, 1–11. [CrossRef]
135. Jaroszewski, J.W.; Kaplan, O.; Cohen, J.S. Action of gossypol and rhodamine 123 on wild type and multidrug-resistant MCF-7 human breast cancer cells: 31P nuclear magnetic resonance and toxicity studies. *Cancer Res.* **1990**, *50*, 6936–6943.
136. Lim, H.A.; Kim, J.H.; Kim, J.H.; Sung, M.K.; Kim, M.K.; Park, J.H.; Kim, J.S. Genistein induces glucose-regulated protein 78 in mammary tumor cells. *J. Med. Food* **2006**, *9*, 28–32. [CrossRef]
137. Uifalean, A.; Schneider, S.; Gierok, P.; Ionescu, C.; Iuga, C.A.; Lalk, M. The impact of soy isoflavones on MCF-7 and MDA-MB-231 breast cancer cells using a global metabolomic approach. *Int. J. Mol. Sci.* **2016**, *17*, 1443. [CrossRef]

138. Azevedo, C.; Correia-Branco, A.; Araujo, J.R.; Guimaraes, J.T.; Keating, E.; Martel, F. The chemopreventive effect of the dietary compound kaempferol on the MCF-7 human breast cancer cell line is dependent on inhibition of glucose cellular uptake. *Nutr. Cancer* **2015**, *67*, 504–513. [CrossRef]
139. Jung, K.H.; Lee, J.H.; Quach, C.H.T.; Paik, J.Y.; Oh, H.; Park, J.W.; Lee, E.J.; Moon, S.H.; Lee, K.H. Resveratrol suppresses cancer cell glucose uptake by targeting reactive oxygen species-mediated hypoxia-inducible factor-1alpha activation. *J. Nucl. Med.* **2013**, *54*, 2161–2167. [CrossRef]
140. Jia, L.; Huang, S.; Yin, X.; Zan, Y.; Guo, Y.; Han, L. Quercetin suppresses the mobility of breast cancer by suppressing glycolysis through Akt-mTOR pathway mediated autophagy induction. *Life Sci.* **2018**, *208*, 123–130. [CrossRef]
141. Li, L.J.; Li, G.W.; Xie, Y. Regulatory effects of glabridin and quercetin on energy metabolism of breast cancer cells. *Zhongguo Zhong Yao Za Zhi* **2019**, *44*, 3786–3791. [PubMed]
142. Wei, R.; Mao, L.; Xu, P.; Zheng, X.; Hackman, R.M.; Mackenzie, G.G.; Wang, Y. Suppressing glucose metabolism with epigallocatechin-3-gallate (EGCG) reduces breast cancer cell growth in preclinical models. *Food Funct.* **2018**, *9*, 5682–5696. [CrossRef] [PubMed]
143. Nelson, J.A.; Falk, R.E. Phloridzin and phloretin inhibition of 2-deoxy-D-glucose uptake by tumor cells in vitro and in vivo. *Anticancer Res.* **1993**, *13*, 2293–2299. [PubMed]
144. Niedzwiecki, A.; Roomi, M.W.; Kalinovsky, T.; Rath, M. Anticancer efficacy of polyphenols and their combinations. *Nutrients* **2016**, *8*, 552. [CrossRef] [PubMed]
145. Silva, C.; Correia-Branco, A.; Andrade, N.; Ferreira, A.C.; Soares, M.L.; Sonveaux, P.; Stephenne, J.; Martel, F. Selective pro-apoptotic and antimigratory effects of polyphenol complex catechin:lysine 1:2 in breast, pancreatic and colorectal cancer cell lines. *Eur. J. Pharmacol.* **2019**, *859*, 172533. [CrossRef] [PubMed]
146. Zhang, W.; Liu, Y.; Chen, X.; Bergmeier, S.C. Novel inhibitors of basal glucose transport as potential anticancer agents. *Bioorg. Med. Chem. Lett.* **2010**, *20*, 2191–2194. [CrossRef]
147. Siddiqui, F.A.; Prakasam, G.; Chattopadhyay, S.; Rehman, A.U.; Padder, R.A.; Ansari, M.A.; Irshad, R.; Mangalhara, K.; Bamezai, R.N.K.; Husain, M.; et al. Curcumin decreases Warburg effect in cancer cells by down-regulating pyruvate kinase M2 via mTOR-HIF1alpha inhibition. *Sci. Rep.* **2018**, *8*, e8323. [CrossRef]
148. Jin, J.; Qiu, S.; Wang, P.; Liang, X.; Huang, F.; Wu, H.; Zhang, B.; Zhang, W.; Tian, X.; Xu, R.; et al. Cardamonin inhibits breast cancer growth by repressing HIF-1alpha-dependent metabolic reprogramming. *J. Exp. Clin. Cancer Res.* **2019**, *38*, e377. [CrossRef]
149. Shahruzaman, S.H.; Mustafa, M.F.; Ramli, S.; Maniam, S.; Fakurazi, S.; Maniam, S. The cytotoxic properties of Baeckea frutescens branches extracts in eliminating breast cancer cells. *Evid. Based Complement. Alternat. Med.* **2019**, *2019*, e9607590. [CrossRef]
150. Hernandez, J.F.; Uruena, C.P.; Cifuentes, M.C.; Sandoval, T.A.; Pombo, L.M.; Castaneda, D.; Asea, A.; Fiorentino, S. A Petiveria alliacea standardized fraction induces breast adenocarcinoma cell death by modulating glycolytic metabolism. *J. Ethnopharmacol.* **2014**, *153*, 641–649. [CrossRef]
151. Zhu, S.; Wei, L.; Lin, G.; Tong, Y.; Zhang, J.; Jiang, X.; He, Q.; Lu, X.; Zhu, D.D.; Chen, Y.Q. Metabolic alterations induced by Kudingcha lead to cancer cell apoptosis and metastasis inhibition. *Nutr. Cancer* **2019**, 1–12. [CrossRef] [PubMed]
152. Jung, C.Y.; Rampal, A.L. Cytochalasin B binding sites and glucose transport carrier in human erythrocyte ghosts. *J. Biol. Chem.* **1977**, *252*, 5456–5463. [PubMed]
153. Keller, K.; Mueckler, M. Different mammalian facilitative glucose transporters expressed in Xenopus oocytes. *Biomed. Biochim. Acta* **1990**, *49*, 1201–1203. [PubMed]
154. Cho, Y.S.; Lee, J.H.; Jung, K.H.; Park, J.W.; Moon, S.H.; Choe, Y.S.; Lee, K.H. Molecular mechanism of (18)F-FDG uptake reduction induced by genipin in T47D cancer cell and role of uncoupling protein-2 in cancer cell glucose metabolism. *Nucl. Med. Biol.* **2016**, *43*, 587–592. [CrossRef]
155. Pan, Y.; Zheng, Q.; Ni, W.; Wei, Z.; Yu, S.; Jia, Q.; Wang, M.; Wang, A.; Chen, W.; Lu, Y. Breaking glucose transporter 1/pyruvate kinase M2 glycolytic loop is required for cantharidin inhibition of metastasis in highly metastatic breast cancer. *Front. Pharmacol.* **2019**, *10*, e590. [CrossRef]
156. Jiao, L.; Wang, S.; Zheng, Y.; Wang, N.; Yang, B.; Wang, D.; Yang, D.; Mei, W.; Zhao, Z.; Wang, Z. Betulinic acid suppresses breast cancer aerobic glycolysis via caveolin-1/NF-kappaB/c-Myc pathway. *Biochem. Pharmacol.* **2019**, *161*, 149–162. [CrossRef]
157. Singh, S.V.; Singh, K. Cancer chemoprevention with dietary isothiocyanates mature for clinical translational research. *Carcinogenesis* **2012**, *33*, 1833–1842. [CrossRef]

158. Xiao, D.; Powolny, A.A.; Singh, S.V. Benzyl isothiocyanate targets mitochondrial respiratory chain to trigger reactive oxygen species-dependent apoptosis in human breast cancer cells. *J. Biol. Chem.* **2008**, *283*, 30151–30163. [CrossRef]
159. Roy, R.; Hahm, E.R.; White, A.G.; Anderson, C.J.; Singh, S.V. AKT-dependent sugar addiction by benzyl isothiocyanate in breast cancer cells. *Mol. Carcinog.* **2019**, *58*, 996–1007. [CrossRef]
160. Calder, P.C. Mechanisms of action of (n-3) fatty acids. *J. Nutr.* **2012**, *142*, 592–599. [CrossRef]
161. Mouradian, M.; Kikawa, K.D.; Dranka, B.P.; Komas, S.M.; Kalyanaraman, B.; Pardini, R.S. Docosahexaenoic acid attenuates breast cancer cell metabolism and the Warburg phenotype by targeting bioenergetic function. *Mol. Carcinog.* **2015**, *54*, 810–820. [CrossRef] [PubMed]
162. Krishnan, A.V.; Feldman, D. Mechanisms of the anti-cancer and anti-inflammatory actions of vitamin D. *Annu. Rev. Pharmacol. Toxicol.* **2011**, *51*, 311–336. [CrossRef] [PubMed]
163. Santos, J.M.; Khan, Z.S.; Munir, M.T.; Tarafdar, K.; Rahman, S.M.; Hussain, F. Vitamin D3 decreases glycolysis and invasiveness, and increases cellular stiffness in breast cancer cells. *J. Nutr. Biochem.* **2018**, *53*, 111–120. [CrossRef]
164. Sylvester, P.W.; Akl, M.R.; Malaviya, A.; Parajuli, P.; Ananthula, S.; Tiwari, R.V.; Ayoub, N.M. Potential role of tocotrienols in the treatment and prevention of breast cancer. *Biofactors* **2014**, *40*, 49–58. [CrossRef]
165. Parajuli, P.; Tiwari, R.V.; Sylvester, P.W. Anticancer effects of gamma-tocotrienol are associated with a suppression in aerobic glycolysis. *Biol. Pharm. Bull.* **2015**, *38*, 1352–1360. [CrossRef]
166. Noguchi, C.; Kamitori, K.; Hossain, A.; Hoshikawa, H.; Katagi, A.; Dong, Y.; Sui, L.; Tokuda, M.; Yamaguchi, F. D-Allose Inhibits Cancer Cell Growth by Reducing GLUT1 Expression. *Tohoku J. Exp. Med.* **2016**, *238*, 131–141. [CrossRef]
167. Wu, K.H.; Ho, C.T.; Chen, Z.F.; Chen, L.C.; Whang-Peng, J.; Lin, T.N.; Ho, Y.S. The apple polyphenol phloretin inhibits breast cancer cell migration and proliferation via inhibition of signals by type 2 glucose transporter. *J. Food Drug. Anal.* **2018**, *26*, 221–231. [CrossRef]
168. Calvaresi, E.C.; Hergenrother, P.J. Glucose conjugation for the specific targeting and treatment of cancer. *Chem. Sci.* **2013**, *4*, 2319–2333. [CrossRef]
169. Cao, J.; Cui, S.; Li, S.; Du, C.; Tian, J.; Wan, S.; Qian, Z.; Gu, Y.; Chen, W.R.; Wang, G. Targeted cancer therapy with a 2-deoxyglucose-based adriamycin complex. *Cancer Res.* **2013**, *73*, 1362–1373. [CrossRef]
170. Sztandera, K.; Dzialak, P.; Marcinkowska, M.; Stanczyk, M.; Gorzkiewicz, M.; Janaszewska, A.; Klajnert-Maculewicz, B. Sugar modification enhances cytotoxic activity of PAMAM-Doxorubicin conjugate in glucose-deprived MCF-7 cells—Possible role of GLUT1 transporter. *Pharm. Res.* **2019**, *36*, e140. [CrossRef]
171. Lin, Y.S.; Tungpradit, R.; Sinchaikul, S.; An, F.M.; Liu, D.Z.; Phutrakul, S.; Chen, S.T. Targeting the delivery of glycan-based paclitaxel prodrugs to cancer cells via glucose transporters. *J. Med. Chem.* **2008**, *51*, 7428–7441. [CrossRef] [PubMed]
172. Liu, P.; Lu, Y.; Gao, X.; Liu, R.; Zhang-Negrerie, D.; Shi, Y.; Wang, Y.; Wang, S.; Gao, Q. Highly water-soluble platinum(II) complexes as GLUT substrates for targeted therapy: Improved anticancer efficacy and transporter-mediated cytotoxic properties. *Chem. Commun. Camb.* **2013**, *49*, 2421–2423. [CrossRef] [PubMed]
173. Macintyre, A.N.; Gerriets, V.A.; Nichols, A.G.; Michalek, R.D.; Rudolph, M.C.; Deoliveira, D.; Anderson, S.M.; Abel, E.D.; Chen, B.J.; Hale, L.P.; et al. The glucose transporter Glut1 is selectively essential for CD4 T cell activation and effector function. *Cell Metab.* **2014**, *20*, 61–72. [CrossRef] [PubMed]
174. Fiaschi, T.; Marini, A.; Giannoni, E.; Taddei, M.L.; Gandellini, P.; de Donatis, A.; Lanciotti, M.; Serni, S.; Cirri, P.; Chiarugi, P. Reciprocal metabolic reprogramming through lactate shuttle coordinately influences tumor-stroma interplay. *Cancer Res.* **2012**, *72*, 5130–5140. [CrossRef] [PubMed]
175. Sheng, H.; Tang, W. Glycolysis inhibitors for anticancer therapy: A review of recent patents. *Recent Pat. Anticancer Drug Discov.* **2016**, *11*, 297–308. [CrossRef] [PubMed]
176. Flaig, T.W.; Gustafson, D.L.; Su, L.J.; Zirrolli, J.A.; Crighton, F.; Harrison, G.S.; Pierson, A.S.; Agarwal, R.; Glode, L.M. A phase I and pharmacokinetic study of silybin-phytosome in prostate cancer patients. *Investig. New Drugs* **2007**, *25*, 139–146. [CrossRef]
177. Raez, L.E.; Papadopoulos, K.; Ricart, A.D.; Chiorean, E.G.; Dipaola, R.S.; Stein, M.N.; Lima, C.M.R.; Schlesselman, J.J.; Tolba, K.; Langmuir, V.K.; et al. A phase I dose-escalation trial of 2-deoxy-D-glucose alone or combined with docetaxel in patients with advanced solid tumors. *Cancer Chemother. Pharmacol.* **2013**, *71*, 523–530. [CrossRef]

178. Jose, C.; Bellance, N.; Rossignol, R. Choosing between glycolysis and oxidative phosphorylation: A tumor's dilemma? *Biochim. Biophys. Acta* **2011**, *1807*, 552–561. [CrossRef]
179. Lee, Y.J.; Lee, G.J.; Yi, S.S.; Heo, S.H.; Park, C.R.; Nam, H.S.; Cho, M.K.; Lee, S.H. Cisplatin and resveratrol induce apoptosis and autophagy following oxidative stress in malignant mesothelioma cells. *Food Chem. Toxicol.* **2016**, *97*, 96–107. [CrossRef]
180. Shi, Y.; Liu, S.; Ahmad, S.; Gao, Q. Targeting key transporters in tumor glycolysis as a novel anticancer strategy. *Curr. Top. Med. Chem.* **2018**, *18*, 454–466. [CrossRef]
181. Garcia-Aranda, M.; Redondo, M. Immunotherapy: A challenge of breast cancer treatment. *Cancers* **2019**, *11*, 1822. [CrossRef] [PubMed]
182. Mochel, F.; Hainque, E.; Gras, D.; Adanyeguh, I.M.; Caillet, S.; Heron, B.; Roubertie, A.; Kaphan, E.; Valabregue, R.; Rinaldi, D.; et al. Triheptanoin dramatically reduces paroxysmal motor disorder in patients with GLUT1 deficiency. *J. Neurol. Neurosurg. Psychiatry* **2016**, *87*, 550–553. [CrossRef] [PubMed]

9

Gigantol Targets Cancer Stem Cells and Destabilizes Tumors via the Suppression of the PI3K/AKT and JAK/STAT Pathways in Ectopic Lung Cancer Xenografts

Nattanan Losuwannarak [1,2], Arnatchai Maiuthed [1], Nakarin Kitkumthorn [3], Asada Leelahavanichkul [4], Sittiruk Roytrakul [5] and Pithi Chanvorachote [1,2,*]

1 Cell-Based Drug and Health Product Development Research Unit, Faculty of Pharmaceutical Sciences, Chulalongkorn University, Bangkok 10330, Thailand; los.nattanan@hotmail.com (N.L.); m.arnatchai@gmail.com (A.M.)
2 Department of Pharmacology and Physiology, Faculty of Pharmaceutical Sciences, Chulalongkorn University, Bangkok 10330, Thailand
3 Department of Oral Biology, Faculty of Dentistry, Mahidol University, Bangkok 10400, Thailand; nakarinkit@gmail.com
4 Department of Microbiology, Faculty of Medicine, Chulalongkorn University, Bangkok 10330, Thailand; a_leelahavanit@yahoo.com
5 Proteomics Research Laboratory, 113 Thailand Science Park, Phahonyothin Road, Khlong 1, Khlong Luang, Pathum Thani 12120, Thailand; sittiruk@biotec.or.th
* Correspondence: pithi_chan@yahoo.com

Abstract: Lung cancer has long been recognized as an important world heath concern due to its high incidence and death rate. The failure of treatment strategies, as well as the regrowth of the disease driven by cancer stem cells (CSCs) residing in the tumor, lead to the urgent need for a novel CSC-targeting therapy. Here, we utilized proteome alteration analysis and ectopic tumor xenografts to gain insight on how gigantol, a bibenzyl compound from orchid species, could attenuate CSCs and reduce tumor integrity. The proteomics revealed that gigantol affected several functional proteins influencing the properties of CSCs, especially cell proliferation and survival. Importantly, the PI3K/AKT/mTOR and JAK/STAT related pathways were found to be suppressed by gigantol, while the JNK signal was enhanced. The in vivo nude mice model confirmed that pretreatment of the cells with gigantol prior to a tumor becoming established could decrease the cell division and tumor maintenance. The results indicated that gigantol decreased the relative tumor weight with dramatically reduced tumor cell proliferation, as indicated by Ki-67 labeling. Although gigantol only slightly altered the epithelial-to-mesenchymal and angiogenesis statuses, the gigantol-treated group showed a dramatic loss of tumor integrity as compared with the well-grown tumor mass of the untreated control. This study reveals the effects of gigantol on tumor initiation, growth, and maintain in the scope that the cells at the first step of tumor initiation have lesser CSC property than the control untreated cells. This study reveals novel insights into the anti-tumor mechanisms of gigantol focused on CSC targeting and destabilizing tumor integrity via suppression of the PI3K/AKT/mTOR and JAK/STAT pathways. This data supports the potential of gigantol to be further developed as a drug for lung cancer.

Keywords: gigantol; AKT; JAK/STAT; cancer stem cell; tumor maintenance; tumor density; lung cancer; proteomics

---

1. Introduction

A new paradigm shift in the field of cancer cell biology is being driven by the concept of a key cancer cell population controlling the whole tumor, termed "cancer stem cells (CSCs)" [1]. CSCs from various types of cancers share a number of conservation properties, such as self-renewal ability, the generation of multiple types of differentiated cancer cells to drive tumor growth and heterogeneity, and resistance to chemotherapy via an upsurge of the DNA repair system and drug efflux transporter [2]. Therapeutic strategies targeting CSCs, including CSC direct eradication, CSC differentiation into tumor bulk cells, deletion of the supportive signals from a CSC niche, and suppression of CSC pathways, could lead to effective cancer therapy [3].

In lung adenocarcinoma, CSCs from patients were found to be less than 1.5% of the whole tumor cell population [4], but this small subpopulation was still substantial for tumorigenesis and tumor relapse [5]. The key driving pathways of CSCs, such as the PI3K/AKT/mTOR and JAK/STAT3 signals, were found to be significantly increased in cancers with high CSC properties, and hence investigations of many small molecules targeting such pathways are ongoing in clinical trials [6,7]. Protein kinase B (PKB) or AKT, which is, in fact, frequently upregulated in lung cancer plays a key role in cell survival and proliferation [8]. The activation of AKT was shown to be related with cisplatin resistance in lung cancer cells [9]. The roles of AKT on the properties of CSCs and their survival have been demonstrated in several key studies [10,11]. Likewise, signal transducer and activator of transcription 3 (STAT3) activation has been associated with poor prognosis as well as augmented CSCs [12]. A higher level of phosphorylated STAT3 (active STAT3) contributed to epithelial-to-mesenchymal transition (EMT) as well as increased CSC-like phenotypes of non-small cell lung cancer cells (NSCLCs), while the inhibition of STAT3 caused the opposite effects [13]. Instead of bulk non-CSC tumor clearance, the targeting of AKT and STAT3 is believed to be a promising anti-cancer strategy that could lead to the tumor collapse and prevention of the relapse of the disease [14,15].

Recently, natural compounds from plants have garnered increasing attention either as potential drugs or lead compounds in drug discovery research [16,17]. The key benefits of natural compounds are the abundance of plants, compound diversity, and cost effectiveness. In focusing on CSCs and tumor growth inhibition, previous studies have reported the promising activities of the bibenzyl derivative chrysotoxine in the suppression of AKT and Src [18]. In vivo studies further revealed that the bibenzyl derivative moscatilin reduced tumor volumes of lung and esophageal cancer xenografts [19,20]. Gigantol, a bibenzyl compound, is one of the polyphenolic components frequently found in traditional Chinese medicine, and has been shown to have several pharmacological effects, e.g., anti-inflammatory, amelioration of diabetic nephropathy and cataract, and anti-cancer [21–23]. The structure of gigantol consists of a bibenzyl core (Figure 1A). In vitro studies reported that gigantol triggered the apoptotic cell death of lung cancer cell lines but was not toxic to keratinocytes [24].

Our previous studies revealed several effects of noncytotoxic concentrations of gigantol on NSCLCs [25–28]. Pretreatment of 5 to 20 μM of gigantol showed a reduction of the tumor-forming capacity of NSCLCs, represented by significantly suppressing the anchorage-independent growth. In addition, with a single pretreatment of gigantol, the ability of cancer cells to form spheroids, a critical hallmark of CSCs, was abundantly suppressed [25]. These data indicated that the cancer cells had lost their self-renewal capability, which was confirmed by Western blot results showing the downregulation of octamer-binding transcription factor 4 (Oct 4) and Nanog, essential transcription factors for self-renewal and CSC-like phenotype maintenance [25]. Altogether, gigantol has the potential to attenuate tumorigenesis. However, certain information regarding the tumor growth attenuation mechanism and key evidence in animal models are still required. In this study, a subcutaneous xenograft model, as well as proteomic analysis of tumor growth regulatory pathways, were performed to help illustrate a clearer picture of how gigantol could suppress lung cancer.

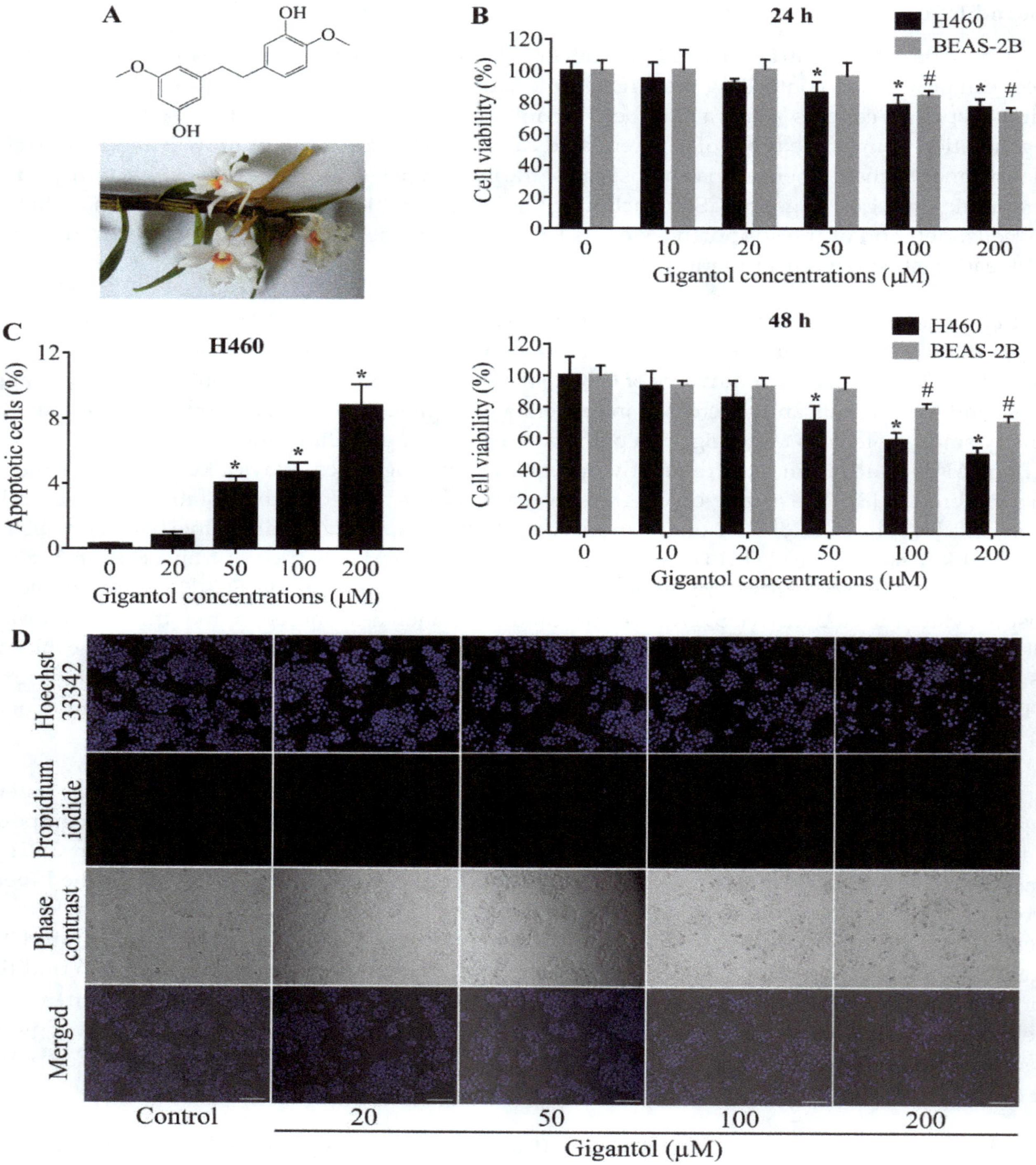

Figure 1. (**A**) Gigantol structure and the plant specimen, Dendrobium draconis Rchb.f. (**B**) Graphs showing the percentages of H460 and BEAS-2B cells viability. Both cell lines were treated with 0 to 200 μM of gigantol or vehicle for 24 to 48 h and then analyzed by MTT assay for cell viability. The percentages of viable cells were compared to their untreated controls. (**C**) Graph showing the percentages of apoptotic cell death after 24 h of gigantol exposure. Necrotic cells could not be detected. (**D**) Photographs of Hoechst 33342, Propidium iodide (PI), and phase contrast fields showing cancer cells morphologies after 24 h of gigantol treatment, the scale bars represent 100 μm and the magnification is 100×. Each experiment was performed in biological triplicates, * indicates $p < 0.05$ as compared with untreated group of H460, # indicates $p < 0.05$ as compared with untreated group of BEAS-2B (one-way ANOVA, Dunnett's test).

2. Results

2.1. Determination of Noncytotoxic Concentrations of Gigantol

Treatment of human NSCLCs H460 with 10 to 20 μM of gigantol for 24 and 48 h had a nonsignificant effect on survival of the cells, while a significant reduction of cell survival could be first detected in response to gigantol at a concentration of 50 μM (Figure 1B). Moreover, cell viability evaluation revealed that gigantol exhibited less toxicity to human lung epithelial cells BEAS-2B as compared with lung cancer cells. Confirmation of cell death, either via apoptosis or necrosis, was detected under a fluorescent microscope after staining with Hoechst 33342 and propidium iodide (PI), as described in the Materials and Methods section. The nuclear staining results revealed that condensed and fragmented nuclei of apoptosis cells could be observed only in the cells treated with gigantol at 200 μM. It is worth indicating that treatment with gigantol at all concentrations (0 to 200 μM) caused no necrosis (Figure 1C,D). Noncytotoxic concentrations of gigantol (0 to 20 μM) were used in subsequent experiments.

2.2. Functional Classification and Enrichment Analysis of the Down- and Upregulated Proteins in Gigantol-Treated Cells

In total, 4351 proteins were identified from the control cells, while 3745 proteins were identified from the gigantol-treated cells. The protein lists from the control and gigantol-treated cells were input to a Venn diagram and 2373 proteins (54.54%) were identified as being only from the control cells, 1767 proteins (47.18%) only from the gigantol-treated cells, and 1978 proteins from both groups (Figure 2A). The protein lists that were uniquely found in the control or gigantol-treated cells were subjected to further bioinformatic analysis (the lists of proteins are in Table S1).

The down- and upregulated protein lists were categorized into three ontologies, molecular function, biological process, and cellular component using Panther software (conducted on 8 October 2019). The most overrepresented molecular functions were binding (38.3% down- and 35.6% upregulated proteins) and catalytic activity (32.0% down- and 35.6% upregulated proteins) (Figure 2B). The most overrepresented biological process categories were cellular process (31.8% down- and 32.6% upregulated proteins), and metabolic process (21.0% down- and 19.8% upregulated proteins) (Figure 2C). The most overrepresented cellular component categories were cell (39.4% down- and 40.2% upregulated proteins) and organelle (33.6% down- and 32.2% upregulated proteins) (Figure 2D).

The two protein lists were input to Enrichr software to identify the enriched biological processes associated with the down- and upregulated proteins after treating with gigantol (conducted on 8 October 2019). Enrichment terms from the Gene Ontology (GO) biological process of downregulated proteins in gigantol-treated cells are involved in macromolecule biosynthesis, DNA-templated transcription, gene expression, protein phosphorylation, cytoskeleton organization, and telomere maintenance. In contrast, enrichment biological processes of upregulated proteins in gigantol-treated cells are involved in intracellular signal transduction, protein phosphorylation, gene expression, and protein biosynthesis processes (Table 1; The full lists of the enriched biological processes of down- and upregulated proteins altered by gigantol are in Tables S2 and S3).

2.3. Protein–Protein Interaction Networks of the Down- and Upregulated Proteins in Gigantol-Treated Cells

Kinases are vital enzymes that regulate intracellular signaling. Several oncogenes and tumor suppressor genes are kinase enzymes or proteins linked to protein kinase activity. Therefore, the proteins that linked to the GO term "protein phosphorylation (GO:0006468)" obtained from Enrichr were subjected to protein-protein interaction network analysis with the Search Tool for Retrieval of Interacting Genes/Proteins (STRING) database in order to determine the significant kinase pathways affected by gigantol.

Table 1. First 10 ranking enrichment terms from the GO biological process of down- and upregulated proteins in gigantol-treated cells.

Term	Overlap	*p*-Value
enriched biological processes associated with the down-regulated proteins		
regulation of cellular macromolecule biosynthetic process (GO:2000112)	129/632	2.65×10^{-10}
regulation of nucleic acid-templated transcription (GO:1903506)	121/608	4.65×10^{-9}
protein phosphorylation (GO:0006468)	97/471	2.82×10^{-8}
regulation of transcription, DNA-templated (GO:0006355)	254/1599	3.09×10^{-7}
regulation of gene expression (GO:0010468)	174/1038	9.47×10^{-7}
phosphorylation (GO:0016310)	76/387	5.61×10^{-6}
protein autophosphorylation (GO:0046777)	41/176	1.44×10^{-5}
cytoskeleton organization (GO:0007010)	29/127	$3.49E \times 10^{-4}$
membrane depolarization during action potential (GO:0086010)	13/39	3.58×10^{-4}
regulation of telomere maintenance (GO:0032204)	10/26	4.67×10^{-4}
enriched biological processes associated with the up-regulated proteins		
regulation of intracellular signal transduction (GO:1902531)	62/423	4.82×10^{-5}
protein phosphorylation (GO:0006468)	67/471	6.24×10^{-5}
ribosomal large subunit biogenesis (GO:0042273)	16/64	1.02×10^{-4}
cyclic purine nucleotide metabolic process (GO:0052652)	10/31	2.17×10^{-4}
regulation of gene expression (GO:0010468)	124/1038	2.75×10^{-4}
nucleotide biosynthetic process (GO:0009165)	9/27	3.40×10^{-4}
DNA replication checkpoint (GO:0000076)	7/17	3.59×10^{-4}
RNA splicing, via transesterification reactions with bulged adenosine as nucleophile (GO:0000377)	37/237	4.55×10^{-4}
regulation of mRNA processing (GO:0050684)	9/29	6.19×10^{-4}
mRNA processing (GO:0006397)	42/284	6.22×10^{-4}

The 97 proteins that were downregulated and 67 proteins that were upregulated in gigantol-treated cells obtained from the GO term "protein phosphorylation (GO: 0006468)" were separately input to the STRING software (conducted on 8 October 2019). The resulting networks were presented (Figure 3A,C), and the significant nodes were determined from both the down- and upregulated protein lists. The top 10% of the downregulated proteins that had the most protein interactions were the following: MTOR, PIK3CA, JAK1, JAK2, PIK3CD, ERBB2, CHEK1, IGF1R, PTK2, ALK, and JAK3. Whereas, the top 10% of the upregulated proteins that had the most protein interactions were the following: AKT1, MAPK1, ABL1, MAPK8, CDK2, and PAK2.

The significant nodes of downregulated proteins were then analyzed for the pathways involved in CSCs using STRING, as shown in Figure 3A. According to the Kyoto Encyclopedia of Genes and Genomes (KEGG) pathway database (https://www.genome.jp/kegg/), the significant proteins that were downregulated by gigantol treatment were involved primarily in the PI3K/AKT and JAK/STAT signaling pathways (Figure 3B). These pathways were indicated as signaling pathways regulating the pluripotency of stem cells. Whereas, the significant nodes of the upregulated proteins were related to the ErbB signaling pathway, which supported the CSCs' properties (Figure 3D). Interestingly, gigantol was previously shown to potentially suppress cancer cells growth, anoikis-resistance, and cancer stemness [25–27]. Regarding the data, the downregulated kinase proteins that were affected by gigantol treatment were linked to the many well-known pathways associated with tumorigenesis and CSC maintenance.

We further confirmed that the gigantol target pathways were crucial for CSC maintenance. The list of proteins involved in CSC regulation was extracted from the KEGG pathway database, using the term "hsa04550: Signaling pathways regulating pluripotency of stem cells—Homo sapiens (human)", and mapped with our H460 proteomic profiles (conducted on 28 October 2019.). In total, 50 proteins were represented in the KEGG pathway, 12 proteins were significantly upregulated, 20 proteins were significantly downregulated, and 18 proteins were not significantly altered by gigantol (Figure 4A). Remarkably, the downregulated proteins affected by gigantol were mostly linked to the PI3K/AKT and JAK/STAT pathways (protein lists of the two pathways were obtained from KEGG pathway database "hsa04151: PI3K-AKT signaling pathway—Homo sapiens (human)" and "hsa04630: JAK-STAT signaling pathway—Homo sapiens (human)"; conducted on 28 October 2019.). Nevertheless, the levels of proteins belonging to the Wnt pathway, another pathway related to CSCs, were not significantly changed.

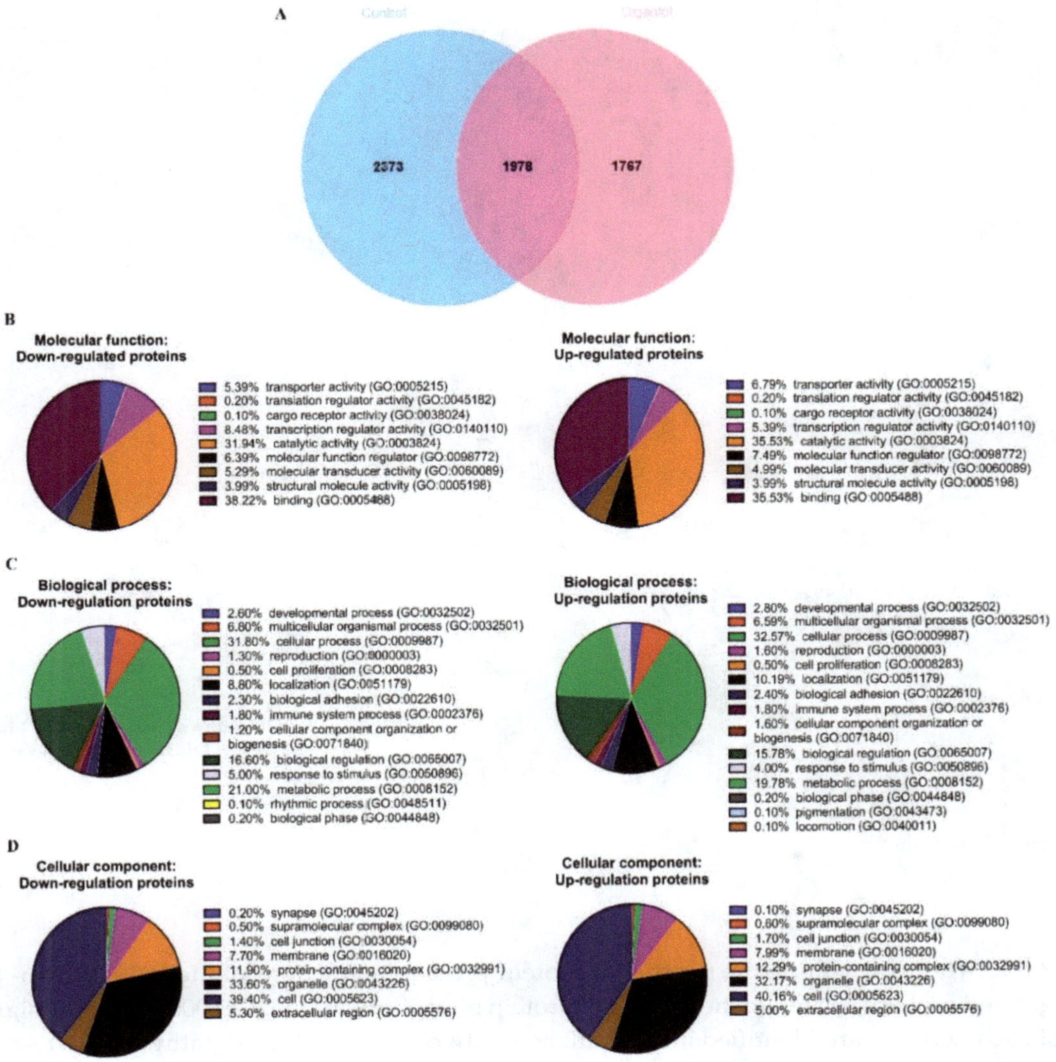

Figure 2. H460 cells were treated with 20 μM of gigantol or its vehicle (0.004% DMSO) for 24 h before the whole-cell lysates were collected. The experiment was performed in biological triplicates. (**A**) Venn diagram showing the difference in proteins expressions between the control and gigantol-treated H460 cells. Three functional classifications of the 2373 down- and 1767 upregulated proteins affected by gigantol treatment using Panther software: (**B**) molecular function, (**C**) biological process, and (**D**) cellular component.

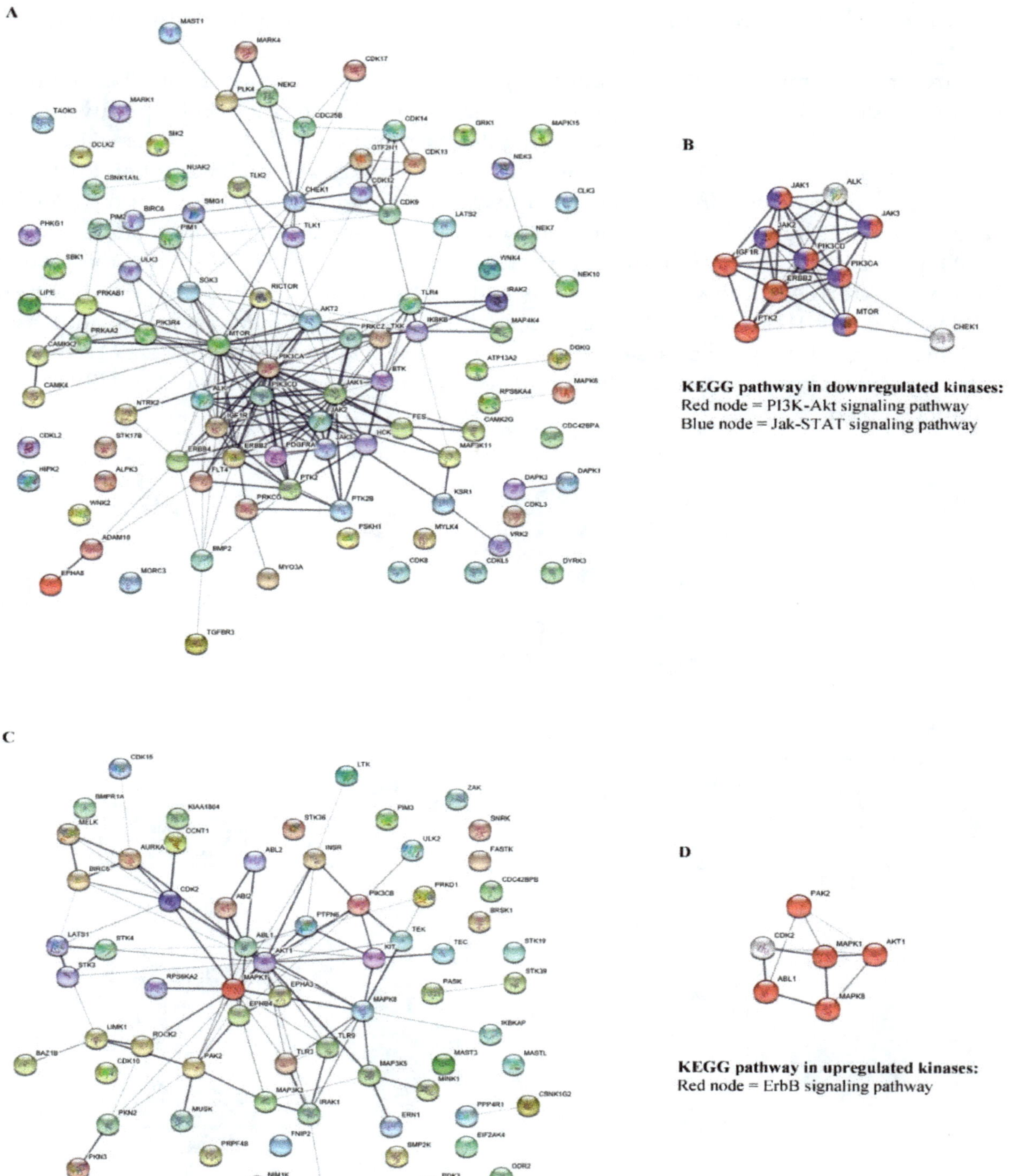

Figure 3. Networks presenting the functional protein-protein interactions of the (**A**) 97 down- and (**C**) 67 upregulated proteins related to the GO term "protein phosphorylation" (GO:0006468). The significant nodes of each network are identified and rebuilt as a network of CSC linked pathways. (**B**) According to the KEGG pathways database, significant nodes of the downregulated proteins were labeled with red for the PI3K-AKT signaling pathway (hsa04151) with FDR 4.08e−13 and blue for the JAK-STAT signaling pathway (hsa04630) with false discovery rate (FDR) 2.80e−09. (**D**) Significant nodes of upregulated proteins were labeled with red for the ErbB signaling pathway (hsa04012) with FDR 1.28×10^{-9}

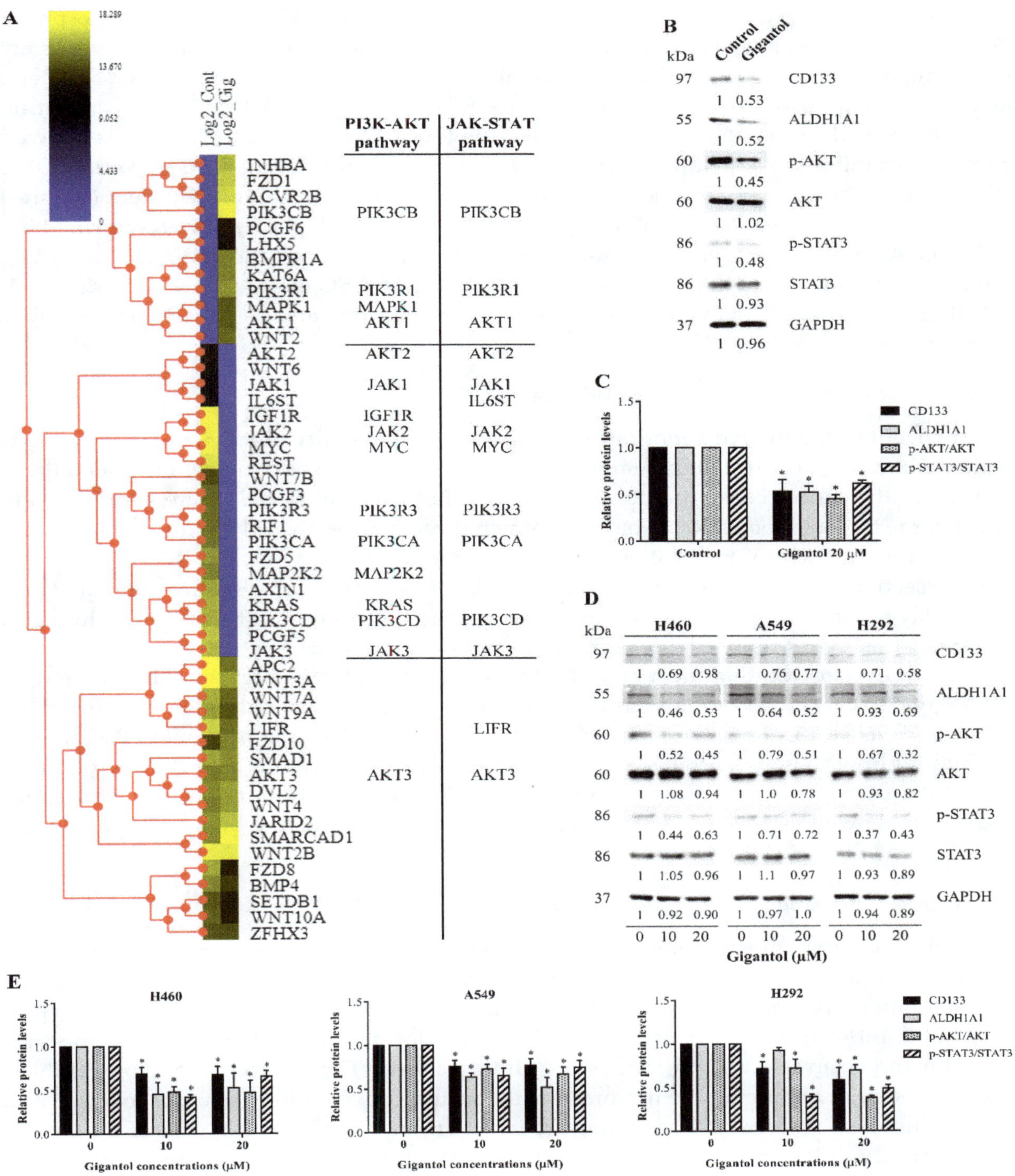

Figure 4. (**A**) Heatmap representing the levels of proteins associated with the signaling pathways regulating the pluripotency of stem cells in the control and gigantol-treated H460 cells (left and right columns of the heatmap, respectively). Proteins belonging to each pathway are listed to the right. (**B**) CSC markers and key kinases of AKT and STAT3 were determined by Western blotting and (**C**) the immunoblot signal intensities were quantified by densitometry. The uncropped protein bands are in Figure S2 (S2A: The protein bands from Figure 4B; S2B: The protein bands from Figure 4D). (**D**) The effects of gigantol on AKT, STATS3, and CSC markers were confirmed in two other NSCLC cell lines, A549 and H292, and (**E**) the relative protein levels were quantified. The mean data from each experiment was normalized to the GAPDH results. The experiment was performed biologically triplicated. Data represent the means ± SD ($n = 3$) * indicates $p < 0.05$ as compared with the control group (student's t-test).

To confirm, the key proteins of PI3K/AKT and JAK/STAT pathways including AKT, phosphorylated Akt (S473), STAT3, phosphorylated STAT3 (S727), and CSC markers were determined by Western blot analysis using the same cell population of proteomics and xenograft experiments. The band density of active form of Akt (phosphorylated AKT) and active STAT3 (phosphorylated STAT3) was normalized with their own total forms in order to determine the levels of activation. The results showed that gigantol could inhibit the activation of AKT and STAT3. In addition, the CSC makers (CD133 and ALHD1A1) were found to be significantly reduced in response to gigantol treatment (Figure 4B,C). Moreover, the effect of gigantol on PI3K/AKT, JAK/STAT, and CSC markers was confirmed in other NSCLC cells (A549 and H292 cells) (Figure 4D,E). It was quite clear that the PI3K/AKT and JAK/STAT signaling pathways were the target pathways of gigantol on CSC maintenance in NSCLCs. It was possible that gigantol could show some effects on tumor formation and its integrity in vivo by means of CSC suppression.

2.4. *Gigantol Negatively Regulates Tumor Cell Growth in Vivo*

The concept of the in vivo xenograft was to compare the ability to form and maintain a tumor between the untreated control and gigantol-treated H460 cells. This experiment revealed the effects of gigantol on the cancer cells whether the CSC or other survival signals were suppressed by the treatment at the time of inoculation. The pretreatment procedure excluded the direct anticancer effect of the compound on the tumor cell after mice implantation.

After injection of lung cancer cells into two flanks of each mouse, most mice generated palpable tumors on day seven and most control tumors had reached their endpoint size on day 13. Figure 5A demonstrates that every mouse had a similar growth rate (indicated by body weight) in a normal range. The results showed that most gigantol-treated tumors were lighter than their paired control tumors (Figure 5B,C). However, the average weights of the tumors were only slightly different (control group mean = 966 ± 154.4 mg, gigantol group mean = 698 ± 154.5 mg, $n = 5$, $p = 0.255$, Student's t-test). Tumor growth rates varied between the mice, but the mean tumor growth rates of the control and gigantol groups were not different (Figure 5D,E). The dissected tumor densities were compared, and the results showed that the gigantol groups had lower tumor densities than their paired untreated controls (Figure 5F).

2.5. *Histological Observation Showed Lower Viable Tumor Areas in the Gigantol-Treated Tumors*

Having shown that gigantol pretreatment caused tumors with a lesser density as compared with the untreated control, we wish to emphasize this phenomenon as previous studies have indicated that changes in tumor density, as indicated by CT imaging showing a loss of tumor mass, can be a potential assessment for anti-cancer drug action [29,30]. Cross-section slices of the tumors were co-stained by hematoxylin and eosin (H&E), and, then, were photographed. The macro-morphology of the tumor structure was similar among all the tumors (small nodules packed within a tumor lobe, surrounded with fibrous tissues), whereas the percentage of intact and non-viable tumor cells of the two groups were dramatically different. Figure 6 demonstrates that while the control tumors exhibited a dense viable tumor mass, the gigantol tumors showed a substantial loss of tumor mass, as indicated by a hollowing with the magenta staining of cells or pale pink cells without nuclear staining.

2.6. *Gigantol Suppresses Tumor Cells Proliferation but not Tumor Vasculature.*

Two pairs of tumors were selected for Ki-67 and α-smooth muscle actin (α-SMA) immunohistochemistry (IHC) staining. The hot spots and cold spots of Ki-67 positive cells are shown in Figure 7A. The mean percentage of Ki-67 positive cells of the control group was 62.45 ± 0.3951 and that of the gigantol-treated group was 49.49 ± 0.7348 (p-value = 0.0041, Student's t-test, $n = 2$, Figure 7B).

The α-SMA signals from cancer cells in all tumors were so low that they could not be scored (Figure 7C). This result indicated that both the control and gigantol groups had a low level of mesenchymal-like phenotypes. Figure 7D presents mature vessels covered by pericytes. The number of vessels per area detected by α-SMA staining was similar in all the tumors.

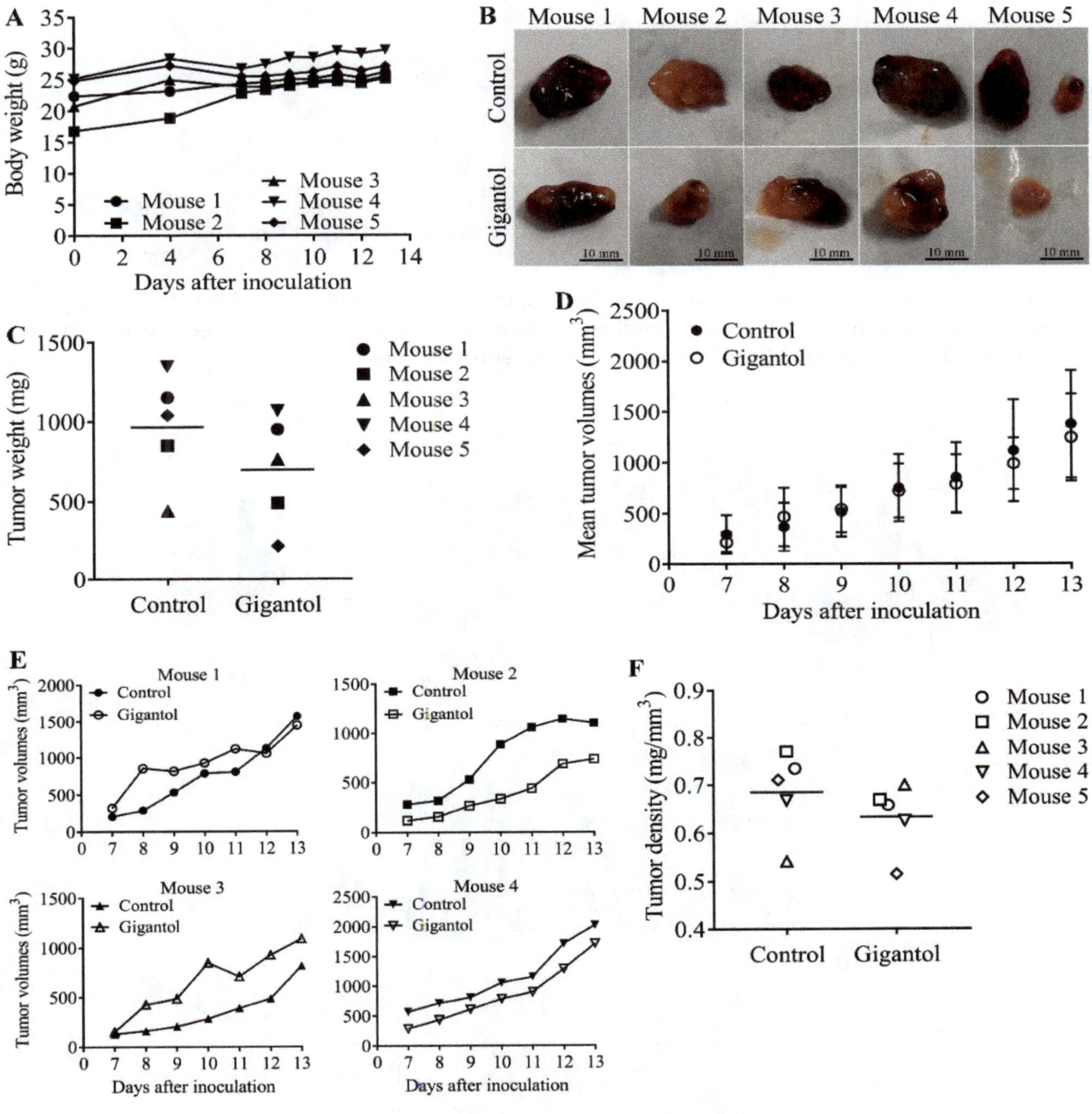

Figure 5. (**A**) Graph showing mice body weights starting at the day of cancer cell inoculation. There was no significant change of the body weights until the day of termination. (**B**) Untreated (upper row) and gigantol-treated (lower row) tumors were dissected and photographed at day 13 after inoculation. Scale bars represent 10 mm in length. (**C**) Graph showing grouped means of the control and gigantol tumor weights. The 5 different markers represent each pair of tumors. The gigantol-treated tumors had lower tumor weights as compared with their own control tumors, except for mouse 3. (**D**) Graph presenting the mean growth rate of the control and gigantol groups. (**E**) Four graphs demonstrating the individual tumor growth rate of each mouse (tumor growth of mouse 5 could not be accomplished because the gigantol-treated tumor was not palpable and measured until the day of termination). (**F**) Tumor density was calculated as weight by volume. The horizon lines represent means of each group.

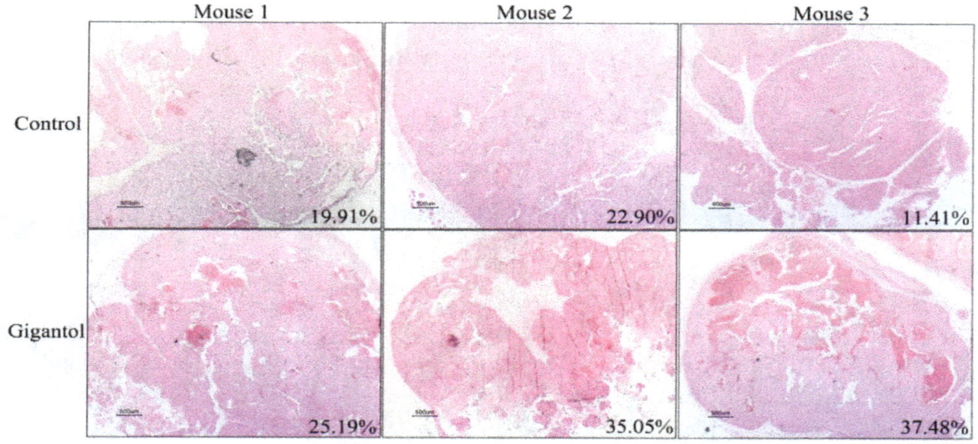

Figure 6. Hematoxylin and eosin staining showing intratumor morphology (20×). Percentages of necrotic areas as compared with their total areas are shown at the lower-right edge of each picture. Scale bars at the lower-left edge of each picture represent 500 μm lengths.

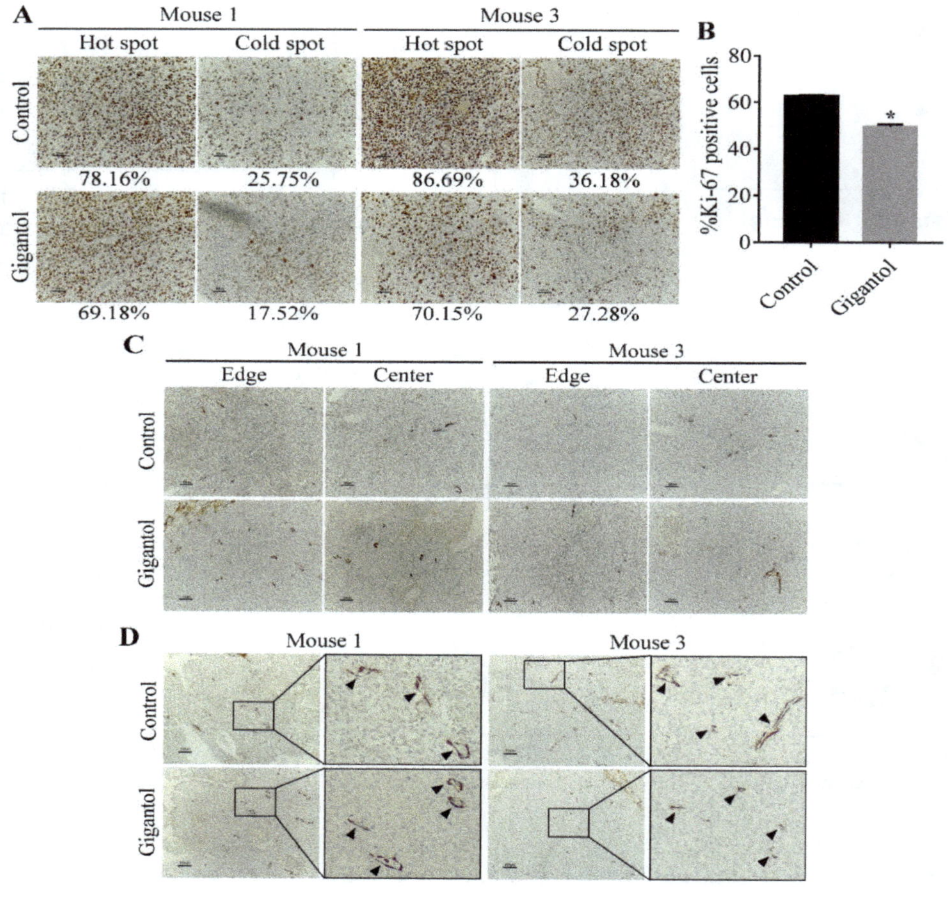

Figure 7. (**A**) Immunohistochemistry (IHC) staining demonstrating 200-fold magnified pictures of hot spots and cold spots from the control and gigantol-treated tumors. The percentages of Ki-67 positive cells as compared with total cells are displayed under their pictures. (**B**) Graph showing the means of %Ki-67 positive cells. The gigantol-treated tumors have lower Ki-67 positive cells than the control tumors. * indicates $p < 0.05$ as compared with the control group (Student's *t*-test). (**C**) α-SMA IHC staining of cancer cells in both edge and center areas of tumors showing no difference of signal levels (200×). The numbers of mature tumor vessels per areas between the control and gigantol groups were not different. (**D**) Pictures showing vessel distribution among the tumor mass (100×). Arrow indicates a vessel (400×).

3. Discussion

According to the increasing trend of cancer incidence and mortality, the development of novel anti-cancer therapies is highly needed. Among malignant tumors, lung cancer has been shown to be the main cause of cancer-related mortality and treatment failure [31], leading to the requirement for effective therapeutic options. Previous studies have reported the potential anti-cancer activities of gigantol, one of the most widely studied bibenzyls. Gigantol has exhibited cytotoxicity against various types of cancer cells, such as breast, liver, and lung cancer cells [24,32,33]. Moreover, gigantol could attenuate certain aggressive phenotypes that bring about tumor progression and metastasis, including proliferation, migration, invasion, anoikis-resistance, and anchorage-independent growth [25–28].

Proteomics analysis (Figure S1).demonstrated that PI3K/AKT/mTOR and JAK/STAT were among the most affected proteins in response to gigantol treatment. The key kinases belonging to the PI3K/AKT/mTOR axis, including phosphoinositide 3-kinases (PI3Ks, α and δ isoforms) and mammalian target of rapamycin (mTOR), were significantly decreased in the gigantol-treated cells (Figure 3A,B). Both isoforms of PI3K can activate phosphatidylinositol (3,4,5)-trisphosphate (PIP3), an upstream activator of AKT [34]. In addition, PI3K can trigger an AKT-independent mechanism, which transduces signals through serine/threonine-protein kinase Sgk3 (SGK3) and mTOR complex 2 (mTORC2) [35]. Consistently, our proteomic results showed the suppression of key proteins of the PI3K-mediated AKT-independent pathway, such as PIK3CA, PIK3CD, SGK3, MTOR, and RICTOR, which were simultaneously downregulated (Table S1).

Janus kinase 1 and 2 (JAK1 and JAK2) are transducers of the heteromeric receptors of interleukin 6 and 10 (IL-6 and IL-10), which activate signal transducer and activator of transcription 3 (STAT3). STAT3 was shown to mediate cancer cell survival, proliferation, angiogenesis, and metastasis, as well as maintaining the CSC phenotypes [7,36]. Although the STAT3 protein could not be detected in our proteomic profiles due to its low abundance, its downstream target genes, including cyclin D1 and c-Myc, were downregulated [12] (Table S1). JAK3 is an upstream regulator of STAT5 and STAT6. An accumulating data exercise revealed that inhibition of the JAK3 signaling could reduce cancer progression [37]. It is possible that the suppression of JAK/STAT signaling by gigantol should attenuate CSC in lung cancer. In addition, the mitogen-activated protein kinase 8 (MAPK8) or c-Jun N-terminal kinase (JNK) protein level was found to be induced by gigantol treatment (Figure 3D). JNK plays a role in controlling cancer cell death. The activation of JNK is necessary for intrinsic and extrinsic apoptosis, and autophagic cell death [38]. JNK signaling has been reported as a vital molecular mechanism of many anti-cancer-agents-induced cancer cell death and inactivation of such a protein led to cancer cell resistance to death stimuli [39,40]. An early upregulation of JNK by gigantol before the cancer cells encountered the stressful conditions in the tumor possibly led to stress induced JNK hyperactivation, which subsequently promoted the expression of proapoptotic proteins [38].

Recent evidence has suggested that CSCs functions as a seed of tumors. Not only do the CSCs use their ability of self-renewal and differentiation for tumor establishing, but also implicate cancer progression, metastasis, and disease relapse [1]. Regarding this matter, our previous work unraveled new information that gigantol could suppress CSC activity and discontinue their role in maintaining tumor [2,41]. This finding is quite in agreement with the previous study indicating that CSCs play a key role in tumor maintenance. This study revealed the effect of gigantol of PI3K/AKT and JAK/STAT3 suppression on the tumor initiation, growth, and maintenance based on the concept that the cells at the first step of tumor initiation had lesser CSC property than the control untreated cells.

In this study, the lung cancer cells were treated with a noncytotoxic concentration of gigantol prior to inoculation into mice subcutaneous skins. The same populations of gigantol-treated cells were subjected to proteomics. This experimental design displays the clear mechanism of gigantol treatment in attenuation of the CSC-supportive PI3K/AKT/mTOR and JAK/STAT3 signals at the time of tumor initiation. Although this experiment used only a single treatment with low dose, gigantol could inhibit the tumor growth rate (Figure 5E). Tumors from the gigantol-pretreated cells had lower weights and densities (Figure 5C,F). Furthermore, the histological tumor integrity was determined.

Previous studies have either demonstrated or proposed that the tumor density can be a promising assessment of anti-cancer drug evaluation as they have given more accuracy on the assessment of an anti-cancer drug response and have contributed to better treatment outcomes [29,30,42]. We observed the cross-sectional histology of the tumors to assess the integrity of intact cell viable areas as compared with the cell death areas as recommended in the guideline [43]. Interestingly, our results indicated that most of the gigantol-treated tumors had a dramatic loss of tumor mass as compared with those of the untreated controls (Figure 6). Consistently, the intratumor structure and tumor phenotype of Ki-67 labeling showed that the gigantol-treated tumors had lower proliferative cancer cells (Figure 7A,B). However, we found that the EMT properties of cancer cells observed by α-SMA staining was not altered by treatment with gigantol (Figure 7C). Also, the angiogenic capability of both groups of tumors was not different (Figure 7D). The phenotypic observation revealed that the pretreatment with gigantol did not have an effect on tumor neoangiogenesis. Further investigation on gigantol-mediated stromal cell-induced angiogenesis is thus suggested.

This study was designed in a manner of a pharmacological study that minimized the confounding factors in the system and focused on the effect of gigantol on the cancer cells. We could assume from the results that gigantol treatment altered the tumor-promoting activities of the cells prior to the process of tumor inoculation and such alteration attenuated the ability of the cancer cell to grow and maintain a tumor, resulting in a reduced tumor mass with viable cancer cell loss. Although our results helped us scope the direct action of the compound on NSCLCs, further investigation is necessary, including the injection of the substance into a tumor or animal after tumor formation to gain more insights.

4. Materials and Methods

4.1. Cell Line Cultures

Human NSCLC H460 and normal bronchus epithelial cell BEAS-2B lines were purchased from the American Type Culture Collection (Manassas, VA, USA) and were cultured in Roswell Park Memorial Institute (RPMI) 1640 medium and Dulbecco's modified Eagle medium (DMEM), respectively, supplemented with 10% fetal bovine serum, 2 mM L-glutamine, and 100 units/mL each of penicillin and streptomycin in a humidified atmosphere with 5% CO_2 at 37 °C.

4.2. Animals

Six-week old male BALB/cAJcl nude mice were purchased from Nomura Siam International (Samut Prakan, Thailand). Five mice were maintained in one cage under strictly hygiene housing with controlled temperature (23 ± 2 °C) and light/dark cycle (12 h light/12 h dark) at the Animal House of Faculty of Medicine, Chulalongkorn University. The study was approved by the Institutional Animal Care and Use Committee of the Faculty of Medicine, Chulalongkorn University, Bangkok, Thailand (ethical reference number CULAC 001/2561). Animal welfare and experimental procedures were strictly carried out in accordance with The Eighth Edition of the Guide for the Care and Use of Laboratory Animals (NRC 2011) [44]. All efforts were made to minimize animals' suffering and to reduce the number of animals used.

4.3. Chemicals and Reagents

Gigantol was extracted from stems of Dendrobium draconis Rchb.f., as previously described [45] and dissolved in dimethylsulfoxide (DMSO) at the indicated working concentrations. 3-(4,5-Dimethylthiazol-2-yl) 2,5-diphenyltetrazolium bromide (MTT), Hoechst 33342, propidium iodide (PI), bovine serum albumin (BSA), dimethyl sulfoxide (DMSO), cocktail protease inhibitor, hematoxylin, and eosin were purchased from Sigma chemical, Inc. (Chemical Express, Bangkok, Thailand). RPMI-1640 medium, DMEM, phosphate buffer saline (PBS), glutamine, penicillin, and streptomycin were purchased from Gibco company (Gibthai, Bangkok, Thailand). Primary antibodies against CD133, ALDH1A1, total AKT, phosphorylated AKT (Ser473), total STAT3, phosphorylated STAT3

(Ser727), and GAPDH, horseradish peroxidase labeled secondary antibodies, and RIPA lysis buffer were purchase from Cell Signaling Technology (Theera Trading, Bangkok, Thailand). Pentobarbital sodium injection was purchased from Ceva Sante Animal (VET AGRITECH, Nonthaburi, Thailand). 3,3′-Diaminobenzidine tetrahydrochloride hydrate was purchased from TCI Co., LTD (Chemical Express, Bangkok, Thailand). Primary antibodies of Ki-67 and α-SMA and matched secondary antibodies were purchased from DAKO (Medicare Supply, Bangkok, Thailand).

4.4. Cell Viability Assay

In order to elucidate the possible tumor suppression activity of gigantol, first, we selected the concentrations of the compound that caused no toxicity to the cancer cells. Cell viability was determined by plating cells at a density of 10,000 cells per well in 96-well plates. The cells were allowed to adhere overnight, medium was removed, and medium with various concentrations of gigantol (0 to 200 μM) or 0.1% DMSO was added. After 24 to 48 h of treatment, the number of viable cells were measured with the use of MTT assay. Medium was aspirated and 0.4 mg/mL of MTT in PBS was added to each well. The plate was then incubated at 37 °C, 5% CO2 for 3 h. Afterwards, the resulting formazan crystal was dissolved in 100 μL of DMSO and subjected to a 570 nm absorbance reading via a microplate reader (ClarioStar, BMG Labtech, Germany). The assay was performed biological triplicate.

4.5. Cell Death Determination Assay

Nuclear co-staining with Hoechst 33342 and propidium iodide (PI) was used to determine apoptotic and necrotic cell death. Cells were treated with gigantol as described in cell viability assay. Then, cells were incubated with 10 μM of Hoechst 33342 and 5 μM PI for 30 min at 37 °C. Cells were visualized and imaged under a fluorescence microscope (Nikon eclipse Ts2 with Nikon DS Fi3 camera). Apoptotic cell could be detected by Hoechst 33342 nuclear staining, showing condensed nucleus and fragmented nuclei of apoptotic bodies. Necrotic cell could be detected by PI staining.

4.6. Sample Preparation

H460 cells were treated with 20 μM gigantol or 0.01% DMSO (vehicle) for 24 h. The cells were lysed with 0.5% SDS. Total protein amount collected from each sample was measured with Lowry assay with bovine serum albumin as a standard [46]. Equal protein amount from 3 independent biological samples were pooled. Fifty micrograms of protein from control or gigantol treated cells were subjected to in-solution digestion. Samples were completely dissolved in 10 mM ammonium bicarbonate (AMBIC), reduced disulfide bonds using 5 mM dithiothreitol (DTT) in 10 mM AMBIC at 60 °C for 1 h and alkylation of sulfhydryl groups by using 15 mM Iodoacetamide (IAA) in 10 mM AMBIC, at room temperature for 45 min in the dark. For digestion, samples were mixed with 50 ng/μL of sequencing grade trypsin (1:20 ratio) (Promega, Walldorf, Germany) and incubated at 37 °C overnight. Prior to LC-MS/MS analysis, the digested samples must be dried and protonated with 0.1% formic acid before injection into LC-MS/MS.

4.7. Liquid Chromatography-Tandem Mass Spectrometry (LC-MS/MS)

The LC-MS/MS was used to determine the quantification of the peptides from the digested samples. The tryptic peptide samples were prepared for injection into an Ultimate3000 Nano/Capillary LC System (Thermo Scientific, Gloucester, UK) coupled to a Hybrid quadrupole Q-Tof impact II™ (Bruker Daltonics, Coventry, UK) equipped with a Nano-captive spray ion source. Briefly, peptides were enriched on a μ-Precolumn 300 μm i.d. × 5 mm C18 Pepmap 100, 5 μm, 100 A (Thermo Scientific, UK), separated on a 75 μm I.D. × 15 cm and packed with Acclaim PepMap RSLC C18, 2 μm, 100Å, nanoViper (Thermo Scientific, UK). Solvent A and B containing 0.1% formic acid in water and 0.1% formic acid in 80% acetonitrile, respectively, were supplied on the analytical column. A gradient of 5% to 55% solvent B was used to elute the peptides at a constant flow rate of 0.30 μL/min for 30 min. Electrospray ionization was carried out at 1.6 kV using the CaptiveSpray. Mass spectra (MS) and

MS/MS spectra were obtained in the positive-ion mode over the range (m/z) 150–2200 (Compass 1.9 software, Bruker Daltonics).

4.8. Bioinformatics and Data Analysis

MaxQuant 1.6.6.0 was used to quantify the proteins in individual samples using the Andromeda search engine to correlate MS/MS spectra to the Uniprot Homo sapiens database [47]. The following parameters were used for data processing: maximum of two miss cleavages, mass tolerance of 20 ppm for main search, trypsin as digesting enzyme, carbamidomethylation of cysteine as fixed modification, and the oxidation of methionine and acetylation of the protein N-terminus as variable modifications. Only peptides with a minimum of 7 amino acids, as well as at least one unique peptide, were required for protein identification. Only proteins with at least two peptides, and at least one unique peptide, were considered as being identified and used for further data analysis.

The gene list enrichment analysis was conducted using Enrichr software (https://amp.pharm.mssm.edu/Enrichr/) [48]. Protein organization and biological action was investigated conforming to protein analysis through evolutionary relationships (Panther software; http://pantherdb.org/) protein classification [49]. A Venn diagram (analyzed by jVenn software; http://jvenn.toulouse.inra.fr/app/index.html) was used to show the differences between protein lists originating from different differential analyses [50]. The Search Tool for Retrieval of Interacting Genes/Proteins (STRING) software version 11 (https://string-db.org/cgi/input.pl) was used to analyze the common and the forecasted functional interaction networks between identified proteins [51]. Cytoscape 3.7.2 (https://cytoscape.org/) was utilized to analyze the significant nodes from protein–protein interaction networks [52]. The significant nodes analysis was modified from Rezaei-Tavirani (2017) [53]. The degree values, which were determined by an amount of interacted proteins with the node, were analyzed and the top 10% of the nodes based on degree value were selected as significant nodes. The heatmap visualization and statistical analyses were conducted using the MultiExperiment Viewer (MeV) in the TM4 suite software (http://mev.tm4.org/#/welcome) [54].

4.9. Western Blot Analysis

Cells were lysed with RIPA lysis buffer containing 20 mM Tris-HCl (pH 7.5), 150 mM NaCl, 1 mM Na_2EDTA, 1 mM EGTA, 1% NP-40, 1% sodium deoxycholate, 2.5 mM sodium pyrophosphate, 1 mM beta-glycerophosphate, 1 mM Na_3VO_4, 1 μg/mL leupeptin, and cocktail protease inhibitor mixture for 30 minutes on ice. The protein contents of the cell lysates were evaluated by Lowry assay. Samples with equal amounts of protein (60 μg) were run in the SDS-PAGE before they were transferred onto 0.45 mm nitrocellulose membranes (Bio-Rad, Hercules, California, United States). Transferred membranes were blocked for 1 h in 5% non-fat dry milk in Tris-buffered saline with Tween 20 (25mM Tris-HCl, pH 7.5, 125 mM NaCl, and 0.05% Tween 20) and incubated overnight with specific primary antibodies against CD133, ALDH1A1, total AKT, phosphorylated AKT (Ser473), total STAT3, phosphorylated STAT3 (Ser727), and GAPDH. Membranes were washed three times with Tris-buffered saline with Tween 20 and incubated with appropriate horseradish peroxidase labeled secondary antibodies for 2 h at room temperature. The immune complexes were detected by Clarity and Clarity Max ECL Western Blotting Substrates (Bio-Rad) and imaged with ImageQuant LAS 4000 biomolecular imager (GE Healthcare, Chicago, Illinois, United States).

4.10. Subcutaneous Tumor Xenograft Procedure

The scheme of experimental design is shown in Figure 8. The human NSCLCs were prepared prior to the tumor establishment. The H460 cells were cultured in medium with 20 μM of gigantol or vehicle for 48 h (5 individual sets of cancer cell cultures). Then, the 70% confluent monolayer lung cancer cells were trypsinized, suspended in Hank's saline buffer solution and counted by TC20 automated cell counter (Bio-Rad). Each cell suspension was adjusted to a concentration of viable

5×106 cells per 100 μL. The cancer cell suspensions were kept on ice and rapidly transferred to an in vivo subcutaneous xenograft operation.

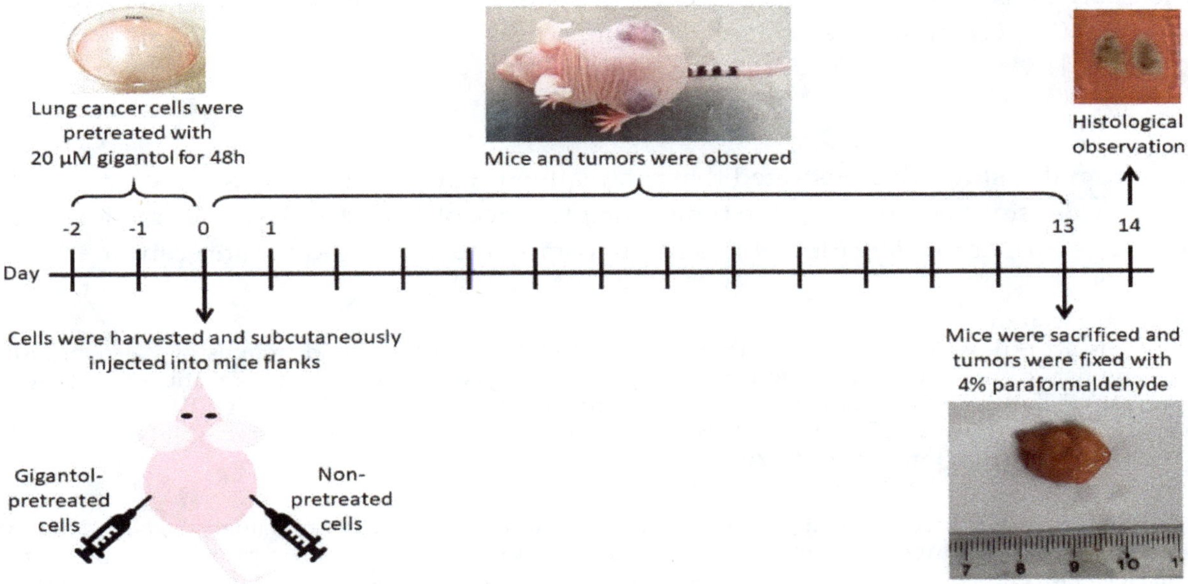

Figure 8. Scheme showing the in vivo experimental procedures.

To minimize variation between animal bodies, one mouse was assigned to bear both control and its paired gigantol-treated tumor. One flank of a mouse was inoculated subcutaneously with viable 5×106 cells of untreated cells and another flank with gigantol pretreated cells. Mice were weighed, and the tumors were observed every 2 days. When a tumor was palpable, the mouse would be observed daily. Vernier Caliper was used to measure the most length and its own orthogonal most width of each tumor. Tumor volumes were calculated by the formula (length × width × width)/2. Tumor growth rates were verified by means of plotting calculated tumor volumes by days. Mice were not exposed to gigantol throughout the experiment. Once control or treatment tumor reached its endpoint size (20 mm in diameter), the tumor-bearing mouse was euthanized by intraperitoneal injection of pentobarbital sodium solution (>150 mg/kg) [55] and then the tumors were dissected, washed with ice-cold PBS, weighed, and photographed with a ruler. The tumors were weighed and immediately fixed with 4% paraformaldehyde for 24 h. Tumors were embedded in paraffin blocks, sliced and stained with hematoxylin and eosin (H&E) for further histologic observation. Necrotic and total areas of tumor slices were determined using ImageJ software [56].

4.11. *Immunohistochemistry Staining of Ki-67 and α-SMA*

Two pairs of tumor slides were selected for staining with Ki-67 (dilution 1:300) and α-smooth muscle actin (α-SMA, dilution 1:100) antibodies and, then, were visualized by incubation with 3,3′-diaminobenzidine. Slides were observed under a brightfield microscope (Nikon eclipse E600 with Nikon DXM1200F camera).

The level of Ki-67 assessment was modified from Jang (2017) [57]. Areas with the highest (hot spot) and the lowest (cold spot) numbers of positive cells (indicated by dark brown staining in nucleus) were selected and the percentages of the positive cells as compared with total cells were calculated. Averages of %Ki-67 positive cells were calculated from the summed total and Ki-67 positive cells from all hot spots and cold spots of the two mice.

α-SMA, a marker of mesenchymal phenotype, was used to detect cancer cells with EMT-like phenotype, endothelial cells, and vascular pericytes [58]. For angiogenesis determination, edge and center areas of each tumor were selected and the number of mature blood vessels (indicated by circular lining of cells labeled with high signal of α-SMA) were counted.

4.12. Statistical Analysis

One-way analysis of variance (one-way ANOVA) and student's *t*-test were performed to conduct statistical analysis (GraphPad Prism 7.0). Data were expressed as mean ± standard deviation (SD) and values of $p < 0.05$ were indicative of significant differences.

5. Conclusions

Data from this study demonstrated that pretreatment with gigantol can suppress tumor growth, reduce tumor density, and attenuate the tumor maintenance of NSCLCs. This information can benefit and encourage further investigation of this useful compound to be used for anti-cancer approaches.

Supplementary Materials:
Figure S1: The workflow for proteomics analysis, Figure S2: The uncropped images of Western blot bands, Table S1: The lists of proteins which were downregulated, upregulated, and not significantly altered by the effects of gigantol, Table S2: GO biological process enrichment analysis results of the significantly downregulated proteins from Enrichr software, Table S3: GO biological process enrichment analysis results of the significantly upregulated proteins from Enrichr software.

Author Contributions: Conceptualization, P.C.; data curation, N.L. and P.C.; formal analysis, N.L., N.K., and S.R.; funding acquisition, P.C.; investigation, N.L.; methodology, P.C., N.L., and A.M.; project administration, P.C.; resources, P.C., S.R., and A.L.; supervision, P.C., S.R., and A.L.; validation, N.L., A.M., N.K., and P.C.; visualization, N.L.; writing—original draft, P.C. and N.L.; writing—review and editing, P.C. and N.L.

Acknowledgments: The authors would like to thank Boonchoo Sritularak for offering orchid extract, Yodying Yingchutrakul for LC-MS/MS technical support, and Panomwat Amornphimoltham for in vivo experiment support. In addition, the authors would like to acknowledge the Pharmaceutical Research Instrument Center, Faculty of Pharmaceutical Sciences, Chulalongkorn University for providing equipment.

References

1. Ayob, A.Z.; Ramasamy, T.S. Cancer stem cells as key drivers of tumour progression. *J. Biomed. Sci.* **2018**, *25*, 20. [CrossRef] [PubMed]
2. Batlle, E.; Clevers, H. Cancer stem cells revisited. *Nat. Med.* **2017**, *23*, 1124–1134. [CrossRef] [PubMed]
3. Garber, K. Cancer stem cell pipeline flounders. *Nat. Rev. Drug Discov.* **2018**, *17*, 771–773. [CrossRef] [PubMed]
4. Carney, D.; Gazdar, A.; Bunn, J.P.; Guccion, J. Demonstration of the stem cell nature of clonogenic tumor cells from lung cancer patients. *Stem Cells* **1982**, *1*, 149–164. [PubMed]
5. Gomez-Casal, R.; Bhattacharya, C.; Ganesh, N.; Bailey, L.; Basse, P.; Gibson, M.; Epperly, M.; Levina, V. Non-small cell lung cancer cells survived ionizing radiation treatment display cancer stem cell and epithelial-mesenchymal transition phenotypes. *Mol. Cancer* **2013**, *12*, 94. [CrossRef] [PubMed]
6. Papadimitrakopoulou, V. Development of PI3K/AKT/mTOR pathway inhibitors and their application in personalized therapy for non-small-cell lung cancer. *J. Thorac. Oncol.* **2012**, *7*, 1315–1326. [CrossRef] [PubMed]
7. Loh, C.Y.; Arya, A.; Naema, A.F.; Wong, W.F.; Sethi, G.; Looi, C.Y. Signal Transducer and Activator of Transcription (STATs) Proteins in Cancer and Inflammation: Functions and Therapeutic Implication. *Front. Oncol.* **2019**, *9*, 48. [CrossRef]
8. Lawlor, M.A.; Alessi, D.R. PKB/AKT. *J. Cell Sci.* **2001**, *114*, 2903.
9. Wang, M.; Liu, Z.M.; Li, X.C.; Yao, Y.T.; Yin, Z.X. Activation of ERK1/2 and AKT is associated with cisplatin resistance in human lung cancer cells. *J. Chemother.* **2013**, *25*, 162–169. [CrossRef]
10. Oo, A.K.K.; Calle, A.S.; Nair, N.; Mahmud, H.; Vaidyanath, A.; Yamauchi, J.; Khayrani, A.C.; Du, J.; Alam, M.J.; Seno, A.; et al. Up-Regulation of PI 3-Kinases and the Activation of PI3K-AKT Signaling Pathway in Cancer Stem-Like Cells Through DNA Hypomethylation Mediated by the Cancer Microenvironment. *Transl. Oncol.* **2018**, *11*, 653–663. [CrossRef]

11. Hambardzumyan, D.; Becher, O.J.; Rosenblum, M.K.; Pandolfi, P.P.; Manova-Todorova, K.; Holland, E.C. PI3K pathway regulates survival of cancer stem cells residing in the perivascular niche following radiation in medulloblastoma in vivo. *Genes Dev.* **2008**, *22*, 436–448. [CrossRef] [PubMed]
12. Galoczova, M.; Coates, P.; Vojtesek, B. STAT3, stem cells, cancer stem cells and p63. *Cell. Mol. Biol. Lett.* **2018**, *23*, 12. [CrossRef] [PubMed]
13. Song, L.; Rawal, B.; Nemeth, J.A.; Haura, E.B. JAK1 activates STAT3 activity in non-small-cell lung cancer cells and IL-6 neutralizing antibodies can suppress JAK1-STAT3 signaling. *Mol. Cancer Ther.* **2011**, *10*, 481–494. [CrossRef] [PubMed]
14. Bahmad, H.F.; Mouhieddine, T.H.; Chalhoub, R.M.; Assi, S.; Araji, T.; Chamaa, F.; Itani, M.M.; Nokkari, A.; Kobeissy, F.; Daoud, G.; et al. The AKT/mTOR pathway in cancer stem/progenitor cells is a potential therapeutic target for glioblastoma and neuroblastoma. *Oncotarget* **2018**, *9*, 33549–33561. [CrossRef] [PubMed]
15. Shibata, M.; Hoque, M.O. Targeting Cancer Stem Cells: A Strategy for Effective Eradication of Cancer. *Cancers* **2019**, *11*, 732. [CrossRef] [PubMed]
16. Chanvorachote, P.; Chamni, S.; Ninsontia, C.; Phiboonchaiyanan, P.P. Potential Anti-metastasis Natural Compounds for Lung Cancer. *Anticancer Res.* **2016**, *36*, 5707–5717. [CrossRef] [PubMed]
17. Shin, S.A.; Moon, S.Y.; Kim, W.Y.; Paek, S.M.; Park, H.H.; Lee, C.S. Structure-Based Classification and Anti-Cancer Effects of Plant Metabolites. *Int. J. Mol. Sci.* **2018**, *19*, 2651. [CrossRef]
18. Bhummaphan, N.; Pongrakhananon, V.; Sritularak, B.; Chanvorachote, P. Cancer Stem Cell-Suppressing Activity of Chrysotoxine, a Bibenzyl from *Dendrobium pulchellum*. *J. Pharmacol. Exp. Ther.* **2018**, *364*, 332–346. [CrossRef]
19. Tsai, A.C.; Pan, S.L.; Liao, C.H.; Guh, J.H.; Wang, S.W.; Sun, H.L.; Liu, Y.N.; Chen, C.C.; Shen, C.C.; Chang, Y.L.; et al. Moscatilin, a bibenzyl derivative from the India orchid *Dendrobrium loddigesii*, suppresses tumor angiogenesis and growth in vitro and in vivo. *Cancer Lett.* **2010**, *292*, 163–170. [CrossRef]
20. Chen, W.K.; Chen, C.A.; Chi, C.W.; Li, L.H.; Lin, C.P.; Shieh, H.R.; Hsu, M.L.; Ko, C.C.; Hwang, J.J.; Chen, Y.J. Moscatilin Inhibits Growth of Human Esophageal Cancer Xenograft and Sensitizes Cancer Cells to Radiotherapy. *J. Clin. Med.* **2019**, *8*, 187. [CrossRef]
21. Won, J.H.; Kim, J.Y.; Yun, K.J.; Lee, J.H.; Back, N.I.; Chung, H.G.; Chung, S.A.; Jeong, T.S.; Choi, M.S.; Lee, K.T. Gigantol isolated from the whole plants of *Cymbidium goeringii* inhibits the LPS-induced iNOS and COX-2 expression via NF-kappaB inactivation in RAW 264.7 macrophages cells. *Planta Med.* **2006**, *72*, 1181–1187. [CrossRef] [PubMed]
22. Wu, J.; Li, X.; Wan, W.; Yang, Q.; Ma, W.; Chen, D.; Hu, J.; Chen, C.O.; Wei, X. Gigantol from *Dendrobium chrysotoxum* Lindl. Binds and inhibits aldose reductase gene to exert its anti-cataract activity: An in vitro mechanistic study. *J. Ethnopharmacol.* **2017**, *198*, 255–261. [CrossRef] [PubMed]
23. Chen, M.F.; Liou, S.S.; Hong, T.Y.; Kao, S.T.; Liu, I.M. Gigantol has Protective Effects against High Glucose-Evoked Nephrotoxicity in Mouse Glomerulus Mesangial Cells by Suppressing ROS/MAPK/NF-kappaB Signaling Pathways. *Molecules* **2018**, *24*, 80. [CrossRef] [PubMed]
24. Charoenrungruang, S.; Chanvorachote, P.; Sritularak, B.; Pongrakananon, V. Gigantol-induced apoptosis in lung cancer cell through mitochondrial-dependent pathway. *Thai J. Pharm. Sci.* **2014**, *38*, 67–73.
25. Bhummaphan, N.; Chanvorachote, P. Gigantol Suppresses Cancer Stem Cell-Like Phenotypes in Lung Cancer Cells. *Evid. Based Complement. Altern. Med.* **2015**, *2015*, 836564. [CrossRef]
26. Charoenrungruang, S.; Chanvorachote, P.; Sritularak, B.; Pongrakhananon, V. Gigantol, a bibenzyl from *Dendrobium draconis*, inhibits the migratory behavior of non-small cell lung cancer cells. *J. Nat. Prod.* **2014**, *77*, 1359–1366. [CrossRef]
27. Unahabhokha, T.; Chanvorachote, P.; Sritularak, B.; Kitsongsermthon, J.; Pongrakhananon, V. Gigantol Inhibits Epithelial to Mesenchymal Process in Human Lung Cancer Cells. *Evid. Based Complement. Altern. Med.* **2016**, *2016*, 4561674. [CrossRef]
28. Unahabhokha, T.; Chanvorachote, P.; Pongrakhananon, V. The attenuation of epithelial to mesenchymal transition and induction of anoikis by gigantol in human lung cancer H460 cells. *Tumor Biol.* **2016**, *37*, 8633–8641. [CrossRef]
29. Faivre, S.; Zappa, M.; Vilgrain, V.; Boucher, E.; Douillard, J.Y.; Lim, H.Y.; Kim, J.S.; Im, S.A.; Kang, Y.K.; Bouattour, M.; et al. Changes in tumor density in patients with advanced hepatocellular carcinoma treated with sunitinib. *Clin. Cancer Res.* **2011**, *17*, 4504–4512. [CrossRef]

30. Hale, M.D.; Nankivell, M.G.; Mueller, W.; West, N.P.; Stenning, S.P.; Wright, A.I.; Treanor, D.; Langley, R.E.; Ward, L.C.; Allum, W.H.; et al. The relationship between tumor cell density in the pretreatment biopsy and survival after chemotherapy in OE02 trial esophageal cancer patients. *J. Clin. Oncol.* **2014**, *32* (Suppl. 3), 49. [CrossRef]
31. Siegel, R.L.; Miller, K.D.; Jemal, A. Cancer statistics, 2018. *CA Cancer J. Clin.* **2018**, *68*, 7–30. [CrossRef] [PubMed]
32. Chen, H.; Huang, Y.; Huang, J.; Lin, L.; Wei, G. Gigantol attenuates the proliferation of human liver cancer HepG2 cells through the PI3K/AKT/NF-kappaB signaling pathway. *Oncol Rep* **2017**, *37*, 865–870. [CrossRef] [PubMed]
33. Yu, S.; Wang, Z.; Su, Z.; Song, J.; Zhou, L.; Sun, Q.; Liu, S.; Li, S.; Li, Y.; Wang, M.; et al. Gigantol inhibits Wnt/beta-catenin signaling and exhibits anticancer activity in breast cancer cells. *BMC Complement. Altern. Med.* **2018**, *18*, 59. [CrossRef] [PubMed]
34. Thorpe, L.M.; Yuzugullu, H.; Zhao, J.J. PI3K in cancer: Divergent roles of isoforms, modes of activation and therapeutic targeting. *Nat. Rev. Cancer* **2015**, *15*, 7–24. [CrossRef] [PubMed]
35. Lien, E.C.; Dibble, C.C.; Toker, A. PI3K signaling in cancer: Beyond AKT. *Curr. Opin. Cell Biol.* **2017**, *45*, 62–71. [CrossRef] [PubMed]
36. Johnson, D.E.; O'Keefe, R.A.; Grandis, J.R. Targeting the IL-6/JAK/STAT3 signalling axis in cancer. *Nat. Rev. Clin. Oncol.* **2018**, *15*, 234–248. [CrossRef] [PubMed]
37. Valle-Mendiola, A.; Weiss-Steider, B.; Rocha-Zavaleta, L.; Soto-Cruz, I. IL-2 enhances cervical cancer cells proliferation and JAK3/STAT5 phosphorylation at low doses, while at high doses IL-2 has opposite effects. *Cancer Investig.* **2014**, *32*, 115–125. [CrossRef]
38. Dhanasekaran, D.N.; Reddy, E.P. JNK-signaling: A multiplexing hub in programmed cell death. *Genes Cancer* **2017**, *8*, 682–694.
39. Hu, L.; Zhang, T.; Liu, D.; Guan, G.; Huang, J.; Proksch, P.; Chen, X.; Lin, W. Notoamide-type alkaloid induced apoptosis and autophagy via a P38/JNK signaling pathway in hepatocellular carcinoma cells. *RSC Adv.* **2019**, *9*, 19855–19868. [CrossRef]
40. Bai, Y.; Liu, X.; Qi, X.; Liu, X.; Peng, F.; Li, H.; Fu, H.; Pei, S.; Chen, L.; Chi, X.; et al. PDIA6 modulates apoptosis and autophagy of non-small cell lung cancer cells via the MAP4K1/JNK signaling pathway. *EBioMedicine* **2019**, *42*, 311–325. [CrossRef]
41. Fukunaga-Kalabis, M.; Roesch, A.; Herlyn, M. From cancer stem cells to tumor maintenance in melanoma. *J. Investig. Dermatol.* **2011**, *131*, 1600–1604. [CrossRef] [PubMed]
42. Yang, D.; Woodard, G.; Zhou, C.; Wang, X.; Liu, Z.; Ye, Z.; Li, K. Significance of different response evaluation criteria in predicting progression-free survival of lung cancer with certain imaging characteristics. *Thorac. Cancer* **2016**, *7*, 535–542. [CrossRef] [PubMed]
43. Lencioni, R.; Llovet, J.M. Modified RECIST (mRECIST) assessment for hepatocellular carcinoma. *Semin. Liver Dis.* **2010**, *30*, 52–60. [CrossRef] [PubMed]
44. *Guide for the Care and Use of Laboratory Animals—Portuguese Edition*; The National Academies Press: Washington, DC, USA, 1996; p. 130.
45. Sritularak, B.; Anuwat, M.; Likhitwitayawuid, K. A new phenanthrenequinone from *Dendrobium draconis*. *J. Asian Nat. Prod. Res.* **2011**, *13*, 251–255. [CrossRef] [PubMed]
46. Lowry, O.H.; Rosebrough, N.J.; Farr, A.L.; Randall, R.J. PROTEIN MEASUREMENT WITH THE FOLIN PHENOL REAGENT. *J. Biol. Chem.* **1951**, *193*, 265–275.
47. Tyanova, S.; Temu, T.; Cox, J. The MaxQuant computational platform for mass spectrometry-based shotgun proteomics. *Nat. Protoc.* **2016**, *11*, 2301–2319. [CrossRef]
48. Kuleshov, M.V.; Jones, M.R.; Rouillard, A.D.; Fernandez, N.F.; Duan, Q.; Wang, Z.; Koplev, S.; Jenkins, S.L.; Jagodnik, K.M.; Lachmann, A.; et al. Enrichr: A comprehensive gene set enrichment analysis web server 2016 update. *Nucleic Acids Res.* **2016**, *44*, W90–W97. [CrossRef] [PubMed]
49. Mi, H.; Muruganujan, A.; Ebert, D.; Huang, X.; Thomas, P.D. PANTHER version 14: More genomes, a new PANTHER GO-slim and improvements in enrichment analysis tools. *Nucleic Acids Res.* **2019**, *47*, D419–D426. [CrossRef]
50. Bardou, P.; Mariette, J.; Escudié, F.; Djemiel, C.; Klopp, C. jvenn: An interactive Venn diagram viewer. *BMC Bioinform.* **2014**, *15*, 293. [CrossRef] [PubMed]

51. Szklarczyk, D.; Gable, A.L.; Lyon, D.; Junge, A.; Wyder, S.; Huerta-Cepas, J.; Simonovic, M.; Doncheva, N.T.; Morris, J.H.; Bork, P.; et al. STRING v11: Protein-protein association networks with increased coverage, supporting functional discovery in genome-wide experimental datasets. *Nucleic Acids Res.* **2019**, *47*, D607–D613. [CrossRef]
52. Shannon, P.; Markiel, A.; Ozier, O.; Baliga, N.S.; Wang, J.T.; Ramage, D.; Amin, N.; Schwikowski, B.; Ideker, T. Cytoscape: A software environment for integrated models of biomolecular interaction networks. *Genome Res.* **2003**, *13*, 2498–2504. [CrossRef] [PubMed]
53. Rezaei-Tavirani, M.; Rezaei-Taviran, S.; Mansouri, M.; Rostami-Nejad, M.; Rezaei-Tavirani, M. Protein-Protein Interaction Network Analysis for a Biomarker Panel Related to Human Esophageal Adenocarcinoma. *Asian Pac. J. Cancer Prev.* **2017**, *18*, 3357–3363. [PubMed]
54. Howe, E.A.; Sinha, R.; Schlauch, D.; Quackenbush, J. RNA-Seq analysis in MeV. *Bioinformatics* **2011**, *27*, 3209–3210. [CrossRef] [PubMed]
55. Leary, S. AVMA Guidelines for the Euthanasia of Animals: 2013 Edition. American Veterinary Medical Association. Journal of the American Veterinary Medical Association 2013. Available online: https://www.avma.org/KB/Policies/Documents/euthanasia.pdf (accessed on 8 October 2019).
56. Schneider, C.A.; Rasband, W.S.; Eliceiri, K.W. NIH Image to ImageJ: 25 years of image analysis. *Nat. Methods* **2012**, *9*, 671–675. [CrossRef] [PubMed]
57. Jang, M.H.; Kim, H.J.; Chung, Y.R.; Lee, Y.; Park, S.Y. A comparison of Ki-67 counting methods in luminal Breast Cancer: The Average Method vs. the Hot Spot Method. *PLoS ONE* **2017**, *12*, e0172031. [CrossRef] [PubMed]
58. Lee, H.W.; Park, Y.M.; Lee, S.J.; Cho, H.J.; Kim, D.H.; Lee, J.I.; Kang, M.S.; Seol, H.J.; Shim, Y.M.; Nam, D.H.; et al. Alpha-smooth muscle actin (ACTA2) is required for metastatic potential of human lung adenocarcinoma. *Clin. Cancer Res.* **2013**, *19*, 5879–5889. [CrossRef] [PubMed]

10

XIAP as a Target of New Small Organic Natural Molecules Inducing Human Cancer Cell Death

Diego Muñoz [1,2], Martina Brucoli [3], Silvia Zecchini [4], Adrian Sandoval-Hernandez [1], Gonzalo Arboleda [5], Fabian Lopez-Vallejo [1], Wilman Delgado [1], Matteo Giovarelli [4], Marco Coazzoli [4], Elisabetta Catalani [6], Clara De Palma [7], Cristiana Perrotta [4], Luis Cuca [1], Emilio Clementi [4,7,8] and Davide Cervia [6,*]

1 Departamento de Química, Facultad de Ciencias, Universidad Nacional de Colombia, Bogotá 111321, Colombia; drmunozc@unal.edu.co (D.M.); agsandovalh@unal.edu.co (A.S.-H.); fhlopezv@unal.edu.co (F.L.-V.); wadelgadoa@unal.edu.co (W.D.); lecucas@unal.edu.co (L.C.)
2 Facultad de Ciencias, Universidad de Ciencias Aplicadas y Ambientales, Bogotá 111166, Colombia
3 Tumour Cell Death Laboratory, Cancer Research UK Beatson Institute, Glasgow G61 1BD, UK; 2310786B@student.gla.ac.uk
4 Department of Biomedical and Clinical Sciences "Luigi Sacco" (DIBIC), Università degli Studi di Milano, 20157 Milano, Italy; silvia.zecchini@unimi.it (S.Z.); matteo.giovarelli@unimi.it (M.G.); marco.coazzoli@unimi.it (M.C.); cristiana.perrotta@unimi.it (C.P.); emilio.clementi@unimi.it (E.C.)
5 Grupo de Muerte Celular, Instituto de Genética, Universidad Nacional de Colombia, Bogotá 111321, Colombia; gharboledab@unal.edu.co
6 Department for Innovation in Biological, Agro-food and Forest systems (DIBAF), Università degli Studi della Tuscia, 01100 Viterbo, Italy; ecatalani@unitus.it
7 Unit of Clinical Pharmacology, University Hospital "Luigi Sacco"-ASST Fatebenefratelli Sacco, 20157 Milano, Italy; clara.depalma@asst-fbf-sacco.it
8 Scientific Institute IRCCS "Eugenio Medea", 23842 Bosisio Parini, Italy
* Correspondence: d.cervia@unitus.it

Abstract: X-linked inhibitor of apoptosis protein (XIAP) is an emerging crucial therapeutic target in cancer. We report on the discovery and characterisation of small organic molecules from *Piper* genus plants exhibiting XIAP antagonism, namely erioquinol, a quinol substituted in the 4-position with an alkenyl group and the alkenylphenols eriopodols A–C. Another isolated compound was originally identified as gibbilimbol B. Erioquinol was the most potent inhibitor of human cancer cell viability when compared with gibbilimbol B and eriopodol A was listed as intermediate. Gibbilimbol B and eriopodol A induced apoptosis through mitochondrial permeabilisation and caspase activation while erioquinol acted on cell fate via caspase-independent/non-apoptotic mechanisms, likely involving mitochondrial dysfunctions and aberrant generation of reactive oxygen species. In silico modelling and molecular approaches suggested that all molecules inhibit XIAP by binding to XIAP-baculoviral IAP repeat domain. This demonstrates a novel aspect of XIAP as a key determinant of tumour control, at the molecular crossroad of caspase-dependent/independent cell death pathway and indicates molecular aspects to develop tumour-effective XIAP antagonists.

Keywords: phytochemicals; small organic agents; *Piper eriopodon*, alkenylphenols; human cancer cells; cell death; apoptosis; caspase-independent cell death; XIAP antagonists; XIAP-BIR3 domain

---

1. Introduction

The characterisation of small molecules (whose molecular weight does not exceed 900 Daltons) with well-defined chemical structures is a good approach to develop new therapeutic agents in proliferative, infectious, or neurodegenerative disorders [1–5]. Natural products possess enormous structural and chemical diversity that cannot be matched by any synthetic libraries of small molecules and continue to show a great translational potential [6–10]. In some cases, the complex chemical composition of some natural products has made difficult their isolation, structure elucidation and characterisation, thus prompting the search of new efficient synthetic pathways. In recent years the interest in the fundamental understanding of natural products and their engineered variants has been strongly renewed [6].

The simple active chemical structures of phenolic compounds from plants make them optimal lead candidates because of their broad biological activity, especially the protective, anti-oxidant and anti-tumour effects [11–14]. Plants of the genus *Piper* (Piperaceae family), are a very common food resource in neotropical forests and are widely used to obtain culinary spices. *Piper* genus constitutes one major class of medicinal plants and contains a valuable resource of phenolic bioactive compounds [15–21]. Among them, piplartine, hydroxychavicol, 4-nerodlidylcatechol and gibbilimbols A–D displayed potent cytotoxic/anti-tumoural effects in a variety of human cancer cells in vitro and in vivo [19,22–29].

Apoptosis, a closely regulated programmed cell death mechanism, is an essential process to maintain tissue homeostasis and its escape it is one of the hallmarks of cancer [30]. Substantial advances have been made on apoptosis-based anti-cancer therapeutics [31]. The most potent human IAP currently identified is the X-linked inhibitor of apoptosis protein (XIAP), a 57 kDa protein with three zinc-binding baculovirus IAP repeat (BIR) domains (BIR 1–3) which may also have actions additional to regulation of apoptosis [32]. The anti-apoptotic function of XIAP is antagonised by the second mitochondria-derived activator of caspases or direct IAP binding protein with low pI (Smac/DIABLO), a mitochondria protein released during apoptosis. The key role of XIAP and its potential clinical relevance is well established in tumours and several XIAP inhibitors have been developed or discovered as cytotoxic agents [32–43]. Despite different small molecules that inhibit XIAP have been identified and are moving through the pipeline of clinical development, the need of new ones to refine further therapeutic approaches based on XIAP antagonism is undeniable in translational research [41].

Herein we wish to report the discovery and chemical/biological characterisation of novel natural small compounds from *Piper* genus. Furthermore, a deeper insight into their cell death mechanism in human cells provides a proof-of-concept study of their pharmaceutical potential as antagonists of XIAP that may open important insights on XIAP as a suitable turning point for multiple cellular pathways.

2. Results and Discussion

2.1. Structural Identification of New Piper Genus-Derived Compounds

The chemical structures of compounds isolated from leaves of *P. eriopodon* (Figure 1A) were identified by interpretation of their corresponding high resolution electrospray ionisation mass spectrometry (HRESIMS), ^{1}H- and ^{13}C-NMR (nuclear magnetic resonance) spectral data, including attached proton test (APT), correlated spectroscopy (COSY), heteronuclear multiple quantum coherence (HMQC) and heteronuclear multiple bond correlation (HMBC) experiments, as well as by comparison of the spectral data with those reported in the literature.

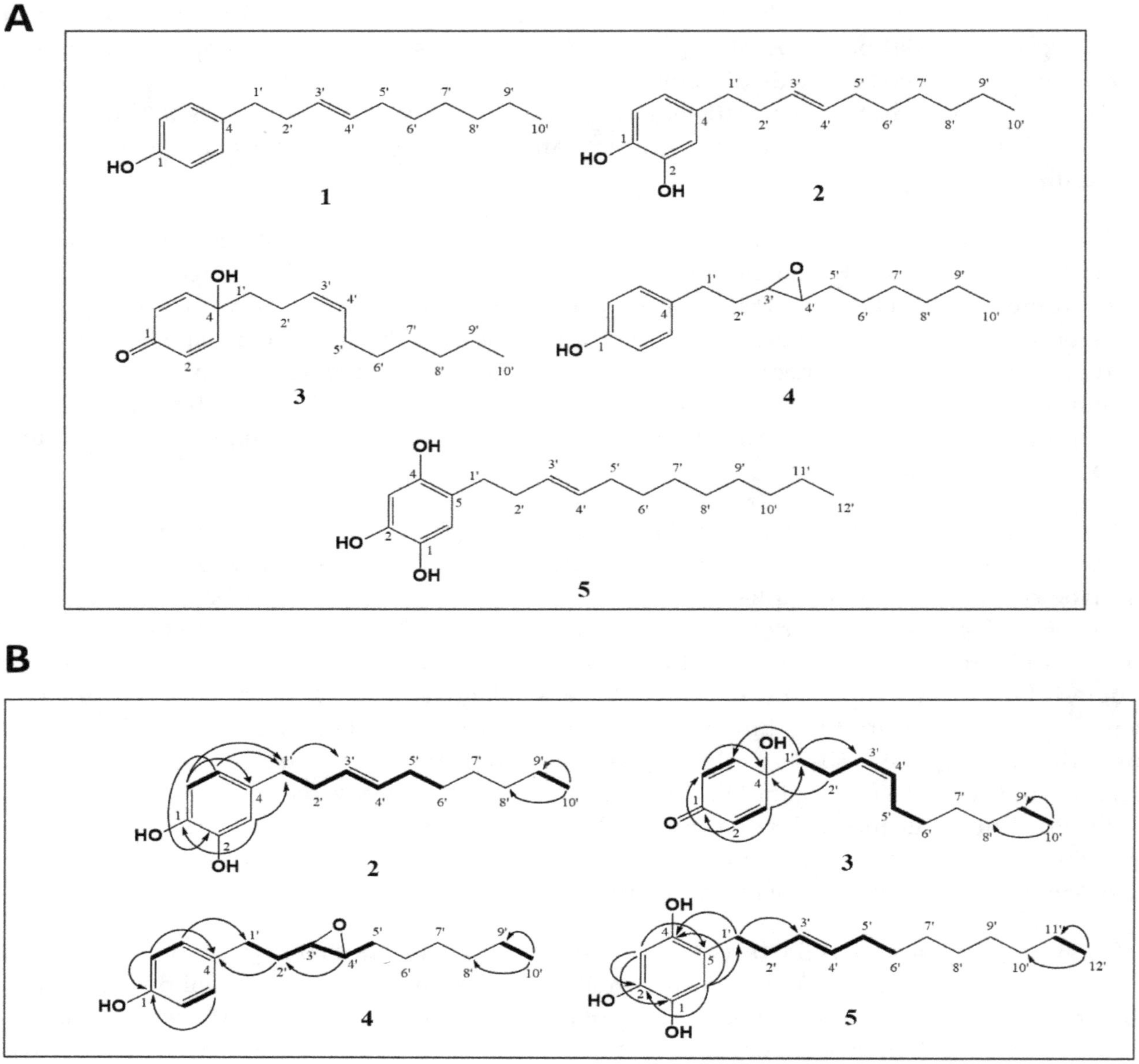

Figure 1. Identification of new *Piper* genus-derived compounds. (**A**) Structures of compounds 1–5. (**B**) Key correlated spectroscopy (COSY) (bold) and heteronuclear multiple bond correlation (HMBC) (H→C) for compounds **2–5**.

Compound 1 (Figure S1, Tables S1 and S2) was obtained as colorless oil and identified unequivocally as gibbilimbol B ((*E*)-4-(dec-3′-enyl)phenol) [19].

Compound 2 (Figure S2, Tables S1 and S2) was obtained as pale yellow oil. The molecular formula for compound **2** was established as $C_{16}H_{24}O_2$ based on the HRESIMS peak at *m/z* 247.1706 [M-H]$^-$ (calcd. 247.1703). The ^{1}H- NMR spectrum showed clear signals for a 1,2,4-trisubstituted aromatic ring δH 6.77 (1H, d, *J* = 7.6 Hz, H-6), 6.71 (1H, s, H-3), 6.60 (1H, d, *J* = 7.5 Hz, H-5) and an alkenyl fragment. The ^{13}C-NMR spectrum showed ten signals, practically the same as the alkenyl chain of gibbilimbol B, including the double bond position in C-3′, which was confirmed by correlations observed in both COSY and HMBC experiments (Figure 1B). Based on the ^{13}C-NMR chemical shifts of the allylic carbons δ_C 34.6 (C-2′) and δ_C 32.6 (C-5′), the configuration of the double bond for compound 2 was assigned as *E* [18], by comparison with the ^{13}C-NMR chemical shift of the allylic carbons in the *E* analogue gibbilimbol B (δ_C 34.6 (C-2′) and δ_C 32.6 (C-5′)), which differed significantly from the chemical shift values reported for the *Z* analogue climacostol [δ_C 33.2 (C-1′) and δ_C 27.3 (C-4′)] [44].

Thus, the chemical structure of compound **2** was elucidated as (*E*)-4-(dec-3′-enyl)benzene-1,2-diol and it was given the common name of eriopodol A.

Compound **3** (Figure S3, Tables S1 and S2) was obtained as clear oil and its molecular formula was deduced as $C_{16}H_{24}O_2$ from the HRESIMS spectrum, which exhibited a molecular ion peak at *m/z* 247.1706 $[M-H]^-$ (calcd. 247.1703). The ^{1}H-NMR spectrum for compound 3 showed signals for an alkenyl chain and two signals in δH 6.11 (2H, d, J = 9.94 Hz) and 6.81(2H, d, J = 9.96 Hz). The ^{13}C-NMR spectrum for compound **3** showed signals for an α-β unsaturated carbonyl in δ_C 185.9, an oxygenated quaternary carbon in δ_C 69.6 and ten signals for the typical side chain of the alkenyl fragment. Based on the correlations observed in COSY and HMBC experiments (Figure 1B), the structure of 3 was determined as a quinol derivative, substituted in the 4-position with an alkenyl group. The position and geometry of the double bond of compound 3 was assigned by comparing the chemical shift values of the allylic carbons δ_C 32.4 (C-2′) and δ_C 26.6 (C-5′) as explained above for eriopodol A. The geometry of compound 3 was determined as *Z* and its chemical structure was elucidated as (Z)-4-(dec-3′-enyl)-4-hydroxycyclohexa-2,5-dien-1-one. The common name of erioquinol was then assigned.

Compound 4 (Figure S4, Tables S1 and S2) was obtained as pale yellow oil. The molecular formula for compound 4 was confirmed to be $C_{16}H_{24}O_2$ based on the HRESIMS peak at *m/z* 247.1715 $[M-H]^-$ (calcd. 247.1703). The ^{1}H-NMR and ^{13}C-NMR spectra of compound 4 showed almost the same chemical shifts as the alkenylphenol gibbilimbol B, but without the unsaturated signal in the ^{1}H-NMR spectrum. Therefore, the carbons C-3′ and C-4′ showed chemical shifts in δ_C 59.6 (C-3′) and δ_C 58.6 (C-4′), corresponding two oxygenated methines from an epoxide group, which was confirmed with COSY and HMBC experiments (Figure 1B). The structure of compound **4** was elucidated as 4-(3′,4′-epoxydecenyl)phenol and the common name of eriopodol B was assigned.

Compound 5 (Figure S5, Tables S1 and S2) was obtained as pale yellow amorphous solid (m.p. 138.5 °C). The molecular formula for compound **5** was established as $C_{18}H_{28}O_3$ based on the HRESIMS peak at *m/z* 291.1973 $[M-H]^-$ (calcd. 291.1966). The NMR data for compound **5** were very close to those of eriopodol A, although it contains one additional hydroxyl group in the benzene ring and two additional carbons at the end of the alkenyl chain (Figure 1B). The position and geometry of the double bound for compound **5** was assigned as explained above. The structure of compound **5** was elucidated as (*E*)-5-(dodec-3′-enyl)benzene-1,2,4-triol and the common name of eriopodol C was assigned.

Taken together, phytochemical investigation of leaves from P. eriopodon yielded four new alkenyl derivatives and one known compound. In particular, erioquinol is a new quinol substituted in the 4-position with an alkenyl group and eriopodols A-C correspond to new alkenylphenols. The known isolated compound was originally identified as gibbilimbol B, from the medicinal plant P. gibbilimbum [19] and, more recently, from P. malacophyllum [21] and P. eriopodon [29]. The simple chemical structure of alkenylphenols are characterised by hydroxylated benzenes, substituted by side alkyl chains of different lengths with at least one double bond, generally with E geometry. Alkenylphenols with different reported biological properties, such as antibacterial, anti-parasitic, anti-inflammatory and cytotoxic activities, are widely found in the Piper genus [17,19–21,45]. Quinols are 4-hydroxycyclohexa-2,5-dien-1-ones which rarely occur as derivatives of some natural products [46–48]. An important feature of quinols substituted in the 4-position with aryl groups, is that they represent a class of potent anti-tumour molecules with activities against colon, renal, and breast cancer cells [49–51].

2.2. *Piper Genus-Derived Compounds Exhibit Cytotoxic Effects*

Several recent studies in glioblastoma and breast cancer cells have reported that extracts or active compounds isolated from *Piper* genus possess anti-tumoural/pro-apoptotic properties [52–61]. In order to assess whether the compounds we isolated could be developed further for therapeutic applications, we tested their cytotoxic action in the human cancer cells, U373 (glioblastoma astrocytoma) and MCF7 (breast adenocarcinoma) cell lines, since they are widely used as suitable in vitro models of cancer research. We first examined the effects of gibbilimbol B, eriopodols A–C, and erioquinol on cell viability. Gibbilimbol B was used as a reference compound of *Piper* genus derivatives, since its cytotoxic action has been previously tested in various tumour cells, including MCF7 [19,29]. In our experiments, cell viability was analysed by 3-(4,5-dimethylthiazol-2-yl)-2,5-diphenyltetrazolium bromide (MTT) assay after treatment with previously mentioned compounds at increasing concentrations for 24 h. As shown in Figure 2, a concentration-dependent inhibition of MTT absorbance was observed for all compounds with an IC_{50} (the concentration producing half the maximum inhibition) ranging from 1.78 to 31.91 μg/mL; the rank order of potencies was: erioquinol > eriopodol A > eriopodol C > gibbilimbol B > eriopodol B and erioquinol > eriopodol A > eriopodol C/gibbilimbol B > eriopodol B for U373 and MCF7 cells, respectively (Table 1). Their effects were maximal (E_{max}—concentration producing the maximum effect—nearly 100% inhibition) between 10–100 μg/mL.

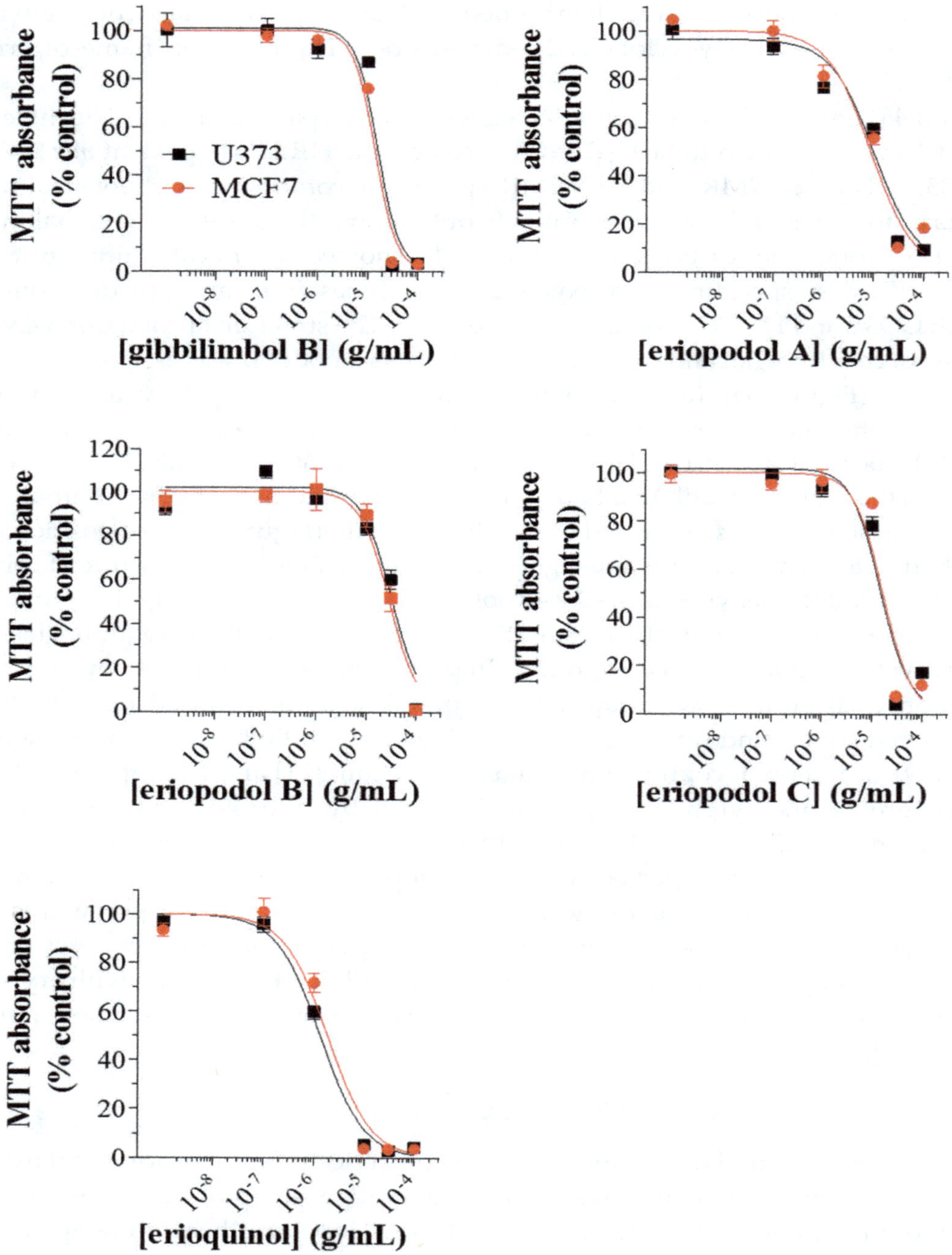

Figure 2. *Piper* genus-derived compounds exhibit cytotoxic effects in human cancer cells. U373 and MCF7 cells were treated with increasing concentrations of gibbilimbol B, eriopodol A, eriopodol B, eriopodol C,

and erioquinol for 24 h before 3-(4,5-dimethylthiazol-2-yl)-2,5-diphenyltetrazolium bromide (MTT) assay. Results are expressed by setting the absorbance of the reduced MTT in the respective control (vehicle-treated) samples, i.e., absence of compounds, as 100%. The data points are representative of four independent experiments.

Table 1. Inhibitory effects of *Piper* genus-derived compounds on human cancer cell viability.

Compound	IC_{50} (μg/mL)	
	U373 Cells	MCF7 Cells
Gibbilimbol B	16.79	16.44
Eriopodol A	11.12	10.12
Eriopodol B	31.91	29.36
Eriopodol C	14.30	16.30
Erioquinol	1.78	2.63

3-(4,5-dimethylthiazol-2-yl)-2,5-diphenyltetrazolium bromide (MTT) assay was performed treating cells for 24 h in the absence (vehicle) or in the presence of increasing concentrations of *Piper* genus-derived compounds. The results have been obtained in four independent experiments.

Eriopodol A and erioquinol were selected for further investigation, as they displayed the most potent inhibitory effects on cell viability. Gibbilimbol B (available in high quantity) was also included. When compared with gibbilimbol B [29], the higher cytotoxic effect of eriopodol A and erioquinol (24 h), was also shown by MTT assays using additional cell lines, like human A549 lung (IC_{50} of eriopodol A and erioquinol: 6.12 and 2.65 μg/mL, respectively) and PC-3 prostate (IC_{50} of eriopodol A and erioquinol: 1.84 and 2.21 μg/mL, respectively) cancer cells, further confirming enhanced pharmacological activity of these new *Piper* genus derivatives (Figure 3A).

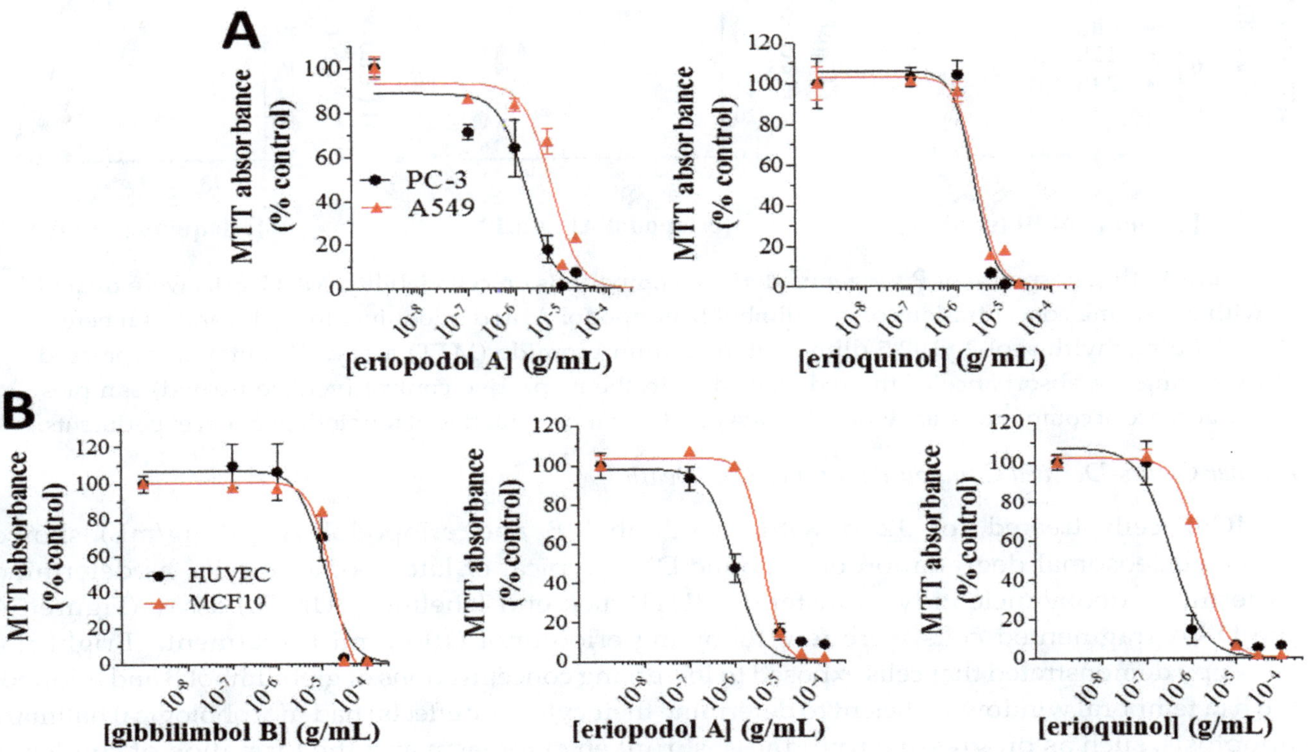

Figure 3. *Piper* genus-derived compounds exhibit cytotoxic effects in cancer and non-transformed human cells. **(A)** PC-3/A549 cells were treated with increasing concentrations of eriopodol A and erioquinol while

(**B**) human umbilical vein endothelial cells (HUVEC)/MCF10 cells were treated with increasing concentrations of gibbilimbol B, eriopodol A, and erioquinol, for 24 h before 3-(4,5-dimethylthiazol-2-yl)-2,5-diphenyltetrazolium bromide (MTT) assay. Results are expressed by setting the absorbance of the reduced MTT in the respective control (vehicle-treated) samples, i.e., absence of compounds, as 100%. The data points are representative of four independent experiments.

Similar results were obtained in human umbilical vein endothelial cells (HUVEC) (IC_{50} of 24 h gibbilimbol B, eriopodol A, and erioquinol: 11.49, 0.99, and 0.36 μg/mL, respectively) and the non-tumourigenic human breast MCF10 cells (IC_{50} of 24 h gibbilimbol B, eriopodol A, and erioquinol: 17.11, 4.27, and 1.70 μg/mL, respectively) (Figure 3B). The fact that the potency of the compounds was even slightly higher in these non-transformed/high proliferating cells suggests that their effects are not necessarily correlated to the cancerous origin of cells, in agreement with other small molecules we have recently characterised [62]. On the other hand, many cytotoxic compounds, including chemotherapy agents, are specifically designed to primarily affect rapidly proliferating cells, and many "normal" cells are also highly proliferative, such as cells in the bone marrow. The possibility that *Piper* genus-derived compounds preferentially affect high proliferating vs. low proliferating cells remains to be elucidated.

We then measured the concentration-dependent inhibition of MTT absorbance at increasing times of exposure in MCF7 cells, used as reference cell line. Our results indicated that the potency of gibbilimbol B did not substantially change (IC_{50}-6 h: 20.31 μg/mL; 12 h: 27.36 μg/mL; 24 h: 16.44 μg/mL) while the potency of eriopodol A increased at 24 h (IC_{50} - 6 h: 31.19 μg/mL; 12 h: 32.75 μg/mL; 24 h: 11.13 μg/mL) (Figure 4). Of interest, the potency of erioquinol was greater than gibbilimbol B and eriopodol A at each time-point, even increasing over time (IC_{50}-6 h: 14.72 μg/mL; 12 h: 4.25 μg/mL; 24 h: 1.93 μg/mL). These comparative data indicate that erioquinol is the most potent compound with faster kinetics when compared with gibbilimbol B; eriopodol A has a somewhat intermediate behavior.

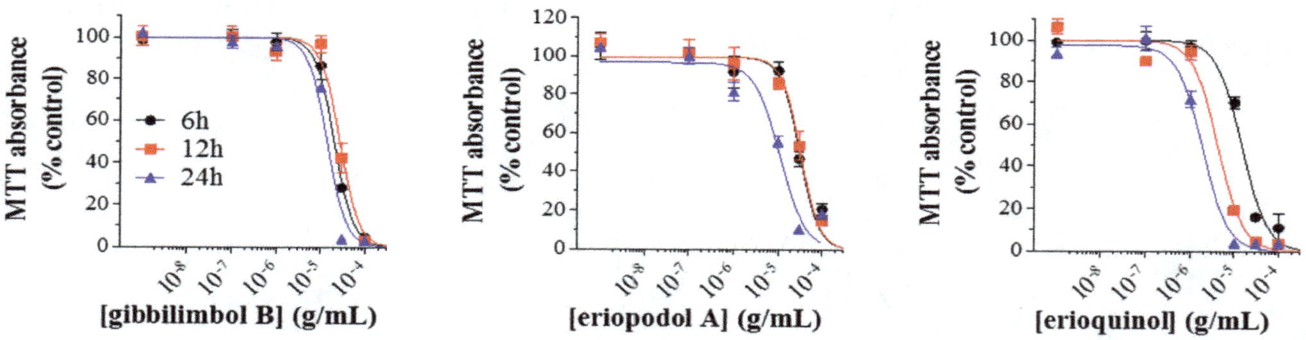

Figure 4. Time-response of *Piper* genus-derived compounds on cell viability. MCF7 cells were treated with increasing concentrations of gibbilimbol B, eriopodol A, and erioquinol for 6, 12, and 24 h before 3-(4,5-dimethylthiazol-2-yl)-2,5-diphenyltetrazolium bromide (MTT) assay. Results are expressed by setting the absorbance of the reduced MTT in the respective control (vehicle-treated) samples, i.e., absence of compounds, as 100%. The data points are representative of four independent experiments.

2.3. *Piper* Genus-Derived Compounds Induce Cell Death

MCF7 cells treated for 12 h with gibbilimbol B and eriopodol A (30 μg/mL) showed an inter-nucleosomal degradation of genomic DNA typical of late apoptotic cells, as determined by a terminal deoxynucleotidyl transferase dUTP nick end labeling (TUNEL) assay (Figure 5A), while DNA fragmented cells were few following erioquinol (10 μg/mL) treatment. Bright field microscopy demonstrated that cells exposed to increasing concentrations of gibbilimbol B and eriopodol A at 6 h (a temporal window sufficient to determine their cytotoxic effects) had morphological hallmarks of apoptosis, such as progressive roundness, shrunken cytoplasm and the formation of condensed nuclei (Figure 5B). In contrast, cells treated with erioquinol displayed a translucent cytoplasm and no overall nuclei condensation. Of interest, 4′,6-diamidine-2′-phenylindole dihydrochloride (DAPI) staining clearly revealed the nuclei of cells undergoing apoptosis in the presence of gibbilimbol B and eriopodol A (30 μg/mL) for 6 h, while erioquinol (10 μg/mL) treatment was associated with the appearence of multinucleated cells (Figure 5C). Accordingly, when analysed by flow cytometry using Annexin V and propidium iodide (PI) staining, MCF7 cells treated with erioquinol showed a progressive and marked increase of membrane disruption, as shown by early positivity to both Annexin V and PI staining, while the typical early apoptotic pattern, evidenced as Annexin V^{+}/PI^{-} was almost undetectable over time (Figure 5D).

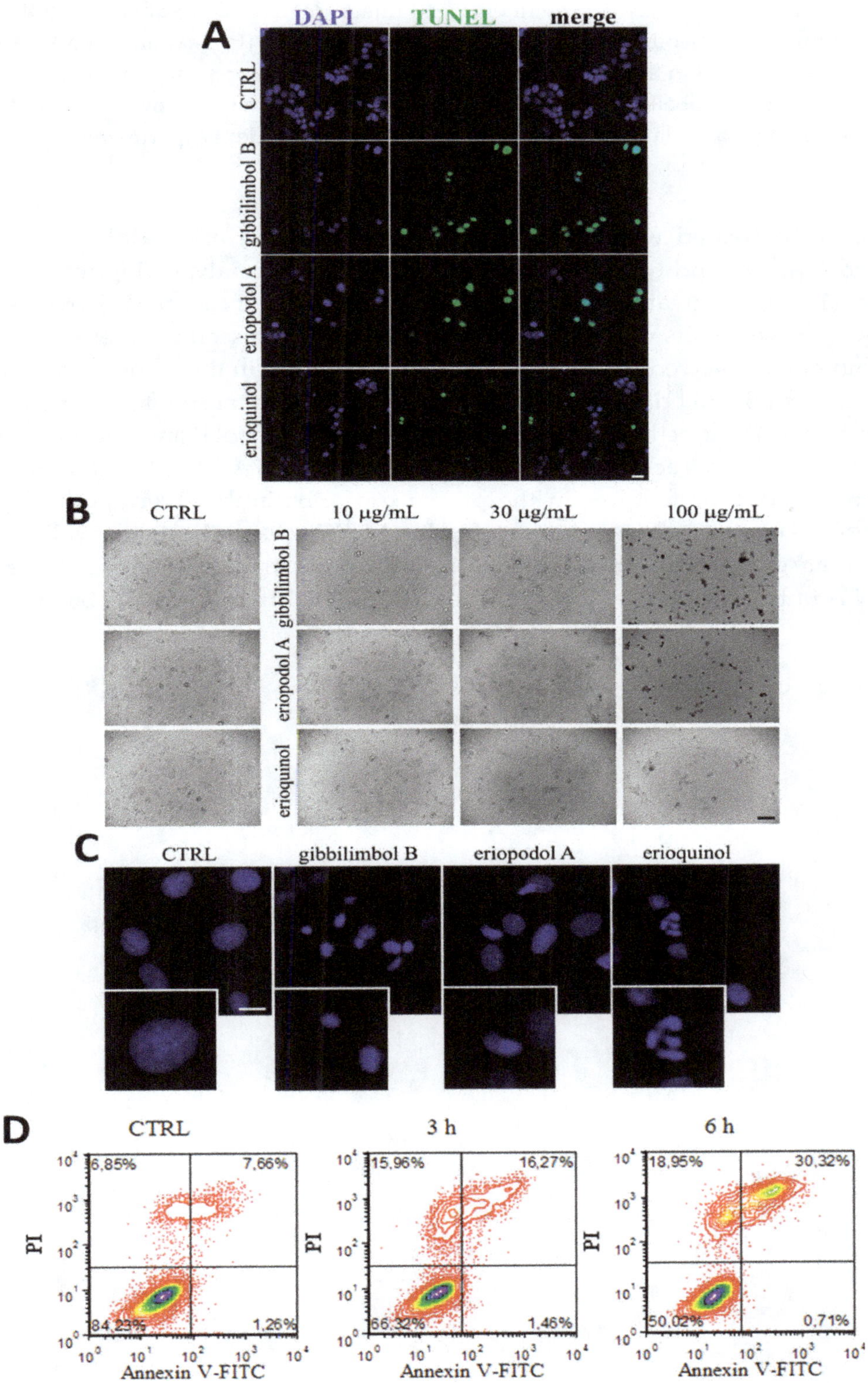

Figure 5. *Piper* genus-derived compounds induce cell death. (**A**) terminal deoxynucleotidyl transferase

dUTP nick end labeling (TUNEL) staining of MCF7 cells treated for 12 h in the absence (CTRL, control) and in the presence of gibbilimbol B/eriopodol A (30 μg/mL) or erioquinol (10 μg/mL). 4′,6-diamidine-2′-phenylindole dihydrochloride (DAPI) was used for nuclei detection. Scale bar = 50 μm. (**B**) Bright field microscopy of MCF7 cells treated for 6 h in the absence (CTRL) and in the presence of gibbilimbol B, eriopodol A, or erioquinol at increasing concentrations. Scale bar = 100 μm. (**C**) 4′,6-diamidine-2′-phenylindole dihydrochloride (DAPI) staining of MCF7 cells treated for 6 h in the absence (CTRL) and in the presence of gibbilimbol B/eriopodol A (30 μg/mL) or erioquinol (10 μg/mL). Scale bar = 10 μm. Lower panels represent enlarged image details. (**D**) Evaluation by flow cytometry of Annexin V-fluorescein isothiocyanate(FITC)/propidium iodide (PI) staining in MCF7 cells treated in the absence (CTRL) and in the presence of 10 μg/mL erioquinol, for 3 and 6 h. Quadrants are drawn, and relative proportion of labelled cells is indicated. The events shown in the lower left-hand quadrant are unlabeled cells. Images and data are representative of four independent experiments.

In addition, cells treated with 30 μg/mL gibbilimbol B and eriopodol A displayed activation of caspase 9 and 7 at 3 h and 6 h, as showed by western blot analysis (Figure 6A,B). On the other hand, erioquinol (10 μg/mL) treated cells did not display any sign of caspase 7 activity even at later time point (Figure 6C). These results were confirmed by immunofluorescence experiments. Indeed, a time-dependent and intensive cleaved-caspase 7 staining was detected in the cytoplasm of MCF7 cells in the presence of gibbilimbol B and eriopodol A while positive cells were absent following the administration of erioquinol (Figure 6D). The activation of caspase 7 by 6 h gibbilimbol B and eriopodol A (30 μg/mL) but not erioquinol (10 μg/mL) was achieved also in U373 cells (Figure 7A). The fact that these cells displayed apoptotic and non-apoptotic features in the presence of gibbilimbol B/eriopodol A and erioquinol, respectively (Figure 7B), similarly to what obtained in MCF7 cells, indicate that cell death mechanisms of the compounds are comparable among cell lines. Accordingly, the activation of caspase 7 by gibbilimbol B and eriopodol A but not erioquinol was observed also in MCF10 cells (Figure S6A).

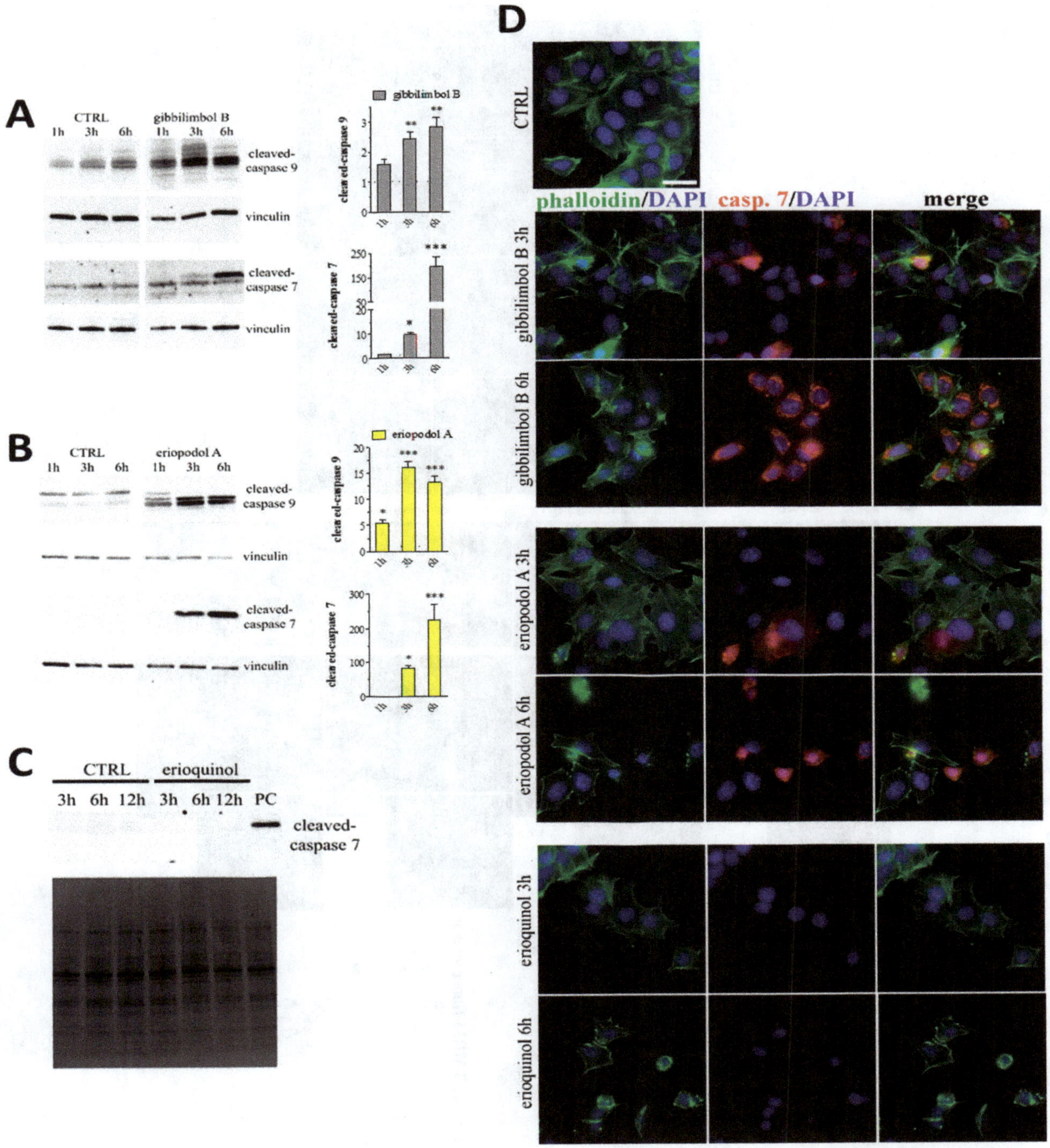

Figure 6. *Piper* genus-derived compounds induce cell death. Western blot analysis of cleaved-caspase 9 and 7 in MCF7 cells treated for increasing times in the absence (CTRL, control) and in the presence of (**A**) gibbilimbol B or (**B**) eriopodol A. Vinculin was used as internal standard. Right panels: densitometric analysis expressed as fold change of CTRL. Images and data are representative of three-five independent experiments. * $p < 0.01$, ** $p < 0.001$, and *** $p < 0.0001$ relative to CTRL. (**C**) Western blot analysis of cleaved-caspase 7 in MCF7 cells treated for increasing times in the absence (CTRL) and in the presence of 10 μg/mL erioquinol. The stain-free gel was used as loading control. Images are representative of three independent experiments. PC: positive control. (**D**) Immunofluorescence imaging of cleaved-caspase 7 (punctate red pattern) in MCF7 cells treated for 3 and 6 h in the absence (CTRL) and in the presence of gibbilimbol B/eriopodol A (30 μg/mL) or erioquinol (10 μg/mL). 4′,6-diamidine-2′-phenylindole dihydrochloride (DAPI) (blue) and phalloidin (green) were used for nuclei and cytoskeleton detection, respectively. Images are representative of four independent experiments. Scale bar = 25 μm.

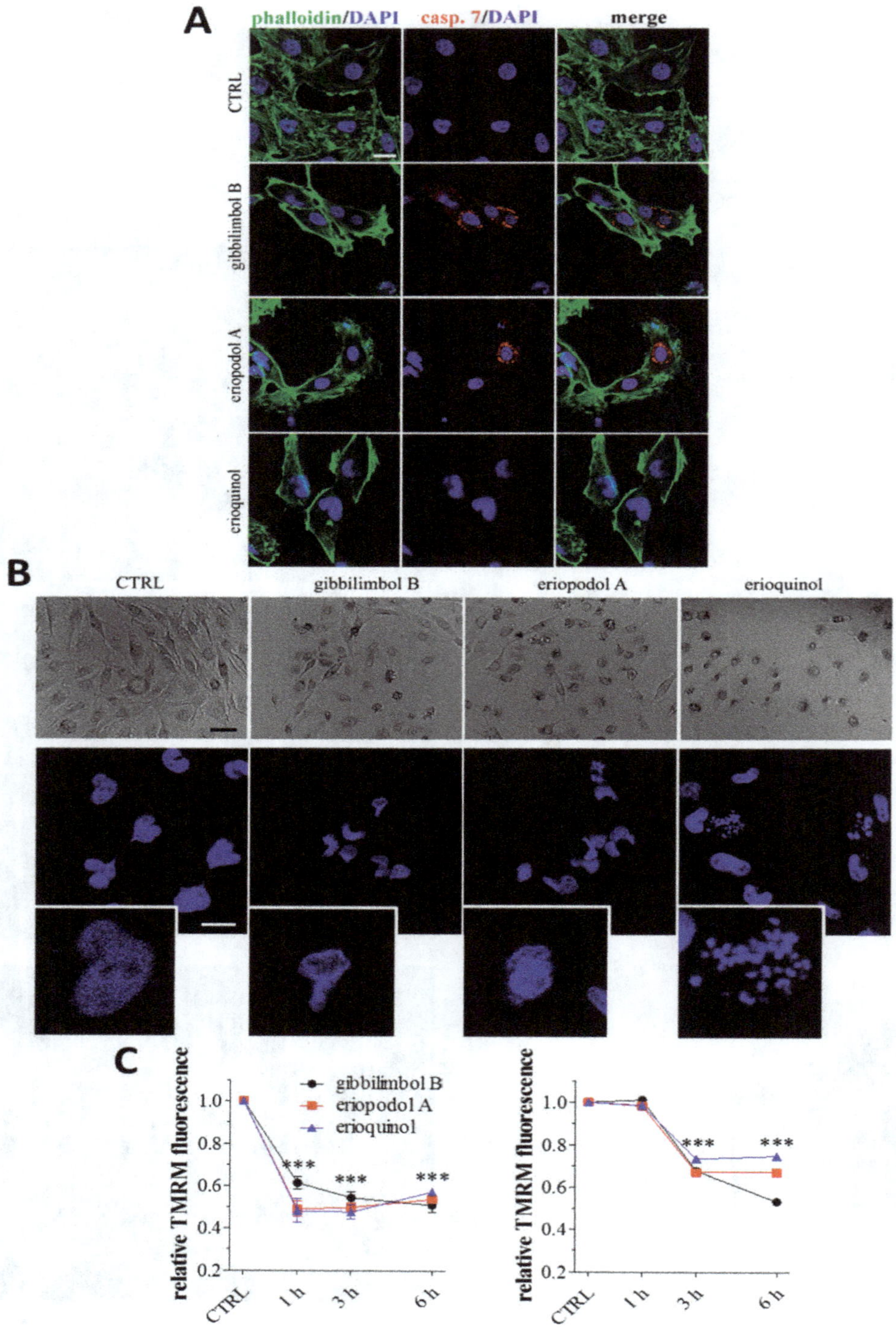

Figure 7. *Piper* genus-derived compounds induce cell death and mitochondrial dysfunction. (**A**) Immunofluorescence (confocal) imaging of cleaved-caspase 7 (punctate red pattern) in U373 cells treated for 6 h in the absence (CTRL, control) and in the presence of gibbilimbol B/eriopodol A (30 μg/mL) or erioquinol (10 μg/mL). 4′,6-diamidine-2′-phenylindole dihydrochloride (DAPI) (blue) and phalloidin (green) were used for nuclei and cytoskeleton detection, respectively. Scale bar = 25 μm. (**B**) Bright field microscopy (upper panels) and DAPI staining (lower panels) of U373 cells treated for 6 h in the absence (CTRL) and in the presence of of gibbilimbol B/eriopodol A (30 μg/mL) or erioquinol (10 μg/mL). Scale bars = 50 μm (bright field) and 10 μm (DAPI). Lower panels represent enlarged image details. (**C**) Quantitative analysis of tetramethylrhodamine methyl ester (TMRM) fluorescence changes over time in MCF7 (left panel) and U373 (righ panel) cells in the absence (CTRL) and in the presence of gibbilimbol B/eriopodol A (30 μg/mL) or erioquinol (10 μg/mL). Results are expressed by setting TMRM fluorescence in the respective control (vehicle-treated) samples, i.e., absence of compounds, as 1. *** $p < 0.0001$ relative to CTRL. Images and data are representative of four independent experiments.

In order to better describe the mechanism behind the activity of the compounds, we investigated mitochondria functionality with tetramethylrhodamine methyl ester (TMRM), a red fluorescent dye that is sequestered by active mitochondria. Of note, MCF7 and U373 cells treated for increasing time with 30 µg/mL gibbilimbol B/eriopodol A or 10 µg/mL erioquinol presented a comparable decrease in TMRM fluorescence vs. control, with MCF7 cells full responding within 1 h (Figure 7C). This indicates low mitochondria membrane potential likely associated to the destabilisation of the mitochondrial membrane systems.

The fact that the three compounds similarly induce mitochondria membrane permeabilisation both in MCF7 and U373 cells, was further confirmed by the subcellular location of cytochrome c. As shown in Figure 8A,B, 3 h administration of gibbilimbol B/eriopodol/erioquinol induced an alteration in the cytochrome c staining pattern from mitochondrial (co-localisation with COX IV, a marker for mitochondria), to a more cytosolic distribution (presence of many clusters which did not overlap with COX IV), indicating a release of cytochrome c from the dysfunctional mitochondria.

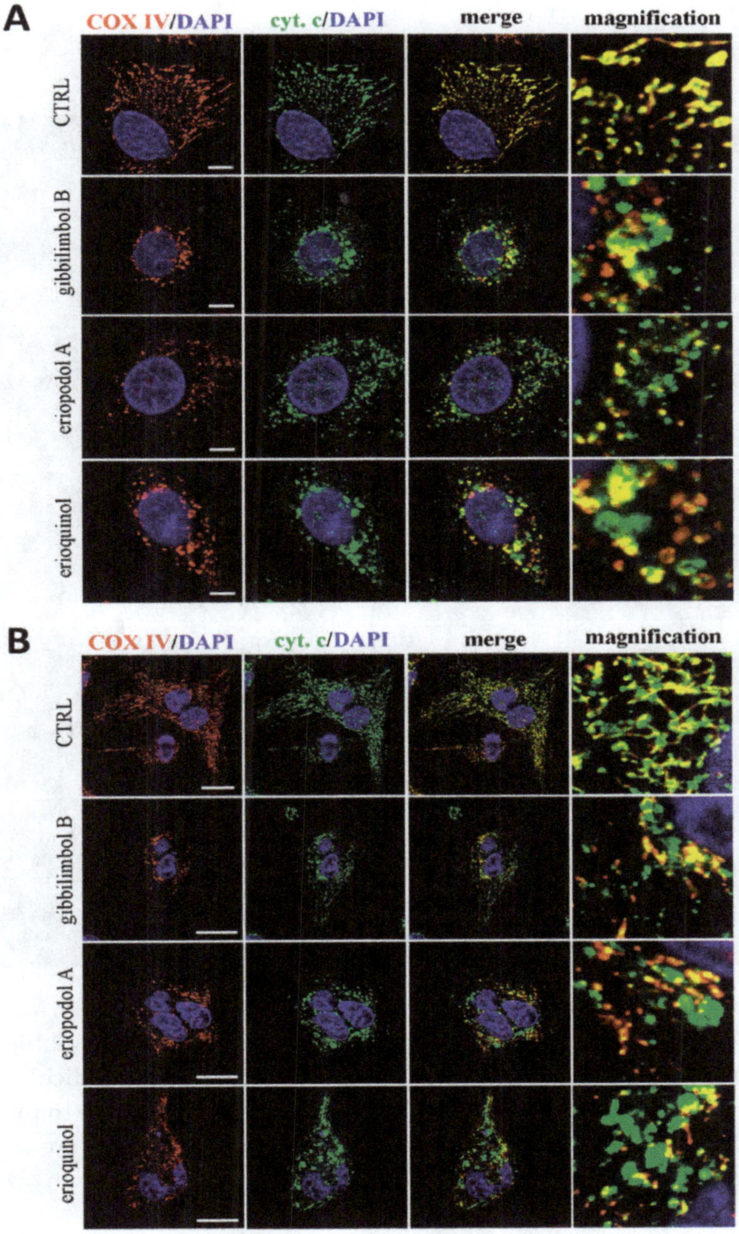

Figure 8. Confocal microscopy for co-localisation of cytochrome c with mitochondria. (**A**) MCF7 and

(**B**) U373 cells were treated for 3 h in the absence (CTRL, control) and in the presence of gibbilimbol B/eriopodol A (30 µg/mL) or erioquinol (10 µg/mL). Cells were then stained for cytochrome c (green) and the mitochondrial marker COX IV). 4′,6-diamidine-2′-phenylindole dihydrochloride (DAPI) (blue) was used for nuclei detection. The images are representative of three independent experiments. Scale bars: 10 µm (MCF7) and 25 µm (U373). Panels on the right represent enlarged image details.

Damaged mitochondria are considered as the main source of reactive oxygen species (ROS) which play major roles in the fate of cancer cells [63]. Noteworthily, MCF7 and U373 cells staining with 2′-7′dichlorofluorescin diacetate (DCFH-DA), a permeant fluorogenic dye cell reagent that measures hydroxyl, peroxyl and other ROS activity, revealed that erioquinol effect (10 µg/mL, 6 h) is characterised by marked accumulation of ROS, which are absent in cells treated with gibbilimbol B and eriopodol A (30 µg/mL, 6 h) (Figure 9A,B). Together with lack of caspase activation, aberrant ROS production is another divergence between gibbilimbol B/eriopodol A and erioquinol-induced cell death. In this respect, erioquinol is likely inducing a robust mitochondrial stress which results in ROS production and release into the cytoplasm.

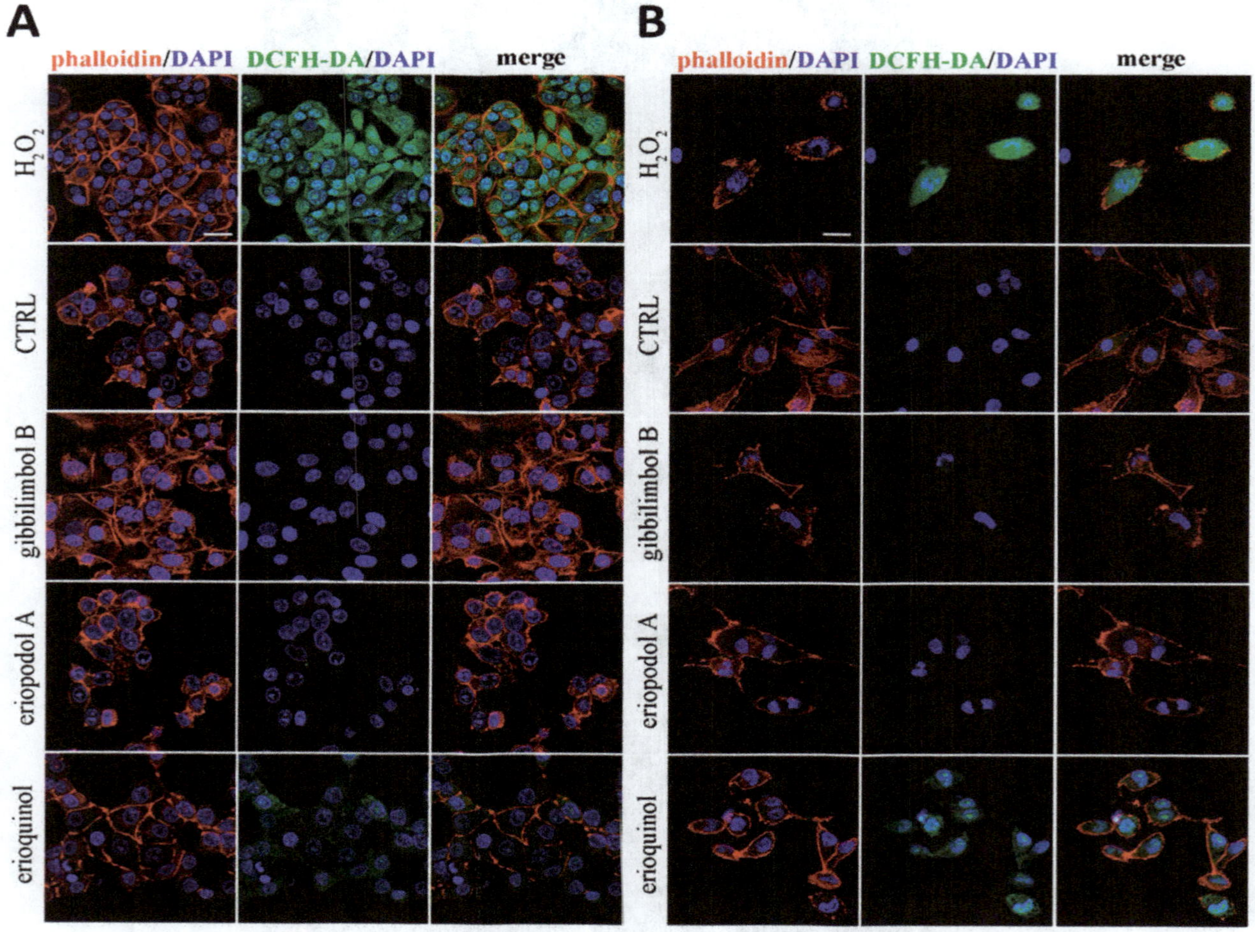

Figure 9. Confocal microscopy for reactive oxygen species (ROS) detection. (**A**) MCF7 and (**B**) U373 cells were treated for 6 h in the absence (CTRL, control) and in the presence of gibbilimbol B/eriopodol A (30 µg/mL) or erioquinol (10 µg/mL). Cells were then stained for ROS (2′-7′dichlorofluorescin diacetate - DCFH-DA, green). 4′,6-diamidine-2′-phenylindole dihydrochloride (DAPI) (blue) and phalloidin (red) were used for nuclei and cytoskeleton detection, respectively. The images are representative of three independent experiments. Scale bar: 25 µm.

Finally we confirmed as apoptotic the effect of gibbilimbol B and eriopodol A by inhibiting their cytotoxic activity with the pan-caspase inhibitor Z-VAD-(OMe)-FMK. As displayed by MTT assays (Figure 10A), the loss of cell viability in MCF7 cells treated with 30 µg/mL gibbilimbol B and eriopodol A was significantly inhibited when 50 μM Z-VAD-(OMe)-FMK was simultaneously added to the 6 h treatment protocol, demonstrating the dependency on caspases of the two compounds. However, the simultaneous addition of Z-VAD-(OMe)-FMK did not affect the activity of 10 μg/mL erioquinol. Taken together our data data demonstrate that gibbilimbol B and eriopodol A effectively induced intrinsic apoptosis triggered by mitochondrial membrane permeabilisation, release of cytochrome c, an early induction of initiator caspase 9, and a consecutive activation of effector caspase 7. Erioquinol, although it affects comparably mitochondrial functions, appears to act in a different manner, i.e., involving mitochondrial ROS release and non-apoptotic/caspase-independent mechanisms. Caspase-independent cell death was first described to affect mitochondria potential, and eventually mitochondrial outer membrane permeabilisation [64], although not followed by caspase activation. Those features resemble the outcome of erioquinol treatment.

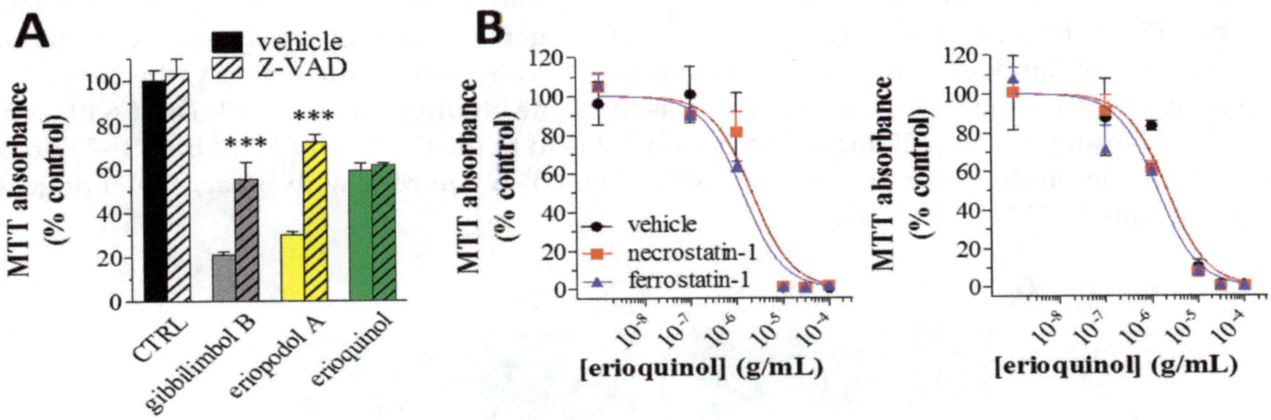

Figure 10. *Piper* genus-derived compounds induce caspase-dependent and independent loss of cell viability. (**A**) MCF7 cells were cultured in the absence (CTRL, control) and in the presence of 30 μg/mL gibbilimbol B/eriopodol A or 10 μg/mL erioquinol for 6 h, before 3-(4,5-dimethylthiazol-2-yl)-2,5-diphenyltetrazolium bromide (MTT) assay. The pan-caspase inhibitor Z-VAD-(OMe)-FMK (50 μM) or its vehicle were used as well. Results are expressed by setting the absorbance of the reduced MTT in the CTRL, as 100%. Data are representative of four-twelve independent experiments. *** $p < 0.0001$ relative to the respective compound alone, i.e., + Z-VAD vehicle. (**B**) MCF7 (left panel) and U373 (right panel) cells were treated with increasing concentrations of erioquinol for 24 h before MTT assay. Erioquinol was administered both in the absence (vehicle) or in the presence of 50 μM necrostatin-1 and 10 μM ferrostatin-1 (2 h pre-treatment), a necroptosis and ferroptosis inhibitor, respectively. Results are expressed by setting the absorbance of the reduced MTT in the control samples (absence of erioquinol) as 100%. The data points are representative of four independent experiments.

Several forms of regulated cell death manifest with a morphology different from apoptosis [65,66], and many compounds from nature source can induce non-apoptotic programmed cell death in cancer cells [67]. Among them, necroptosis can be partially rescued by the receptor-interacting serine-threonine kinase 1 inhibitor necrostatin-1 and ferroptosis by ferrostatin-1, an inhibitor of lipid peroxidation. We thus treated MCF7 and U373 cells with increasing concentrations of erioquinol (24 h) with or without 50 μM necrostatin-1 and 10 μM ferrostatin-1 (2 h pre-treatment). As shown in Figure 10B, the concentration-dependent inhibition of MTT absorbance did not change, suggesting erioquinol-induced death was independent from necroptosis and ferroptosis, two cell death pathways known to be caspase-independent [65,66]. ROS were recently linked to a caspase-independent form of cell death, which cannot be rescue by necrostatin-1 or ferrostatin-1 treatment, and therefore not imputable to either necroptosis or ferroptosis [68]. Treatment with erioquinol might lead to a similar cascade of events, although additional work is required to fully characterise the role of ROS and the cell death process induced by this *Piper* genus-derived compound.

2.4. XIAP as a Molecular Target of Piper Genus-Derived Compounds

XIAP-mediated inhibition of apoptosis goes through its reversible binding to active caspase-9, via its BIR3 domain, and caspase-3/7 when stabilised to XIAP-BIR2 domain [69–71]. It has been also demonstrated that XIAP controls different pathways functionally uncoupled to caspases, leading to the possibility that XIAP system might control cell death/survival through multiple mechanisms [32,34,72–82].

Embelin, a natural benzoquinone with potential therapeutic interest, has been isolated from the fruit of the *Embelia* ribes and discovered through molecular docking analysis of over 8200 molecules as a potent small molecule XIAP inhibitor that binds to the XIAP-BIR3 domain [83–86]. It should be noted that embelin displays chemical features similar to those of erioquinol, eriopodol A, and gibbilimbol B [83]. We assessed if erioquinol, eriopodol A, and gibbilimbol B are able to bind to the XIAP-BIR3 domain in a similar way of embelin. Using molecular docking analysis and molecular dynamics simulations for embelin and isolated new compounds, it was found the structural basis of the predicted interactions with the BIR3 domain of XIAP. Figure 11A provides a general view of the docked conformations obtained for gibbilimbol B, eriopodol A, erioquinol, and embelin. Interestingly, the binding site for gibbilimbol B, eriopodol A, and erioquinol is the same binding site of embelin and with similar energy and binding mode. All docked compounds fits in to the P1, P2 and P3 of the P1–P4 pockets reported for the binding site of the XIAP-BIR3 domain in complex with Smac, the endogenous antagonist ligand of IAPs [35,87,88].

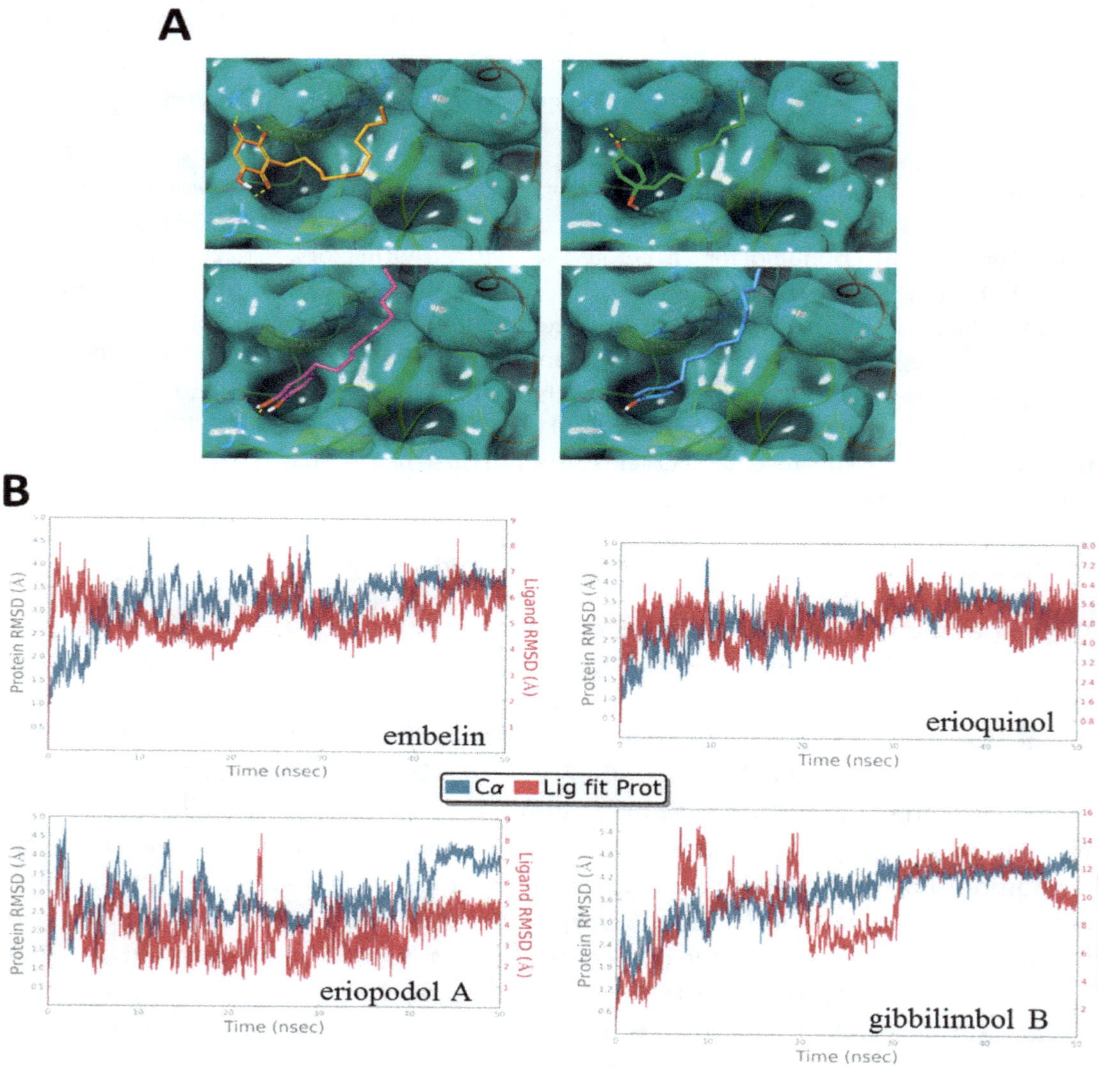

Figure 11. *Cont.*

C

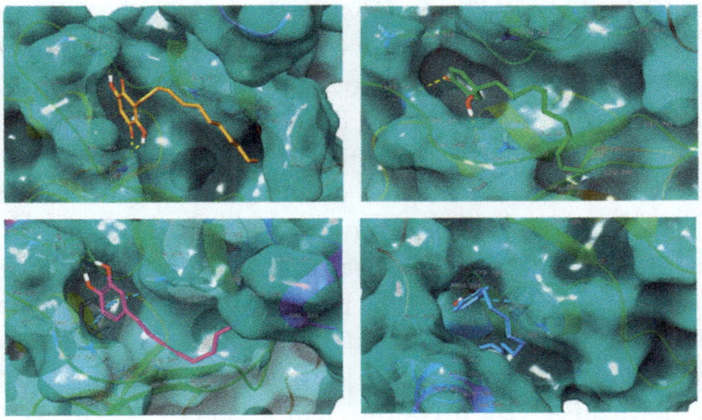

Figure 11. X-linked inhibitor of apoptosis protein (XIAP) as a molecular target of *Piper* genus-derived compounds. (**A**) Molecular docking and (**C**) dynamics analysis of embelin (orange), erioquinol (green), eriopodol A (purple) and gibbilimbol B (blue) in complex with the baculovirus IAP repeat (BIR)-3 domain of XIAP (PDB code 5C83). Interacting residues are displayed in wireframe, hydrogen bonds are displayed in yellow dot lines and π-π stacking interactions are displayed in blue dot lines. (**B**) Protein-ligand root mean square deviation (RMSD) trajectory of the atomic positions for ligands (red, Lig fit Prot) and the receptor (blu, Cα positions) BIR-3 domain of XIAP, for the dynamics trajectory of 50 ns.

Experimental structures of the XIAP-BIR3 domain in different complexes with embelin, Smac or Smac mimetics and non-peptidomimetics small molecules, revealed that residues GLY306, THR308, GLU314, TRP323 and TYR324 are crucial residues involved in the interaction with the BIR3 domain of XIAP [35,41,86,89]. The results of the docking experiments show a possible binding mode for gibbilimbol B, eriopodol A, and erioquinol. Accordingly, the phenolic ring of gibbilimbol B and eriopodol A forms hydrogen bonds with LYS311 and GLU314 (Figure 11A), the quinol ring of erioquinol forms three hydrogen bonds with THR308, LYS322, and TRP323, while residues GLY306, LEU307, TRP323, and TYR324 of the XIAP-BIR3 domain forms hydrophobic interactions with the tail of the alkenyl derivatives.

In addition, molecular dynamics simulations for 50 ns were carried out to assess the stability of the protein-ligand complexes between the docked compounds and the BIR3 domain of XIAP. The stability of the modelled complex of alkenyl derivatives and embelin was confirmed during the period of simulation by little variations in the root mean square deviation (RMSD) trajectory (Figure 11B). Although some changes were observed in the interacting residues of XIAP BIR-3 domain after molecular dynamics simulations (Figure S7), the preferred location of the binding mode for all evaluated ligands were maintained in the pockets P1-P4 of BIR-3 domain of XIAP during the period of simulation (Figure 11C). Also, the binding mode obtained in the docking and dynamics simulations for embelin are according to the interactions pattern determined experimentally by NMR studies in the XIAP-embelin complex, which revealed that TRP323 of the BIR3 domain of XIAP are crucial in the binding of embelin [86]. These findings strongly suggest the highly stable complex formation between the BIR-3 domain of XIAP and the alkenyl derivatives.

XIAP is highly expressed in different human tumour cells and cancer specimens from patients and plays an important role in conferring chemoresistance [33,90]. Because XIAP blocks apoptosis at the downstream effector phase, where multiple signalling events may converge, it represents an attractive molecular target for the design of new anti-cancer drugs [32–41,43]. Two broad approaches have been taken to develop clinical inhibitors of XIAP—antisense oligonucleotides, targeting the entire protein, and small molecule inhibitors, binding a single domain. Small molecule inhibitors offer the potential of more rapid inhibition of their target in vivo and more predictable duration of action [34,41]. Among the small molecule phytochemicals, the XIAP inhibitor embelin exhibited cytotoxic activity in various human tumoural cells, including breast cancer [83–86,91]. In addition, the withaferin-A induced cytotoxicity in human breast cancer cells was associated with suppression of XIAP protein [92] and berberine was shown to induce apoptosis in tumours, likely through the inhibition of XIAP [93]. The just mentioned molecular modelling of our new molecules binding to XIAP-BIR3 domain drove us to examine if they shared a similar activity with already described XIAP inhibitors. With the aim of understanding the role of XIAP in the cell death phenotype, we first determined if our cellular model is anyhow affected by XIAP depletion. Using the Lipofectamine reagent, MCF7 cells were transiently transfected with a XIAP-specific or a scrambled targeting siRNA. When treated with 50 nM of siRNA for 24 h, the protein levels of XIAP markedly decreased to ca. 45% compared to control siRNA transfected samples (Figure 12A) indicating a partial depletion of XIAP. In agreement with previous indications [94–96], the outcome in viability of XIAP knockdown in MCF7 cells, which showed a significant reduction (ca. 40%) in MTT absorbance upon depletion of XIAP (Figure 12B), led us to the conclusion that MCF7 cells depend on XIAP for survival since death mechanisms are neutralised by physiological levels of XIAP. We then tried to add clues on the involvement of XIAP in the cytotoxic effect of *Piper* genus-derived compounds. As shown in Figure 12B, XIAP downregulation in MCF7 cells significantly enhanced the toxicity, as measured by MTT absorbance, of 6 h administration of gibbilimbol B (30 μg/mL), eriopodol A (30 μg/mL) and erioquinol (10 μg/mL) indicating their combined action with XIAP siRNA in inhibiting cell viability. Since 100% knockdown was never achieved with siRNA technique (the absence of detectable XIAP after siRNA transfection, i.e., by XIAP siRNA at 100 nM for 24 h, paralleled the increase of cleaved-caspase 7 levels and the complete loss of MCF7 cell viability (Figure S6D and data not shown)), it is reasonable to assume that that the effects of gibbilimbol B/eriopodol A/erioquinol on the residual XIAP protein in the siRNA-treated cells further induced MCF7 cell death. On the other hand, similar results (additive effect) would be achieved if the compounds target cytotoxic pathways other than XIAP. However, although this is not a formal biological evidence, the simplest explanation of the combined action is a XIAP-mediated mechanism accounting for, at least in part, the cytotoxicity of our new compounds. Accordingly, the positive effects of gibbilimbol B and eriopodol A on caspase 7 activity robustly increased after XIAP silencing (Figure 12C). Downregulation of XIAP by siRNA is known to sensitise human breast cancer cells to death mediated by different chemical agents [94,97]. Finally, using real-time PCR and western blot assays to measure XIAP expression, we found that cell exposure to gibbilimbol B, eriopodol A, and erioquinol at increasing times did not significantly modify mRNA (Figure 12D) and protein levels (Figure 12E) of XIAP. Overall, our data exclude a role of gibbilimbol B/eriopodol A/erioquinol on the regulation of XIAP expression but rather are consistent with the antagonism of XIAP activity through their binding to XIAP-BIR3 domain.

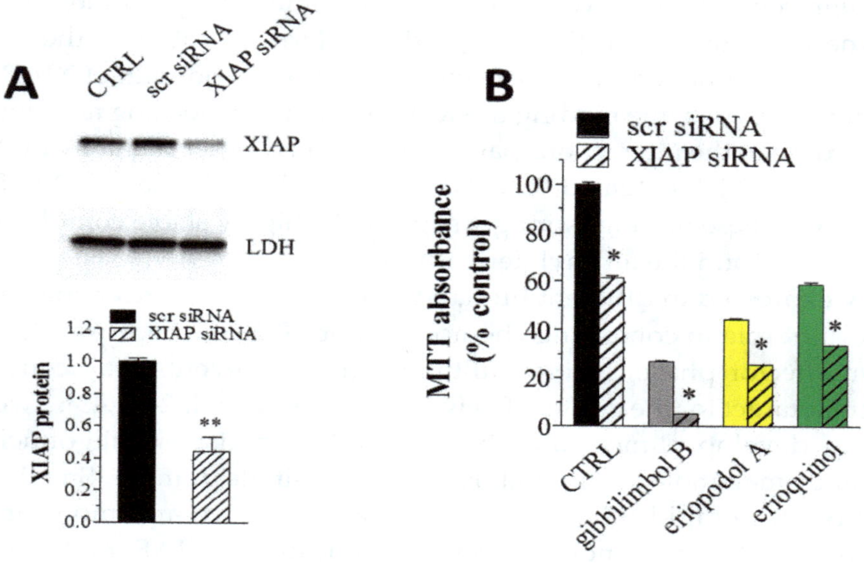

Figure 12. *Cont.*

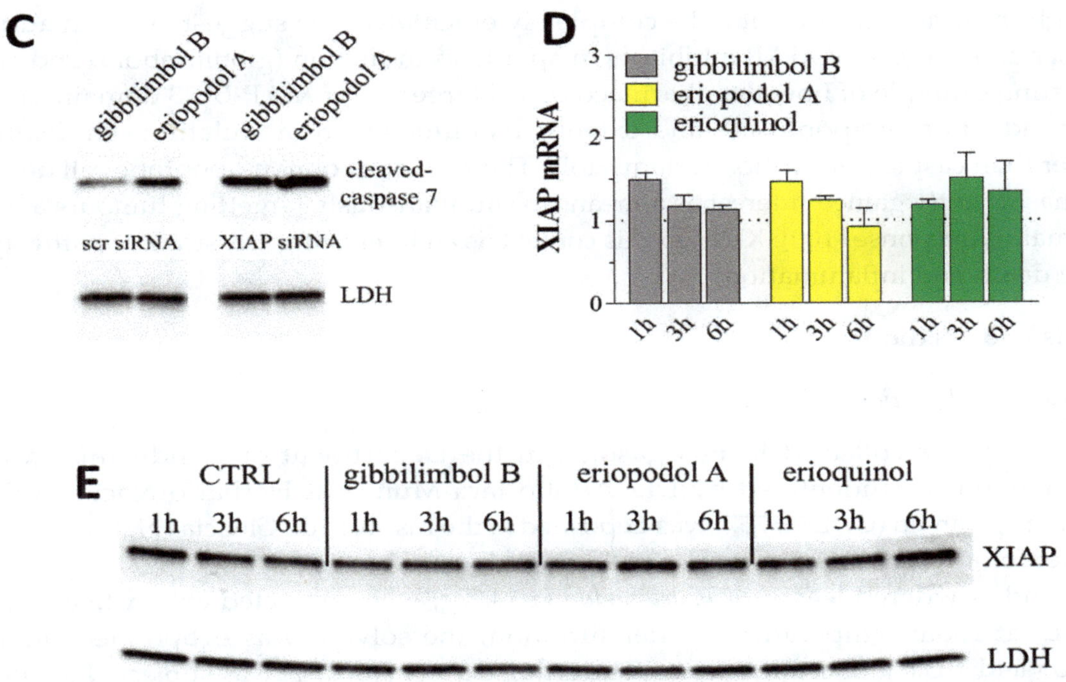

Figure 12. X-linked inhibitor of apoptosis protein (XIAP) as a molecular target of *Piper* genus-derived compounds. (**A**) Western blot analysis of XIAP in MCF7 cells both untransfected (CTRL, control) or transfected for 24 h with a XIAP-specific and scrambled targeting (scr) siRNA (50 nM). Lactate dehydrogenase (LDH) was used as internal standard. Low panel: densitometric analysis expressed as fold change of scr siRNA. Images and data are representative of three independent experiments. **P < 0.001 relative to scr siRNA. (**B**) MCF7 cells were transfected for 24 h with a XIAP-specific or scr siRNA (50 nM) and then cultured in the absence (CTRL) and in the presence of 30 µg/mL gibbilimbol B/eriopodol A or 10 µg/mL erioquinol for 6 h, before 3-(4,5-dimethylthiazol-2-yl)-2,5-diphenyltetrazolium bromide (MTT) assay. Results are expressed by setting the absorbance of the reduced MTT in the scr siRNA CTRL, as 100%. Data are representative of three independent experiments. * $p < 0.0001$ relative to the respective scr siRNA. (**C**) Western blot analysis of cleaved-caspase 7 in MCF7 cells transfected for 24 h with a XIAP-specific or scr siRNA (50 nM) and then cultured in the presence of 30 µg/mL gibbilimbol B and eriopodol A for 6 h. LDH was used as internal standard. Images are representative of three independent experiments. (**D**) Real-time PCR and (**E**) Western blot analysis of XIAP mRNA and protein expression, respectively, in MCF7 cells treated for increasing times in the absence (CTRL) and in the presence of 30 µg/mL gibbilimbol B/eriopodol A or 10 µg/mL erioquinol. β-actin (PCR) and LDH (Western blot) were used as internal standards. PCR results are expressed as fold change of respective CTRL, set as 1. Images and data are representative of three independent experiments.

Since escape from apoptosis is one of the preeminent features of cancer, pharmacological interest in targeting endogenous apoptosis inhibitors, such as B-cell lymphoma (BCL)-2 and IAPs family members, has been constant [32–43,82,98,99]. The efforts, including clinical trials, directed towards identifying small molecules inhibitors of the BCL-2 family of proteins and promote apoptosis with the so-called BH3 mimetics, that mimic the action of certain BH3-only proteins [98], proved the releasing of "apoptosis brakes" as a winning strategy to induce primary cell death in cancer or to sensitise tumour to chemotherapy. Differently to BCL-2 family members, IAPs, and in particular XIAP, have a late role in the apoptotic timeline, and they target already active caspases to prevent cell death. The structural data surrounding the interaction between the BIR3 domain of XIAP and caspases suggest that small molecules that bind the BIR3 pocket of XIAP could mimic the action of Smac and inhibit the interaction between XIAP and caspase [34,41]. Interestingly its multi-domain structure makes XIAP a component of multiple cellular pathways, not only the ones leading to apoptosis. XIAP versatility has been highlighted in inflammation and inflammatory cell death, such as necroptosis [32,79–82].

Even though these aspects are yet to be completely elucidated, we suggest here - in addition to the widely described activity of XIAP inhibitors in apoptosis induction (gibbilimbol B and eriopodol A)—an interesting example of how the pharmacological targeting of XIAP-BIR3 domain can go beyond the simple induction of apoptosis—and extends its influence in modulating cell death signalling events other than caspase-activation (erioquinol). The relevance of non-apoptotic cell death in cancer treatment has recently gained interest as a means to simultaneously targetting tumours and enhancing the inflammatory response [100]; XIAP, in this context, is an interesting crossroad of pathways involved in both cell death and inflammation.

3. Materials and Methods

3.1. Extraction and Isolation of Natural Compounds

P. eriopodon was collected in Fusagasuga, in the Department of Cundinamarca (Colombia). The plant material was identified by Dr. Adolfo Jara Muñoz at Herbario Nacional Colombiano and a voucher specimen (COL516757) was deposited at the Instituto de Ciencias Naturales, Universidad Nacional de Colombia.

Dried and powdered leaves of *P. eriopodon* (1.14 Kg) were extracted exhaustively with ethanol 96% (3 × 5L) at room temperature. After filtration, the solvent was evaporated under reduced pressure, to yield 103.6 g of crude extract. The crude extract (100.0 g) was subjected to silica gel flash chromatography and eluted with a step gradient of toluene/ethyl acetate (0:100, 20:80, 40:60, 60:40, 80:20 and 0:100 (V/V)) to afford eight fractions. Fraction 1 (34.2 g) was chromatographed over silica gel, eluting with a mixture of a three-phase *n*-hexane/dichloromethane/ethyl acetate (25:70:5) solvent system to afford ten fractions (A to J). Fraction E (10.0 g) was chromatographed over Sephadex LH-20 (4.5 × 45 cm, *n*-hexane/chloroform/methanol, 2:2:1) to give six fractions (E1 to E6). In agreement with a previous report [29], compound **1** (7.93 g) was obtained from fraction E3, after column chromatography on Sephadex LH-20 (4.5 × 30 cm, *n*-hexane/acetone/methanol, 2:2:1). Fraction E4 (974.6 mg) was submitted to column chromatography on Sephadex LH-20 (4.0 × 20 cm, *n*-hexane/acetone/methanol, 2:2:1) to yield six fractions (E4.1 to E4.6). Compound **3** (33.2 mg) was obtained from fraction E4.4 (378.8 mg) through Sephadex LH-20 (2.0 × 25 cm, *n*-hexane/acetone/methanol, 2:2:1) and silica gel column chromatography eluted with *n*-hexane/acetone 8:2. Fraction E5 (2.19 g) was subjected to column chromatography on silica gel using a mixture of toluene/ethyl acetate (9:1) to afford ten fractions (E5.1 to E5.10). Fraction E5.3 (153.2 mg) was purified by flash chromatography to yield compound 4 (20.0 mg).

Fraction 2 (8.0 g) was submitted to silica gel column chromatography eluted with *n*-hexane/ethyl acetate 8:2, yielding seven fractions (K–Q). Fraction Q was subjected to flash chromatography eluted with dichloromethane/acetone (7:3) to yield six fractions (Q1–Q6). Fraction Q3 (1.44 g) was subjected to column chromatography over Sephadex LH-20 (4.0 x 20 cm, hexane/acetone/methanol, 2:2:1) to afford six fractions (Q3.1 to Q3.6). Fraction Q3.4 (239.4 mg) was chromatographed over Sephadex LH-20 (4.0 × 20 cm, hexane/chloroform/methanol, 2:2:1) and then purified by silica gel column chromatography eluted with *n*-hexane/acetone (7:3) to yield compound **5** (4.0 mg). Fraction Q6 (570.5 mg) was subjected to flash chromatography eluted with *n*-hexane/acetone 7:3 to afford seven fractions (Q6.1–Q6.7). Compound **2** (166.0 mg) was obtained from fraction Q6.1.

3.2. General Chemical Methods

Flash chromatography was carried out with silica gel (230–400 mesh; Merck, Darmastadt, Germany), column chromatography was performed using silica gel (70–230 mesh; Merck) and Shepadex® LH20 (Sigma-Aldrich, St. Louis, MO, USA), analytical thin layer chromatography was performed using precoated silica gel plates 60 F_{254} (0.25 mm, Merck). ^{1}H and ^{13}C NMR 1D and 2D (COSY, HMQC and HMBC) spectra, were recorded on an Avance 400 spectrometer (Bruker, Millerica, MA, USA) at 400 MHz for ^{1}H and 100 MHz for ^{13}C using the solvent peaks as internal references, the spectra were recorded in $CDCl_3$ and MeOD (Merck). High-resolution mass data were collected on an Accurate-Mass quadrupole Time-of-Flight (q-TOF) (Agilent Technologies, Santa Clara, CA, USA) mass spectrometer, ESI negative mode, Nebuliser 50 (psi), Gas Flow 10 L/min, Gas Temp 350 °C. Fragmentor 175 V, Skimmer 75 V, Vpp 750 V.

3.3. *Cell Culture and Chemicals*

Human U373 glioma, MCF7 breast cancer, A549 lung cancer and PC-3 prostate cancer cells were grown in Dulbecco's Modified Eagle Medium (DMEM), supplemented with 10% foetal bovine serum, 2 mM glutamine, 100 U/mL penicillin/streptomycin, at 37 °C in a humidified atmosphere containing 5% CO_2 (logarithmic growth phase, routine passages every 3 days). The human breast epithelial cell line MCF10 was cultured in DMEM/F12 Ham's Mixture supplemented with 5% horse serum, epithelial growth factor 20 ng/mL, insulin 10 µg/mL, hydrocortisone 0.5 mg/mL, cholera toxin 100 ng/mL, and 100 U/mL penicillin/streptomycin. HUVEC were grown in EGM-2 Endothelial Cell Growth Medium-2 BulletKit (Lonza, Basel, Switzerland), according to the manufacturer's protocol.

Foetal bovine serum, horse serum, glutamine and penicillin/streptomycin were obtained from Euroclone (Milano, Italy). TMRM was purchased from ThermoFisher Scientific (Waltham, MA, USA) while necrostatin-1 and ferrostatin-1 were obtained from Santa Cruz Biotechnology (Dallas, TX, USA). Where not indicated, the reagents were purchased from Sigma-Aldrich.

3.4. *MTT Assay*

U373, MCF7, A549, PC-3, HUVEC, and MCF10 cell viability was determined by MTT assay using published protocols [101–105]. MTT absorbance was quantified spectrophotometrically using a Glomax Multi Detection System microplate reader (Promega, Milano, Italy).

3.5. *TUNEL Assay*

Using published protocols [106,107], MCF7 or U373 cells cultured in 120-mm coverslips were fixed in 4% paraformaldehyde in 0.1 M phosphate buffer (PB), pH 7.4, for 10 min. The TUNEL method (DeadEnd Fluorometric TUNEL System, Promega) was used to assay apoptosis, according to the manufacturer's protocol. DAPI (nuclei detection) staining was also performed.

3.6. *Immunofluorescence Microscopy Analysis*

Using published protocols [106,108], MCF7 or U373 cells cultured in 120-mm coverslips were fixed in 4% paraformaldehyde in 0.1 M PB, pH 7.4, for 10 min. Cells were pre-incubated for 1 h min with 5% of normal goat serum (Life Technologies, Monza, Italy) in 0.1 M PB (pH 7.4) containing 0.1% Triton X-100, before overnight incubation with the rabbit monoclonal anti-cleaved caspase 7 (Cell Signaling Technology, Danvers, MA, USA). In double-label immunofluorescence experiments, the mouse monoclonal anti-cytochrome c primary antibody (Cell Signaling Technology) was used in conjunction with the rabbit monoclonal primary antibody directed to COX IV (Cell Signaling Technology). For fluorescence detection, coverslips were stained with the appropriate Alexa Fluor secondary antibodies (Life Technologies) and mounted on glass slides in a ProLong Gold Antifade Mountant (Life Technologies). DAPI and/or fluorescein phalloidin (cytoskeleton detection) staining was also used. Cells were analysed with a DMI4000 B automated inverted microscope equipped with a DCF310 digital camera (Leica Microsystems, Wetzlar, Germany). When indicated, confocal imaging was performed with a TCS SP8 System (Leica Microsystems). Image acquisitions were controlled by the Leica Application Suite X.

3.7. *Annexin V Staining*

MCF7 cells were incubated with 5 µg/mL Annexin V-fluorescein isothiocyanate (FITC) to assess the phosphatidylserine exposure on the outer leaflet of the plasma membrane, and 5 µg/mL PI

(DNA-binding probe) to exclude necrotic cells in binding buffer (10 mM HEPES, 140 mM NaCl, 2.5 mM $CaCl_2$) [109]. Cell staining was analysed by Gallios Flow Cytometer (Beckman-Coulter, Brea, CA, USA) and the software FCS Express 4 (De Novo System, Portland, OR, USA).

3.8. Western Blotting

Using published protocols [107,110,111], MCF7 and MCF10 cells were homogenised in RIPA lysis buffer, supplemented with a cocktail of protease inhibitors (cOmplete; Roche Diagnostics, Milano, Italy). Equal amounts of proteins were separated by 4–20% SDS-polyacrylamide gel electrophoresis (Criterion TGX Stain-free precast gels and Criterion Cell system; Bio-Rad, Hercules, CA, USA) and transferred onto nitrocellulose membrane using a Bio-Rad Trans-Blot Turbo System. When indicated, the membranes were probed using the rabbit monoclonal anti-cleaved caspase 7 and anti-XIAP (Cell Signaling Technology) primary antibodies. After the incubation with the appropriate horseradish-peroxidase-conjugated secondary antibody (Cell Signaling Technology), bands were visualised using the Clarity Western ECL substrate with a ChemiDoc MP imaging system (Bio-Rad). To monitor for potential artefacts in loading and transfer among samples in different lanes, the blots were routinely treated with the Restore Western Blot Stripping Buffer (ThermoFisher Scientific) and re-probed with the goat anti-Lactate dehydrogenase (LDH)-A (Santa Cruz Biotechnology) and the mouse anti-vinculin primary antibodies. The stain-free gel was used as loading control as well. When appropriated, bands were quantified for densitometry using the Bio-Rad Image Lab software.

3.9. Mitochondrial Membrane Potential Analysis

Using published protocols [112], mitochondria of MCF7 and U373 cells were labeled using TMRM, a voltage-sensitive cationic lipophilic dye, partitioning and accumulating in the mitochondrial matrix based upon the Nernst equation. After treatments, cells were trypsinised, counted and incubated with 100 nM TMRM for 30 min at 37 °C. Fluorescence was measured by using a Glomax Multi Detection System microplate reader (Promega), excitation wavelength: 525 nm; emission wavelength: 580–640 nm). After background subtraction, the data were normalised on cell number.

3.10. Measurement of ROS

MCF7 or U373 cells cultured in 120-mm coverslips were exposed to 30 μM DCFH-DA (0.1 M PB, pH 7.4) and fixed in 4% paraformaldehyde for 20 min. For fluorescence detection, coverslips were mounted on glass slides and observed with a laser-scanning confocal microscope (TCS SP8 System and Application suite X, Leica Microsystems). DAPI and fluorescein phalloidin (nuclei and cytoskeleton detection, respectively) staining was also used.

3.11. Molecular Modeling

AutoDock4 was used to carry out the molecular docking. The Protein Data Bank crystallographic structure PDB 5C83 was considered as receptor model [87]. The preparation of the macromolecule was made with PyMOL (version 2.0, PyMol Molecular Graphics, Schrodinger, New York, NY, USA) System) and XIAP-BIR3 domain was selected as receptor [113]. Energy maps was established with Autogrid4 involving all atom types. After 25 million of energy evaluations in the binding pocket and using a grid of 50 × 50 × 50 points, all conformations of the ligand were clustered according to the energy and conformations. The docking results were visualised using the computational program Maestro 11.6. The molecular dynamics simulations were carried out with Desmond simulation package of Maestro (Desmond Molecular Dynamics System; D. E. Shaw Research, New York, NY, USA, 2016) using the OPLS 2005 force field parameters. A solvated system (TIP3P) and a predefined model for electrically neutral system (physiological concentrations of monovalent ions, NaCl 0.15 M) were used in an orthorhombic box and maintained at constant temperature of 300 K for all simulations. The dynamics simulations were analysed using the Simulation Interaction Diagram tool of Desmond package, monitoring the behaviour and stability of simulations by RMSD of the ligand and protein atom positions in time.

3.12. RNA Interference

Gene silencing of XIAP in MCF7 cells was performed as previously published [106]. Briefly, according to the manufacturer's protocol, iBONI siRNA Pool (Riboxx, Radebeul, Germany) targeting human XIAP were mixed to Lipofectamine RNAiMax transfection reagent (Life Technologies). iBONI siRNA Pool negative control (Riboxx) (scrambled targeting siRNAs) was also used. The mix was added to cultured MCF7 cells at a siRNA concentration of 50 nM for 24 h.

3.13. Real-Time PCR

The analysis of mRNA expression was performed as previously described [106,114,115]. Briefly, total RNA from MCF7 cells was extracted with the High Pure RNA Isolation Kit (Roche Applied Science, Mannheim, Germany), according to the manufacturer's protocol. First-strand cDNA was generated from 1 μg of total RNA using iScript Reverse Transcription Supermix (Bio-Rad). Primer pairs (Eurofins Genomics, Milano, Italy) for XIAP (NM_001167; forward ACCGTGCGGTGCTTTAGTT, reverse TGCGTGGCACTATTTTCAAGATA) and β-actin (NM_001101; forward ATAGCACAGCCTGGATAGCAACGTAC, reverse CACCTTCTACAAT GAGCTGCGTGTG) were designed to hybridise to unique regions of the appropriate gene sequence. PCR was performed using SsoAdvanced Universal SYBR Green Supermix and the CFX96 Touch Real-Time PCR Detection System (Bio-Rad). The fold change was determined relative to the selected control sample after normalising to β-actin (internal standard) by the formula $2^{-\Delta\Delta CT}$.

3.14. Statistics

Statistical significance of raw data between the groups in each experiment was evaluated using unpaired Student's *t*-test (single comparisons) or one-way ANOVA followed by the Newman-Keuls post-test (multiple comparisons). The IC_{50} and E_{max} concentration were determined by non-linear regression curve analysis of the concentration-effect responses. Potency values among concentration-response curves were compared with the F-test. Data belonging from different experiments were represented and averaged in the same graph. The GraphPad Prism software package (GraphPad Software, San Diego, CA, USA) was used. The results were expressed as means ± standard error of mean (SEM) of the indicated n values.

4. Conclusions

This study adds to the renewed biological interest in natural derived compounds, by presenting a chemical and biological characterisation of new small organic molecules derived from *Piper* genus plants. Following a recent preliminary report of gibbilimbol B as cytotoxic in breast cancer cell lines, we explored this observation by comparing it to similarly structured new molecules. Erioquinol that appeared to be the most potent compound versus gibbilimbol B and eriopodol A was listed as an intermediate. A more detailed investigation of the biological mechanism behind these molecules' activity in shaping cell viability revealed induction of caspase-dependent apoptosis following exposure of tumour cells to gibbilimbol B and eriopodol A and, interestingly, display of caspase-independent/non-apoptotic features in cell treated with erioquinol. In silico modelling and molecular approaches gave us a first preliminary insight into the molecular target of *Piper* genus compounds, the anti-apoptotic protein XIAP (Figure 13). Of note, an already identified XIAP inhibitor shared structural and binding similarities with them. The appeal of XIAP as a therapeutic target in cancer is not restricted to inhibition of apoptosis, but comprehends the regulation of other cellular physiological aspects, such as control of caspase-independent cell death. The molecular signature behind our observation opens important implications to further dissect the role of XIAP and for the development of novel XIAP antagonists for cancer treatment.

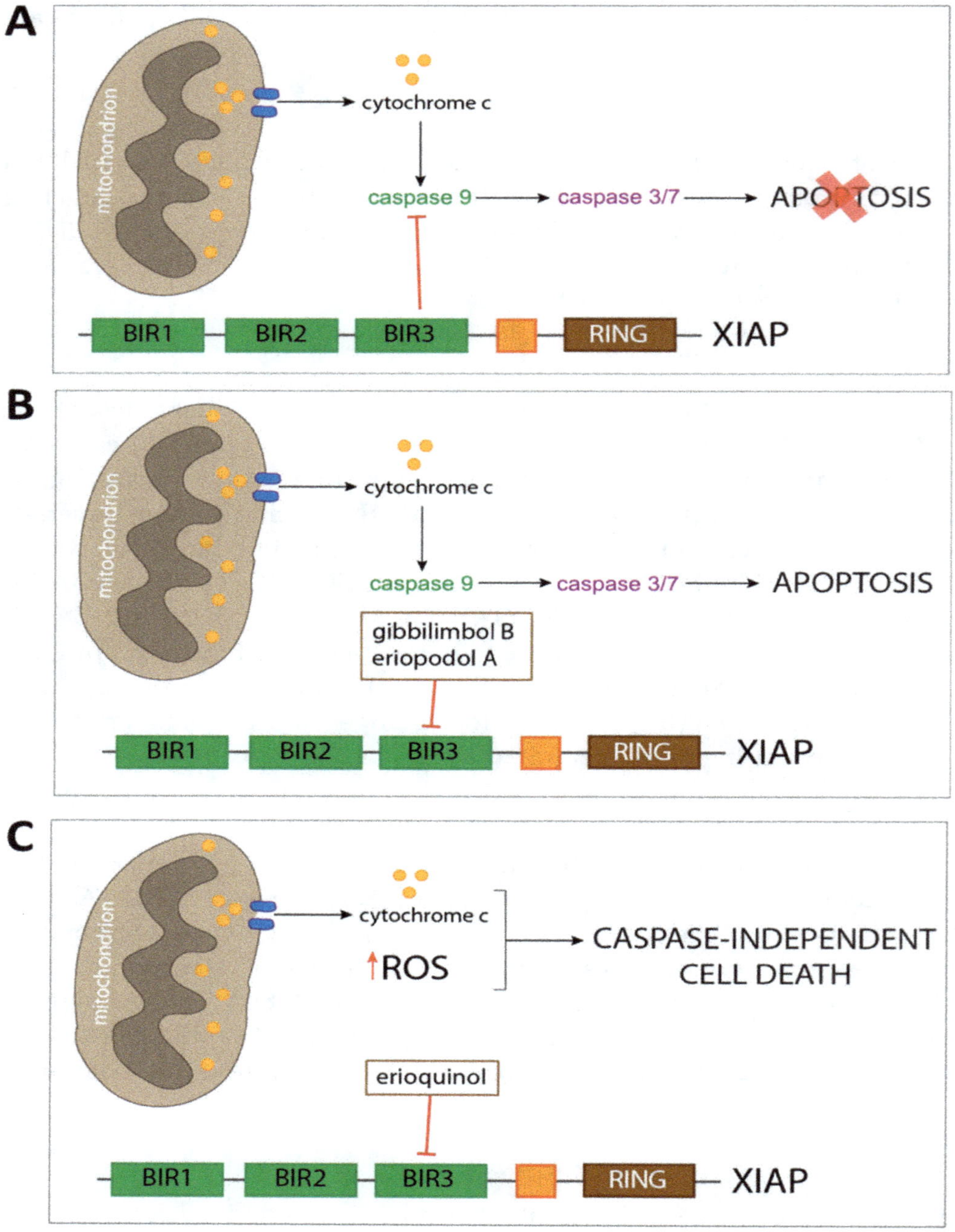

Figure 13. Schematic picture depicting cell death mechanisms of *Piper* genus-derived compounds. Escape of both intrinsic and extrinsic apoptosis is a common feature of cancer cells. (**A**) This hallmark is often carried out by overexpressing anti-apoptotic proteins, such as X-linked inhibitor of apoptosis protein (XIAP), which prevents the execution of apoptosis by binding of its baculovirus IAP repeat (BIR) 3 domain to already active initiator caspase 9. In order to counteract this resistance to cell death, several cancer pharmacological therapies have the aim of removing the 'molecular brakes' to apoptosis sensitising cancer cell to undergo loss of viability. The approach we described includes the use of three compounds from *Piper* genus plants which were predicted to bind XIAP-BIR3 domain. (**B**) Two of the compounds (gibbilimbol B and eriopodol A) were shown to induce a classical pro-apoptotic response, including mitochondrial outer membrane polarisation, release of cytochrome c, and subsequent activation of both initiator and effector caspases. (**C**) Despites triggering a similar response at the mitochondria level, erioquinol does not act through the apoptotic machinery, and results in a caspase-independent cell death characterised by cytoplasmic reactive oxygen species (ROS) accumulation.

Supplementary Materials:
Figure S1: NMR spectroscopy (400 MHz, $CDCl_3$) and HRESIMS of compound 1, Figure S2: NMR spectroscopy (400 MHz, $CDCl_3$) and HRESIMS of compound 2, Figure S3: NMR spectroscopy (400 MHz, $CDCl_3$) and HRESIMS of compound 3, Figure S4: NMR spectroscopy (400 MHz, $CDCl_3$) and HRESIMS of compound 4, Figure S5: NMR spectroscopy (400 MHz, $CDCl_3$) and HRESIMS of compound 5, Figure S6: Western blot, Figure S7: Protein-ligand interactions fraction for evaluated ligands and X-linked inhibitor of apoptosis protein (XIAP) baculovirus IAP repeat (BIR)-3 domain during the molecular dynamics trajectory of 50 ns, Table S1: ^{1}H NMR (400 MHz) data for compounds 1–4 in $CDCl_3$ and compound 5 in MeOD, Table S2: ^{13}C NMR (100 MHz) data for compounds 1–4 in $CDCl_3$ and compound 5 in MeOD.

Author Contributions: D.M.: design and conception of the experimental plan and analysis work, isolation and characterisation of the compounds, acquisition analysis and interpretation of human cell data, in silico analysis, contribution to article writing. M.B., S.Z.: design, acquisition, analysis and interpretation of human cell data, contribution to the experimental plan and article writing. F.L.-V.: in silico analysis, contribution to the supervision of the experiments, interpretation and processing of the results. A.S-H., M.G., M.C., E.C. (Elisabetta Catalani): acquisition and processing of the results, contribution to the experimental plan. C.D.P., C.P., E.C. (Emilio Clementi): contribution to the design, conception and interpretation of human cell results, contribution to article writing. G.A., W.D., L.C.: supervision of the experiments and interpretation of the results, contribution to article writing. D.C.: conception and coordination of the experimental and analysis work, supervision of human cell experiments, analysis/interpretation and processing of data, article writing. All authors provided critical feedback, edited and approved the final manuscript.

Acknowledgments: We are grateful to Francesca Proietti Serafini (University of Tuscia, Viterbo, Italy) for the help with viability cell assays and to Debora Parolin (University of Milan, Milano, Italy) for HUVEC supply.

References

1. Gurevich, E.V.; Gurevich, V.V. Therapeutic potential of small molecules and engineered proteins. *Handb. Exp. Pharmacol.* **2014**, *219*, 1–12.
2. Cheng, B.; Yuan, W.E.; Su, J.; Liu, Y.; Chen, J. Recent advances in small molecule based cancer immunotherapy. *Eur. J. Med. Chem.* **2018**, *157*, 582–598. [CrossRef]
3. Huck, B.R.; Kotzner, L.; Urbahns, K. Small Molecules Drive Big Improvements in Immuno-Oncology Therapies. *Angew. Chem. Int. Ed. Engl.* **2018**, *57*, 4412–4428. [CrossRef]
4. Schiavone, S.; Trabace, L. Small Molecules: Therapeutic Application in Neuropsychiatric and Neurodegenerative Disorders. *Molecules* **2018**, *23*, 411. [CrossRef]
5. Dhanak, D.; Edwards, J.P.; Nguyen, A.; Tummino, P.J. Small-Molecule Targets in Immuno-Oncology. *Cell Chem. Biol.* **2017**, *24*, 1148–1160. [CrossRef]
6. Shen, B. A New Golden Age of Natural Products Drug Discovery. *Cell* **2015**, *163*, 1297–1300. [CrossRef]
7. Nobili, S.; Lippi, D.; Witort, E.; Donnini, M.; Bausi, L.; Mini, E.; Capaccioli, S. Natural compounds for cancer treatment and prevention. *Pharmacol. Res.* **2009**, *59*, 365–378. [CrossRef]
8. Harvey, A.L.; Edrada-Ebel, R.; Quinn, R.J. The re-emergence of natural products for drug discovery in the genomics era. *Nat. Rev. Drug Discov.* **2015**, *14*, 111–129. [CrossRef]
9. Newman, D.J.; Cragg, G.M. Natural Products as Sources of New Drugs from 1981 to 2014. *J. Nat. Prod.* **2016**, *79*, 629–661. [CrossRef]
10. Catalani, E.; Proietti Serafini, F.; Zecchini, S.; Picchietti, S.; Fausto, A.M.; Marcantoni, E.; Buonanno, F.; Ortenzi, C.; Perrotta, C.; Cervia, D. Natural products from aquatic eukaryotic microorganisms for cancer therapy: Perspectives on anti-tumour properties of ciliate bioactive molecules. *Pharmacol. Res.* **2016**, *113*, 409–420. [CrossRef]
11. Carocho, M.; Ferreira, I.C. The role of phenolic compounds in the fight against cancer—A review. *Anticancer Agents Med. Chem.* **2013**, *13*, 1236–1258. [CrossRef]
12. Guerra, A.R.; Duarte, M.F.; Duarte, I.F. Targeting Tumor Metabolism with Plant-Derived Natural Products: Emerging Trends in Cancer Therapy. *J. Agric. Food Chem.* **2018**, *66*, 10663–10685. [CrossRef]

13. Jafari, S.; Saeidnia, S.; Abdollahi, M. Role of natural phenolic compounds in cancer chemoprevention via regulation of the cell cycle. *Curr. Pharm. Biotechnol.* **2014**, *15*, 409–421. [CrossRef]
14. Tungmunnithum, D.; Thongboonyou, A.; Pholboon, A.; Yangsabai, A. Flavonoids and Other Phenolic Compounds from Medicinal Plants for Pharmaceutical and Medical Aspects: An Overview. *Medicines* **2018**, *5*, 93. [CrossRef]
15. Parmar, V.S.; Jain, S.C.; Gupta, S.; Talwar, S.; Rajwanshi, V.K.; Kumar, R.; Azim, A.; Malhotra, S.; Kumar, N.; Jain, R.; et al. Polyphenols and alkaloids from Piper species. *Phytochemistry* **1998**, *49*, 1069–1078. [CrossRef]
16. Xiang, C.P.; Shi, Y.N.; Liu, F.F.; Li, H.Z.; Zhang, Y.J.; Yang, C.R.; Xu, M. A Survey of the Chemical Compounds of Piper spp. (Piperaceae) and Their Biological Activities. *Nat. Prod. Commun.* **2016**, *11*, 1403–1408. [CrossRef]
17. Valdivia, C.; Marquez, N.; Eriksson, J.; Vilaseca, A.; Munoz, E.; Sterner, O. Bioactive alkenylphenols from Piper obliquum. *Bioorg. Med. Chem.* **2008**, *16*, 4120–4126. [CrossRef]
18. Yang, S.X.; Sun, Q.Y.; Yang, F.M.; Hu, G.W.; Luo, J.F.; Wang, Y.H.; Long, C.L. Sarmentosumols A to F, new mono- and dimeric alkenylphenols from Piper sarmentosum. *Planta Med.* **2013**, *79*, 693–696. [CrossRef]
19. Orjala, J.; Mian, P.; Rali, T.; Sticher, O. Gibbilimbols A-D, cytotoxic and antibacterial alkenylphenols from Piper gibbilimbum. *J. Nat. Prod.* **1998**, *61*, 939–941. [CrossRef]
20. Yoshida, N.C.; Benedetti, A.M.; dos Santos, R.A.; Ramos, C.S.; Batista, R.; Yamaguchi, L.F.; Kato, M.J. Alkenylphenols from Piper dilatatum and P. diospyrifolium. *Phytochem. Lett.* **2018**, *25*, 136–140. [CrossRef]
21. De Oliveira, A.; Mesquita, J.T.; Tempone, A.G.; Lago, J.H.G.; Guimaraes, E.F.; Kato, M.J. Leishmanicidal activity of an alkenylphenol from Piper malacophyllum is related to plasma membrane disruption. *Exp. Parasitol.* **2012**, *132*, 383–387. [CrossRef] [PubMed]
22. Bezerra, D.P.; Pessoa, C.; de Moraes, M.O.; Saker-Neto, N.; Silveira, E.R.; Costa-Lotufo, L.V. Overview of the therapeutic potential of piplartine (piperlongumine). *Eur. J. Pharm. Sci.* **2013**, *48*, 453–463. [CrossRef] [PubMed]
23. D'Sousa Costa, C.O.; Araujo Neto, J.H.; Baliza, I.R.S.; Dias, R.B.; Valverde, L.F.; Vidal, M.T.A.; Sales, C.B.S.; Rocha, C.A.G.; Moreira, D.R.M.; Soares, M.B.P.; et al. Novel piplartine-containing ruthenium complexes: Synthesis, cell growth inhibition, apoptosis induction and ROS production on HCT116 cells. *Oncotarget* **2017**, *8*, 104367–104392. [CrossRef] [PubMed]
24. Piska, K.; Gunia-Krzyzak, A.; Koczurkiewicz, P.; Wojcik-Pszczola, K.; Pekala, E. Piperlongumine (piplartine) as a lead compound for anticancer agents—Synthesis and properties of analogues: A mini-review. *Eur. J. Med. Chem.* **2018**, *156*, 13–20. [CrossRef] [PubMed]
25. Benfica, P.L.; Avila, R.I.; Rodrigues, B.D.S.; Cortez, A.P.; Batista, A.C.; Gaeti, M.P.N.; Lima, E.M.; Rezende, K.R.; Valadares, M.C. 4-Nerolidylcatechol: Apoptosis by mitochondrial mechanisms with reduction in cyclin D1 at G0/G1 stage of the chronic myelogenous K562 cell line. *Pharm. Biol.* **2017**, *55*, 1899–1908. [CrossRef] [PubMed]
26. Cortez, A.P.; de Avila, R.I.; da Cunha, C.R.; Santos, A.P.; Menegatti, R.; Rezende, K.R.; Valadares, M.C. 4-Nerolidylcatechol analogues as promising anticancer agents. *Eur. J. Pharmacol.* **2015**, *765*, 517–524. [CrossRef] [PubMed]
27. Gundala, S.R.; Yang, C.; Mukkavilli, R.; Paranjpe, R.; Brahmbhatt, M.; Pannu, V.; Cheng, A.; Reid, M.D.; Aneja, R. Hydroxychavicol, a betel leaf component, inhibits prostate cancer through ROS-driven DNA damage and apoptosis. *Toxicol. Appl. Pharmacol.* **2014**, *280*, 86–96. [CrossRef] [PubMed]
28. Hemamalini, V.; Velayutham, D.P.M.; Lakshmanan, L.; Muthusamy, K.; Sivaramakrishnan, S.; Premkumar, K. Inhibitory potential of Hydroxychavicol on Ehrlich ascites carcinoma model and in silico interaction on cancer targets. *Nat. Prod. Res.* **2018**, 1–6. [CrossRef]
29. Munoz, D.R.; Sandoval-Hernandez, A.G.; Delgado, W.A.; Arboleda, G.H.; Cuca, L.E. In vitro anticancer screening of Colombian plants from Piper genus (Piperaceae). *J. Pharmacogn. Phytother.* **2018**, *10*, 174–181.
30. Hanahan, D.; Weinberg, R.A. Hallmarks of cancer: The next generation. *Cell* **2011**, *144*, 646–674. [CrossRef]
31. Pfeffer, C.M.; Singh, A.T.K. Apoptosis: A Target for Anticancer Therapy. *Int. J. Mol. Sci.* **2018**, *19*, 448. [CrossRef] [PubMed]
32. Lalaoui, N.; Vaux, D.L. Recent advances in understanding inhibitor of apoptosis proteins. *F1000Research* **2018**, *7*. [CrossRef] [PubMed]

33. Rathore, R.; McCallum, J.E.; Varghese, E.; Florea, A.M.; Busselberg, D. Overcoming chemotherapy drug resistance by targeting inhibitors of apoptosis proteins (IAPs). *Apoptosis* **2017**, *22*, 898–919. [CrossRef] [PubMed]
34. Schimmer, A.D.; Dalili, S.; Batey, R.A.; Riedl, S.J. Targeting XIAP for the treatment of malignancy. *Cell Death Differ.* **2006**, *13*, 179–188. [CrossRef]
35. Tamanini, E.; Buck, I.M.; Chessari, G.; Chiarparin, E.; Day, J.E.H.; Frederickson, M.; Griffiths-Jones, C.M.; Hearn, K.; Heightman, T.D.; Iqbal, A.; et al. Discovery of a Potent Nonpeptidomimetic, Small-Molecule Antagonist of Cellular Inhibitor of Apoptosis Protein 1 (cIAP1) and X-Linked Inhibitor of Apoptosis Protein (XIAP). *J. Med. Chem.* **2017**, *60*, 4611–4625. [CrossRef]
36. Sun, H.; Stuckey, J.A.; Nikolovska-Coleska, Z.; Qin, D.; Meagher, J.L.; Qiu, S.; Lu, J.; Yang, C.Y.; Saito, N.G.; Wang, S. Structure-based design, synthesis, evaluation, and crystallographic studies of conformationally constrained Smac mimetics as inhibitors of the X-linked inhibitor of apoptosis protein (XIAP). *J. Med. Chem.* **2008**, *51*, 7169–7180. [CrossRef]
37. Fakler, M.; Loeder, S.; Vogler, M.; Schneider, K.; Jeremias, I.; Debatin, K.M.; Fulda, S. Small molecule XIAP inhibitors cooperate with TRAIL to induce apoptosis in childhood acute leukemia cells and overcome Bcl-2-mediated resistance. *Blood* **2009**, *113*, 1710–1722. [CrossRef] [PubMed]
38. Vogler, M.; Walczak, H.; Stadel, D.; Haas, T.L.; Genze, F.; Jovanovic, M.; Bhanot, U.; Hasel, C.; Moller, P.; Gschwend, J.E.; et al. Small molecule XIAP inhibitors enhance TRAIL-induced apoptosis and antitumor activity in preclinical models of pancreatic carcinoma. *Cancer Res.* **2009**, *69*, 2425–2434. [CrossRef]
39. Dean, E.J.; Ward, T.; Pinilla, C.; Houghten, R.; Welsh, K.; Makin, G.; Ranson, M.; Dive, C. A small molecule inhibitor of XIAP induces apoptosis and synergises with vinorelbine and cisplatin in NSCLC. *Br. J. Cancer* **2010**, *102*, 97–103. [CrossRef]
40. Obexer, P.; Ausserlechner, M.J. X-linked inhibitor of apoptosis protein—A critical death resistance regulator and therapeutic target for personalized cancer therapy. *Front. Oncol.* **2014**, *4*, 197. [CrossRef]
41. Cong, H.; Xu, L.; Wu, Y.; Qu, Z.; Bian, T.; Zhang, W.; Xing, C.; Zhuang, C. Inhibitor of Apoptosis Protein (IAP) Antagonists in Anticancer Agent Discovery: Current Status and Perspectives. *J. Med. Chem.* **2019**. [CrossRef]
42. Fulda, S. Promises and Challenges of Smac Mimetics as Cancer Therapeutics. *Clin. Cancer Res.* **2015**, *21*, 5030–5036. [CrossRef] [PubMed]
43. Schimmer, A.D.; Welsh, K.; Pinilla, C.; Wang, Z.; Krajewska, M.; Bonneau, M.J.; Pedersen, I.M.; Kitada, S.; Scott, F.L.; Bailly-Maitre, B.; et al. Small-molecule antagonists of apoptosis suppressor XIAP exhibit broad antitumor activity. *Cancer Cell* **2004**, *5*, 25–35. [CrossRef]
44. Masaki, M.E.; Harumoto, T.; Terazima, M.N.; Miyake, A.; Usuki, Y.; Iio, H. Climacostol, a defense toxin of the heterotrich ciliate Climacostomum virens against predators. *Tetrahedron Lett.* **1999**, *40*, 8227–8229. [CrossRef]
45. Varela, M.T.; Dias, R.Z.; Martins, L.F.; Ferreira, D.D.; Tempone, A.G.; Ueno, A.K.; Lago, J.H.G.; Fernandes, J.P.S. Gibbilimbol analogues as antiparasitic agents-Synthesis and biological activity against Trypanosoma cruzi and Leishmania (L.) infantum. *Bioorg. Med. Chem. Lett.* **2016**, *26*, 1180–1183. [CrossRef] [PubMed]
46. Carreno, M.C.; Gonzalez-Lopez, M.; Urbano, A. Oxidative de-aromatization of para-alkyl phenols into para-peroxyquinols and para-quinols mediated by oxone as a source of singlet oxygen. *Angew. Chem. Int. Ed.* **2006**, *45*, 2737–2741. [CrossRef]
47. Freitas, G.C.; Batista, J.M.; Franchi, G.C.; Nowill, A.E.; Yamaguchi, L.F.; Vilcachagua, J.D.; Favaro, D.C.; Furlan, M.; Guimaraes, E.F.; Jeffrey, C.S.; et al. Cytotoxic non-aromatic B-ring flavanones from Piper carniconnectivum C. DC. *Phytochemistry* **2014**, *97*, 81–87. [CrossRef] [PubMed]
48. Nishino, C.; Kobayashi, K.; Fukushima, M. Halleridone, a cytotoxic constituent from Cornus controversa. *J. Nat. Prod.* **1988**, *51*, 1281–1282. [CrossRef]
49. Bradshaw, T.D.; Matthews, C.S.; Cookson, J.; Chew, E.H.; Shah, M.; Bailey, K.; Monks, A.; Harris, E.; Westwell, A.D.; Wells, G.; et al. Elucidation of thioredoxin as a molecular target for antitumor quinols. *Cancer Res.* **2005**, *65*, 3911–3919. [CrossRef]
50. Berry, J.M.; Bradshaw, T.D.; Fichtner, I.; Ren, R.; Schwalbe, C.H.; Wells, G.; Chew, E.H.; Stevens, M.F.; Westwell, A.D. Quinols as novel therapeutic agents. 2.(1) 4-(1-Arylsulfonylindol-2-yl)-4-hydroxycyclohexa-2,5-dien-1-ones and related agents as potent and selective antitumor agents. *J. Med. Chem.* **2005**, *48*, 639–644. [CrossRef]
51. McCarroll, A.J.; Bradshaw, T.D.; Westwell, A.D.; Matthews, C.S.; Stevens, M.F. Quinols as novel therapeutic agents. 7.1 Synthesis of antitumor 4-[1-(arylsulfonyl-1H-indol-2-yl)]-4-hydroxycyclohexa-2,5-dien-1-ones by Sonogashira reactions. *J. Med. Chem.* **2007**, *50*, 1707–1710. [CrossRef] [PubMed]

52. Abu Bakar, A.; Akhtar, M.N.; Mohd Ali, N.; Yeap, S.K.; Quah, C.K.; Loh, W.S.; Alitheen, N.B.; Zareen, S.; Ul-Haq, Z.; Shah, S.A.A. Design, Synthesis and Docking Studies of Flavokawain B Type Chalcones and Their Cytotoxic Effects on MCF-7 and MDA-MB-231 Cell Lines. *Molecules* **2018**, *23*, 616. [CrossRef] [PubMed]
53. Sriwiriyajan, S.; Sukpondma, Y.; Srisawat, T.; Madla, S.; Graidist, P. (-)-Kusunokinin and piperloguminine from Piper nigrum: An alternative option to treat breast cancer. *Biomed. Pharm.* **2017**, *92*, 732–743. [CrossRef] [PubMed]
54. Sriwiriyajan, S.; Ninpesh, T.; Sukpondma, Y.; Nasomyon, T.; Graidist, P. Cytotoxicity Screening of Plants of Genus Piper in Breast Cancer Cell Lines. *Trop. J. Pharm. Res.* **2014**, *13*, 921–928. [CrossRef]
55. Fan, L.; Cao, X.; Yan, H.; Wang, Q.; Tian, X.; Zhang, L.; He, X.; Borjihan, G.; Morigen. The synthetic antihyperlipidemic drug potassium piperate selectively kills breast cancer cells through inhibiting G1-S-phase transition and inducing apoptosis. *Oncotarget* **2017**, *8*, 47250–47268. [CrossRef] [PubMed]
56. Park, M.J.; Lee, D.E.; Shim, M.K.; Jang, E.H.; Lee, J.K.; Jeong, S.Y.; Kim, J.H. Piperlongumine inhibits TGF-beta-induced epithelial-to-mesenchymal transition by modulating the expression of E-cadherin, Snail1, and Twist1. *Eur. J. Pharmacol.* **2017**, *812*, 243–249. [CrossRef] [PubMed]
57. De Souza Grinevicius, V.M.; Kviecinski, M.R.; Santos Mota, N.S.; Ourique, F.; Porfirio Will Castro, L.S.; Andreguetti, R.R.; Gomes Correia, J.F.; Filho, D.W.; Pich, C.T.; Pedrosa, R.C. Piper nigrum ethanolic extract rich in piperamides causes ROS overproduction, oxidative damage in DNA leading to cell cycle arrest and apoptosis in cancer cells. *J. Ethnopharmacol.* **2016**, *189*, 139–147. [CrossRef]
58. Deng, Y.; Sriwiriyajan, S.; Tedasen, A.; Hiransai, P.; Graidist, P. Anti-cancer effects of Piper nigrum via inducing multiple molecular signaling in vivo and in vitro. *J. Ethnopharmacol.* **2016**, *188*, 87–95. [CrossRef]
59. Da Nobrega, F.R.; Ozdemir, O.; Nascimento Sousa, S.C.S.; Barboza, J.N.; Turkez, H.; de Sousa, D.P. Piplartine Analogues and Cytotoxic Evaluation against Glioblastoma. *Molecules* **2018**, *23*, 1382. [CrossRef]
60. Abdul Rahman, A.; Jamal, A.R.; Harun, R.; Mohd Mokhtar, N.; Wan Ngah, W.Z. Gamma-tocotrienol and hydroxy-chavicol synergistically inhibits growth and induces apoptosis of human glioma cells. *BMC Complement. Altern. Med.* **2014**, *14*, 213. [CrossRef]
61. Subramanian, U.; Poongavanam, S.; Vanisree, A.J. Studies on the neuroprotective role of Piper longum in C6 glioma induced rats. *Investing. New Drugs* **2010**, *28*, 615–623. [CrossRef] [PubMed]
62. Buonanno, F.; Catalani, E.; Cervia, D.; Proietti Serafini, F.; Picchietti, S.; Fausto, A.M.; Giorgi, S.; Lupidi, G.; Rossi, F.V.; Marcantoni, E.; et al. Bioactivity and Structural Properties of Novel Synthetic Analogues of the Protozoan Toxin Climacostol. *Toxins* **2019**, *11*, 42. [CrossRef] [PubMed]
63. Moloney, J.N.; Cotter, T.G. ROS signalling in the biology of cancer. *Semin. cell Dev. Biol.* **2018**, *80*, 50–64. [CrossRef] [PubMed]
64. Tait, S.W.; Green, D.R. Caspase-independent cell death: Leaving the set without the final cut. *Oncogene* **2008**, *27*, 6452–6461. [CrossRef]
65. Galluzzi, L.; Kepp, O.; Chan, F.K.; Kroemer, G. Necroptosis: Mechanisms and Relevance to Disease. *Annu. Rev. Pathol.* **2017**, *12*, 103–130. [CrossRef] [PubMed]
66. Green, D.R. The Coming Decade of Cell Death Research: Five Riddles. *Cell* **2019**, *177*, 1094–1107. [CrossRef] [PubMed]
67. Ye, J.; Zhang, R.; Wu, F.; Zhai, L.; Wang, K.; Xiao, M.; Xie, T.; Sui, X. Non-apoptotic cell death in malignant tumor cells and natural compounds. *Cancer Lett.* **2018**, *420*, 210–227. [CrossRef]
68. Holze, C.; Michaudel, C.; Mackowiak, C.; Haas, D.A.; Benda, C.; Hubel, P.; Pennemann, F.L.; Schnepf, D.; Wettmarshausen, J.; Braun, M.; et al. Oxeiptosis, a ROS-induced caspase-independent apoptosis-like cell-death pathway. *Nat. Immunol.* **2018**, *19*, 130–140. [CrossRef] [PubMed]
69. Chai, J.; Shiozaki, E.; Srinivasula, S.M.; Wu, Q.; Datta, P.; Alnemri, E.S.; Shi, Y. Structural basis of caspase-7 inhibition by XIAP. *Cell* **2001**, *104*, 769–780. [CrossRef]
70. Shiozaki, E.N.; Chai, J.; Rigotti, D.J.; Riedl, S.J.; Li, P.; Srinivasula, S.M.; Alnemri, E.S.; Fairman, R.; Shi, Y. Mechanism of XIAP-mediated inhibition of caspase-9. *Mol. Cell* **2003**, *11*, 519–527. [CrossRef]
71. Suzuki, Y.; Nakabayashi, Y.; Nakata, K.; Reed, J.C.; Takahashi, R. X-linked inhibitor of apoptosis protein (XIAP) inhibits caspase-3 and -7 in distinct modes. *J. Biol. Chem.* **2001**, *276*, 27058–27063. [CrossRef] [PubMed]
72. Jung, S.; Li, C.; Duan, J.; Lee, S.; Kim, K.; Park, Y.; Yang, Y.; Kim, K.I.; Lim, J.S.; Cheon, C.I.; et al. TRIP-Br1 oncoprotein inhibits autophagy, apoptosis, and necroptosis under nutrient/serum-deprived condition. *Oncotarget* **2015**, *6*, 29060–29075. [CrossRef] [PubMed]

73. Lewis, J.; Burstein, E.; Reffey, S.B.; Bratton, S.B.; Roberts, A.B.; Duckett, C.S. Uncoupling of the signaling and caspase-inhibitory properties of X-linked inhibitor of apoptosis. *J. Biol. Chem.* **2004**, *279*, 9023–9029. [CrossRef] [PubMed]
74. Burstein, E.; Ganesh, L.; Dick, R.D.; van De Sluis, B.; Wilkinson, J.C.; Klomp, L.W.; Wijmenga, C.; Brewer, G.J.; Nabel, G.J.; Duckett, C.S. A novel role for XIAP in copper homeostasis through regulation of MURR1. *EMBO J.* **2004**, *23*, 244–254. [CrossRef] [PubMed]
75. Sanna, M.G.; da Silva Correia, J.; Ducrey, O.; Lee, J.; Nomoto, K.; Schrantz, N.; Deveraux, Q.L.; Ulevitch, R.J. IAP suppression of apoptosis involves distinct mechanisms: The TAK1/JNK1 signaling cascade and caspase inhibition. *Mol. Cell Biol.* **2002**, *22*, 1754–1766. [CrossRef] [PubMed]
76. Lewis, E.M.; Wilkinson, A.S.; Davis, N.Y.; Horita, D.A.; Wilkinson, J.C. Nondegradative ubiquitination of apoptosis inducing factor (AIF) by X-linked inhibitor of apoptosis at a residue critical for AIF-mediated chromatin degradation. *Biochemistry* **2011**, *50*, 11084–11096. [CrossRef] [PubMed]
77. Levkau, B.; Garton, K.J.; Ferri, N.; Kloke, K.; Nofer, J.R.; Baba, H.A.; Raines, E.W.; Breithardt, G. xIAP induces cell-cycle arrest and activates nuclear factor-kappaB: New survival pathways disabled by caspase-mediated cleavage during apoptosis of human endothelial cells. *Circ. Res.* **2001**, *88*, 282–290. [CrossRef] [PubMed]
78. Mufti, A.R.; Burstein, E.; Csomos, R.A.; Graf, P.C.; Wilkinson, J.C.; Dick, R.D.; Challa, M.; Son, J.K.; Bratton, S.B.; Su, G.L.; et al. XIAP Is a copper binding protein deregulated in Wilson's disease and other copper toxicosis disorders. *Mol. Cell* **2006**, *21*, 775–785. [CrossRef] [PubMed]
79. Wicki, S.; Gurzeler, U.; Wei-Lynn Wong, W.; Jost, P.J.; Bachmann, D.; Kaufmann, T. Loss of XIAP facilitates switch to TNFalpha-induced necroptosis in mouse neutrophils. *Cell Death Dis.* **2016**, *7*, e2422. [CrossRef] [PubMed]
80. Yabal, M.; Jost, P.J. XIAP as a regulator of inflammatory cell death: The TNF and RIP3 angle. *Mol. Cell. Oncol.* **2015**, *2*, e964622. [CrossRef] [PubMed]
81. Yabal, M.; Muller, N.; Adler, H.; Knies, N.; Gross, C.J.; Damgaard, R.B.; Kanegane, H.; Ringelhan, M.; Kaufmann, T.; Heikenwalder, M.; et al. XIAP restricts TNF- and RIP3-dependent cell death and inflammasome activation. *Cell Rep.* **2014**, *7*, 1796–1808. [CrossRef] [PubMed]
82. Lawlor, K.E.; Feltham, R.; Yabal, M.; Conos, S.A.; Chen, K.W.; Ziehe, S.; Grass, C.; Zhan, Y.; Nguyen, T.A.; Hall, C.; et al. XIAP Loss Triggers RIPK3- and Caspase-8-Driven IL-1beta Activation and Cell Death as a Consequence of TLR-MyD88-Induced cIAP1-TRAF2 Degradation. *Cell Rep.* **2017**, *20*, 668–682. [CrossRef] [PubMed]
83. Poojari, R. Embelin—A drug of antiquity: Shifting the paradigm towards modern medicine. *Expert Opin. Investig. Drugs* **2014**, *23*, 427–444. [CrossRef] [PubMed]
84. Ko, J.H.; Lee, S.G.; Yang, W.M.; Um, J.Y.; Sethi, G.; Mishra, S.; Shanmugam, M.K.; Ahn, K.S. The Application of Embelin for Cancer Prevention and Therapy. *Molecules* **2018**, *23*, 621. [CrossRef] [PubMed]
85. Prabhu, K.S.; Achkar, I.W.; Kuttikrishnan, S.; Akhtar, S.; Khan, A.Q.; Siveen, K.S.; Uddin, S. Embelin: A benzoquinone possesses therapeutic potential for the treatment of human cancer. *Future Med. Chem.* **2018**, *10*, 961–976. [CrossRef] [PubMed]
86. Nikolovska-Coleska, Z.; Xu, L.; Hu, Z.; Tomita, Y.; Li, P.; Roller, P.P.; Wang, R.; Fang, X.; Guo, R.; Zhang, M.; et al. Discovery of embelin as a cell-permeable, small-molecular weight inhibitor of XIAP through structure-based computational screening of a traditional herbal medicine three-dimensional structure database. *J. Med. Chem.* **2004**, *47*, 2430–2440. [CrossRef]
87. Chessari, G.; Buck, I.M.; Day, J.E.; Day, P.J.; Iqbal, A.; Johnson, C.N.; Lewis, E.J.; Martins, V.; Miller, D.; Reader, M.; et al. Fragment-Based Drug Discovery Targeting Inhibitor of Apoptosis Proteins: Discovery of a Non-Alanine Lead Series with Dual Activity Against cIAP1 and XIAP. *J. Med. Chem.* **2015**, *58*, 6574–6588. [CrossRef]
88. Jin, X.; Lee, K.; Kim, N.H.; Kim, H.S.; Yook, J.I.; Choi, J.; No, K.T. Natural products used as a chemical library for protein-protein interaction targeted drug discovery. *J. Mol. Graph. Model.* **2018**, *79*, 46–58. [CrossRef]
89. Johnson, C.N.; Ahn, J.S.; Buck, I.M.; Chiarparin, E.; Day, J.E.H.; Hopkins, A.; Howard, S.; Lewis, E.J.; Martins, V.; Millemaggi, A.; et al. A Fragment-Derived Clinical Candidate for Antagonism of X-Linked and Cellular Inhibitor of Apoptosis Proteins: 1-(6-[(4-Fluorophenyl)methyl]-5-(hydroxymethyl)-3,3-dimethyl-1H,2H,3H-pyrrolo[3,2-b]pyridin-1-yl)-2-[(2R,5R)-5-methyl-2-([(3R)-3-methylmorpholin-4-yl]methyl)piperazin-1-yl]ethan-1-one (ASTX660). *J. Med. Chem.* **2018**, *61*, 7314–7329.
90. Kashkar, H. X-linked inhibitor of apoptosis: A chemoresistance factor or a hollow promise. *Clin. Cancer Res.* **2010**, *16*, 4496–4502. [CrossRef]

91. Shah, P.; Djisam, R.; Damulira, H.; Aganze, A.; Danquah, M. Embelin inhibits proliferation, induces apoptosis and alters gene expression profiles in breast cancer cells. *Pharmacol. Rep.* **2016**, *68*, 638–644. [CrossRef] [PubMed]
92. Hahm, E.R.; Singh, S.V. Withaferin A-induced apoptosis in human breast cancer cells is associated with suppression of inhibitor of apoptosis family protein expression. *Cancer Lett.* **2013**, *334*, 101–108. [CrossRef] [PubMed]
93. Liu, J.; Zhang, X.; Liu, A.; Liu, S.; Zhang, L.; Wu, B.; Hu, Q. Berberine induces apoptosis in p53-null leukemia cells by down-regulating XIAP at the post-transcriptional level. *Cell. Physiol. Biochem.* **2013**, *32*, 1213–1224. [CrossRef] [PubMed]
94. Lima, R.T.; Martins, L.M.; Guimaraes, J.E.; Sambade, C.; Vasconcelos, M.H. Specific downregulation of bcl-2 and xIAP by RNAi enhances the effects of chemotherapeutic agents in MCF-7 human breast cancer cells. *Cancer Gene Ther.* **2004**, *11*, 309–316. [CrossRef] [PubMed]
95. Sensintaffar, J.; Scott, F.L.; Peach, R.; Hager, J.H. XIAP is not required for human tumor cell survival in the absence of an exogenous death signal. *BMC Cancer* **2010**, *10*, 11. [CrossRef] [PubMed]
96. Zhang, Y.; Wang, Y.; Gao, W.; Zhang, R.; Han, X.; Jia, M.; Guan, W. Transfer of siRNA against XIAP induces apoptosis and reduces tumor cells growth potential in human breast cancer in vitro and in vivo. *Breast Cancer Res. Treat* **2006**, *96*, 267–277. [CrossRef] [PubMed]
97. Foster, F.M.; Owens, T.W.; Tanianis-Hughes, J.; Clarke, R.B.; Brennan, K.; Bundred, N.J.; Streuli, C.H. Targeting inhibitor of apoptosis proteins in combination with ErbB antagonists in breast cancer. *Breast Cancer Res. BCR* **2009**, *11*, R41. [CrossRef] [PubMed]
98. Montero, J.; Letai, A. Why do BCL-2 inhibitors work and where should we use them in the clinic? *Cell Death Differ.* **2018**, *25*, 56–64. [CrossRef] [PubMed]
99. Delbridge, A.R.; Strasser, A. The BCL-2 protein family, BH3-mimetics and cancer therapy. *Cell Death Differ.* **2015**, *22*, 1071–1080. [CrossRef]
100. Giampazolias, E.; Zunino, B.; Dhayade, S.; Bock, F.; Cloix, C.; Cao, K.; Roca, A.; Lopez, J.; Ichim, G.; Proics, E.; et al. Mitochondrial permeabilization engages NF-kappaB-dependent anti-tumour activity under caspase deficiency. *Nat. Cell Biol.* **2017**, *19*, 1116–1129. [CrossRef] [PubMed]
101. Armani, C.; Catalani, E.; Balbarini, A.; Bagnoli, P.; Cervia, D. Expression, pharmacology, and functional role of somatostatin receptor subtypes 1 and 2 in human macrophages. *J. Leukoc. Biol.* **2007**, *81*, 845–855. [CrossRef] [PubMed]
102. Cervia, D.; Martini, D.; Garcia-Gil, M.; Di Giuseppe, G.; Guella, G.; Dini, F.; Bagnoli, P. Cytotoxic effects and apoptotic signalling mechanisms of the sesquiterpenoid euplotin C, a secondary metabolite of the marine ciliate *Euplotes crassus*, in tumour cells. *Apoptosis* **2006**, *11*, 829–843. [CrossRef] [PubMed]
103. Cervia, D.; Garcia-Gil, M.; Simonetti, E.; Di Giuseppe, G.; Guella, G.; Bagnoli, P.; Dini, F. Molecular mechanisms of euplotin C-induced apoptosis: Involvement of mitochondrial dysfunction, oxidative stress and proteases. *Apoptosis* **2007**, *12*, 1349–1363. [CrossRef] [PubMed]
104. Perrotta, C.; Buldorini, M.; Assi, E.; Cazzato, D.; De Palma, C.; Clementi, E.; Cervia, D. The thyroid hormone triiodothyronine controls macrophage maturation and functions: Protective role during inflammation. *Am. J. Pathol.* **2014**, *184*, 230–247. [CrossRef]
105. Di Giuseppe, G.; Cervia, D.; Vallesi, A. Divergences in the Response to Ultraviolet Radiation Between Polar and Non-Polar Ciliated Protozoa: UV Radiation Effects in Euplotes. *Microb. Ecol.* **2011**, *63*, 334–338. [CrossRef] [PubMed]
106. Perrotta, C.; Buonanno, F.; Zecchini, S.; Giavazzi, A.; Proietti Serafini, F.; Catalani, E.; Guerra, L.; Belardinelli, M.C.; Picchietti, S.; Fausto, A.M.; et al. Climacostol reduces tumour progression in a mouse model of melanoma via the p53-dependent intrinsic apoptotic programme. *Sci. Rep.* **2016**, *6*, 27281. [CrossRef] [PubMed]
107. Bizzozero, L.; Cazzato, D.; Cervia, D.; Assi, E.; Simbari, F.; Pagni, F.; De Palma, C.; Monno, A.; Verdelli, C.; Querini, P.R.; et al. Acid sphingomyelinase determines melanoma progression and metastatic behaviour via the microphtalmia-associated transcription factor signalling pathway. *Cell Death Differ.* **2014**, *21*, 507–520. [CrossRef]
108. Zecchini, S.; Proietti Serafini, F.; Catalani, E.; Giovarelli, M.; Coazzoli, M.; Di Renzo, I.; De Palma, C.; Perrotta, C.; Clementi, E.; Buonanno, F.; et al. Dysfunctional autophagy induced by the pro-apoptotic natural compound climacostol in tumour cells. *Cell Death Dis.* **2019**, *10*, 10. [CrossRef]

109. Assi, E.; Cervia, D.; Bizzozero, L.; Capobianco, A.; Pambianco, S.; Morisi, F.; De Palma, C.; Moscheni, C.; Pellegrino, P.; Clementi, E.; et al. Modulation of Acid Sphingomyelinase in Melanoma Reprogrammes the Tumour Immune Microenvironment. *Mediat. Inflamm* **2015**, *2015*, 370482. [CrossRef]
110. Cervia, D.; Assi, E.; De Palma, C.; Giovarelli, M.; Bizzozero, L.; Pambianco, S.; Di Renzo, I.; Zecchini, S.; Moscheni, C.; Vantaggiato, C.; et al. Essential role for acid sphingomyelinase-inhibited autophagy in melanoma response to cisplatin. *Oncotarget* **2016**, *7*, 24995–25009. [CrossRef]
111. Perrotta, C.; De Palma, C.; Clementi, E.; Cervia, D. Hormones and immunity in cancer: Are thyroid hormones endocrine players in the microglia/glioma cross-talk? *Front. Cell. Neurosci.* **2015**, *9*, 236. [CrossRef] [PubMed]
112. Vantaggiato, C.; Castelli, M.; Giovarelli, M.; Orso, G.; Bassi, M.T.; Clementi, E.; De Palma, C. The Fine Tuning of Drp1-Dependent Mitochondrial Remodeling and Autophagy Controls Neuronal Differentiation. *Front. Cell. Neurosci.* **2019**, *13*, 120. [CrossRef] [PubMed]
113. Pfisterer, P.H.; Wolber, G.; Efferth, T.; Rollinger, J.M.; Stuppner, H. Natural products in structure-assisted design of molecular cancer therapeutics. *Curr. Pharm. Des.* **2010**, *16*, 1718–1741. [CrossRef] [PubMed]
114. Cazzato, D.; Assi, E.; Moscheni, C.; Brunelli, S.; De Palma, C.; Cervia, D.; Perrotta, C.; Clementi, E. Nitric oxide drives embryonic myogenesis in chicken through the upregulation of myogenic differentiation factors. *Exp. Cell Res.* **2014**, *320*, 269–280. [CrossRef] [PubMed]
115. Cervia, D.; Catalani, E.; Belardinelli, M.C.; Perrotta, C.; Picchietti, S.; Alimenti, C.; Casini, G.; Fausto, A.M.; Vallesi, A. The protein pheromone Er-1 of the ciliate Euplotes raikovi stimulates human T-cell activity: Involvement of interleukin-2 system. *Exp. Cell Res.* **2013**, *319*, 56–67. [CrossRef] [PubMed]

Permissions

All chapters in this book were first published by MDPI; hereby published with permission under the Creative Commons Attribution License or equivalent. Every chapter published in this book has been scrutinized by our experts. Their significance has been extensively debated. The topics covered herein carry significant findings which will fuel the growth of the discipline. They may even be implemented as practical applications or may be referred to as a beginning point for another development.

The contributors of this book come from diverse backgrounds, making this book a truly international effort. This book will bring forth new frontiers with its revolutionizing research information and detailed analysis of the nascent developments around the world.

We would like to thank all the contributing authors for lending their expertise to make the book truly unique. They have played a crucial role in the development of this book. Without their invaluable contributions this book wouldn't have been possible. They have made vital efforts to compile up to date information on the varied aspects of this subject to make this book a valuable addition to the collection of many professionals and students.

This book was conceptualized with the vision of imparting up-to-date information and advanced data in this field. To ensure the same, a matchless editorial board was set up. Every individual on the board went through rigorous rounds of assessment to prove their worth. After which they invested a large part of their time researching and compiling the most relevant data for our readers.

The editorial board has been involved in producing this book since its inception. They have spent rigorous hours researching and exploring the diverse topics which have resulted in the successful publishing of this book. They have passed on their knowledge of decades through this book. To expedite this challenging task, the publisher supported the team at every step. A small team of assistant editors was also appointed to further simplify the editing procedure and attain best results for the readers.

Apart from the editorial board, the designing team has also invested a significant amount of their time in understanding the subject and creating the most relevant covers. They scrutinized every image to scout for the most suitable representation of the subject and create an appropriate cover for the book.

The publishing team has been an ardent support to the editorial, designing and production team. Their endless efforts to recruit the best for this project, has resulted in the accomplishment of this book. They are a veteran in the field of academics and their pool of knowledge is as vast as their experience in printing. Their expertise and guidance has proved useful at every step. Their uncompromising quality standards have made this book an exceptional effort. Their encouragement from time to time has been an inspiration for everyone.

The publisher and the editorial board hope that this book will prove to be a valuable piece of knowledge for researchers, students, practitioners and scholars across the globe.

List of Contributors

Nethaji Muniraj, Sumit Siddharth and Dipali Sharma
Department of Oncology, Johns Hopkins University School of Medicine and the Sidney Kimmel Comprehensive Cancer Center at Johns Hopkins, Baltimore, MD 21231, USA

Feroza K. Choudhury, G. Lavender Hackman and Alessia Lodi
Department of Nutritional Sciences, College of Natural Sciences, The University of Texas at Austin, Austin, TX 78712, USA
Department of Pediatrics, Dell Medical School, The University of Texas at Austin, Austin, TX 78723, USA

Stefano Tiziani
Department of Nutritional Sciences, College of Natural Sciences, The University of Texas at Austin, Austin, TX 78712, USA
Department of Pediatrics, Dell Medical School, The University of Texas at Austin, Austin, TX 78723, USA
Department of Oncology, Dell Medical School, The University of Texas at Austin, Austin, TX 78723, USA

Simone Sampaolo
Department of Advanced Medical and Surgical Sciences, 2nd Division of Neurology, Center for Rare Diseases and InterUniversity Center for Research in Neurosciences, University of Campania "Luigi Vanvitelli", Via Sergio Pansini, 5 80131 Naples, Italy

Lorena Perrone
Department of Advanced Medical and Surgical Sciences, 2nd Division of Neurology, Center for Rare Diseases and InterUniversity Center for Research in Neurosciences, University of Campania "Luigi Vanvitelli", Via Sergio Pansini, 5 80131 Naples, Italy
Department of Chemistry and Biology, University Grenoble Alpes, 38400 Saint-Martin-d'Hères, France

Mariarosa Anna Beatrice Melone
Department of Advanced Medical and Surgical Sciences, 2nd Division of Neurology, Center for Rare Diseases and InterUniversity Center for Research in Neurosciences, University of Campania "Luigi Vanvitelli", Via Sergio Pansini, 5 80131 Naples, Italy
Sbarro Institute for Cancer Research and Molecular Medicine, Department of Biology, Temple University, BioLife Building (015-00)1900 North 12th Street, Philadelphia, PA 19122-6078, USA

Ammad Ahmad Farooqi
Institute of Biomedical and Genetic Engineering (IBGE), Islamabad 54000, Pakistan

Marina Pinheiro, Andreia Granja and Salette Reis
LAQV, REQUIMTE, Departamento de Ciências Químicas, Faculdade de Farmácia, Universidade do Porto, 4050-313 Porto, Portugal

Fulvia Farabegoli
Department of Pharmacy and Biotechnology (FaBiT), University of Bologna, 40126 Bologna, Italy

Rukset Attar
Department of Obstetrics and Gynecology, Yeditepe University, Ata¸sehir/˙Istanbul 34755, Turkey

Uteuliyev Yerzhan Sabitaliyevich
Department of Health Policy and Health Care Development, Kazakh Medical University of Continuing Education, Almaty 050004, Kazakhstan

Baojun Xu
Food Science and Technology Program, Beijing Normal University-Hong Kong Baptist University United International College, Zhuhai 519087, China

Aamir Ahmad
Department of Medicine, University of Alabama at Birmingham, Birmingham, AL 35205, USA

Emiliano Montalesi, Manuela Cipolletti, Patrizio Cracco, Marco Fiocchetti and Maria Marino
Department of Science, University Roma Tre, Viale Guglielmo Marconi 446, I-00146 Roma, Italy

Joanna Xuan Hui Goh
Biofunctional Molecule Exploratory (BMEX) Research Group, School of Pharmacy, Monash University Malaysia, Bandar Sunway 47500, Selangor Darul Ehsan, Malaysia

Loh Teng-Hern Tan
Novel Bacteria and Drug Discovery (NBDD) Research Group, Microbiome and Bioresource Research Strength, Jeffrey Cheah School of Medicine and Health Sciences, Monash University Malaysia, Bandar Sunway 47500, Selangor Darul Ehsan, Malaysia
Institute of Biomedical and Pharmaceutical Sciences, Guangdong University of Technology, Guangzhou 510006, China

Joo Kheng Goh
School of Science, Monash University Malaysia, Jalan Lagoon Selatan, Bandar Sunway 47500, Selangor Darul Ehsan, Malaysia

Kok Gan Chan
Division of Genetics and Molecular Biology, Institute of Biological Sciences, Faculty of Science, University of Malaya, Kuala Lumpur 50603, Malaysia
International Genome Centre, Jiangsu University, Zhenjiang 212013, China

Priyia Pusparajah
Medical Health and Translational Research Group, Jeffrey Cheah School of Medicine and Health Sciences, Monash University Malaysia, Bandar Sunway 47500, Selangor, Malaysia

Bey-Hing Goh
Biofunctional Molecule Exploratory (BMEX) Research Group, School of Pharmacy, Monash University Malaysia, Bandar Sunway 47500, Selangor Darul Ehsan, Malaysia
Asian Centre for Evidence Synthesis in Population, Implementation and Clinical Outcomes (PICO), Health and Well-being Cluster, Global Asia in the 21st Century (GA21) Platform, Monash University Malaysia, Bandar Sunway, 47500, Malaysia

Learn-Han Lee
Novel Bacteria and Drug Discovery (NBDD) Research Group, Microbiome and Bioresource Research Strength, Jeffrey Cheah School of Medicine and Health Sciences, Monash University Malaysia, Bandar Sunway 47500, Selangor Darul Ehsan, Malaysia
Asian Centre for Evidence Synthesis in Population, Implementation and Clinical Outcomes (PICO), Health and Well-being Cluster, Global Asia in the 21st Century (GA21) Platform, Monash University Malaysia, Bandar Sunway, 47500, Malaysia

Sònia Palomeras, Santiago Ruiz-Martínez and Teresa Puig
New Therapeutic Targets Laboratory (TargetsLab)-Oncology Unit, Department of Medical Sciences, Faculty of Medicine, University of Girona, 17003 Girona, Spain

Joaquim Ciurana
Product, Process and Production Engineering Research Group (GREP), Department of Mechanical Engineering and Industrial Construction, University of Girona, 17003 Girona, Spain

Emma Polonio-Alcalá
New Therapeutic Targets Laboratory (TargetsLab)-Oncology Unit, Department of Medical Sciences, Faculty of Medicine, University of Girona, 17003 Girona, Spain
Product, Process and Production Engineering Research Group (GREP), Department of Mechanical Engineering and Industrial Construction, University of Girona, 17003 Girona, Spain

Daniel Torres-Oteros
Department of Nutrition, Food Sciences and Gastronomy, School of Pharmacy and Food Sciences, Food Torribera Campus, University of Barcelona, E-08921 Santa Coloma de Gramanet, Spain

Joana Relat
Department of Nutrition, Food Sciences and Gastronomy, School of Pharmacy and Food Sciences, Food Torribera Campus, University of Barcelona, E-08921 Santa Coloma de Gramanet, Spain
Institute of Nutrition and Food Safety of the University of Barcelona (INSA-UB), E-08921 Santa Coloma de Gramenet, Spain
CIBER Physiopathology of Obesity and Nutrition (CIBER-OBN), Instituto de Salud Carlos III, E-28029 Madrid, Spain

Marta Planas and Lidia Feliu
LIPPSO, Department of Chemistry, University of Girona, 17003 Girona, Spain

Ana M. Barbosa
Instituto de Ciências Biomédicas Abel Salazar, University of Porto, 4169-007 Porto, Portugal

Fátima Martel
Unit of Biochemistry, Department of Biomedicine, Faculty of Medicine, University of Porto, 4200-319 Porto, Portugal
Instituto de Investigação e Inovação em Saúde, University of Porto, 4200-135 Porto, Portugal

Arnatchai Maiuthed
Cell-Based Drug and Health Product Development Research Unit, Faculty of Pharmaceutical Sciences, Chulalongkorn University, Bangkok 10330, Thailand

Nattanan Losuwannarak and Pithi Chanvorachote
Cell-Based Drug and Health Product Development Research Unit, Faculty of Pharmaceutical Sciences, Chulalongkorn University, Bangkok 10330, Thailand
Department of Pharmacology and Physiology, Faculty of Pharmaceutical Sciences, Chulalongkorn University, Bangkok 10330, Thailand

Nakarin Kitkumthorn
Department of Oral Biology, Faculty of Dentistry, Mahidol University, Bangkok 10400, Thailand

Asada Leelahavanichkul
Department of Microbiology, Faculty of Medicine, Chulalongkorn University, Bangkok 10330, Thailand

Sittiruk Roytrakul
Proteomics Research Laboratory, 113 Thailand Science Park, Phahonyothin Road, Khlong 1, Khlong Luang, Pathum Thani 12120, Thailand

Adrian Sandoval-Hernandez, Fabian Lopez-Vallejo, Wilman Delgado and Luis Cuca
Departamento de Química, Facultad de Ciencias, Universidad Nacional de Colombia, Bogotá 111321, Colombia

Diego Muñoz
Departamento de Química, Facultad de Ciencias, Universidad Nacional de Colombia, Bogotá 111321, Colombia
Facultad de Ciencias, Universidad de Ciencias Aplicadas y Ambientales, Bogotá 111166, Colombia

Martina Brucoli
Tumour Cell Death Laboratory, Cancer Research UK Beatson Institute, Glasgow G61 1BD, UK

Silvia Zecchini, Matteo Giovarelli, Marco Coazzoli and Cristiana Perrotta
Department of Biomedical and Clinical Sciences "Luigi Sacco" (DIBIC), Università degli Studi di Milano, 20157 Milano, Italy

Gonzalo Arboleda
Grupo de Muerte Celular, Instituto de Genética, Universidad Nacional de Colombia, Bogotá 111321, Colombia

Davide Cervia and Elisabetta Catalani
Department for Innovation in Biological, Agro-food and Forest systems (DIBAF), Università degli Studi della Tuscia, 01100 Viterbo, Italy

Clara De Palma
Unit of Clinical Pharmacology, University Hospital "Luigi Sacco"-ASST Fatebenefratelli Sacco, 20157 Milano, Italy

Emilio Clementi
Department of Biomedical and Clinical Sciences "Luigi Sacco" (DIBIC), Università degli Studi di Milano, 20157 Milano, Italy
Unit of Clinical Pharmacology, University Hospital "Luigi Sacco"-ASST Fatebenefratelli Sacco, 20157 Milano, Italy
Scientific Institute IRCCS "Eugenio Medea", 23842 Bosisio Parini, Italy

Index

A

Adenocarcinoma, 16, 20, 59, 103, 107, 114, 132, 144, 146, 148, 168, 171, 185, 189, 207, 211

Angiogenesis, 16, 51, 61, 76, 79, 98, 100, 103, 108, 113-114, 118-120, 126-127, 129, 133, 143, 153, 164, 167, 176, 188, 199-200, 203, 205

Anti-cancer Drug, 1, 64, 196, 200

Anti-proliferative Effect, 31, 50, 53, 103, 107-108

Anticancer, 1, 3, 14, 21-23, 29-31, 40-41, 43, 57, 59-60, 63-64, 75, 79-82, 84, 88, 92, 95, 121, 124, 127, 132-133, 135, 142, 146-150, 152-154, 167, 169, 171, 175-177, 179-181, 185-187, 196, 205-206, 231-233

Anticancer Effect, 30, 40, 88, 95, 167, 171, 196

Anticancer Properties, 171

Anticancer Therapy, 43, 142, 152, 186, 232

Apoptosis, 1, 3-9, 12-23, 29-32, 39-44, 48, 50-54, 57-61, 66-67, 70-72, 76-80, 84, 91, 93, 96, 98, 100, 102-107, 110-113, 117, 119, 121, 124-127, 131, 133, 136-137, 142, 147-149, 153-155, 199, 205-206, 208-209, 214, 221-227, 229-236

Autophagy, 5, 7-8, 15, 20-21, 31, 42-43, 50-53, 59-61, 77, 80, 108, 110-112, 121, 125-126, 142, 149, 167, 178, 185, 187, 206, 234, 236-237

B

Bioavailability, 8, 12, 16, 22, 25, 29, 46, 54-57, 62-63, 72, 74-75, 82, 84, 95-96, 98, 114, 116-118, 120, 127-128, 146, 177

Blood-brain Barrier, 46, 62

Brain Cancer, 46-47

Breast Cancer, 1, 3-9, 11-23, 29, 31-32, 39-41, 43-45, 57-58, 64, 66, 71, 74-75, 77, 79-85, 92-97, 99, 118, 121, 127, 129, 133, 142-143, 147-159, 163-165, 167-171, 175-176, 178-187, 206-207, 211, 223-224, 227, 229, 234, 236

Breast Carcinoma, 15, 18, 20-23, 57, 168

C

Cancer Cell, 1, 4-6, 15, 17, 19-23, 29-33, 39-40, 42-43, 48, 50-51, 57-59, 72, 78-79, 81, 85, 92-93, 96-97, 103, 111-112, 121-124, 129, 131, 147-148, 150-159, 163-165, 167-171, 175, 179-186, 189, 197, 205, 208, 213, 229-230, 233-234

Cancer Progression, 5, 13, 48, 50, 67, 77-78, 98, 112, 114, 120, 127, 151, 158, 165, 180, 199

Cardiovascular Disease, 14, 24

Cascade, 6, 9, 48, 59, 64-65, 84-85, 92-93, 110, 221, 235

Cell Cycle, 7-9, 15-16, 20, 22, 29-31, 39-41, 44, 50-51, 53-54, 57, 59, 74, 77, 98, 100, 102-107, 109-110, 119, 121, 124-125, 131, 142, 149, 154, 157, 167, 178, 181-182, 232, 234

Cell Death, 1, 5-6, 14-15, 18, 21-22, 31-32, 39, 42-44, 52-53, 57-59, 70-71, 77, 79, 85, 93, 97, 110-111, 125-126, 135-136, 142, 149, 157, 176, 182, 185, 189-191, 199-201, 206, 208-209, 214-218, 220-222, 224-226, 229-230, 233-236

Cell Growth, 1, 5-6, 23, 25-26, 31, 43, 51-54, 79, 81, 102, 109, 112, 122, 124, 131, 133, 153-154, 164, 168-169, 171, 179, 181, 183, 185-186, 196, 227, 232

Cell Lines, 4, 15, 17, 20-21, 29-31, 40, 50, 52-53, 61, 64, 97, 102-106, 109-111, 113-114, 121, 123, 127, 144, 151-159, 163, 165, 167-171, 175, 179, 181-183, 185, 189-190, 195, 211, 213, 216, 229, 234

Cell Metabolism, 39, 57, 152, 164, 171, 184, 186

Cell Proliferation, 4, 9, 20, 25, 31, 43, 49-50, 53, 92-93, 96, 98, 100, 103-104, 109-110, 112-113, 117, 122, 124, 129, 135-136, 143-144, 153-155, 157-158, 164-165, 167, 180-181, 183, 188

Central Nervous System, 46, 51-54, 56, 61, 117, 129

Chemoprevention, 5, 7, 15, 17, 19, 40, 57, 59, 74, 80, 82, 95, 98-99, 102-103, 107, 110, 112, 114, 116, 119-120, 126, 130, 170-171, 184-185, 232

Chemotherapy, 4, 7-9, 12, 14, 21, 74-75, 83, 85, 99, 117, 119, 129, 142, 150, 152, 154, 163-164, 178, 182-183, 189, 206, 214, 225, 233

Chromatography, 96, 102, 115, 119, 122-123, 128, 130, 201, 226

Clinical Practice, 46, 56, 119

Clinical Trial, 11-12, 24, 31, 82

Colorectal Cancer, 21, 29, 31, 41, 65-66, 69-71, 77-80, 94, 98-100, 102, 108, 118, 120, 122-124, 126-127, 185

Curcumin, 1, 7-8, 11-13, 20-22, 26, 29-31, 33, 38, 41, 49, 51-52, 54-55, 57-60, 62, 64, 76, 118, 130, 169, 173, 185

Cytotoxic Effect, 22, 30, 32, 36, 49, 134-135, 156, 168-169, 175, 213, 224

Cytotoxicity, 8, 16, 32, 41, 53, 61, 104-106, 132, 134-135, 142, 153, 175, 199, 224, 234

D

Demethylation, 101, 109, 116

Diabetes, 12, 45, 99, 117, 121, 129, 155, 171, 179

Drug-resistant, 15, 22, 51, 66, 71, 81-82

E

Energy Metabolism, 25, 33, 48-49, 133, 150, 152, 158, 176, 180, 182, 185

F

Fatty Acids, 36, 38, 133, 136, 151, 171, 186

Flavonoid, 6, 39, 61, 99-100, 114, 121-124, 127, 129, 133, 167, 169

G

Gefitinib Resistant, 132, 134-138, 140-141, 144

Gemcitabine, 8, 70, 79, 148-149

Gliomas, 46, 51, 54

Glucose Metabolism, 43-44, 49, 57, 148, 153, 156-157, 180-182, 184-185

Glucose Transport, 29, 40, 150-151, 153-155, 158, 169, 176-177, 179-180, 184-185

Glucose Uptake, 29-30, 32-33, 35, 37-38, 40, 48-50, 57-58, 150-158, 163-165, 167-171, 173, 175-180, 183-185

Glycolysis, 30, 32-36, 38, 40-42, 44-45, 48-50, 151, 153, 156, 158, 167-171, 176-181, 183-187

Glycolytic Pathway, 50, 151, 154-155

H

Honokiol, 1, 4-5, 13, 16-17

Hydroxyl, 48, 51, 102, 115, 211, 220

I

Immunoblotting, 134, 137

L

Lactate Production, 29-30, 50, 153, 155-156, 163, 165, 167-171, 173

Leptin, 4, 6, 17-19, 107, 113-114, 127

Lung Cancer, 11-12, 29, 35, 40-41, 59, 68-69, 71, 75, 78-80, 83, 99, 118, 121, 129, 132-133, 142, 146-150, 169, 188-189, 191, 196, 199, 202, 204-206, 227

M

Magnolol, 4, 16

Metabolic Pathway, 25, 32, 45, 158, 177

Molecular Target, 58, 152, 222-223, 225, 229, 233

N

Natural Compounds, 14, 39, 41, 44, 46, 58, 116, 142, 146, 149-150, 153, 167, 170, 177, 189, 205, 226, 231, 234

Necrosis, 23, 40, 42-43, 50, 95, 106, 110, 125, 191

Neurofibromas, 46-47, 54

Nobiletin, 98-103, 117, 121-124, 126-131

O

Obesity, 6, 12, 19, 99, 117, 129, 132, 143, 181

Oral Cancer, 5-6, 19, 64, 76-77, 129

Oxidation, 32, 50-51, 59, 150, 167, 202

Oxidative Stress, 14, 30, 37, 40, 46, 48, 50-51, 54-55, 58, 65, 74, 96, 122, 126, 153, 187, 236

P

Paclitaxel, 1, 8, 21, 29, 32, 52, 60, 74, 81, 84-85, 88, 90-93, 95-96, 121, 126, 153-155, 157, 175, 182, 186

Pancreatic Cancer, 6, 19, 31, 41, 43, 58, 70, 79, 143, 149

Pharmacokinetics, 12, 24, 43, 72, 82, 114, 118, 128

Phosphofructokinase, 26, 30, 152

Polyphenols, 4, 11, 16, 19-20, 23, 44, 46, 48-52, 54-60, 62, 66, 78, 81, 83-84, 93, 96, 99-100, 120, 123, 127, 142-143, 148, 167, 169, 177, 184-185, 232

Prognosis, 46, 52, 60, 114, 123, 133, 147, 150, 152, 164-165, 171, 189

Protein Kinase, 4-5, 9, 16, 22, 50, 64, 89, 113, 121, 127, 152, 154, 156, 158, 168, 189, 191, 199

Q

Quercetin, 29, 49-53, 57-58, 61, 64, 77, 80, 92, 97, 110, 118, 168, 180, 185

R

Reactive Oxygen Species, 5, 15, 18, 31, 36-37, 40, 49-50, 57-59, 78, 113, 125, 151, 185-186, 208, 220, 230

S

Schwannomas, 46-47, 54

Signaling Pathway, 11-12, 16, 20, 22, 30, 41, 43-44, 52-53, 59-61, 64, 70, 77, 79, 125, 133, 142-143, 146, 149, 156, 158, 179, 181, 192-194, 204, 206

Spleen, 116-117

T

Transmembrane, 70, 143, 151, 155, 164

Tumor Cell, 15, 30-31, 39, 56, 61, 79, 126, 154, 165, 175, 179, 188-189, 196, 206, 236

Tumor Suppressor, 4, 6, 17, 22, 48, 54, 67, 71-72, 78, 158, 164, 184, 191

Tumorigenesis, 5, 31, 35, 52, 109, 112, 121, 123, 151, 158, 179, 181, 189, 193

Printed in the USA
CPSIA information can be obtained
at www.ICGtesting.com
LVHW080046211023
761596LV00010BA/1927

9 781646 475216